Inflammation, Aging and Cancer

Mahin Khatami

Inflammation, Aging and Cancer

Biological Injustices to Molecular Village of Immunity that Guard Health

Springer

Mahin Khatami
Bethesda, Maryland, USA

ISBN 978-3-319-66473-6 ISBN 978-3-319-66475-0 (eBook)
https://doi.org/10.1007/978-3-319-66475-0

Library of Congress Control Number: 2017953871

Printed on acid-free paper

This Springer imprint is published by Springer Nature
The registered company is Springer International Publishing AG
The registered company address is: Gewerbestrasse 11, 6330 Cham, Switzerland

To the loving memories of my parents
Kazem and Badri-Zaman Khatami

And

In honor and memory of millions of patients who lost precious lives to wrongful approaches to cancer research and treatment.

It is recognized that current cancer epidemic is an induced disease of Twentieth Century, facilitated by medical/cancer establishment for corporate profit.

Contents

About the Author

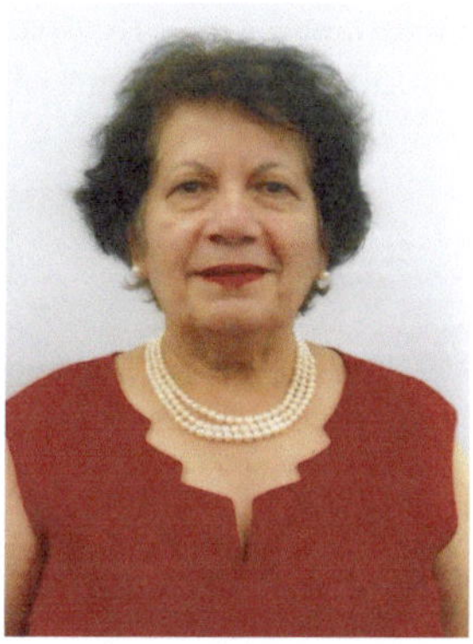

Professor Mahin Khatami immigrated to the USA in 1969. She completed her PhD in Molecular Biology from the University of Pennsylvania (UPA, 1980) after completion of a master's degree in Biochemistry at State University of New York (SUNY), Buffalo. Her BS in Chemistry and MS in Science Education were from Iran. Her postdoctoral research was in the fields of physiology (UVA), protein chemistry (proteomics), and immunology at Fox Chase Cancer Center and UPA. In the 1980s, as a research faculty at UPA, she was involved in two major collaborative projects—molecular/cellular biology of diabetes complications (retinopathy, maculopathy, and neuropathy) and experimental models of acute and chronic ocular inflammatory diseases—as well as biology of muscle development and supervisory activities. At UPA, Dr. Khatami became the most productive academician in the USA—she published 39 scientific articles in refereed journals and book chapters and over 60 abstracts in conference proceedings in the first decade of her junior academic career.

In 1998, Dr. Khatami joined the National Cancer Institute (NCI), the National Institutes of Health (NIH). As Program Director (HSA), she was involved in concept development for molecular diagnosis and prevention of cancer, review of large clinical trials such as Prostate-Lung-Colorectal-Ovarian (PLCO) Cancer Screening Trials, and the utilization of patients' biospecimen (biological samples). Her earlier studies on models of inflammatory diseases that resulted in multistep tumorigenesis and angiogenesis became accidental discoveries and intimately relevant to cancer research and clinical studies. She submitted a series of novel proposals for cancer molecular diagnosis, prevention, and design of clinical trials based on important roles of inflammation in cancer science. Her challenging efforts to promote the role of inflammation in cancer research initially met with severe oppositions, denials, and rejections of submitted proposals and lectures by NCI decision makers. However, in the last couple of decades, it seems that these efforts awakened the entire cancer community within and outside NIH. Despite the hostile environment at NCI/NIH, in 2005, Khatami published two articles and an NCI-Invention on standardizing cancer biomarkers criteria (data elements) as a foundation for a cancer biomarkers database (Fed. Reg.). In 2005, NCI/CCR initiated a program for inflammation and cancer research for which Khatami submitted a comprehensive proposal as an extension of her pioneering studies. Numerous funded projects, symposia, and networks are currently focused on various basic research and models of immunotherapy or clinical trials.

Before retiring at the professor level, Dr. Khatami was Director of the Innovative Molecular Analysis Technology (IMAT) Program, and Assistant Director for Technology Program Development at OTIR/OD/NCI/NIH. She continues to analyze and integrate relevant data and extend her original discoveries into novel concepts for cancer science and design of biological roadmaps for disease processes. These efforts are reflected in her recent publications and this monograph. Her goal is to offer the medical community better rational for systematic and cost-effective approaches to solving the century-old cancer mystery, including development of universal vaccines for a healthier society.

Chapter 1
Introduction to Interrelated Biology of Age-Associated Chronic Diseases and Cancer: Chronic Inflammation, a Common Denominator in Morbidity and Mortality

We could certainly slow the aging process down if it had to work its way through Congress

Will Rogers

Abstract The biological events that regulate the body's multi-organ systems from conception to development and through adulthood and aging process are fascinating molecular communications between immune and non-immune systems. The highly organized interdependent network of signals and chemical interactions (crosstalk) among the organ systems such as immune cells, vasculature, neuronal, metabolic hormonal pathways constitute the body's effective immunity that defend the body against any intrinsic or extrinsic components that are perceived hazardous. Body's protection against all unwanted elements was originally conceptualized as the theory of immune surveillance that also defined control of cancer growth; by Sir Mc Farland Burnet in 1957. Disturbance of the orchestrated crosstalk in immunity by frequent exposures to various immune disruptors, including pathogen-specific vaccines and aging process can cause retardation of various interrelated communications in susceptible tissues and initiation of mild or severe health conditions. In this introductory chapter we overviewed the topics that are detailed separately throughout the book. It is suggested that policy makers and professionals in decision making roles in medical sciences to return to common sense and logics that our Forefathers used to serve the public. Future directions in medical cancer research are suggested to be systematical studies of oxidative stress initiating events that disturb the effective immunity (immune surveillance) toward multistep disease processes.

Keywords Age-associated chronic diseases • American health status • Answer to cancer • Antigen overload • Autoimmune diseases • Biological heterogeneity • Cancer financial toxicity • Cancer/medical establishment • Clinical trials • Colitis • Congress • Early immune dysfunction • Effective immunity • Healthy aging • Historical neglected observations • Host-pathogen interactions and synergies • Hypertension • Immune disrupters • Immune-privileged • Immune-responsive •

M. Khatami, *Inflammation, Aging and Cancer*,
https://doi.org/10.1007/978-3-319-66475-0_1

Infections • Longevity • Morbidity • Mortality • Neurodegenerative • Shotgun research • Signal transduction network • Systematic study • Translational medicine • Tumor virology • Virus-contaminated polio vaccines • War on cancer • Yin–Yang of inflammation

1 Introduction

Fascination with the topic of aging remains the mysterious or mystical subject for scientists, poets and philosophers for centuries. Over the past few decades, the scientific interest in the biology of aging process has accelerated, especially because of the significant increased in the growth rate of the older adult population around the world. Advancing in age is associated with increased risk of developing one or more chronic disabling medical illnesses such as allergies, hypertension, neurodegenerative and autoimmune diseases, adult on-set diabetes and cardiovascular complications, vulnerability to infectious diseases and many site-specific cancers.

Longevity and the rate of susceptibility and severity to chronic and disabling illnesses vary among individuals due to the complex combination of interactions and heterogeneities between the intrinsic and extrinsic factors that would determine the biology of aging. The increased growth rate of healthy older adults around the world suggests that the aging process is not necessarily associated with illnesses; and not all older individuals develop chronic illnesses at the same rate or severity. The degrees of interactions between intrinsic (innate) factors including the genetic make-up of the individual influencing other biological features of immune and non-immune systems (e.g., vasculature, metabolic, hormonal, neuronal and physiological), and response profiles toward immune disruptors or extrinsic factors (e.g., infective agents or exposures to diverse chemical, biological or environmental hazards and life styles) vary among individuals.

To date, our biological information on aging process and chronic diseases are fragmentary, obscure and confusing, due in part to the fact that, except for a small group of decision makers within the medical establishment, majority of scientists work in isolated fields of expertise for a limited durations of funding. It is also noteworthy that despite the fact that there are enormous numbers of published data on a wide range of age-associated topics, the available information is not effectively integrated to make better sense of what data is worth following to benefit the public. Furthermore, the fashionable field of computational biology cannot be expected to provide the intellectual answers to too many biological knowledge gaps and questions that currently exist for connecting the dots on the scattered data. The best evidence for disconnect in understanding the fragmented data comes from the ongoing debates, confusion and misunderstanding of the role of immune/inflammation in the genesis and progression of chronic diseases and cancer (reviewed in 1, 2).

The followings are excerpts and analyses of data on American health status in comparison with other developed nations, from Mirror, Mirror (2014, details in Chap. 5)[1]:

"The United States health care system is the most expensive in the world, but this report and prior editions consistently show the U.S. underperforms relative to other countries on most dimensions of performance. Among the 11 nations studied in this report—Australia, Canada, France, Germany, the Netherlands, New Zealand, Norway, Sweden, Switzerland, the United Kingdom, and the United States—the U.S. ranks last, as it did in the 2010, 2007, 2006, and 2004 editions of Mirror, Mirror. Most troubling, the U.S. fails to achieve better health outcomes than the other countries, and as shown in the earlier editions, the U.S. is last or near last on dimensions of access, efficiency, and equity. In this edition of Mirror, Mirror, *the United Kingdom ranks first, followed closely by Switzerland…..*The U.S. ranks last of 11 nations overall. Findings in this report confirm many of those in the earlier four editions of Mirror, Mirror, with the U.S. still ranking last on indicators of efficiency, equity, and outcomes. The U.K. continues to demonstrate strong performance and ranked first overall, though lagging notably on health outcomes. Switzerland, which was included for the first time in this edition, ranked second overall. In the subcategories, the U.S. ranks higher on preventive care, and is strong on waiting times for specialist care, but weak on access to needed services and ability to obtain prompt attention from primary care physicians. Any attempt to assess the relative performance of countries has inherent limitations. These rankings summarize evidence on measures of high performance based on national mortality data and the perceptions and experiences of patients and physicians. They do not capture important dimensions of effectiveness or efficiency that might be obtained from medical records or administrative data. Patients' and physicians' assessments might be affected by their experiences and expectations, which could differ by country and culture…. Major Findings

- ***Quality***: *The indicators of quality were grouped into four categories: effective care, safe care, coordinated care, and patient-centered care. Compared with the other 10 countries, the U.S. fares best on provision and receipt of preventive and patient-centered care. While there has been some improvement in recent years, lower scores on safe and coordinated care pull the overall U.S. quality score down. Continued adoption of health information technology should enhance the ability of U.S. physicians to identify, monitor, and coordinate care for their patients, particularly those with chronic conditions.*
- ***Access***: *Not surprisingly—given the absence of universal coverage—people in the U.S. go without needed health care because of cost more often than people do in the other countries. Americans were the most likely to say they had access problems related to cost. Patients in the U.S. have rapid access to specialized health care services; however, they are less likely to report rapid access to pri-*

[1] Davis K, Stremikis K, Schoen C, Squires D: *Mirror, Mirror on the Wall, 2014 Update: How the U.S. Health Care System Compares Internationally,* The Commonwealth Fund, June 2014.

mary care than people in leading countries in the study. In other countries, like Canada, patients have little to no financial burden, but experience wait times for such specialized services. There is a frequent misperception that trade-offs between universal coverage and timely access to specialized services are inevitable; however, the Netherlands, U.K., and Germany provide universal coverage with low out-of-pocket costs while maintaining quick access to specialty services.

- ***Efficiency**: On indicators of efficiency, the U.S. ranks last among the 11 countries, with the U.K. and Sweden ranking first and second, respectively. The U.S. has poor performance on measures of national health expenditures and administrative costs as well as on measures of administrative hassles, avoidable emergency room use, and duplicative medical testing. Sicker survey respondents in the U.K. and France are less likely to visit the emergency room for a condition that could have been treated by a regular doctor, had one been available.*
- ***Equity**: The U.S. ranks a clear last on measures of equity. Americans with below-average incomes were much more likely than their counterparts in other countries to report not visiting a physician when sick; not getting a recommended test, treatment, or follow-up care; or not filling a prescription or skipping doses when needed because of costs. On each of these indicators, one-third or more lower-income adults in the U.S. said they went without needed care because of costs in the past year.*
- ***Healthy lives**: The U.S. ranks last overall with poor scores on all three indicators of healthy lives—mortality amenable to medical care, infant mortality, and healthy life expectancy at age 60. The U.S. and U.K. had much higher death rates in 2007 from conditions amenable to medical care than some of the other countries, e.g., rates 25–50% higher than Australia and Sweden. Overall, France, Sweden, and Switzerland rank highest on healthy lives."*

With regard to cancer research and therapy, it is alarmingly disappointing that while over 20 million publications exist on cancer-related topics, the scientists still argue whether inflammation is protective or destructive to the body. The author believes that the reductionist approaches and creation of a double vision for the mission of cancer, by decision makers (establishment, insiders) in cancer community who emphasize to fund too many projects that are claimed as 'targeted' therapies, 'personalized' or 'precision' medicine, are the principal reasons for extremely slow progress and repeated failed outcomes [2].

In preparing this book, attempts were made to discuss some of the known heterogeneities in the biological systems, address pitfalls and shortcomings or misunderstanding of the cancer science and identify the intellectually important knowledge gaps and questions on age-associated chronic diseases with emphasis on cancer biology and treatment. A goal in this effort is to demonstrate that for improving public health decision makers need to move away from the current reductionist views and the irresponsible shut-gun approaches in cancer research and therapy, which have been extremely costly and produced high failure rate outcomes. The overall future proposed directions will be to conduct systematic and logical studies that are cost effective and would lay a foundation to understand cancer biology toward better preventing or treating cancer and benefiting the growing society and the cancer-stricken public.

The chapters in this book were prepared as extensions of the author's discoveries and suggestions that the major known biological theories of aging (genomics, free radicals and immune) are interdependent; and that chronic, persistent or unresolved inflammation (oxidative stress, sub-clinical) is a common denominator in the initiation, progression and manifestation of nearly all age-associated chronic diseases [1, 2]. A focus of the book chapters will be discussing recent definitions and hypotheses on the role of acute and chronic inflammation in health and diseases, based on the analyses and extension of our 'accidental' discoveries that were established in 1980s on experimental models of acute and chronic ocular inflammatory diseases at the University of Pennsylvania. The results of these groundbreaking studies, as summarized below are suggestive of a series of interrelated and systematic findings as the first evidence for a direct link between inflammation-induced distinct developmental phases of immune dysfunction in the direction of tumorigenesis and angiogenesis including demonstration of the early events of immune disruptors-induced altered response profiles in host tissues [1, 2]. The emphasis will be to demonstrate how the altered inherent and natural duality and response dynamics of immune and non-immune systems (e.g., vasculature, metabolic, hormonal and neuronal) facilitate cancerous cells to bypass (escape) immunity for their enhanced growth requirements and invasive characters during cancer metastasis and angiogenesis (Fig. 1.1). The ultimate goal of this undertaking is to demonstrate the serious need for conducting systematic studies of the inherent protective properties of immunity that are altered or lost during aging process as bases for induction of chronic diseases. Future unique opportunities and challenges for cancer research and therapy will also be proposed.

2 Neglected Historical Observations, Theories and Discoveries on the Role of Immunity in Controlling Carcinogenesis

The following sections highlight the neglected century-old fundamental observations and recent theories and discoveries that are intimately relevant to the importance of inflammation in multistep carcinogenesis. Lack of interest to support systematic studies on cancer biology by decision makers (reductionists in medical establishment) who moved away from extending these logical and groundbreaking observations are the principal reasons for very costly cancer-care (cancer financial toxicity to the society) that produced very little to positively influence public health [1–15].

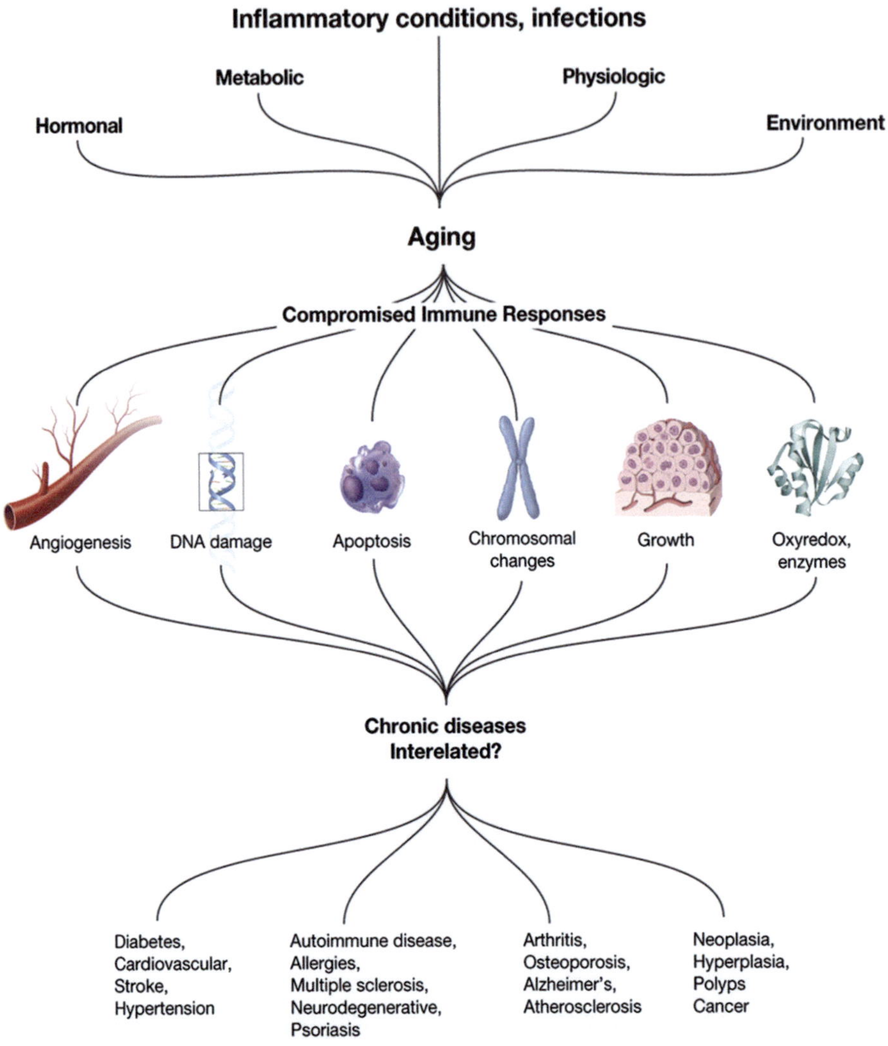

Fig. 1.1 Longevity and oxidative stress are co-morbidity and co-mortality risk factors that increase the incidence of many chronic diseases. Age-induced hormonal, metabolic and physiological changes in the body, impose biological rearrangements in organ systems (biological senescence). Aging also induced minor or major changes in immune cell responses or immunosenescence. Unresolved inflammation together with aging process could adversely and progressively cause DNA damage and chromosomal changes, alteration in vascular function-toning neovascularization or angiogenesis, tissue necrosis or cell growth and changes in oxido-redox status with accumulation of free radicals. Depending on the type and susceptibility of the target tissues manifestation of potentially interrelated diseases such as diabetes and cardiovascular complications, neurodegenerative and autoimmune diseases, arthritis, Alzheimer's, atherosclerosis, as well as neoplasia, hyperplasia or cancer could occur. (Reproduced with permission from Khatami Ref. [1], all rights reserved.)

2.1 Observations by Paul Ehrlich and Ilya Mechinkov in Nineteenth and Twentieth Centuries: Era of Modern Experimental Immunology

At the end of nineteenth century, Ilya Mechnikov discovered the action of phagocytosis and the basis for studying innate immunity. In the same period, Paul Ehrlich hypothesized that antigen and antibody behave as the fit between key and lock; thus establishing the innovative concept of antigen-antibody complementarities and the basis for studying adaptive immunity. Ehrlich and Mechnikov shared the Nobel Prize in 1908 for their pioneering studies in the field of immunity and host defense mechanisms. In 1909, using the newly invented technology of microscope, Ehrlich observed that cancer cells were monitored and destroyed by immune cells [3, 4].

2.2 Contributions of Peyton Rous in 1900s: Era of Tumor Virology. Virus-Causing Cancers

A century ago, in 1910, Peyton Rous reported the first transplantable avian tumor virus of 'spindle-celled sarcoma' a discovery that began the era of tumor virus biology and tumor biology [5]. The avian tumor as Rous reported '*closely resembles the typical mammalian neoplasms that are transplantable*'. Several related studies on comparison of tumor growth in different species (e.g., rat, mouse, dog, fish) presented controversies whether the findings were genuine tumors as they produced different growth characteristics. However, Rous' careful observations on chicken sarcoma became the first evidence for a virus-causing tumor which is transmissible to other individuals [5]. The main factor that was found in similar studies for transmissible chicken leukemia, lymphoma, sarcoma and other neoplasms was a filterable virus [5].

Rous' visionary work demonstrated the cumulative effects of the 'initiators' in carcinogenesis. His concept is now described as the cumulative role of immune disruptors (e.g., pathogens, allergen, chemical, biological and environmental factors) in altering cellular behaviors in the direction of growth promotion.

In 1966, Peyton Rous, at the age of 87 was finally recognized for his novel contributions in the field of tumor virology and was awarded the Nobel Prize in Medicine. Despite his impeccable integrity and exceptional scientific qualities that were ahead of his time for showing the origin of cancer, it took 55 years, the longest period in the history of Nobel Prizes, to be honored for his major discovery. His colleagues noted Rous' impeccable integrity and honesty and exceptionally gifted writing skills on details of his work. Rous shared the award with Charles B. Higgins.

While data on the role of virus-causing cancers existed, half a century prior to injecting the American population with million doses of virus-contaminated polio vaccines in 1955, the decision makers in the establishment proceeded to downplay and ignore the existing data, as well as the serious warnings and findings of a competent microbiologist at NIH (Bernice Eddy, MD) and created the deadly cancer epidemic and other chronic diseases such as neurodegenerative and autoimmune diseases that is destroying the health of baby boomers in America and to some extent around the world [6, 7]. In recent reports, the author described the scientific concerns regarding newly popularized vaccines against human papilloma virus (HPV) for prevention of cervical cancers in young generation. Suffice to note that while a great deal of studies have been devoted on reductionist approaches for identifying details of structure and substructure of viral DNA and expression products and mechanisms of actions of the evolving characteristics for HPVs or other viruses or bacteria (e.g., polio, herpes, AIDS, EBOLA, influenza, measles, hepatitis A, B, meningitis) that behave differently in different susceptible tissues for induction and manifestation of infectious or neurological diseases or cancer, there is a peculiar absence of study to understand what initiate the immune disruptor-,(virus)-induced altered biological properties in the susceptible tissues (host-pathogen interactions and synergies) that lead to manifestation of virus-causing disease processes. We also hypothesized that the exposure to many pathogen-specific vaccines or their particles (recombinant DNA) and adjuvant/ingredients, could impact the homeostasis and dynamics (ecosystem) of the host microorganisms (e.g., GI track, skin), particularly in young adults. Altering the hazard/benefit ratios of body's microbiota may be important contributing factors in the induction of chronic diseases such as allergies, autoimmune or neurodegenerative complications or cancers. Already, mild or moderate chronic health problems have been reported in younger adults who were vaccinated with HPV or other pathogen-specific vaccines (see Chap. 5) [6, 7].

In general, we described that systematic understanding of the effective immunity of host and its protective mechanisms against all internal and external foreign entities, and how to promote the organ systems defense ability, have greater priorities than investing resources on understanding the details of evolving DNA substructures of trillions of viruses for producing vaccines that are potentially hazardous.

2.3 *Burnet (1957): Insightful Theory of Immune Surveillance-Controlling Cancer Cells*

Sir Macfarlane Burnet in a seminal article developed the theory of immune (cancer) surveillance, the body's protective mechanism that controls the growth of microorganisms or cancerous cells [8]. Since the principal content of this book is devoted to extension of the Burnet's theory of immune surveillance, here the original theory of cancer control mechanisms are discussed in more details, along with our recent definitions of acute and chronic inflammation [6–12]. Aspects of the Burnet's theory of immunological selections have been challenged in recent years [9]. As discussed below, the fundamental role of immune surveillance, as well as, the important observations of Ehrlich that were originally documented over a century ago, have been practically ignored and downplayed by the cancer community [1, 2, 6, 7, 10–12].

In his 1957 article [8] Burnet commented that scientists, particularly in USA have "*a strong tendency to concentrate on investigations that may provide leads to (a) to the elaboration of tests for the early diagnosis of cancer, and (b) to its cure by non-surgical means. This has led perhaps to an undue interest in the biochemical aspects and especially the enzymic activities of tumour cells... Scientists may be divided into three groups. There are those, like myself, who believe that at every stage in scientific development it is necessary to provide the best available generalizations as a guide to effective work, both in the application of knowledge to human needs and in the planning of future research. At the other extreme are those who feel that the only valuable scientific activity is to concentrate on some significant facet of knowledge until the facts are incontrovertible and are expressible in some general statement, preferably mathematical in form, that is acceptable to all competent workers...*" [8].

Acknowledging the fundamental observations of Ehrlich [3, 4] and other colleagues, Burnet argued on the requirements for any general theory of cancer to be universally admitted so that "*...the essence of group of phenomena we know as cancer or neoplastic growth is growth of cells free from the normal control exercised by the organism as a whole...Cancer is a negative condition- a manifestation of the breakdown in one or more aspects of the positive control that welds the cells of the body into a single functioning unit-the organism as a whole...The failure in cancer is due not to any weakness of the organism but to a change in the character of the cells rendering them in one way or another insusceptible to the normal control. This statement is self-evident when we consider the phenomena of metastasis and experimental transplantation....*" [8].

Burnet's thoughtful analyses of data from different scientific groups (e.g., Wiess, Mascona, Medawar, Ebert, Green, Stewart, Krebs, Hauschka, Koprowski, Law, Furth, Armitage, Doll, Metcalfe, Fisher, Holloman, Cowdry, Mackay, Habich, Kanzow, Berenblum and Shubik, Weiler, Haddow, Millers, Pollock, etc) of his era who studied in the fields of developmental biology, immunology and cancer, and emphasized the followings:

(a) Embryonic cells dissociation and association, under appropriate tissue cultures and enzymatic assays;
(b) Immunological tolerance capacity, using skin grafts mice models;
(c) Transplant studies in mice and studies of ascites tumors;
(d) Heterogeneity of tumor strains, extending its virulence to other hosts;
(e) Selective survival of mutant cells and resistant to agents provided rational for cellular control "*...the first step is for the cells to become grouped according to kind, aggregating into clusters by a variety of processes which seem to include random encounter, directional migration, and surface interactions. The next process is one of organization within the aggregates and their interaction with clusters of cells of other types to develop the tissue-like appearance... From the point of view of cellular control in its relation to cancer the important aspect of*

these results is the indication that cells of many types are constantly liberating ' self- markers' into the lymph and blood circulations…This is perhaps equivalent to saying that every normal cell in the body is played on by multiple controls, and that more than one of these controls must be abrogated to allow unrestrained or excessive growth …" [8].

The 'multiple controls' in preventing cancer growth that Burnet discussed in 1950s, were later defined as the elaborate signal transduction mechanisms between immune and non-immune (e.g., vasculature, metabolic, hormonal and neuronal) responses of tissues that protect the body against harmful elements, including the growth of cancerous cells that threaten the body's survival [1, 2, 6, 7, 10–12].

In his early visionary approach to control the growth of cancer cells, Burnet explained that "*a small fraction of heteroploid cells in a tumour could be concentrated by propagation in a partially incompatible host. In his* [Hauschka] *view loss of transplantation specificity is a result of immunological selection of cell types with least antigenicity amongst the available chromosomal variants. The possibility that the selection is rather for cell types which are unduly resistant to the destructive action of immunological processes must also be considered. When transplantable tumours are exposed to therapeutic concentrations of radiations or antimetabolites it is the rule to find the eventual appearance of resistant tumour strains… the working hypothesis that the development of malignancy is the result of a biological process in which successive mutations occur in cells capable of continued proliferation, by which a certain advantage is gained. If cell A mutates to A', and A' has a slight advantage over A, there will be a gradual conversion of at least some regions from a population of A to one of A'…with increasing age more and more patches of cells in expendable tissues are the offspring of cells which have undergone more than one mutation in the line of progression to cancer. Perhaps a very clear indication of this is to look at the skin on the back of the hand of an elderly man and note its mosaic of colour and texture...in his* [Cowdry] *summary of the main changes, which include: increased thickness of epidermis in some areas, lessened thickness in others, diminution in hairs, sweat and sebaceous glands, patchy areas of hypo- and hyper- mineralization, occasional marked hypertrophy of single hairs. There are probably invisible mosaics of similar character in many other parts of the ageing body… a cardinal point of the theory that only if a mutation results in the loss of some structure or function by which general control over growth is exercised will the descendants of the mutated cell become sufficiently numerous to produce clinically or chemically detectable effects. The commonest effects will, of course, be those resulting directly from malignant growth of the cell descendants concerned….*" [8].

Burnet further explains that macroglonulinaemia is "*a relatively rare condition found in elderly patients in which the blood contains an abnormal globulin of very high molecular weight. It is always associated with a gross replacement of the bone marrow by lymphocyte-like cells which are clearly neoplastic and which in a small proportion of cases give a blood picture hardly distinguishable from chronic lymphatic leukaemia. Whenever the abnormal proteins from different cases of macro-*

globulinaemia have been compared they have shown sharp individual antigenic differences…" [8].

Acknowledging the concept of Green (1954), on immunological theory of cancer, Burnet further described "*…that the basic reason for failure to grow* [cancer] *in a heterologous strain is the immune response of the new host to the foreign marker antigens in the graft…*" [8].

This was a basic important theory that provided scientists a foundation to start understanding the role of immune surveillance in protecting the body against minor or major injuries or insults such as exposures to pathogens or biological, chemical or environmental hazards or carcinogens that threaten the survival of the body throughout life [1, 2, 10–12].

However, systematic extension and application of these fundamental observations for cancer research and therapy were practically ignored and downplayed by the decision makers in the cancer community for about a century. Instead, the decision makers created reductionist approaches to cancer research and therapy for motives that seem far from conducting effective projects to benefit the patients or to prevent cancer [2, 7, 10–12]. The heavy investment of public and private funds on disproportionate identification of numerous genetic mutations in the chaotic molecular environments of site-specific cancers was recently considered as 'molecular false flags' that are based on false foundations [2, 6, 7, 10]. The best evidence for wrong approaches in cancer research and therapy comes from the repeatedly failed outcomes (90% +/−5, failure rates) of claimed 'targeted' therapies, 'personalized' or 'precision' medicine for solid tumors that are heavily popularized by the might of decision makers, under the banners of 'cancer cure' or 'stand up to cancer' [2, 6, 7, 10].

Even in the last couple of decades that the establishment in the cancer community began to appreciate the role of immunity and inflammation in cancer research and translational medicine, nearly all publications relate to numerous fragmented and shut-gun data on a wide range of studies demonstrating tumors infiltration by leukocytes in experimental models of tumors or human cancers, with inconclusive prognostic values, or high failure rates for therapies [2, 6, 7, 10–22]. In recent years, other governmental agencies, professionals and media have raised serious concerns about the validity and high costs of cancer research and therapy and vaccines [6, 7, 12, 22–27][2,3,4]. As discussed below, in these expensive projects, little serious attempts are demonstrated to understand what are the early steps that change the

---

[2] Medscape December 5, 2011 (Washington DC) reported by Dr. Foji (NCI) 'zero [is] the number of targeted therapies that prolonged survival by 1 year' when compared with conventional treatment.

[3] Bennett, A. (2010) End-of-life warning at $618,616 makes me wonder was it worth it, Mar. 4. Bloomberg News. http://www.bloomberg.com/apps/news?pid=newsarchive&sid=avRFGNF6Qw_w

[4] Berger, E. (2012) Interview with the president of MD Anderson, DePinho in CNBC program, June 1, 2012, http://blog.chron.com/sciguy/2012/06/m-d-anderson-president-goes-on-cnbc-extols-his-own-company.

immune surveillance properties toward loss of its effectiveness to control the growth of cancerous cells, particularly during aging process [1, 2, 6, 7, 10–12].

Examples of fragmented data reported on cancer immunology and therapeutic projects that resulted a cancer financial toxicity, costing trillions of dollars to the public, while producing over 20 millions cancer-related articles and thousands of cancer drugs are outlined below (details in Chaps. 5 and 6):

(a) Types of tumor infiltrated leukocytes [e.g., polymorphonuclear cells (PMNs), natural killer cells (NKs), dendritic cells (DCs), macrophages (MΦs), eosinophils (Eos) and mast cells (MCs), T or B lymphocytes, in site-specific cancers from experimental models of tumors, basic science or clinical studies including identification of numerous biomarkers [1, 2, 6, 7, 24–41].
(b) Ongoing findings of hundreds and thousands of immune and inflammatory factors and mediators [e.g., cytokines/chemokines (e.g., CX3C, CCL2, interleukins, IL-1, IL-2, IL5, IL-8, IL-10, IL-12, IL-17, IL-23, IL-27, M-CSF, GM-CSF), vasoactive components (e.g., histamine), interferons (IFNs/IFN-γ), oxidants (e.g., ROS, RNS, caspases), neurotoxins (e.g., EDN, eotaxin), expression of suppressors or adaptive molecules from innate or adoptive immune cells; subsets/lineage of cells and surface molecules [e.g., CD4 + −CD25+, Th1, Th2, T reg, CD8+/cDC, DC1/Dc2, M1/M2-TAM, FOXP3, myeloid-derived suppressor cells (e.g., MDSC)], immunoglobulins and isotypes and receptor molecules (e.g., IgE- IgEfcR, IgG1/IgG2, IgM, IgA), growth factors expressed from lymphocytes or vasulature components (e.g., NFκb, FGF, VEGF), kinases (e.g., IP3K, MAPKs, thr/serK), toll-like receptors, transforming growth factors or adapter molecules (e.g., TGF-α,β, TLRs, TNF-R, dectins), membrane lipid metabolism and activated enzymes or proteins [e.g., cyclooxygenase, lipooxygenase, prostaglandins/PGs (e.g., PGI2, PGF1α, PGE2), surface glycoproteins, lipoproteins, indoleamine 2,3-dioxygenase (IDO), tryptase, chymase], as well as endless identification of genetic mutations and transcription factors of DNA/RNA, epigenetic components and repair protein/enzyme factors (e.g., p53, p38, ERK, GATA3, STAT3, 4, ALK) or immune checkpoints in experimental models of tumors or human subjects or approaches to clinical trials and immunotherapy or development of pathogen-specific vaccines [1, 2, 9–21, 28–72];
(c) In these efforts, development of numerous specific technologies for detection of specific molecular entities in experimental mouse or rat models for testing, developing, popularizing and utilizing specific networks in the fields of genomics, proteomics, lipidomics, metabolomics, glycomics continue to flood the literature.

The discoveries of these individual molecules accompany reports on mechanisms of actions of related pathways in site-specific cancer microenvironments lay the foundations for drug development and clinical trials with limited scientific visions or values to benefit the public. Furthermore, while the cascades of cancer metastasis to secondary specific organs are relatively understood (see below); systematic studies of multistep carcinogenesis that are the most important events for understanding the loss of cancer control, that could lead to effective detection and prevention as well as, therapy of cancer remain a mystery. In other words, very little efforts have gone to systematically demonstrate the initial events during multistep loss of immune response dynamics (immune surveillance) that could lead to effective monitoring, reversing and controlling cancer cell growth.

2.4 *Biological Cascades Toward Cancer Metastasis: Extension of the Theory of 'Seed and Soil' by Paget (1889)*

The metastatic spread of cancer cells from primary host tissue to distant organs that is the basis for most cancer deaths is the topic of intense investigations. The important original hypothesis by Paget in 1889 [73] which held the test of time by numerous insightful studies on the mechanisms of metastasis from primary tumor sites to secondary specific organs, demonstrate requirements of selective crosstalks between cancer cells (the 'seed') and specific organ microenvironment (the 'soil') [73–77].

However, as stated above, while the mechanisms of cancer metastatic cascades to different secondary sites have been investigated relatively well, very little efforts have gone to conduct systematic studies of understanding how cancer cells escape the monitoring ability of immune surveillance in the first place. It is also noteworthy that despite the relative advancements in understanding the metastatic stages of cancer, finding the 'cure' for solid tumors repeatedly failed the patients, most likely due to wrong approaches for treatments (see below).

2.5 *Contribution of Dvorak (1986): 'Tumors Are Wounds that Do Not Heal'*

In his cogent report that was published prior to recent definitions of inflammation, Dvorak made important molecular analyses of tumor behavior, particularly with regard to blood-derived wound healing properties of coagulation-related components and angiogenesis, comparing tumors with wounds that do not heal [78, 79]. The observation was recently described as unresolved inflammation or the loss of balance between tumoricidal ('Yin') and tumorigenic ('Yang') properties of immunity [1, 2, 11].

Dvorak analyses of data and hypotheses in cancer biology is perhaps among those few insightful contributions that stood the test of time in the past decades, as are the fundamental observations on immunology of carcinogenesis and metastasis reported by Ehrlich and Burnet or Paget (details in Chap. 6).

2.6 'Accidental' Discoveries: Systematic Studies Led to First Evidence on Direct Link Between Inflammation and Tumorigenesis (Khatami et al. 1980s)

In 1980s, working on experimental models of acute and chronic ocular inflammatory diseases, at the University of Pennsylvania, under the direction of John H Rockey (M.D., Ph.D.) we reported a series of findings that later became 'accidental' discoveries and the first series of evidence toward multistep induction of tumorigenesis and angiogenesis.[5] In 1980s, our research team was not involved in cancer research and we had no idea of the importance or significance of these findings until Khatami joined the National Cancer Institute (NCI); the National Institutes of Health (NIH) in 1998. At the Division of Cancer Prevention (DCP/NCI/NIH), the author was given the responsibility for producing molecular concepts for cancer diagnosis and prevention, design of clinical trials and utilization of patient samples for large clinical trials such as prostate-lung-colorectal-ovarian (PLCO) Cancer Screening Trials [6, 7, 10 (NCI documents since 1998)]. A brief background on the challenging efforts of Khatami to promote the role of inflammation in cancer research would be interesting from scientific and human spirit dimensions.

At NCI/NIH, review of numerous published data on cancer-related topics revealed that the results of our 'accidental' discoveries were suggestive of the first series of systematic and interrelated findings in tumor growth as outlined below (details in Chaps. 2, 4 and 6) [1, 2, 80–89] (Figs. 1.2 and 1.3):

(i) First evidence for the early effects of immune disruptors-(antigen-) induced altered immune response dynamics. Briefly, the antigen or immune disruptor was a chemically synthesized fluorescein conjugation to ovalbumin (fluoresceinyl ovalbumin-FLOA). Working at the Department of Ophthalmology at University of Pennsylvania, there was dual purpose for using FLOA as antigen in our experimental models of ocular allergies;

  (a) Diabetic patients who developed retinopathy and treated with fluoresceine dyes (angiography) prior to laser surgery and therapy, often developed allergic conditions. We were interested to understand how the dye influenced immunobiology of the eye.
  (b) The synthesis of covalent conjugation of fluoresceine with ovalbumin (FLOA) was a suitable antigen for studying the effects of immune disruptors in experimental models of acute and chronic ocular inflammatory diseases.

In these studies, early immune responses (within 11 days) upon repeated topical applications of FLOA in conjunctival-associated lymphoid tissues (CALTs) included sensitization of mast cells (MCs), through activation of B lymphocytes by FLOA-specific IgE antibodies, followed by MCs degranulation and release of hista-

[5] In 1980s, the author was also studying the role of glucose toxicity in ocular tissues to understand biology of diabetes complications with focus on retinopathy and maculopathy (examples in Ref. [90–94]). This was a tremendous thought-provoking period for author's professional life and bases for her desire to integrate useful data from multidisciplinary fields of biomedical sciences and extend earlier discoveries to better understand the biology of cancer.

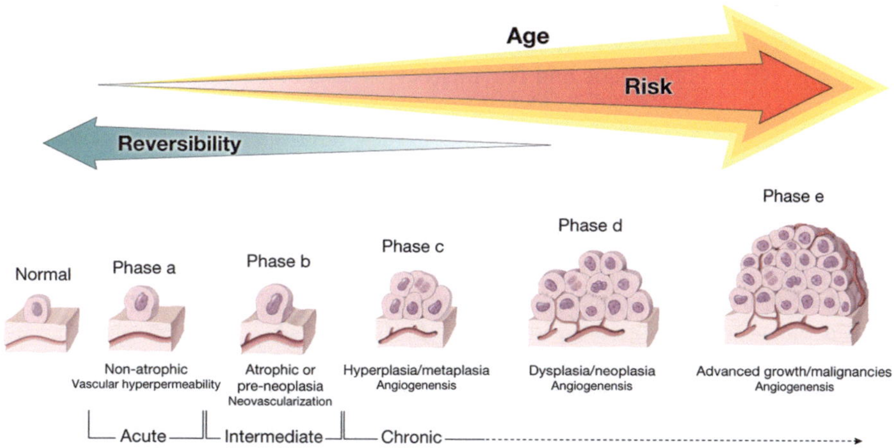

Fig. 1.2 Schematic representation that aging and long-term exposure to inflammatory conditions could increase the risk of immune suppression in direction of cellular growth promotion. Inflammation-induced identifiable phases of immune dysfunction that the author's research group demonstrated on experimental models of ocular allergies (1980's); included phases (**a**); acute reactions causing mast cells (MCs) degranulation, vascular hyperpermeability and tissue edema (reversible); (**b**) intermediate phase; persistent inflammation, tissue atrophy and/or pre-neoplasia along with neovascularization (potentially reversible); (**c**) induction of hyperplasia/neoplasia; progression of immune dysfunction and loss of tissue integrity towards Phases (**d**) and (**e**) in the direction of tumor growth, metastasis and angiogenesis. Reproduced from Khatami [87] with permission. All Rights Reserved

mine and prostaglandins from target/inflamed tissue. Ocular responses often associated with tissue edema, tearing, and vascular hyperpermeability reactions (Fig. 1.2) [80]. In 1980s, these early responses were identified as acute inflammatory reactions toward antigen. In 2014/2015, working as co-author in a multi-authored report on the role of chemical and environmental hazards (immune disruptors), to demonstrate the potential effects of low level carcinogens [88], the author learned with much excitements that the studies that her group reported in 1984 [80] were the first, and the only evidence on the role of immune disruptors in the induction of earliest response profiles in the direction of tumorigenesis (Fig. 1.2).

(ii) The first report on time-course kinetics of inflammation-induced identifiable developmental phases of immune response dynamic alterations toward tumorigenesis and angiogenesis [1, 2, 80–86]. The identified phases included,

  (a) acute inflammation responses (within days);
  (b) intermediate phase (within a couple of months)- induction of desensitization phenomenon, heavy infiltration of eosinophils into tissue epithelium and goblet cells; and
  (c) chronic phases (within 30 months of tissue stimulation)- induction of hyperplasia of lymphoid tissues, activation of macrophages and angiogenesis, epithelial thickening and/or thinning (necrosis or growth) often noted in the same tissue sections, increased MCs degranulation ('leaky' MCs) (details in Chap. 4) (Fig. 1.2).

(iii) Recent analyses of data on these studies further suggested the first evidence for sequential and synergistic interactions between host (local) immune cells (e.g., MCs, goblet cells and B lymphocytes) and those of recruiting immune cells (e.g., activated macrophages or TAMs), in the direction of tissue damage and massive hyperplasia of lymphoid tissues, tumorigenesis and angiogenesis (Fig. 1.2) [2].

(iv) In 2008, acute inflammation was defined for the first time, as the balance between 2 tightly regulated and biologically opposing arms of immunity, termed Yin (apoptosis or tumoricidal) and Yang (wound healing or tumorigenic) event with intimate involvement of vasculature for protecting the body against foreign elements, throughout life ('friend') [11]. Unresolved or chronic inflammation (oxidative stress) was suggested as the loss of balance between Yin and Yang of acute inflammation ('Foe'), causing expression and co-expression of mismatched apoptotic and wound healing factors, creating immunological chaos or immune tsunami, in susceptible target tissue [1, 2, 10–12, 86, 87]. Chronic inflammation was suggested to be the basis for induction of altered immune responses in tissue that could lead to 'mild', 'moderate' or 'severe' immune disorders, influencing the bioenergetics of tissues (mitophagy) and causing instability of chromosomal components (DNA/RNA, epigenetics and repair mechanisms), damage to extra- and intra-cellular membrane components in the direction of chronic diseases or cancer, particularly during aging process (Figs. 1.1 and 1.2) [1, 2, 10–12].

(v) It was hypothesized that inflammation differentially influences the tissues that are immune-privileged (e.g., neuronal tissues, CNS, neuroretina, cornea, reproductive system) or immune-responsive (e.g., squamous or glandular epithelia, endothelia, stroma, vasculature), creating 'immunological chaos' or 'immune tsunami' in the target tissues. Inflammation-induced immunological chaos could switch response profiles in the oxidative stress-sensitive immune-privileged tissues toward necrosis causing the induction of neurodegenerative or autoimmune diseases. On the other hand, in immune-responsive target tissues, chronic inflammation and expression, or co-expression of wound healing and apoptotic factors could create altered (decreased) ratios of Yin vs Yang (tumoricidal vs tumorigenic) of immune responses in the direction of cell growth promotion and initiation of neoplasia, hyperplasia, tumorigenesis, cancer and angiogenesis and metastasis (Fig. 1.3) [1, 2, 10–12, 86, 87].

(vi) In 1999, at DCP/NCI/NIH, Khatami suggested and discussed the potential anti-inflammatory roles of drugs such as aspirin, Captopril and Sulindac for cancer prevention (May 12, 1999, lecture at DCP/NCI/NIH and documents) [85].

(vii) In 2004/2005 an initial project involving standardization of cancer biomarkers using 'data elements' as a foundation of a cancer biomarkers database for oncology research became an NCI-Invention. Abstract of the invention published in Federal Register (2005). A more detailed description of the work was also published in 2007 [41]. This was a needed project, according to the NCI/NIH records.

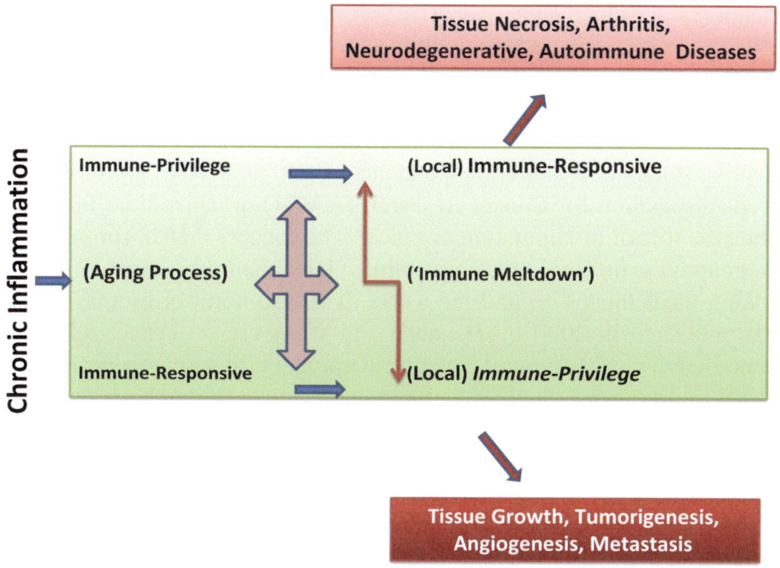

Fig. 1.3 Schematic representation of chronic inflammation-induced immune response shifts ('immune meltdown' or 'immune tsunami') in tissues that are naturally immune—privileged or immune-responsive in the induction of local responsiveness or immune-privilege toward tissue necrosis and/or growth. See text

In 2016, we hypothesized that site-specific cancers are 'severe' (irreversible) forms of cumulative delayed hypersensitivity responses that would induce immunological chaos in favor of growth in target tissues. Shared or special features of growth from fetus development into adulthood and aging processes and carcinogenesis were compared with regard to energy requirements of highly complex function of Yin and Yang (details in Chaps. 2 and 6) [7, 12].

In summary, since 1998, the author submitted a series of concepts and hypotheses on the role of inflammation in carcinogenesis emphasizing that 'inflammatory mediators are ideal targets for detection, prevention and therapy of cancer'; followed by designs of clinical trials; as well as, standardizing cancer biomarkers criteria (data elements) for developing a cancer biomarkers database. In 2006, at the request of the upper management at NCI/NIH, the author also submitted a comprehensive proposal to extend her pioneering studies that were published in 1980s, (Khatami, documents submitted to CCR-Center for Cancer Research, NCI/NIH, 2006).

After heavy opposition, denial, rejection and minimization of the submitted documents, the decision makers in the cancer community decided to fragment the concepts and treat them as many separate ideas apparently for fundraising and career promotional purposes of those who serve at the pleasure of the decision makers with power to control project funding. In the last decade, significantly increased funded projects focus on a wide range of basic research and clinical trials that relate to inflammation and cancer using expensive and specific detection technologies; organizing many networking forums within and outside NCI/NIH. For example, in 2005, NCI management developed a program for inflammation and cancer within Center for Cancer Research (CCR/NCI), for which the author was requested to submit a comprehensive proposal on extension of her groundbreaking studies ([2, 9, 10] scientific documents and correspondence, CCR/NCI/NIH, 2006). In 2003, the American Association for Cancer Research (AACR) organized the first symposia promoting the role of inflammation in cancer. The cancer OMICS (proteomics, lipidomics, genomics, metabolomics, glycomics) have their own separate networking and funding mechanisms around the world. It is also noteworthy that in the book that was published in 2000 by Hanahan and Weinberg on cancer-related topics, there is no mention of the importance of inflammation in carcinogenesis. However, in their 2011 edition, the role of inflammation in cancer research and therapy had a prominent position.

The behaviors of the members of cancer establishment with regard to Khatami's proposed concepts on the fundamental roles of inflammation in cancer research remind us that even the scientific truth often goes through three stages of *'opposition, denial and rejection, and it then becomes a routine and ordinary fact of life'*. Such heavy politics and abuse of power by medical/cancer establishment have been extremely costly to the public. The outcomes of such approaches to cancer science and therapy repeatedly failed patients, cost millions of precious lives and brought financial toxicity to the society, particularly in America. Cancer is the induced disease of twentieth century and has been made as an imaginary problem that is too complex and cannot be solved for the purpose of corporate profit (details in Chap. 5) [6, 7].

Figure 1.4, is the cover page of Time Magazine (2004) showing 'Inflammation' as 'The Silent Killer' involved in all chronic diseases including cancer.

3 Why War on Cancer Will Not End: False Foundation and Visionless/Reductionist Approaches to Cancer Research and Therapy as Bases for Extremely Slow Progress and Financial Toxicity to Society. Might of Power Over Right of Science!

The major reasons for the extremely slow progress in understanding the pathways in multistep diseases or carcinogenesis include:

(a) Absence of systematic approaches in studying the biology of aging and chronic diseases, particularly pathways involved in carcinogenesis. As noted above, while the biological cascades of cancer metastasis have been studied in relative details [73–77]; except for our 'accidental' discoveries on the sequential events that are involved in tumorigenesis and angiogenesis [1, 2, 10–12], very little is known about the early biological events that contribute to immune disruption in the multistep carcinogenesis.

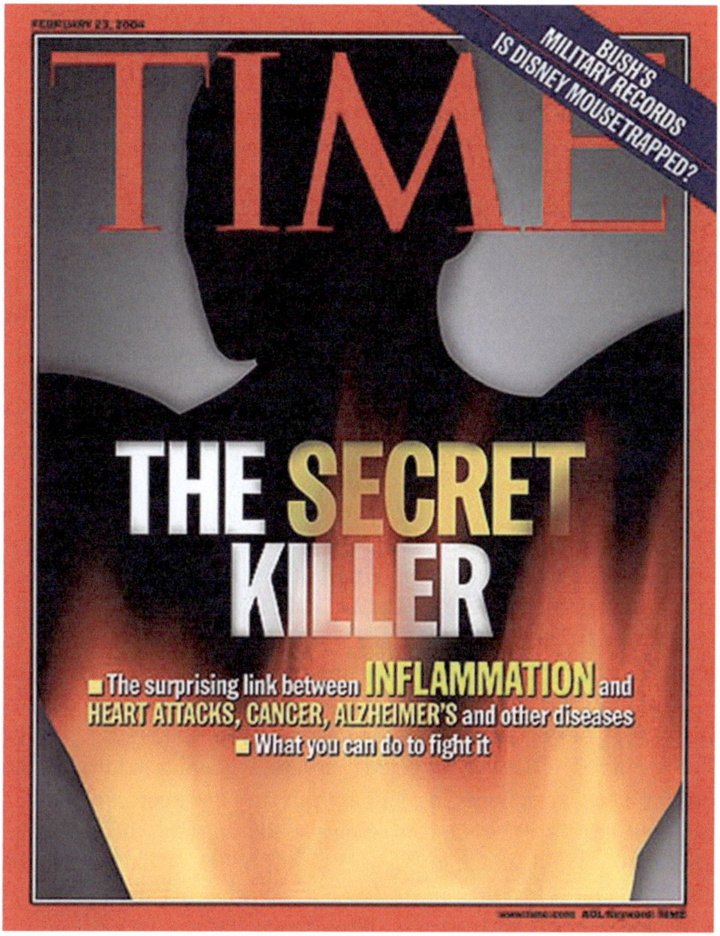

Fig. 1.4 Cover page of Time, 2004 showing inflammation as 'The Secret Killer' of chronic diseases or cancer

(b) Controversies and disconnects in existing biological data within different scientific disciplines, particularly for cancer biology and treatment;
(c) Fundamental knowledge gaps between initiation, progression and manifestation of diseases in susceptible or vulnerable tissues/organs;
(d) Lack of knowledge on cellular composition and nature of susceptibility of organ systems during induction of a specific disease;
(e) Lack of interest or support in understanding the biological heterogeneities of intrinsic and extrinsic interactions between organ systems exposed to harmful agents (immune disruptors) that shift the normal physiology of tissues toward the induction of diseases and manifestations of tissue-specific age-associated chronic illnesses and cancer;

(f) There is a powerful group of decision makers in cancer community, with career longevity of 40–65 years who exclusively decide, popularize, insist and defend too many molecular false flags that are based on false foundations for cancer research and therapy with claims of 'targeted' therapy, 'precision' or 'personalized' medicine as well as pathogen-specific vaccines. The outcomes of these scientifically visionless projects produced failure rates of 90% (+/−5) according to governmental and private organizations [2, 6, 7, 10–12, 22–27].

In the last century, there are too many reports on too many isolated molecules that flood the literature on site-specific cancers [2, 6, 7]. Analyzing data on cost and benefit to the public, one concludes that these efforts are primarily for fundraising purposes and increased power of the establishment in cancer community. There is no intellectually independent evaluation of the funded projects and no clear vision when decision makers support identifying a set of mutated genes, among thousands of others that are identified with specific detection protocols, in the 'molecular cancer tsunami' of site-specific cancers to benefit the public [6, 7].

Another serious concern is that the fragmented published data generated much confusions, misinformation and misunderstanding among cancer researchers. Majority (90% +/−5) of efforts for making therapeutic decisions for solid tumors have failed in the last century [2, 6, 7, 10, 25–27]. Every few years, members of establishment overtly publicize and exaggerate the role of their chosen molecules for cancer research and therapy to the public and policy makers for fundraising purposes. The highly exaggerated promises of 'cure' by decision makers remind us of a 'pie in the sky', or the Congressional debates on 'building bridge (s) to nowhere' [6, 7, 10]. The highly claimed 'targeted' therapies become additional motives to recruit desperate cancer patients in clinical trials and use such drugs (poisons) that have been tested in rats and mice for patients while charging insurance companies and public ([2, 10], details in Chap. 5). The author believes that the visionless decisions and building on shut-gun approaches are the principal sources of high cost of clinical trials and cancer care and more importantly the loss of millions of precious lives. The approaches to develop pathogen-specific vaccines are no different (details in Chaps. 5 and 6).

4 Answer to Cancer: A Case for Inflammation as Common Denominator in Induction of Nearly All Age-Associated Chronic Diseases and Site-Specific Cancers

There is now little dispute that aging process is associated with the combined diminutions (retarded levels or effectiveness) of important hormones and metabolites; related enzymes or receptor molecules and immune responses in organs/tissues, known as the biological and immunological senescence [1, 2] (details in Chaps. 3 and 6). The age-associated intrinsic biological changes are often adversely influenced by accumulation of a wide variety of internal or external stimuli (e.g., antigens/allergens, pathogens/infective agents, senescent cells, immune lymphocyte complexes, oxidized metabolites, chemical, biological or environmental hazards) that would increase the risks of induction of a wide range of chronic diseases, inflammatory conditions or site-specific cancers [1, 2, 10–12, 25, 35–40, 45, 50–55, 81, 82, 84–87]. We proposed that chronic inflammation-induced initiation of multi-step pathways toward tumorigenesis and angiogenesis affect primarily immune-response tissues (e.g., squamous or glandular epithelial cells, endothelial, stroma, mucosal cells). However, in immune-privileged tissues (e.g., CNS, BBB, reproductive organs, neuroretina or asvascular cornea), sustained oxidative stress could switch these oxidative stress-sensitive tissues to be immune responsive causing initiation of neurodegenerative or autoimmune diseases as well as, tumorigenesis [1, 2, 10–12].

Among the principal roles that impaired immunity and inflammatory responses play during aging process and negatively affect health are:

(a) Decreased antigen-processing ability of immune and non-immune systems (e.g., vasculature, metabolism, neuronal) that affect proper responses toward new or old antigen challenges;
(b) Diminished co-stimulatory capability and limited repertoire diversity of immune cells;
(c) Immune response changes that influence vascular dynamics (e.g., vascular toning, hyperpermeability, neovascularization or angiogenesis) causing alterations in the rates or nature of cellular infiltration, proliferation and maturation in host/target tissues. It should be emphasized that vasculature (the body's tree of life), being the gate-keeper of immune cells trafficking to host tissue and crosstalk with cellular or neuronal receptor molecules (e.g., histamine receptors during induction of pain or tissue edema), perhaps play the most important roles in health and in acute and chronic inflammatory diseases, as well as, treatment and drug-delivery to target tissues [1, 2, 6, 7, 10–20, 25, 35–40, 61–68, 81, 82, 84–87].

Accumulating data on epidemiological, clinical and prospective meta- analyses demonstrate a role for inflammation-induced dysregulation of immune cell responses in the genesis and progression of many diseases including:

(a) Severe acute inflammatory diseases such as sepsis, pneumonia, meningitis or major trauma) often leading to multiple organ failures (MOF) or death;
(b) Increased incidence of allergies such as asthma, emphysema, skin and ocular inflammatory conditions, particularly among the older adults, and major health concerns in recent in recent decades around the globe;
(c) Increased risks of a wide range of age-associated chronic illnesses, neurodegenerative and autoimmune diseases such as rheumatoid arthritis, atherosclerosis, dementia, Alzheimer's, multiple sclerosis, hypertension, diabetes, stroke and cardiovascular complications, colitis, gastritis, hepatitis, nephritis, prostatis, pancreatitis, appendicitis, thyroiditis, opthalmitis, Grave's disease, fibromyalgia, Bechet's, esophagitis, neuritis, lupus, Parkinson's, psoriasis;

(d) Numerous circumstantial evidence documented a link between prior injuries, infections or chronic irritations with development of many site-specific soft tissue and solid cancers (e.g., lung, colon/rectal, breast, stomach, cervical, prostate, bladder, liver, gall bladder, appendix, ovarian, thyroid, pancreas, brain, hematologic malignancies).

(e) Clinical and epidemiological data on cancer metastasis suggests that the metastasis is a combined biological, bioenergetics, mechanical and physical phenomena. The metastatic cascades are the complex and extraordinary processes that enable tumor cells to acquire a series of molecular features to develop at distant site ('seed and soil' theory). Many such features include rupturing of the cellular membrane, loss of integrity of cell junctions, migration through extracellular spaces and changes in matrix structures. These processes most likely are due to, in part, cancer cells taking advantage of the inherent duality of immune cells for selective DNA-directed expression of growth and apoptotic factors that would alter the balance between tumoricidal vs tumorigenic properties of immunity. Overall analyses of data on metastatic cascades demonstrate involvement of exaggerated expression of proteolytic enzymes and degradation of intra-and extravasation of B cells for fusion and cloning involving altered activities of plasma and other immune cells, epithelial-mesenchymal transformation and vasculature accompanied by changes in oxidative metabolism and DNA/RNA mutations. Moreover, reports from cell culture and experimental models of tumors, and human cancers show that host and tumor cells merge [1, 2, 10–12, 38–74, 84–87, 95–125] (details in Chap. 6).

Many of the chronic diseases that manifest as distinct and site-specific diseases are potentially interrelated (Figs. 1.1, 1.2 and 1.3). However, how the intrinsic and extrinsic biological heterogeneities in organ systems and their collective responses differentially interact with the age-associated altered hormonal, physiological, metabolic and immunological rearrangements in organ/tissue systems (biological and immunological senescence) in manifestation of disease processes are among important knowledge gaps that require systematic studies [1, 2, 6, 7].

In brief, longevity and accumulation of multiple context-dependent signaling pathways of long-standing inflammation (antigen-load or oxidative stress), including changes in the regulation of stem cell function and site-specific-dependent loss of control switch mechanisms and altered oxidative metabolism are very likely the key initiators (immune disruptors) in the induction of progressive changes in many cellular components toward multistep diseases processes. Important biological changes that collectively contribute to inappropriate signaling pathways toward new stimuli or microbiota, include altered lysosomal activities and loss of control of cellular homeostasis (autophagy), energy production from mitochondrial oxidative metabolism (mitophagy), accumulation of mutations and damages to genetic material (e.g., DNA/RNA, chromosomal proteins, repair mechanisms), other cellular and membrane components (e.g., ribosome, Golgi apparatus) [1, 2, 6, 7, 10–12, 86, 87, 99–124]. Mutations that lead to multistep site-specific cancers often require many years/decades to develop. Furthermore, many initial phases of genetic mutations and damages to chromosomal repair mechanisms are potentially preventable, if details of early events in multistep carcinogenesis were systematically investigated and understood.

Depending on the nature of stimuli, the extent of inflammatory responses, as well as, the site of tissue injury, the spectrum of manifestation of inflammatory conditions/illnesses and/or the mortality and morbidity risks in older adults vary. Therefore, in an inflammatory condition, the nature (quality), quantity, frequency and duration (extent) of tissue exposure to irritants or infective agents, as well as the extent of responses perhaps will determine the outcome of inflammation that is, whether to support cell growth inhibition/arrest (apoptosis) or growth promotion, proliferation and tumorigenesis (Figs. 1.1, 1.2 and 1.3).

5 Assessing Claimed 'Targeted' Therapies, 'Personalized' or 'Precision' Medicine for Solid Tumors

In this section, the following fundamental questions are addressed before assessing the claimed 'targeted' therapies:

1. Why we have not solved cancer biology, or why we have not been able to control cancer after six decades of heavy public and private investment on war against cancer?
2. Except for scientists/professionals who are in decision making roles and direct cancer research and therapy to maintain a profitable enterprise, who would select from hundreds and thousands of molecular chaos of site-specific cancers, any one or 2 or 5 evolving mutated genes or growth factors to inhibit or activate as answer for cancer therapy?
3. Is cancer 'OUTSMARTING' scientists?

An overall evaluation of current cancer therapeutic strategies demonstrates that the cytoreductive and fragmented molecular approaches for therapies, particularly the heavy emphasis on gene mutation-based regimen that are claimed 'targeted' therapies, 'personalized' or 'precision' medicine are conducted on a false foundation (Fig. 1.4). The outcomes on the use of such drugs proven to be poisonous rather than curative for solid tumors; as they substantially aggregate the patient's immune and non-immune system problems that kill them [2, 6, 7, 10–12, 125–131]. The principal/active components of such costly drugs that are used in clinical trials for site-specific solid tumors are potent apoptotic factors (specific growth factor inhibitors) and clearly indicate that the approaches are wrong and unethical as outlined below (details in Chaps. 5 and 6):

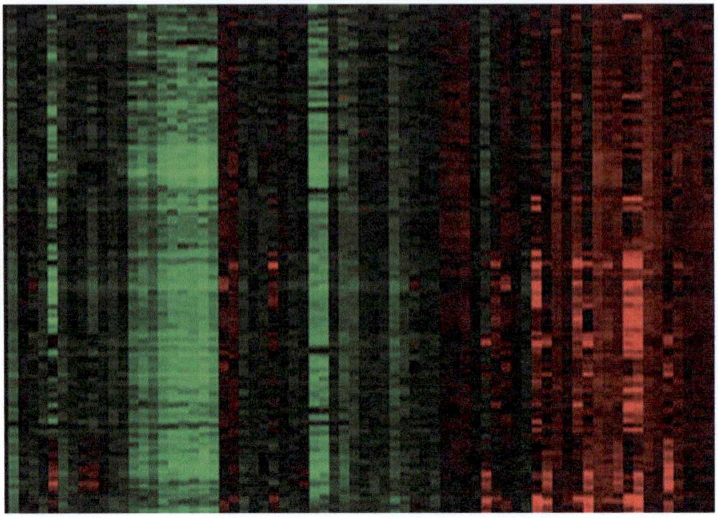

Fig. 1.5 Example of genetic-mutational diagrams, showing an image of identification of thousands of signals that become the bases for development of cancer claimed 'targeted' therapy, 'precision' or 'personalized' medicine. The diagram apparently! shows active or abnormal (*red*) or normal (*green*) genes and the intensity of such signals and anything in between in a site-specific cancer (Source: AACR document 2014. Image of cancer genomic and mutations—Reproduced from AACR meeting announcement (accessed 11/17/2014)

(a) A distorted picture of cancer biology. Research and treatment of cancer are based on molecular false flags and identification of numerous evolving genetic mutations in the cancer 'molecular tsunami', where hundreds or thousands of other dysfunctional molecules exist. Figure 1.5, is an example of image of hundreds of mutations that are identified in site-specific cancer; longer spikes seemingly are selected by one laboratory or another as the choice for drug development;
(b) Poorly designed protocols for safety and efficacy of the drugs that are tested in rats and mice and approved by FDA before clinical trials start;
(c) Drug development strategies basically ignore the importance of compensatory mechanisms of response dynamics. These mutational-derived drugs are specific growth factor inhibitors, or potent apoptotic factors (e.g., antibodies or inhibitors of specific growth factors, kinases or receptor molecules), identified by specific costly technologies in the molecular chaos of site-specific cancers (Fig. 1.5);
(d) Majority of 'targeted' drugs produce serious and life-threatening side effects such as drug-resistance, cancer relapse, cachexia, anorexia, fatigue, sarcopenia, thromboembolism, often leading to multiple organ failure (MOF) and death; symptoms that are associated with potent pathogen-induced acute inflammatory diseases such as sepsis, meningitis, and salmonella poisoning or major trauma.

(e) Another serious concern is the safety or efficacy of drugs. The drugs are tested in animal models such as rats and mice prior to conducting expensive Phase I and II clinical trials.
(f) The outcomes of such approaches produced failure rates of 90% (±5) for solid tumors, according to admission by government and private industry [2, 9, 10, 22–26, 63, 86, 108, 125–130].

The statement made by Payton Rous (Nobel Laureate in Physiology and Medicine) over half a century ago, best describes the current situations in cancer therapy; "*A hypothesis is best known by its fruits. What have been those of the somatic mutation hypothesis? It has resulted in no good thing as concerns the cancer problem, but in much that is bad... Most serious of all the results of the somatic mutation hypothesis has been its effect on research workers. It acts as a tranquilizer on those who believe in it.*" This statement was made decades before the emphasis on genetic mutations was put on steroids! [10].

In summary, the claimed 'targeted' drugs are strong poisons (potent apoptotic agents) that affect not only the function of T and B cells, in the body of an already immune-compromised cancer patient, but cause serious side effects often leading to MOF and death (Fig. 1.6) [2, 6, 7, 10].

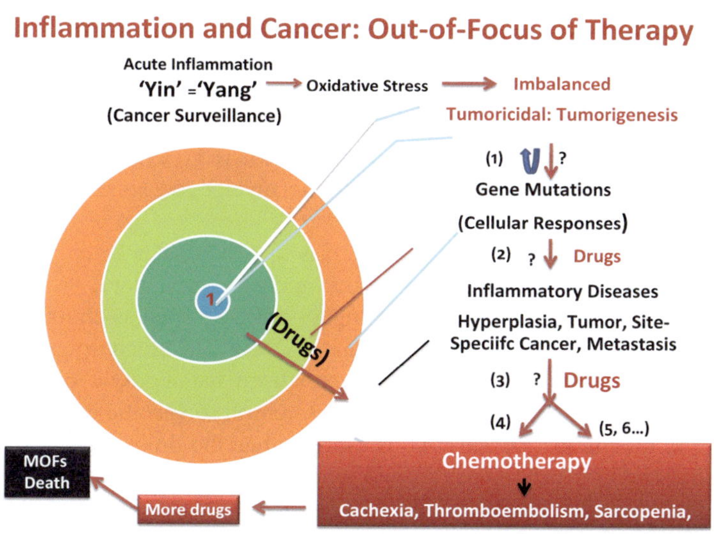

Fig. 1.6 Schematic representation of targeting cancer therapy (Modified from Cell Biochem Biophy Ref. [10] with permission. All right reserved)

6 Heavy Economic Burden to Society on Falsely Designed Clinical Trials that Repeatedly Failed: Cancer Financial Toxicity

Economically, a great proportion of the national and international resources is spent for therapy, hospitalization and long-term care of the older adults that suffer from chronic illnesses, many of which are potentially preventable. For example, in the past six decades, while trillions of dollars were spent on cancer research and therapy, millions of lives were lost to cancer. The outcomes of highly publicized and claimed 'targeted' therapies, 'personalized' or 'precision' medicine produced failure rates of 90% (±5) [2, 6, 7, 10–12, 22–27, 125–128, 131]. In only 1 year (2008), 7.6 million patients lost their lives to cancer; while in the same year, 1.6 trillion dollars were spent on cancer research, drug development, clinical trials and hospitalization of cancer patients, according to official reports by WHO or other governmental and private organizations. Evaluation of life-threatening side effects of drugs clearly demonstrates wrong approaches to cancer science and therapy. The high cost of care for chronic illnesses, particularly for cancer drug development, clinical trials and care, is not sustainable much longer [2, 6, 7, 22–27].

The reductionist approaches to cancer research and treatment options, repeatedly failed patients; cancer became a problem not to be solved. With the tremendous funding that cancer community has received for decades, cancer biology and many other chronic diseases should have been understood, prevented and/or treated years ago if the decision makers who control cancer community did not insist supporting too many out-of-focus projects that failed in translational research and clinical trials. Even the reported limited benefits of 'targeted' therapies on some forms of leukemia occurred when the defective immune cells [e.g., dysfunctional B cells in acute lymphocytic leukemia (ALL) or chronic myelocytic leukemia (CML)] are corrected [2, 6, 7, 10–12].

As noted above, another serious concern is that the cancer drugs are primarily tested for efficacy and safety in test tubes and/or experimental models of site-specific cancers in rats and mice (not in higher primates such as chimpanzees) and approved by the governmental agencies (e.g., FDA in US). Such drugs that worked in mice or rats are standardized and commercialized as the only choices for use in clinical trials. Physicians encourage patients to enroll to specific clinical trials and be subject to treatment. 'Success' is measured when the drugs postpone the death sentence of patients for short durations (3–6 months) before the life-threatening side effects of the drugs kick in to cause cancer relapse, metastasis and multiple organ failure and death [2, 6, 7, 10–12, 125–131].

With the availability of modern technologies, decision makers in the cancer community (government, academia and Big pharma) have become narrowly experts in their fields of 'omics' (e.g., genomic, proteomic, lipidomic, glycomic, metabolomic) and know details of structures and substructures of viruses, bacteria, parasites (microbiotics), carcinogens and endless broken/defective molecules (e.g., somatic mutations of growth or apoptotic factors, enzymes, receptors) or how to inhibit them in experimental models of tumors or clinical trials [6, 7].

Lack of oversight and accountability and abuse of funds on too many out-of-focuses and failed projects made cancer a myth making machine. The war on cancer remains an imaginary problem ('it is too many diseases') to solve. Public deception on cancer science reminds us of the statement that '*The creation and maintenance of public myths exert a powerful influence.*' Philip Zelikow [7].[6]

7 Challenges in Conducting Effective Research and Clinical Trials for Cancer

In general, aside from heavy financial and political motives that prevent an effective solution for cancer research and therapy, the principal scientific challenges and complexities in the designs of effective clinical trials, drug development and formulation of accurate risk assessments in multistep carcinogenesis fall into the following major confounding and interrelated categories:

1. Lack of systematic study on identifying the dynamics of immune and non-immune responses toward a wide range of stimuli (immune disruptors) is perhaps the most serious factor in lack of understanding the biological pathways in aging process and chronic diseases or cancer;
2. Heterogeneities in determining the immune-biological disease outcomes including the extent/duration, nature/potency and route of exposures to immune disruptors and carcinogens and cumulative/additive long-term influence on intrinsic and extrinsic stimuli. Immune disruptors-induced diversities in the rates of dysfunction or extent of activation/deactivation of innate or acquired immune cells are among major knowledge gaps that deserve further studies.
3. Heterogeneities in host (target tissue) immune and non-immune cells composition and related variations in the interactions and potential synergies between resident and recruiting immune or non-immune cells in the direction of disease processes;
4. Heterogeneities in reported outcomes of case-control studies, epidemiologic, prospective or meta-analyses; when risk values are estimated and formulated toward wide ranges of potential hazards or immune disruptors;

There is undisputed fact that the physiology and metabolism (e.g., oxidative metabolism, glucose utilization), immune response profiles (e.g., CMI and HI) at the microenvironmental levels of solid tumors are sufficiently different from the normal tissues from which they arise. Such differences, if studied systematically are expected to provide unique and selective targets for cancer prevention or treatment. However, systematic targeting of tumor physiology and metabolism on molecular

[6] Philip Zelikow was one of the architects behind creation of war against powerless nations.

differences between transformed and untransformed cells has received very little attention compared with the heavy support on shut-gun approaches on identification of too many evolving genetic mutations within the chaotic cancer molecular environment.

Therefore, it is reasonable to propose that designs of logical strategies that would correct or minimize defects in the important function of immune surveillance; the principal protecting (controlling) systems for proper activities of metabolic-physiology-genomic pathways are keys to understanding the biology of aging. The proposed future studies are to consider correcting the defects for the maintenance of balance between 2 biologically opposing arms of acute inflammation; Yin (tumoricidal) vs. Yang (tumorigenic) that intimately involve crosstalk between vasculature, neuronal, hormonal and metabolic activities of organ systems.

8 Concluding Remarks and Proposed Future Directions: Maintenance of Immune Surveillance Key to Healthy Aging

Longevity combined with persistent oxidative stress are likely the co-conspirators in altering the effectiveness of immune surveillance, provided through acute inflammation, a tightly controlled balance between 2 biologically opposing arms (Yin - Yang) of immunity or the crosstalks between immune and non-immune systems. Sustained or unresolved inflammation differentially affects the immune-privileged or immune-responsive tissues in the directions of disease processes. In immune-privileged tissues oxidative stress could lead to induction and progression of tissue necrosis and complications of site-specific diseases such as neurodegenerative or autoimmune diseases; while in immune-responsive tissues, oxidative stress causes cell growth promotion, neoplasia, hyperplasia, polyps, tumorigenesis, angiogenesis and cancer metastasis.

Cancerous cells should be regarded as the intrinsic cellular defects whose oncogenic growth features, within the multilayered organized tissues, are routinely monitored and arrested by the self-terminating protective properties of acute inflammation as any other pathogens, infective agents, senescent and useless cell complexes that are perceived as 'foreign elements' and threaten body's survival. Chronic irritations or sustained injuries to the epithelial or endothelial cells result in exaggerated activation, migration or recruitment of other inflammatory cells to the site of injured tissue that would alter the balance between 'Yin' and 'Yang' properties of immune surveillance. Stimulated phagocytes or lymphocytes can induce exaggerated signals in the direction of altered cellular activities including expression of unresolved growth or apoptotic factors, chromosomal breaks and altered nuclear repair mechanisms, sister chromatid exchanges, increased DNA/RNA damage and mutations and altered energy consumption from defective mitochondria. Loss of effectiveness of immune cellular and humoral factors plays important roles in the production or aggravation of most of tissue responses toward damage.

Proposed future studies in the designs of effective diagnostic, preventive or therapeutic measures are summarized in the following.

1. Systematic studies on the role of unresolved inflammation in the loss of balance between inherent tumoricidal vs tumorigenic (Yin and Yang) protective properties of innate and adaptive immune cells as primary focus in understanding the cancer biology and other chronic diseases.
2. Role of unresolved inflammation or oxidative stress in the induction of immune dysfunction in tissues that are naturally immune-privileged or immune-responsive and could lead to neurodegenerative and autoimmune diseases or cancer.
3. Tissue susceptibility toward oxidative stress in insulin-dependent or insulin-independent tissues for glucose transport.
4. Pathogen-host interaction profiles that include identification of principal response features of pathogen-, allergen-, oxidative stress-induced activation of resident or recruited immune cells in target tissues.
5. Potential reversibility of early stages of inflammation-induced immune dysfunction [e.g., developmental phases of immune dysregulation during acute, intermediate and chronic responses] including altered initial immune response dynamics and cellular chromosomal/genetic material that would lead to cellular growth and induction of hyperplasia, neoplasia/precancer or cancer-malignancy deserve detailed studies.
6. Potential health benefits of antioxidants, anti-inflammatory agents, or sulfhydryl-containing agents (e.g., Amifostine, isothiocyanate, mercaptoethanol, N-acethylcysteine or captopril) or precursors of glutathione on redox-sensitive transcription factors (e.g., NF-kB), leukocyte adherence to be examined at early stages of immune dysfunction for potential promotion and/or stabilization of innate and adaptive immune cells.

The expected outcomes for conducting systematic studies of the role of immune disruptors (hazardous materials) in altering response dynamics of metabolic, neurological and immune systems in the induction of tissue damage and initiation of disease processes including cancer are proposed to be the following (details in Chap. 6):

(a) Improved accuracy of risk assessment formulation for chronic diseases;
(b) Accuracy on cancer diagnosis, minimizing costly over-, or under diagnosis of site-specific cancers;
(c) Effective decision making for prevention strategies of age-associated chronic illnesses and cancer;
(d) Effective designs of drug development for clinical trials and therapy with the goal to minimize life-threatening side effects of drugs.

Developing useful roadmaps on key biological events that govern the biology of aging process is a timely and important undertaking for the scientific community toward improving the health of growing population around the world. A reliable 'roadmap' on major interrelated biological events of aging is expected to provide a

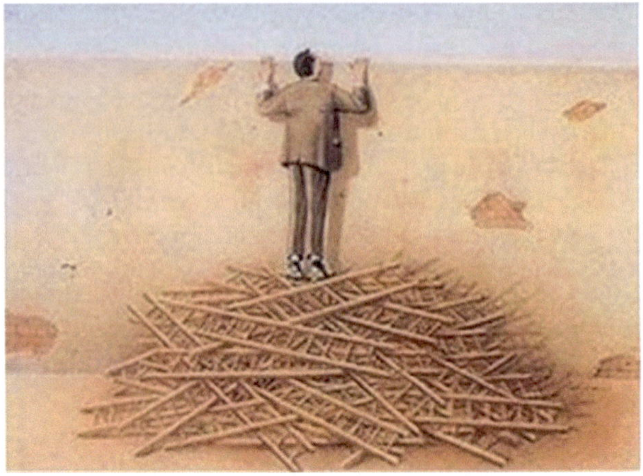

Fig. 1.7 It does not matter how many resources you have, if you don't know how to use them, they will never be enough (Source: Internet)

forum for identification of tremendous biological gaps that currently exist in our knowledge for understanding the chronic health problems. The author believes that the existence of too many fragmented data on a wide range of immunobiological topics is among the important roadblocks for getting a better handle on the complexity of chronic illnesses that is crippling our society.

Author's Personal Note

Vision without action is daydream, action without vision is nightmare. (Japanese proverb)

A closer look at a century of cancer science reveals that highly power structure (system) in medical establishment vs. anti-system and chaos in cancer research and therapy or pathogen-specific vaccines are potent recipes for failed therapeutics that kills patients but generate huge corporate profits [6, 7].

Personally, I believe that pretending or claiming that we are winning the war on cancer is worse than admitting that we are not. Policy makers and professionals in decision making roles are urged to return to common sense and logics that our Forefathers used to serve the public. Otherwise, it does not matter 'how many resources you have, if you don't know (or don't want to know) how to use them, there will never be enough' (Fig. 1.7).

In the last few decades, the largest proportion of the national and international resources are invested for long-term care and hospitalization of the elderly. Cancer therapy and care is particularly the major economic burden in USA and other developed countries [7, 125, 130, 131].

There is a need to move away from shotgun approaches to cancer research and therapy and pay attention to conducting systematic studies to understand the biology of aging process, since most chronic diseases or the multistep carcinogenesis occur during aging. Systematic identification and monitoring of the composition and interactions between host/target tissues and those of recruited cells should provide key information on early events in the loss of immune surveillance whose importance in controlling cancer were documented decades ago. The systematic identification of stages of immune dysfunction would tremendously help scientists to make informed decisions for balancing and promoting the inherent tumoricidal (Yin) and tumorigenic (Yang) properties of immune system, toward formulation of accurate risk assessment, effective preventive and therapeutic approaches with the goal to improve public health.

Personally, I feel it in my bones that the current false foundation in cancer projects that are decided, directed and funded by an elite group of insiders in the cancer community is eroding not only the health values of our society but our commitment to humanity. On behalf of patients around the world it is argued that with appropriate scientific vision and proper disciplines obtaining true scientific and clinical outcomes are achievable, not only for cancer, but also for nearly all chronic disorders and it should not be as costly to achieve better health for the growing society that is free and happy.

Finally, we should remind ourselves that the '*Destiny of human being is determined by love alone.*' Shakespeare

References

1. Khatami M. Inflammation, aging and cancer: tumoricidal vs tumorigenesis of immunity: a common denominator mapping chronic diseases. Cell Biochem Biophys. 2009;55:55–79.
2. Khatami M. Chronic inflammation: synergistic interactions of recruiting macrophages (TAMs) and eosinophils (Eos) with host mast cells (MCs) and tumorigenesis in CALTs. M-CSF, suitable biomarker for cancer diagnosis! Cancers. 2014;6:297–322.
3. Ehrlich P. Uber den jetzigen Stand der Karzinomforschung. Ned Tijdschr Geneeskd. 1909;5:273–90.
4. Lokaj J, John C. [Ilya Ilich Metchnikov and Paul Ehrlich: 1908 Nobel prize winners for their research on immunity] [Article in Czech]. Epidemiol Mikrobiol Immuno. 2008;57:119–24.
5. Rous P. The challenge to man of the neoplastic cell: nobel lecture, December 13, 1966.
6. Khatami M. Safety concerns and hidden agenda behind HPV vaccines: another generation of drug-dependent society? Clin Transl Med. 2016;5(1):46. Epub 2016 Dec 5
7. Khatami M. In Cancer research and therapy: scam of century – promote immunity [Yin-Yang]; 2016. ISBN-10:153043100X; ISBN-13:978-1530431007; Amazon-Createspace pp. 1–166, http://www.createspace.com/6123573.
8. Burnet, M: Cancer: A biological approach. The processes of control. British Med. J. Apr. 6, 1957.
9. Lederberg J. Instructive selection and immunological theory. Immunol Rev. 2002;185:50–3.
10. Khatami M. Unresolved inflammation and cancer: loss of natural immune surveillance as the correct "target" for therapy! Seeing the "elephant" in the light of logic. Cell Biochem Biophys. 2012;62:501–9.
11. Khatami M. "Yin and Yang" in inflammation: duality in innate immune cell function and tumorigenesis. Expert Opin Biol Ther. 2008;8:1461–72.
12. Khatami M. Is cancer a severe delayed hypersensitivity reaction and histamine a blueprint? Clin Transl Med. 2016;5(1):35. doi:10.1186/s40169-016-0108-3. Epub 2016 Aug 23
13. Al-Sarireh B, Eremin O. Tumour-associated macrophages (TAMs): disordered function, immune suppression and progressive tumour growth. J R Coll Surg Edinb. 2000;45:1–16.

14. Liotta LA, Stetler-Stevenson WG. Principles of molecular cell biology of cancer. 4th ed. Philadelphia: JB Lippincott; 1993.
15. Fidler IJ. Selection of successive tumour lines for metastasis. Nat New Biol. 1973;242:148–9.
16. DiCarlo E, Forni G, Lollini PL, Colombo MP, Modesti A, Musiani P. The intriguing role of polymorphonuclear neutrophils in antitumor reactions. Blood. 2001;97:339–45.
17. Weitzman SA, Gordon LI. Inflammation and cancer: role of phagocytic-generated oxidants in carcinogenesis. Blood. 1990;76(4):655–63.
18. Balch CM, Tilden AB, Dougherty PA, Cloud GA, Abo T. Depressed levels of granular lymphocytes with natural killer (NK) cell function in 247 cancer patients. Am Surg. 1983;198:192–9.
19. Daly C, Dube C, Rollins BJ. Chemokine influences on adaptive immunity and malignancies of the immune system. Emst Schering Res Found Workshop. 2004;45:11–30.
20. Hakim FT, Flomerfelt FA, Boyiadzis M, Gress RE. Aging, immunity and cancer. Curr Opin Immunol. 2004;18:151–8.
21. Aspinall R. Age-related changes in the function of T cells. Microsc Res Tech. 2003;62:508–13.
22. Ledford H. Translational research: 4 ways to fix the clinical trial. Nature. 2011;477:526–8.
23. U.S. FDA. Silver Spring (MD): U.S. FDA. Proposal to withdraw approval for the breast cancer indication for bevacizumab (avastin). FDA Public Hearing. June 29, 2011... http://www.fda.gov/downloads/NewsEvents/MeetingsConferencesWorkshops/UCM261697.pdf
24. International Agency for Research on Cancer (IARC). WHO, Press Release, Lyon/London, 3 February 2014.
25. Sledge GW Jr. Anti–vascular endothelial growth factor therapy in breast cancer: game over? J Clin Oncol (ASCO). 2015;33:133–5.
26. Gøtzsche PC. Deadly medicines and organised crime: how big pharma has corrupted health care. London: Radcliffe Publishing; 2013.
27. Neustadt RE, Fineberg HV, editors. The swine flu affair: decision-making on a slippery disease. Washington (DC): National Academies Press; 1978.
28. Eberlein TJ, Rosenstein M, Rosenberg SA. Regression of a disseminated syngeneic solid tumor by systemic transfer of lymphoid cells expanded in interleukin 2. J Exp Med. 1982;156:385–97.
29. Tomita M, Matsuzaki Y, Edagawa M, Shimizu T, Hara M, Onitsuka T. Distribution of mast cells in mediastinal lymph nodes from lung cancer patients. World J Surg Oncol. 2003;1:25.
30. Tobin MJ. Chronic obstructive disease, pollution, pulmonary vascular disease, transplantation, pleural disease, and lung cancer. Am J Respir Crit Care Med. 2000;164:1789.
31. Huovinen E, Kapiro J, Vesterinen E, Koshenvuo M. Mortality of adults with asthma: a prospective cohort study. Thorax. 1997;52:49–54.
32. Vesterinen E, Oukkala E, Timonen T, Aromaa A. Cancer incident among 78000 asmatic patients. Int J Epidemiol. 1993;22:976–82.
33. Le Meur Y, Tesch GH, Hill PA, Mu W, Foti R, Nikolic-Paterson DJ, Atkins RC. Macrophage accumulation at a site of renal inflammation is dependent on the M-CSF/c-fms pathway. J Leukocyte Biol. 2002;72:530–7.
34. Kronenberg M. Toward an understanding of NKT cell biology: progress and paradoxes. Annu Rev Immunol. 2005;23:877–900.
35. Keibel A, Singh V, Sharma MC. Inflammation, microenvironment, and the immune system in cancer progression. Curr Pharm Des. 2009;15:1949–55.
36. Kimura YN, Watari K, Fotovati A, Hosoi F, et al. Inflammatory stimuli from macrophages and cancer cells synergistically promote tumor growth and angiogenesis. Cancer Sci. 2007;98:2009–18.
37. Drayton DL, Liao S, Mounzer RH, Ruddle NH. Lymphoid organ development: from ontology to neogenesis. Nat Immunol. 2006;7:344–53.
38. Montovani A, Ming WJ, Balotta C, Abdeljalil B, Bottazzi B. Origin and regulation of tumor-associated macrophages: the role of tumor-derived chemotactic factor. Biochim Biophys Acta. 1986;865:59–67.

39. Teranishi A, Akada S, Saito S, Hatake K, Morikawa H. Macrophage colony-stimulating factor restored chemotherapy-induced granulocyte dysfunctions: role of Il-8 production by monocytes. Int Immunopharmacol. 2002;2:83–94.
40. Ribatti D, Ennas MD, Vacca A, et al. Tumour vascularity and tryptase-positive mast cells correlate with a poor prognosis in melanomas. Eur J Clin Investig. 2003;33:420–5.
41. Khatami M. Standardizing cancer biomarkers criteria: data elements as a foundation for a database. Inflammatory mediator/M-CSF as model marker. Cell Biochem Biophysics. 2007;47:187–98.
42. Fang J, Seki T, Tetsuya T, Qin H, Liao L, Nakamura H, Maeda H. Protection from inflammatory bowel disease and colitis associated carcinogenesis with4-vinyl-2,6-dimethoxyphenol (canolol) via suppression of oxidative stress. Carcinogenesis. 2013;34:2833–41.
43. Vincent PA, Xiao K, Buckley KM, Kowalczky AP. VE-cadherin: adhesion at arm's length. Am J Physiol Cell Phyiol. 2004;286:C987–97.
44. Vijg J, Hasty P. Aging and p53: getting it straight. A commentary on a recent paper by Gentry and Venkatachalam. Aging Cell. 2005;4:335–8.
45. Krtolica A, Campisi J. Cancer and aging: a model for the cancer promoting effects of the aging stroma. Int J Biochem Cell Biol. 2002;34:1401–14.
46. Vogelstein B, Papadopoulos N, Velculescu VE, Zhou S, Diaz LA Jr, Kinzler KW. Cancer genome landscapes. Science. 2013;339:1546–58.
47. Nash MA, Ferrandina G, Gordinier M, Loercher A, Freedman RS. The role of cytokines in both the normal and malignant ovary. Endocr Relat Cancer. 1999;6:93–107.
48. Maeda H, Sawa T, Yubisui T, Akaike T. Free radical generation from heterocyclic amines by cytochrome b5 reductase in the presence of NADH. Cancer Lett. 1999;143:117–21.
49. Harman D. Ageing: a theory based on free radical and radiation chemistry. J Gerontol. 1956;11:298–300.
50. Farrow B, Sugiyama Y, Chen A, Uffort E, Nealon W, Evers BM. Inflammatory mechanisms contributing to pancreatic cancer development. Ann Surg. 2004;239:763–71.
51. D'Alessio P. Aging and the endothelium. Exp Gerontol. 2004;39:165–71.
52. Meyer KC. Lung infections in aging. Ageing Res Rev. 2004;3:55–67.
53. Knight JA. The biochemistry of aging. Adv Clin Chem. 2000;35:1–62.
54. Kerbel RS, Frost P, Liteplo R, Carlow DA, Elliott BE. Possible epigenetic mechanisms of tumor progression: induction of high frequency heritable but phenotypically unstable changes in the tumorigenesis and metastatic properties of tumor cell population by 5-azacytidine treatment. J Cell Physiol Suppl. 1984;3:87–97.
55. Fulop T Jr, Larbi A, Dupuis G, Pawelec G. Ageing, autoimmunity and arthritis: perturbations of TCR signal transduction pathways with ageing- a biochemical paradigm for the ageing immune system. Arthritis Res Ther. 2003;5:290–302.
56. Krishnamurthy J, Sharpless NE. Stem cells and the rate of living. Cell Stem Cell. 2007;1:9–11.
57. Leslie M. Cell biology. Beyond clotting: the powers of platelets. Science. 2010;328:562–4.
58. Idzko M, Ferrari D, Eltzschig HK. Nucleotide signalling during inflammation. Nature. 2014;509(7500):310–7.
59. Colborn T. A case for revisiting the safety of pesticides: a closer look at neurodevelopment. Environ Health Perspect. 2006;114(1):10–7.
60. Colborn T. Commentary: setting aside tradition when dealing with endocrine disruptors. ILAR J. 2004;45(4):394–400.
61. Colborn T. Neurodevelopment and endocrine disruption. Environ Health Perspect. 2004;112(9):944–9.
62. Weber J. Immune checkpoint proteins: a new therapeutic paradigm for cancer—preclinical background: CTLA-4 and PD-1 blockade. Semin Oncol. 2010;37:430–9.
63. Topalian SL, Hodi FS, Brahmer JR, Gettinger SN, Smith DC, McDermott DF, et al. Safety, activity, and immune correlates of anti–PD-1 antibody in cancer. N Engl J Med. 2012;366:2443–54.

64. Rosenberg SA, Yang JC, Restifo NP. Cancer immunotherapy: moving beyond current vaccines. Nat Med. 2004;10:909–15.
65. Fahmy N, Lazo-Langer A, Lansavichene AL, Paulter SE. Effect of anticoagulants and antiplatelet agents on the efficacy of intravesicle BCG treatment of bladder cancer: a systematic review. Can Urol Assoc J. 2013;7:E740–9.
66. George J, Goldstein E, Abashidze S, Deutsch V, Shmilovich H, Finkelste A, Herz I, Miller H, Keren G. Circulating endothelial progenitor cells in patients with unstable angina: association with systemic inflammation. Eur Heart J. 2004;25:1003–8.
67. Frost P, Kerbel RS, Hunt B, Man S, Pathalk S. Selection of metastatic variants with identifiable karyotypic changes from a nonmetastatic murine tumor after treatment with 2-deoxy-5-azacytidine or hydroxyurea implication for the mechanisms of tumor progression. Cancer Res. 1987;47:2690–5.
68. Zhou Q, Facciponte J, Jin M, Shen Q, Lin Q. Humanized NOD-SCID IL2rg−/− mice as a preclinical model for cancer research and its potential use for individualized cancer therapies. Cancer Lett. 2014;344:13–9.
69. Kirma N, Luthra R, Jones J, Liu Y-G, Nair HB, Mandava U, Tekmal RR. Overexpression of the colony-stimulating factor (CSF-1) and/or its receptor c-fms in mammary glands of transgenic mice results in hyperplasia and tumor formation. Cancer Res. 2004;64:4162–70.
70. Moore MM, Chua W, Charles KA, Clarke SJ. Inflammation and cancer: causes and consequences. Clin Pharmacol Ther. 2010;87:504–8.
71. Pardoll DM. The blockade of immune checkpoints in cancer immunotherapy. Nat Rev Cancer. 2012;12:252–64.
72. Weinberg RA. In the biology of cancer. New York: Garland Science, Taylor and Francis Group; 2007.
73. Paget S. The distribution of secondary growth in cancer of the breast. Lancet. 1889;1:571–3.
74. Fidler IJ. The pathogenesis of cancer metastasis: the ‘seed and soil hypothesis revisited. Nat Rev Cancer. 2003;3:1–6.
75. Nowell PC. The clonal evolution of tumor cell populations. Science. 1976;194:23–8.
76. Weiss L. Metastasis of cancer: a conceptual history from antiquity to the 1990s. Cancer Metastasis Rev. 2000;19:193–400.
77. Rebelles N, Santonja A, Pajares B, Llacer C, Alba E. The seed and soil hypothesis revisited: current state of knowledge of inherited genes on prognosis in breast cancer. Cancer Treat Rev. 2014;40:293–9.
78. Dvorak HF. Tumors: wounds that do not heal. Similarities between tumor stroma generation and wound healing. N Engl J Med. 1986;315:1650–9.
79. Dvorak HF, Detmar M, Claffey KP, Nagy JA, van der Water L, Senger DR. Vascular permeability factor/vascular endothelial growth factor: an important mediator of angiogenesis in malignancy and inflammation. Int Arch Allergy Immunol. 1995;107:233–5.
80. Khatami M, Donnelly JJ, John T, Rockey JH. Vernal conjunctivitis. Model studies in guinea pigs immunized topically with fluoresceinyl ovalbumin. Arch Ophthalmol. 1984;102:1683–8.
81. Khatami M, Donnelly JJ, Rockey JH. Induction and down-regulation of conjunctival type-1 hypersensitivity reactions in guinea pigs sensitized topically with fluoresceinyl ovalbumin. Ophthalmic Res. 1985;17:139–47.
82. Khatami M, Donnelly JJ, Haldar JP, Rockey JH. Massive follicular lymphoid hyperplasia in experimental chronic recurrent allergic conjunctivitis. Arch Ophthalmol. 1989;107:433–8.
83. Haldar JP, Khatami M, Donnelly JJ, Rockey JH. Experimental allergic conjunctivitis: production of different isotypes of antibody by conjunctival-associated lymphoid tissue in culture. Reg Immunol. 1988;1:92–999.
84. Helleboid L, Khatami M, Wei Z-G, Rockey JH. Histamine and prostacyclin: primary and secondary release in allergic conjunctivitis. Invest Ophthalmol Vis Sci. 1991;32:2281–9.
85. Khatami M. Developmental phases of inflammation-induced massive lymphoid hyperplasia and extensive changes in epithelium in an experimental model of allergy. Implications for a direct link between inflammation and carcinogenesis. Am J Ther. 2005;12:117–28.

86. Khatami M. Inflammation, aging and cancer: friend or foe? In: Khatami M, editor. Inflammation, chronic diseases and cancer- cell and molecular biology, immunology and clinical bases. Rejeka: InTech Publishing; 2012. p. 3–30. [978-953-51-0102].
87. Khatami M. Unresolved inflammation: "immune tsunami" or erosion of integrity in immune-privileged and immune-responsive tissues and acute and chronic inflammatory diseases or cancer. Exp Opin Biol Ther. 2011;11:1419–32.
88. Thompson P, Khatami M, Baglole CJ, Sun J, Harris SA, Moon EY, et al. Environmental immune disruptors, inflammation and cancer risk. Carcinogenesis. 2015;36(Suppl 1):S232–53. doi:10.1093/carcin/bgv038. Review
89. Khatami M. Cyclooxygenase inhibitor ketorolac or mast cell stabilizers: immunological challenges in cancer therapy. Letters to the editor. Clin Cancer Res. 2005;11:1350–2.
90. Li W, Khatami M, Robertson G, Shen S, Rockey JH. Non-enzymatic glycosylation of bovine retinal microvessel basement membrane in vitro: kinetic analysis and inhibition of by aspirin. Invest Ophthalmol Vis Sci. 1984;25:884–92.
91. Khatami M, Angeletti RH, Rockey JH. Amino acid sequence adjacent to a sulfhydryl group exposed on illumination of bovine rhodopsin. J Biol Chem. 1981;256:9826–9.
92. Khatami M. Prevention and treatment of diabetes complications. In: Sakamoto N, Alberti KGMM, Hotta N, editors. 1990, p. 649–654.
93. Khatami M, Roel LE, Li W, Rockey JH. Ascorbate regeneration in bovine ocular tissues by NADH-dependent semidehydroascorbate reductase. Exp Eye Res. 1986;43:167–75.
94. Khatami M, Li W, Rockey JH. Kinetics of ascorbate transport by cultured retinal capillary pericytes. Invest Ophthalmol Vis Sci. 1986;27:1665–71.
95. Werling D, Hope JC, Howard CJ, Jungi TW. Differential production of cytokines, reactive oxygen and nitrogen by bovine macrophages and dendritic cells stimulated with toll-like receptor agonists. Immunology. 2004;111:41–52.
96. Udler M, Maja AT, Cebrian A, Brown C, Greenberg D, Shah M, et al. Common germline genetic variation in antioxidant defense genes and survival after diagnosis of breast cancer. J Clin Oncol. 2007;25:3015–23.
97. Ren J-L, Pan J-S, Lu Y-P, Sun P, Han J. Inflammatory signaling and cellular senescence. Cell Signal. 2009;21:378–83.
98. Romanyukha AA, Yashin AI. Age related changes in population of peripheral T cells: towards a model of immunoscenescence. Mech Ageing Dev. 2003;124:433–43.
99. Muller AJ, Sharma MD, Chandler PR, Duhadaway JB, et al. Chronic inflammation that facilitate tumor progression create local immune suppression by inducing indoleamine 2, 3 dioxygenase. Proc Natl Acad Sci. 2008;105:17073–8.
100. Meur YL, Tesch GH, Hill PA, Mu W, Foti R, Nikolic-Paterson DJ, Atkins RC. Monocyte proliferation outside the bone marrow has also been demonstrated in vitro studies using monocytes extracted from peripheral blood and glomeruli. J Leukocyte Biol. 2002;72:530–7.
101. Galli SJ. Biology of disease: new insights into 'the riddle of mast cells'; microenvironmental regulation of mast cell development and phenotypic heterogeneity. Lab Investig. 1990;62:5–33.
102. Schwartz LB. The mast cell. In: Kaplan AP, editor. Allergy, vol.1. Edingurgh: Churchil Livingston; 1985. 1, p. 53–92.
103. Gu L, Tseng S, Horner RM, Tam C, Loda M, Rollins BJ. Control of TH2 polarization by the chemokine monocyte chemoattractant protein-1. Nature. 2000;404:407–11.
104. Valent P, Bettelheim P. Cell surface structures on human basophils and mast cells: biochemical and functional characterization. Adv Immunol. 1992;52:333–423.
105. Serhan CN, Savill J. Resolution of inflammation: the beginning programs to end. Nat Immunol. 2005;6:1191–7.
106. Sethi G, Sung B, Aggarwal BB. TNF: a master switch for inflammation and cancer. Front Biosci. 2008;13:5094–107.
107. Shames DS, Minna JD, Gazdar AF. DNA methylation in health, disease, and cancer. Curr Mol Med. 2007;7:85–102.

108. Florescu A, Amir E, Bouganim N, Clemons M. Immune therapy for breast cancer in 2010-hype or hope? Curr Onco. 2011;18:e9–e18.
109. Rossi DJ, Jamieson CH, Weissman IL. Stem cells and the pathways to aging and cancer. Cell. 2008;132:681–96.
110. Sharpless NE, DePinho RA. Telomeres, stem cells senescence and cancer. J Clin Invest. 2004;113:160–8.
111. Van Zant G, Liang Y. The role of stem cells in aging. Exp Hematol. 2003;31:659–72.
112. Peggs KS, Quezada SA, Allison JP. Cell intrinsic mechanisms of T cell inhibition and application to cancer therapy. Immunol Rev. 2008;224:141–65.
113. Davalos AR, Coppe JP, Campisi J, Desprez PY. Senescent cells as a source of inflammatory factors for tumor progression. Cancer Metastasis Rev. 2010;29:273–83.
114. Hibberd C, Yau JL, Seckl JR. Glucocorticoids and the ageing hippocampus. J Anat. 2000;197(Pt 4):553–62.
115. McGlauchlen KS, Vogel LA. Ineffective humoral immunity in the elderly. Microbes Infect. 2003;5:1279–84.
116. Herrero C, Sebastian C, Marques L, Comalada M, Xaus J, Valledor AF, Lioberas J, Celada A. Immunosenescence of macrophages: reduced MHC class II gene expression. Exp Gerontol. 2002;37:389–94.
117. Lee YS, Kang YS, Lee JS, Nicolova S, Kim JA. Involvement of NADPH oxidase-mediated generation of reactive oxygen species in the apoptotic cell death by capsaicin in Hep G2 human hepatoma cells. Free Radic Res. 2004;38:405–12.
118. Hiyama E, Hiyama K. Telomere and telomerase in stem cells. Br J Cancer. 2007;96:1020–4.
119. Crotzer VL, Blum JS. Cytosol to lysosome transport of intracellular antigens during immune surveillance. Traffic. 2010;9:10–6.
120. Davis BK, Wen H, Ting JP. The inflammasome NLRs in immunity, inflammation and associated disease. Ann Rev Immunol. 2011;29:707–35.
121. Gray LH, Conger AD, Ebert M, Hornsey S, Scott OC. Concentration of oxygen dissolved in tissues at the time of irradiation as a factor in radiotherapy. Brit J Radiol. 1953;26:638–48.
122. Fadok VA, de Cathelineau A, Daleke DL, Henson PM, Bratton DL. Loss of phospholipids asymmetry and surface exposure of phosphatidylserine is required for phagocytosis of apoptotic cell by macrophages and fibroblasts. J Biol Chem. 2001;276:1071–7.
123. Racker E. Bioenergetics and the problem of tumor growth. Am Sci. 1972;60:56–63.
124. Klein L, Hinterberger M, Wirnsberger G, Kyewski B. Antigen presentation in the thymus for positive selection and central tolerance induction. Nat Rev Immunol. 2009;9:833–44.
125. Kamb A, Wee S, Lengauer C. Why is cancer drug discovery so difficult. Nat Rev Drug Discov. 2007;6:115–20.
126. Fojo T, Amiri-Kordestani L, Bates SE. Potential pitfalls of crossover and thoughts on Iniparib in triple negative breast cancer. J Natl Cancer Inst. 2011;103:1738–40.
127. Amiri-Kordestani L, Basseville A, Kurziel K, Fojo AT, Bates SE, Targeting MDR. Trageting MDR in breast and lung cancer: discriminating its potential importance from the failure of drug resistance reversal studies. Drug Resist Updat. 2012;15:50–61. http://jco.ascopubs.org/search?author1=Harold+J
128. Burstein HJ. Bevacizumab for advanced breast cancer: all tied up with a RIBBON? J Clin Oncol. 2011;29:1232–5.
129. Hensley ML. Editorial. Big costs for little gain in ovarian cancer. J Clin Oncol. 2011;29:1230–2.
130. Sinha G. Expensive cancer drugs with modest benefit ignite debate over solutions. J Natl Cancer Inst. 2008;100:1347–9.
131. Lenz HJ, Stintzing S. So much effort, so little progress? J Natl Cancer Inst. 2014;106(10):dju282. https://doi.org/10.1093/jnci/dju282.

Chapter 2
Immune Surveillance in Health and Diseases of Aging: Definitions of Acute and Chronic Inflammation [Yin and Yang]

Abstract Acute inflammation is a secretive success of self-terminating and inherent property of the immune system that protects the host tissue against internal (intrinsic) or external (extrinsic) foreign elements so that the body survive and thrive throughout life. For over a century, a role for inflammation in many acute and chronic diseases such as sepsis, allergies, neurodegenerative and autoimmune diseases, diabetes and cardiovascular complication, Alzheimer's, lupus as well as site-specific cancer has been documented. However, ongoing controversies, debates, misinformation and misunderstanding on the role of inflammation in chronic diseases, particularly cancer research and therapy, continue to be very costly for the society, as ageing population around the world increases. In recent years, Khatami defined acute inflammation as the balance between two tightly regulated and biologically opposing arms, termed 'Yin' (apoptosis, pro-inflammatory, initiation or tumoricidal) and 'Yang' (wound healing, post-inflammatory, termination or tumorigenic) properties of effective immunity (immune surveillance). The self-termination ability of acute inflammation is governed by a complex and precise series of signal transductions and cross communications between immune cells, genetic/epigenetic- neuronal-hormonal-metabolic and physiological responses of tissues toward internal or external hazardous agents (e.g., defective cells or proteins, allergens, pathogens or low level carcinogens) that threaten body's health. The two principal arms (positive and negative control switches) in acute inflammation, 'Yin', is responsible for production of death signals and oxidants to destroy both the enemy and injured host cells, requiring efficient energy from mitochondrial oxidative phosphorylation; while the 'Yang' arm is responsible for simultaneous removal of toxicity and debris and repair or remodeling of host, requiring low energy from glycolysis. Chronic or unresolved inflammation was hypothesized as loss of balance between 'Yin' and 'Yang' of immune responses or exaggerated expression and co-expression of mismatched factors in target host. Oxidative stress and longevity could cause defects in dynamics of innate and adaptive immune cell responses along with molecular, mechanical and physical changes in vascular, neuronal and metabolic integrities and functions leading to dysregulation of response profiles. Oxidative stress-induced altered local or systemic activities of cellular and humoral responses that create antigen burden could result an 'immunological chaos' or 'immune tsunami' and differentially influence architectural integrity and function of immune-

M. Khatami, *Inflammation, Aging and Cancer*,
https://doi.org/10.1007/978-3-319-66475-0_2

responsive or immune-privileged tissues and initiation of chronic diseases. Future research directions and designs of clinical studies are proposed on promotion of homeostasis of immune surveillance, or inherent properties of Yin and Yang of acute inflammation.

Keywords Acute inflammation • Allergen • Antibody • Angiogenesis • Antigen-load • Antigen presenting cells • Apoptosis • ATP hydrolysis • Autophagy • Bacteria • B cells • Bioenergetics • Cancer risk factors • Cell-mediated immunity • Chronic/unresolved inflammation • Dendritic cells • Early immune dysfunction • Effector cells • Effective immunity • Epigenetic modifications • Genetically modified organisms • Growth arrest • Growth promote • Humoral immunity • Immediate hypersensitivity • Immune dysfunction • Immune-privileged • Immune surveillance • Macrophages • Mast cells • Metabolism • Mitochondria • Mitophagy • Multipotentent stem cells • Natural killer cells • Neuronal • Oncosis • Oxidative phosphorylation • Parasites • Pathogen • Phagocytes • Polarization • Programmed cell death • Pro-inflammatory • Post-inflammatory • Pyroptosis • Reactive oxygen species • Redox potential • T cells • Tissue susceptibility • Toll-like receptors • Tumoricidal • Tumorigenic • Vasculature • Viruses • Wound healing • Yin and Yang

1 Introduction

Rudolph Virchow, in the nineteenth century noted that the signs of inflammation were four; *"redness and swelling, with heat & pain"*. In 1909, Ehrlich recorded important observations that tumor cells are recognized and eliminated by immune/inflammatory cells. In 1957, Sir McFarland Burnet developed the important theory of immune surveillance or the body's defense mechanism for controlling cancer growth [1–4]. Since these historical observations, a role for defective inflammatory processes reported in the genesis of many immune disorders, including the severe immediate anaphylactic hypersensitivity or delayed type hypersensitivity (DTH) and variations of defective immune responses (e.g., type I, II, III and IV reactions) [4–17]. The induction of mild or severe hypersensitivity syndromes often involve molecular defects in the dynamics of immune and non-immune cells, including mast cells (MCs), eosinophils (Eos), basophils, B and T lymphocytes, vascular activation, complement cascades and platelets in susceptible tissue. Altered activities of cell-mediated or humoral immunity (CMI, HI) have been reported in a number of potent pathogen-induced acute inflammatory diseases (e.g., sepsis, pneumonia, meningitis) or major trauma; chronic allergies (e.g., asthma, emphysema, skin and ocular inflammatory diseases), immunodeficiency syndromes, bacterial, parasitic or viral infectious diseases (AIDS, tuberculosis, rubella, rabies, measles) [3–5, 11–20]. The role of inflammation in age-associated chronic illnesses such as neurodegenerative and autoimmune diseases, or in hypertension, colitis, gastritis, hepatitis, nephritis, prostatis, pancreatitis, appendicitis, opthalmitis, Bechet's, esophagitis, neuritis, diabetes and other metabolic disorders, cardiovascular complications, stroke, rheumatoid arthritis, atherosclerosis, lupus, psoriasis, Alzheimer's, multiple sclerosis and other immune or metabolic disorders also have been widely reported in the literature [3–5, 21–47]. Regarding the role of inflammation in cancer research and therapy, although for many decades circumstantial evidence reported a role for inflammation in cancer, the decision makers in the cancer community ignored and downplayed these reports including the historically important observations of Ehrlich and Burnet in early twentieth century [1–6, 48–68]. In 1998, Khatami presented compelling evidence, based on extension of her earlier 'accidental' discoveries that were established in 1980s and demonstrated a direct association between inflammation and tumorigenesis to the NCI upper management. The originally submitted concepts including proposal that 'inflammatory mediators are ideal targets for molecular diagnosis, prevention and therapy of many cancers' and related designs of clinical trials, and introduction of several anti-inflammatory agents (i.e., aspirin, Captopril and Sulindac) met with serious opposition, downplay, denials and rejections by the NCI upper management [3–5, 50, 55, 63–68], NCI/NIH documents, since 1998]. However, in the last decade, increasing number of funded projects, networks, symposia and technologies focused on the roles of numerous inflammatory mediators and their influence in cancer research without a vision to conduct such funded programs on systematic bases to understand what inflammation does with regard to cancer and how to prevent or treat it. The many funded projects include molecular markers identification, design of clinical trials, 'targeted' therapies and immunotherapies for soft or solid site-specific cancers such as lung, colon/rectal, breast, prostate, bladder, liver, ovarian, pancreas, brain, lymphoid tissues or leukemia, in experimental models of tumors or cancer clinical trials [3, 4, 37, 60–108].

However, the ongoing debates, controversies, misunderstanding or misinformation on the role of inflammation, whether it is protective in preventing cancer or it causes cancer are among the major reasons for the extremely costly and wrong approaches in cancer immunotherapy with proven failed outcomes [3, 4, 50, 63, 64]. Current modalities and therapies, using anti-inflammatory mediators, hormone replacement therapy and steroids to manage chronic inflammatory diseases, particularly claimed cancer 'targeted' therapies or 'personalized' or 'precision' medicine, often have serious and life-threatening side effects [3, 4, 50, 63–65, 69, 80, 85, 101–109].

Since 1960s, several worthy investigations reported the definitions and classifications on mechanisms of cell death, primarily based on morphological features of tissues and types of cell death or tissue necrosis. The categories of cell death included 'type I', involved in heterophagy; 'type II', associated with autophagy and 'type III', which was not included in morphological categories of any type of digestion and corresponding to apoptosis, as autophagic cell death and necrosis. Cell necrosis defined as a regulated event that played significant role in numerous physiological and pathological activities, including DNA damage, excitotoxins having specific death receptors for binding to death factors such as caspases and other oxidants under special conditions [109–118]. Many investigators also reported the mechanisms of actions of numerous mediators of inflammatory processes and identification of cancer markers; receiving federal and private funding to separately develop networks and technologies in the fields of proteomics, genomics, lipidomics, metabolomics, glycomics searching for hundreds and thousands of molecules and many such molecules were suggested or claimed as molecular targets for cancer research and therapy [3, 4, 37, 55, 63–68, 71, 72, 74–107, 109, 118–128].

However, despite the availability of enormous data on the roles that inflammation play in health and diseases, a clear definition of what acute and chronic inflammation do in maintaining health or initiating diseases, particularly during aging and the development of multistep carcinogenesis has been missing in the literature. With regard to cancer, numerous circumstantial evidence document a role for inflammation in site-specific cancers [3, 4, 37, 60–68, 70–80, 83–109, 125]. However, as noted above, except for the 'accidental' discoveries that we established in 1980s and extended in recent years [3–5, 16, 17, 63, 66–68, 81, 82, 109], direct evidence that oxidative stress (chronic, persistent or recurrent inflammation) is linked to the genesis of benign or malignant tumors/cancers in mammalians has yet to be established. Consequently, little or no information is available on the developmental stages of inflammation-induced altered immune response dynamics that would lead to tumorigenesis or angiogenesis. The author suggests that a major serious obstacle in advancing our efforts to understand the cancer biology and effectively design clinical trials and drug development is intentional lack of interest to systematic understanding of the roles that immune disruptors (intrinsic or extrinsic stimuli) play in the induction of early/initial changes in response dynamics in susceptible tissues (see Chaps. 4 and 6) [3, 4, 63–68, 81, 82, 109].

A major focus of this chapter is to describe the recent definitions of acute and chronic inflammation in health and diseases, with emphasis on multistep carcinogenesis. The original concept that acute inflammation possesses two biologically opposing arms, termed Yin and Yang was introduced in the literature in 2008 (Ref. [66]).[1] The fundamental idea was proposed after detailed analyses of data from a series of our earlier experiments on experimental models of acute and chronic inflammatory diseases that were established in 1980s and resulted in tumorigenesis and angiogenesis, and later became 'accidental' discoveries. Definition of Yin-Yang included review of a large amount of scattered data that intellectually and logically would fit the Yin and Yang arms of self-terminating properties of acute inflammation (immune-surveillance) for maintenance of health (see below). Furthermore, a preliminary roadmap on the role of inflammation in the genesis and progression of age-associated chronic diseases was developed and led to hypotheses that chronic inflammation is a common denominator in the genesis and progression of nearly all

[1] The article that was published in 2008 was originally prepared for and submitted to Nat. Rev. Caner in 2006 (NPG Manuscript Tracking System NY-610A-NPG&MTS); the editor rejected it, claiming their journal was not interested in mast cells. In 2007, the manuscript was submitted to Nat. Rev. Immunol the editor stated that while the manuscript would potentially be of interest to the readership of their journal, a similar topic has been commissioned to someone else!! The topic is now the focus of numerous projects and published articles.

age-associated chronic diseases or site-specific cancers [3–5, 15–17, 50, 55, 63–69, 81, 82, 109].

Currently, numerous important biological knowledge gaps exist in basic understanding of how the protective properties of immunity turn against the body in the direction of multi-phases immune destruction that threaten its survival. A goal for preparing this and other chapters in this book was to address such biological gaps in the context of influence of inflammatory processes in specific target tissues (e.g., immune-responsive or immune-privileged) and the induction and progression of age-associated chronic diseases or site-specific cancers.

The present chapter was an attempt to continue analyses and integration of information on the overall roles that inflammation play in tissue metabolism, neuronal, hormonal, vasculature and immune cells in maintaining health or initiating age-associated chronic diseases or site-specific cancers. Potential interdependence between immune-mediated programmed cell death and other mechanisms of cell death, such as necrosis, pyroptosis, oncosis, and the energy requirements and biological recycling pathways (e.g., authophagy, mitochondria/mitophagy or ribosome/ribophagy) that contribute to the homeostasis of immunity or initiation of diseases will be outlined (details in Chap. 6).

Future proposed studies are directed on systematic understanding of the role of sustained oxidative stress (stimuli, immune disrupters) in alterations of Yin-Yang balance and differential energy requirements of mitochondria in maintenance of health or initiation of disease processes, with emphasis on cancer [109]. The results are anticipated to guide scientists to find logical approaches for developing cost-effective strategies for accurate formulation of risk assessment of diseases, as well as effective prevention, and control of chronic diseases and/or multistep carcinogenesis.

2 Acute Inflammation: Division of Labor in Programmed Cell Death. Protective, Self-Terminating Property of Immune Surveillance. Balancing Growth-Arrest (Yin) and Growth-Promote (Yang) Arms of Immunity

Acute inflammation is part of a biologically amazing complex and secretive success of the body's effective immunity (immune surveillance) that protects the body against unwanted (foreign) elements or immune disruptors that could threaten the body's survival throughout life. Stimulation of the host/target tissue by any intrinsic or extrinsic immune disruptors (stimuli), evokes an inflammatory response; an elaborate and precise signal transduction and crosstalk, between innate and adaptive immune cells and closely facilitated and orchestrated by non-immune pathways, such as the vasculature, metabolic, hormonal and neuronal systems (the entire network is referred to as effective immunity). Stimuli-induced local/host tissue responses are initiated by expression of alarming signals, death factors and receptor molecules from activated immune cells. The processes engage a tightly regulated and sophisticated generation of often thousands or millions of other required chemicals from recruiting and attracting (activating) other inflammatory or non-inflammatory cells via the activation of vasculature, metabolic and neuronal pathways.

Recently, acute inflammation was defined as the inherent immune responses of two biologically and functionally opposing and reversible arms, termed; Yin (pro-inflammatory, initiation, growth-arrest or tumoricidal) and Yang (post-, anti-inflammatory, wound healing, resolution, growth-promote or tumorigenic) responses [66].

To better understand the roles that each arm plays in acute inflammation, the Yin and Yang events are separately described below (Fig. 2.1).

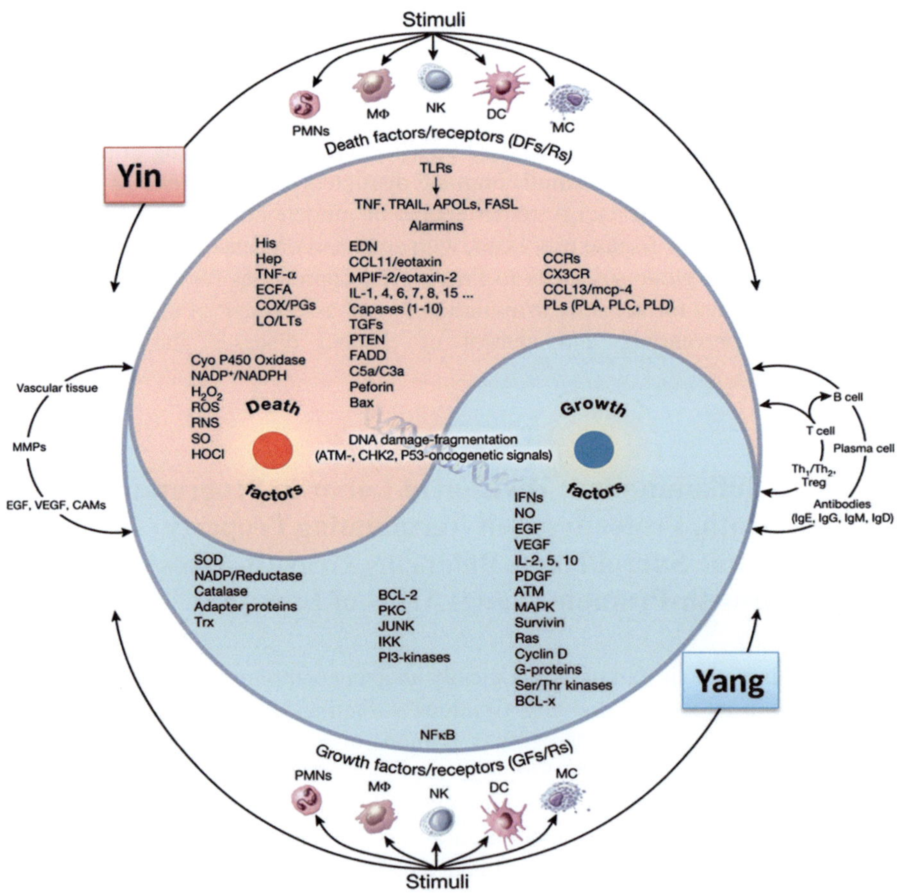

Fig. 2.1 Schematic representation of original definitions of Yin and Yang processes in acute inflammation (Modified with permission from Ref. [66], Exp. Opin. Biol. Ther. 2008. Informa Healthcare, all rights reserved)

2.1 *Yin Phenomenon: Pro-inflammatory or Initiation Stage: Apoptosis, Program Cell Death, Growth-Arresting or Tumoricidal [DRESSED TO KILL!]*

As schematically represented in Fig. 2.1, the overall role in Yin processes is generation of death factors, toxins and oxidants for the purpose of destruction and elimination of foreign components and also destruction of the injured/infected host tissue. Depending on the type of tissue and inflammatory condition, the major responses include a combination of the following interdependent biological events that occur to destroy the unwanted elements and injured tissue (Fig. 2.1) [3, 4, 63–68, 81, 82, 109]:

(i) Stimuli-induced activation of appropriate antigen presenting cells (APCs) within innate and/or adaptive immune system;
(ii) Encounter and recognize the nature of stimuli (e.g., pathogens, allergen, antigens);
(iii) Process of destruction of pathogens/antigens by induction of expression of danger signal molecules and receptors, generation of a wide range of death factors, oxidants and toxins from host activated immune cells and/or recruited cells from vasculature, neuronal or metabolic pathways;
(iv) Induction of stimuli-specific antibodies, surface and receptor molecules and activation of immune cells, aggregation of specific receptors and effector (pharmacological) function;
(v) Changes in oxidative status of tissue, burst of energy in activated immune cells (e.g., MΦs) resulting in ATP hydrolysis from mitochondrial oxidative phosphorylation and generation of ROS and other oxidants and enzymes; changes/increases in intracellular ionic (Na + and/or Ca++) levels needed to destroy/kill cells (lysis of pathogen structure and infected host), disruption of membrane integrity and efflux of required intracellular components;
(vi) Vasculature-derived activation of complement cascade enzymes (e.g.,c1-c5) facilitating cell fixation and perforation/lysis of infective agents and injured host cells;
(vii) Induction of cell/tissue edema, often accompanied by coagulation of plasma proteins/lipids in injured tissue, perhaps as part of 'temporary'/immediate healing (filling) process of the damaged cell/tissue and/or to dilute toxicity;
(viii) Simultaneous initiation of termination processes from polarized cells for healing the tissue and terminating inflammation (Yang events, below).

External and internal hazardous elements (immune disruptors) include a wide range of antigens or allergens (e.g., pollen, ragweed, foodstuff), infective agents/microbiomes, pathogens, carcinogens/mutagens, chemical, biological and environmental hazards. The stimuli include intrinsic or extrinsic changes in the levels of hormones and their functions occurring naturally in aging process or treated individuals with hormones or steroids. Among intrinsic immune disruptors are accumulation of defective, senescent or useless (non-functional) cellular and molecular components [e.g., immune or non-immune cells, B lymphocyte complexes or cancerous cells, damaged chromosomal, genetic and epigenetic materials (mutated DNA/RNA and epigenetic hypo-, hyper methylated molecules, related repair enzymes or repressor molecules), oxidized metabolites (e.g., crystallized uric acid) or accumulation of pathogen-specific particles, use of fetal tissue and adjuvant (e.g., mercury, L-histidine) in vaccines] [3–5, 15–17, 63–68, 81, 82, 109–125].

As depicted in Fig. 2.1, depending on the nature of stimuli, specialized host inflammatory cells, such as innate immune cells (e.g., NKs, MΦs, DCs or MCs), are sensitized or activated and prepared for appropriate responses. Activated host cells also provide signals to activate, mature, differentiate and recruit (infiltrate) other immune cells and blood components through activation of vasculature and expression of precise quantities of required pro-inflammatory mediators, vasoactive agents, oxidants, enzymes or cytokines/chemokines to destroy the unwanted components (Fig. 2.1, Yin processes identified as Death Factors) [3–5, 63–68, 81, 82, 109].

The pro-inflammatory mediators that are expressed during Yin processes (death factors) include toll-like receptors (TLRs), vasoactive components (e.g., histamine), acidic glycoproteins (e.g., heparin), eosinophil chemotactic factor of anaphylaxis (ECFA), CCL11/eotaxin-1, MPIF-2/eotaxin-2, tumor necrosis factor–α (TNF-α), transforming growth factors (TGFs), PTEN, FADD, interleukins (e.g., IL-1β, IL-4, IL-6, IL-8), caspases family of enzymes (caspases 1–10), blood-born complement cascades (e.g., C1-C5), perforin molecules, Bax, prostaglandins (PGs), leukotrienes (LTs), a variety of cytokines and chemokines receptor molecules (e.g., TNFR/TNFSF5, IgE-FcεR, TGFRs, CCL13/mcp-4, CCR family of chemokine receptors, CX3CR1, ILBrA, XCR1/CCXCR1), membrane phospholipases, antibodies (e.g., IgE, IgA, IgG, IgM), NO and genesis of free radicals and oxidants [e.g., reactive oxygen species (ROS), reactive nitrogen species (RNS), superoxide radicals, hydrogen peroxide,…] (Fig. 2.1, Yin) [3–11, 15–17, 63–65, 109] .

The Yin activities often require receptor aggregation and synthesis of immunoglobulins (e.g., IgG to activate myeloid cells or IgE to activate and degranulate MCs). These events also involve activation of membrane enzymes phospholipases (PLs, e.g., PLA, PLC or PLD), sphingosine kinase and metabolism of arachidonic acid [e.g., activation of cyclooxygenase (COX) and lipoxygenase (LO)] pathways and biosynthesis of prostaglandins [(PGs), PGF1α, PGI2, PGE2 and leukotrienes (LTs, LTA, LTC) and thromboxanes (TXs)] to produce the required pharmacological effects [3–5, 15–17, 63, 66–68, 81, 82, 109, 125–128].

In the list of immune disruptors or antigens that potentially increase the risk of chronic diseases, the genetically engineered or modified food products, genetically modified organisms (GMOs) should be included. These and other components of preserved foods or environmental hazards, as well as pathogen-specific vaccines, are likely important contributors of the reported increasing risks of allergies (or perhaps cancers) among both older and younger individuals in America in the last couple of decades [63–65, 125]. GMOs (e.g., corn, soybean products, cotton, fruits) are bacteria-crops, and considered 'transgenic', herbicide and insecticide resistant foods. They have long shelf lives and are marketed for animal and/or human consumption. Recent articles discuss controversies regarding the health benefits, ethics, biotechnologies and environmental challenges of such products for human or animal use [129–134]. The digested modified proteins of the GMO foods are likely antigen burden for the immune system. Like the pathogen-specific vaccines, the genomic components or amino acids of bacteria-derived GMO products may interfere with body' ecosystem of microbiomes in the gastrointestinal tract and potentially lead to a wide range of health conditions (details Chaps. 5 and 6). Currently, the health concerns of consumption of GMO foods are expressed primarily for the American population compared with other developed nations. That is because the United States is the major producer and consumer of genetically engineered foods. These products are heavily endorsed and publicized by a powerful lobbying group who minimizes and ignores the potential adverse influence of these health hazards for human.

2.2 *Yang Phenomenon: Post-inflammatory or Termination/ Resolution of Acute Inflammation (Wound Healing, Growth-Promoting, Tissue Repair, Tumorigenic). Host Revival!*

The Yang (termination, post-inflammatory, wound healing, growth promote or tumorigenic) arm of acute inflammation is responsible for neutralizing the toxicity of death factors and oxidants that are generated in Yin events and to resolve and terminate the inflammation. The overall activities involved in Yang processes include the following steps [3, 4, 50, 63–68, 81, 82, 109]:

(i) Simultaneous polarization of immune cells that signal for immune suppression. The polarization of immune cells include generation of mature DCs (DC2, TADC), induction of M2 (TAM) phenotypes, induction of regulatory T (Treg) or memory cells for expression of appropriate growth factors and antioxidants from activated immune cells, and/or recruited cells from vasculature. Yang events are often facilitated by hormonal, neuronal and metabolic pathways that signal for immune suppression.
(ii) Removal/expel and/or dilution of the unwanted components and oxidants by production of tears, mucus secretion from goblet cells, or influx of plasma proteins to the site of injury;
(iii) Induction of signals for generation of reducing power to offset the oxidative status of injured tissues. In this process expression of several inhibitors of apoptosis, decoy receptor molecules (e.g., TNFRdr), immune suppressor interleukins (e.g., IL-1dR or IRAK-M), interferons and growth factors, antioxidants and enzymes are involved to reduce/inhibit energy consumption within mitochondria via inhibition of ATPase activities creating 'temporary' hypoxic condition for expression of growth factors (e.g., HIF1-VEGF), induction of kinases (mTOR/PI3K/AKT) for growth promotion and repair of the injured host tissue (anabolic events);

(iv) Resolution and termination of inflammation for repairing and/or remodeling of the injured host tissue also involve neovascularization or angiogenesis under hypoxic conditions to resolve injury and return tissue to normal function;

Therefore, the Yang phase involves simultaneous activation of appropriate anti-inflammatory pathways to precisely neutralize and remove the toxicity generated during the pro-inflammatory (Yin) response processes and to heal and repair or remodel the injured host tissue and terminate the inflammation (Figs. 2.1 and 2.2). As depicted in Fig. 2.1 (Yang), a wide range of signals from activated immune and non-immune cells induce expression of growth factors and inhibitors of oxidative materials and generation of reducing powers to terminate the inflammation [3, 4, 63–68, 81, 82, 109].

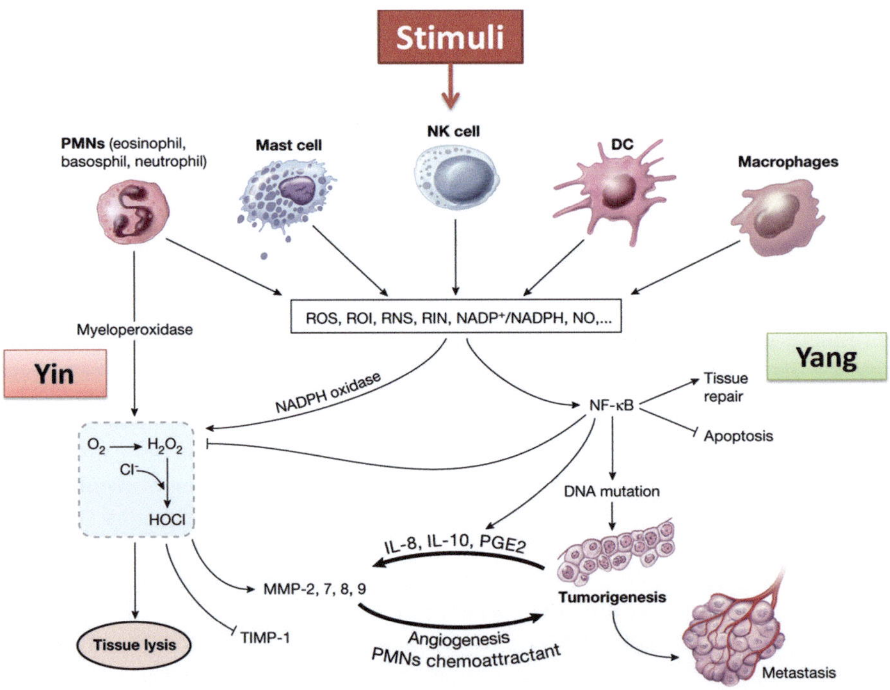

Fig. 2.2 Schematic representation of acute inflammatory responses during Yin (apoptosis) and Yang (wound healing). Stimuli-induced activation of immune cells such as polymorphonuclear, mast cells, natural killer cells, dendritic cells or macrophages lead to generation of oxidants such as reactive oxygen species and intermediates (ROS, ROI), reactive nitrogen species and intermediate (RNS or RIN), increased ratio of $NADP^+/NADPH$, nitric oxide (NO) by activation of enzymes such as NADPH oxidase to produce precise quantity of toxic material that lead to lysis of pathogen and host tissue as well as induction of vascular hyperpermeability. The Yin events simultaneously signal for production of anti-oxidants and growth factors to neutralize the toxicity generated in Yin. The figure depicts that continued stimulation of tissue would change the balance between Yin and Yang of acute inflammation in favor of cell growth and induction of cancer, angiogenesis and metastasis (Modified from Khatami (Ref. [67]) all rights reserved)

Again, depending on the nature, potency and type of stimulation, extent of tissue injury and/or the composition of host immune and non-immune cells, the wound healing pathways involve appropriate expression of growth promoting factors such as lymphocyte-derive nuclear factor (NF-kB) and receptor molecules, BCL-2, protein kinases (e.g., PKC, PI3 kinase-related kinases and mutated-ATM, MAPK family, JUNK, IKK, Ataxia Telangiectasia), synthesis of related receptor molecules, inhibitors of pro-inflammatory mediators (decoy receptors), immune suppressor factors, or inhibition of oxidative components [e.g., histaminases, iNOS, cytosolic or mitochondrial super-oxide dismutases (SODs), catalase, fibroblast growth factor (FGF), vascular endothelial growth factor (VEGF), metalloproteases (MMPs), chemokines or cytokines [e.g., interferons (IFNs), interleukins (ILs)…] (Figs. 2.1 and 2.2) [3–5, 15–25, 37, 63, 66–68, 72, 80–128, 135–175].

Therefore, the principal function of post-inflammatory responses in Yang is to:

(i) Neutralize and/or remove death factors and toxins from the injured target tissue;
(ii) Provide the required growth factors and reducing powers that would repair any damage or scar (tissue necrosis) caused by expression of pro-inflammatory responses in Yin processes;
(iii) Switch from high energy to low energy consumption, shutting down mitochondrial oxidative phosphorylation, ATP utilization from glycolysis (Warburg effect);
(iv) Repair and remodel the cellular DNA damage, tumor suppressor genes (e.g., p53) and genomic integrity in the target tissue;
(v) Resolution and termination of inflammation;

2.3 *Contribution of Non-immune Systems in Acute Inflammation in Balancing Yin-Yang*

To accomplish its protective and self-terminating role, acute inflammation through Yin and Yang processes, induces a complex, well-orchestrated, elaborate and precise chemical signal communications between mediators of innate and adaptive immune cells that are intimately facilitated by vasculature, metabolic, hormonal and neuronal responses. The following sections briefly incorporate the contributions of intracellular components such as mitochondria, ER and ribosomal activities during completion and/or clearance of byproducts of inflammatory responses. Analyses and integration of large amount of scattered data from basic and clinical research on complex biological rules are helpful for initiating a roadmap on the importance of maintenance of effective immunity for protecting health [3–6, 15–17, 47, 58, 63–66, 71, 79–82, 84, 103, 109, 113–122, 126, 136–151, 157–195]. The integration of such data also provides opportunities to identify major biological gaps as well as insights into correcting and delaying the age-, and oxidative stress-induced alterations of effective immunity toward preventing or delaying initiation of multistep diseases (details in Chap. 6). The overall analyses and integration of data will also reveal important knowledge gaps that are suggested to be major obstacles in advancing the goals of effective disease prevention and/or therapeutic approaches.

Examples of major interrelated biological activities that are likely to contribute to self-terminating properties of Yin-Yang of acute inflammation (immune surveillance) are outlined below (detailed in Chap. 6) [3–6, 15–17, 47, 58, 63–66, 71, 79–82, 84, 103, 109, 113–122, 126, 136–151, 157–195] (Figs. 2.1, 2.2 and 2.3).

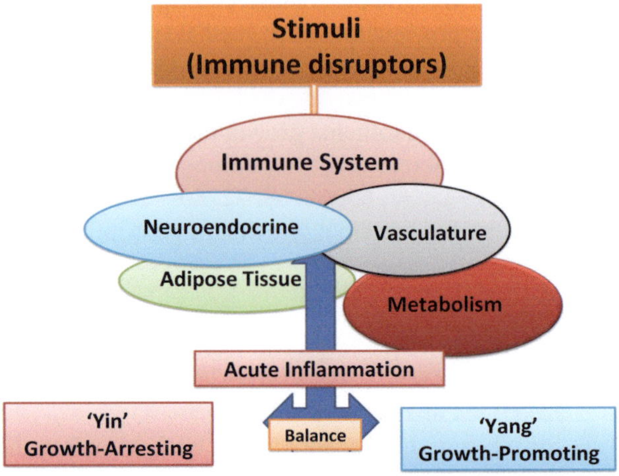

Fig. 2.3 Role of immune and non-immune systems in acute inflammation. Maintaining balance between Yin (growth-arresting) and Yang (growth-promoting) arms of immunity is through activation of immune cells assisted by vasculature, metabolic and neuronal pathways including contribution from adipose tissue (Modified from Khatami [4] InTech Publishing)

2.3.1 Bioenergetics of Yin ['Dressed to Kill'] -Role of Mitochondria

During Yin responses (the 'dressed to kill' phase of acute inflammation), burst of oxygen and production of high energy released from mitochondria of activated immune cells (e.g., MΦs, NKs, MCs, DCs, T or B cells) are required. It is not clear to what extent activated non-immune cells (e.g., epithelium, mucus-secreting cells or vascular endothelium) contribute to the host production of high energy at this phase of inflammation. The rapid generation of free energy requirements comes from oxidative phosphorylation of mitochondria via activation of ATPase that hydrolyze ATP.

Hydrolysis of ATP rapidly lowers cellular ATP/ADP/AMP ratios and changes (increases) influx of [Ca++] and mobilization and intracellular [Na+], resulting in increased host oxido-redux potential. The high energy production temporarily decreases the tissue reducing powers (e.g., NADH/NAD$^+$ or NADPH/NADP+, glutathione recycling pathways) and allows generation of reactive oxygen species (ROS), reactive nitrogen species (RNS), NO, superoxide radicals and activate oxidizing enzymes (e.g., caspases, NADPH oxidase, myeloperoxidase, membrane metalloproteases). The increased levels of oxidants in tissue are perhaps signals that would further facilitate increased vasculature hyperpermeability and activation and infiltration of other immune cells and/or blood complement cascades contribution during lysing pathogens and injured host tissue. As noted above, the biological events in Yin are often initiated by induction of pathogen (stimuli)-specific danger molecules or TLRs (TRL 1–11). The events in Yin are further accompanied by expression of hun-

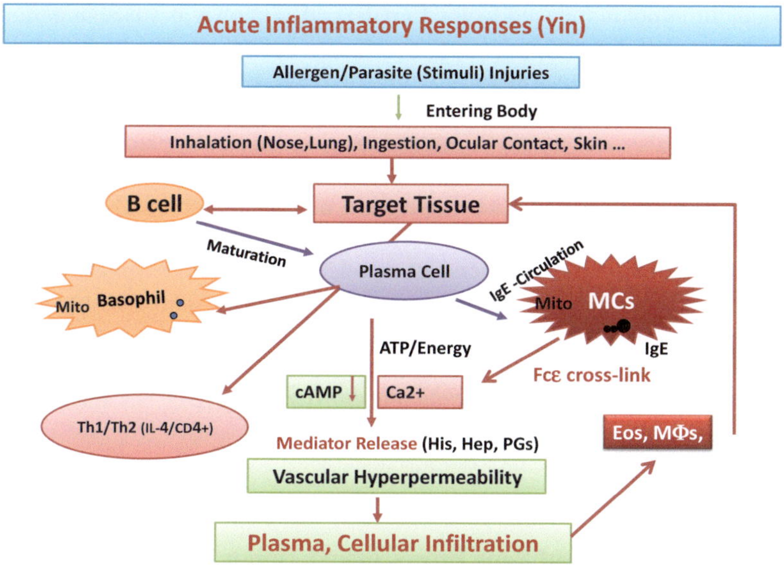

Fig. 2.4 Schematic representation of steps involved in acute (immediate) hypersensitivity responses, primarily Yin (pro-inflammatory) events. It depicts the three major stages of sensitization, activation and effector (pharmacological) function of tissues, involving primarily mast cells (MCs). See text

dreds of respective adaptor and surface molecules or expression of oxidative enzymes or release of vasoactive components (e.g., histamine) and interleukins (e.g., IL-1) or prostaglandins (PGF1α) that activates other tissue components (e.g., nuclear membrane, DNA/RNA, cytoplasmic, membrane lipid, ion transport). These steps are suggested to be simultaneous and well orchestrated for the purpose of destroying pathogens and the injured tissues in Yin responses (Figs. 2.1, 2.2 and 2.4). See text.

2.3.2 Shift/Reversal of Energy Consumption and Metabolism in Yang ('Revival' of Host from Death')

Following killing of the foreign elements, the injured host tissue needs to simultaneously recover and repair by biological activities that possess opposite properties (growth-promote) from the growth-arrest actions of Yin pathways. As schematically represented in Figs. 2.1 and 2.2, the Yang responses ('recovery from death') involve simultaneous shift in oxidative metabolism by polarization of immune and non-immune systems for wound healing of injured tissue. The Yang events require switching away from high energy production of oxidative phosphorylation (shutting down mitochondrial function) to aerobic glycolysis (Warburg effect), a condition that also occurs in tumor microenvironment during tumor growth. Polarized immune cells (e.g., MΦs in M2 or TAMs phenotypes, degranulated or 'leaky' MCs, DC2 or TADCs) signal for induction of hypoxic conditions (impaired mitochondria) and expression of hypoxia induced factor 1 (HIF1), also known as vascular endothelial growth factor (VEGF) and induction of neovascularization. The high energy ATP level that is spent during Yin causes mitochondria to conserve/reduce oxidative metabolism for its TCA cycle intermediates and anabolic/catabolic homeostasis. Events in Yang also accompany simultaneous generation of reducing powers, anti-oxidants and growth factors from activation of adrenal (production of cortisol) and/or thyroid (immune suppression by thyroxine, thyrotropin or TSH) glands. Among numerous important metabolites that are likely involved in Yang, are the activation of adenosine deaminase and generation of adenosine monophosphate (AMP) and related surface molecule CD 73, a key event in energy reversal for facilitating termination of inflammation and recovery of tissue. The AMP signaling is perhaps needed for ATP synthesis from aerobic glycoslysis and expression of growth factors and enzymes such as PI3 kinase, PKC, reducing enzymes (e.g., SODs, catalase) or FGF, VEGF and membrane proteases to promote growth under hypoxic conditions (Figs. 2.1 and 2.2).

2.3.3 Shared Features of Yang Processes and Tumor Growth

As noted above, there are shared features between metabolism of activated immune cells, under oxidative stress, and growth of tumor cells. For example, both Yang processes and tumor growth utilize aerobic glycolysis (Warburg effect) for wound healing (termination of cell death or growth). Similarly, several growth promoting factors (e.g., mTOR/PI3 Kinase, MAPKinase, PKC, VEGF, FGF, IFNs, NFkB…) or other immune suppressors and growth promoting angiogenic factors are involved in Yang events as well as during tumor cell growth (Figs. 2.1 and 2.2, Yang arm of acute inflammation). In 1986, Dvorak suggested that tumors are wound that do not heal [51]. This cogent observation stood the test time in cancer research. However, even recent review of the literature does not seem to differentiate the metabolic and bioenergetic requirements of Yin vs. Yang processes in acute inflammation or the Warburg phenomena in tumor growth [63, 109, 179]. Recently, the author hypothesized that the oxidative phosphorylation in mitochondria (during Yin) and the aerobic glycolysis (Warburg effect) in cytosol (during Yang) use differential energy requirements for the 'duality' that effective immunity has for self-terminating function of acute inflammation [63, 109]. In other words, upon tissue stimulation, the activated immune cells first engage in rapid generation of free energy (ATP) by utilizing the oxidative phosphorylation from mitochondria, that otherwise is needed for tricarboxylic acid (TCA) cycle intermediates and biosynthesis of lipids, related enzymes and homeostasis of mitochondrial energy power for cells. Providing rapid energy (ATP hydrolysis) from oxidative metabolism, enables immune cells (e.g., M1, tumoricidal phenotype of MΦs) to produce pro-inflammatory mediators and generate needed toxicity for killing/destroying pathogens or foreign elements (Fig. 2.1 Yin arm). However, Yang responses that are involved in resolution of inflammation simultaneously use activated/polarized immune cells (e.g., M2 or TAMs phenotype) with growth promoting features. The

Yang responses shift to low energy requirements from aerobic glycolysis (Warburg effect) and under hypoxic condition, which signals for expression of HIF1 (VEGF), in the neighborhood of hypoxic neovasculature, for the purpose of resolveing and terminating inflammation, repairing or remodeling and returning target tissue to resting status. The energy shifts away from mitochondrial ATP hydrolysis during Yang also enable the tissue to correct Yin-induced rise in tricarboxylic acid (TCA) cycle intermediates (e.g., succinate, fumarate) and reduced production of ROS in mitochondria.

However, it is suggested that sustained oxidative stress or persistent unresolved inflammation increases utilization of aerobic glycolysis (Warburg effect) for energy consumption due to overwhelming/exhaustion of oxidative phosphorylation pathways and the need for production of wound healing factors to terminate inflammation. The validity of this hypothesis seems supported by findings that angiogenesis and hypoxic conditions are primary features in tumor microenvironment and inflammatory diseases. One should also keep in mind that oxidative stress and aging retard the effectiveness of immunity to fight new antigens, perhaps as the result of loss of tightly regulated Yin and Yang processes toward necrosis and/or tissue growth promotion and ineffectiveness in energy homeostasis (Fig. 2.2) (details in Chaps. 3, 4 and 6).

2.3.4 Activation of Vasculature

Being the gatekeeper of the immune cell trafficking, vasculature has the most crucial function in facilitating both, the Yin (tumoricidal) and Yang (tumorigenic) processes by expression of precise quantities of death and growth factors. Activation of vascular tissue often involves activation of complement cascades (e.g., C3, C5 enzymes) to assist perforation and lysis of infective agents and/or damaged host (Yin); release of granules from platelets and expression of required amounts of growth factors (e.g., PDGF, EGF, VEGF, MMPs, CAMs) (Yang) for completion of Yin and Yang processes (Figs. 2.1, 2.2, 2.3 and 2.4). In addition, vascular endothelial cells provide receptor molecules for vasoactive components (e.g., histamine, heparin) that contribute to vascular hyperpermeability, cell adhesion, infiltration of immune cells, influx of plasma proteins, induction of edema and coagulation of plasma proteins to potentially facilitate ‘temporary’ wound healing [3–5, 11, 24, 56–60, 63, 72, 74, 87, 95, 96, 99, 100, 109, 155], (Figs. 2.1 and 2.4).

2.3.5 Activation of Neuronal and Endocrine Systems

Expression of several other factors and receptors for inflammatory mediators such as histamine receptors and hormones, metabolites or neuropeptides such as serotonin, adrenalin/ norepinephrine or cortisol contributes to the induction of pain and wound healing processes, respectively, during inflammatory reactions (details in Chap. 6) [3, 4, 63, 109, 177, 178, 180–187, 190, 191].

2.3.6 Role of Adipose Tissue in Inflammation

Immunologically, adipose tissue is a large and active tissue composed of innate and adaptive immune cells, such as B and T cells, MΦs and neutrophils. The polarized or subtype forms of such cells play important roles in immune surveillance, or induction of metabolic diseases such as insulin- resistant, hyperglycemia of diabetes or obesity. Adipose tissue perhaps contributes directly or indirectly in the induction of other diseases such as atherosclerosis, cardiovascular complications or cancer. Inflammatory mediators such as IL-6 and receptor molecule activation are linked to insulin-insufficiency and deterioration of glucose homeostasis in adipose tissue and a shift in MΦs polarization that results in expression of IL-4 and increased susceptibility to lipopolysaccharide (LPS)-induced endotoxemia [63, 171, 173, 192–194].

2.4 Mission and Outcomes of Acute Inflammation (Yin-Yang) or Effective Immunity (Immune Surveillance)

The principal mission of an inflammatory process (Yin and Yang) is twofold:

(a) To encounter, recognize, process, destroy and eliminate the external or internal foreign elements that may harm the target/host tissue; and
(b) To neutralize the death factors and oxidants and remove toxins that is present in the host cell and to repair the damaged cells and terminates inflammation.

The time course kinetics for induction and termination (resolution) of an inflammatory condition often depend on the quality and/or severity of an inflammatory condition. With the exception of non-specific or minimal tissue stimulation (e.g., acid burn or minor injuries), the major outcomes of an inflammatory reaction include:

(a) Synthesis of allergen/pathogen-specific antibodies and receptor molecules;
(b) Increased synthesis of memory B and T cells (T reg);
(c) Upon tissue exposure to the same types of stimuli, the 'initiated' immune system can unleash appropriate responses (e.g., expression of antigen-specific antibodies) to destroy unwanted foreign elements and terminate inflammation.

In summary, effective immunity that protects the body against all potential harms plays a crucially important, exact and justifying role in health. Acute inflammation possesses two opposing biological properties characterized as (Yin) that is responsible for production of death signals to destroy both the enemy and the injured host cells; and (Yang) that is responsible for removal of toxicity and debris generated in target tissue and to repair and remodel the host and resolve inflammation (Figs. 2.1, 2.2, 2.3, and 2.4).

3 Sequence of Events in Immediate Hypersensitivity Reactions

The exact time course kinetics and mechanisms of actions of responses involved in inflammatory processes are not fully understood. Overall analyses of relevant data on sequences of events occurring during immediate type 1 (acute) hypersensitivity reactions in host tissues whose prominent immune cells are MCs and lymphoid tissues [e.g., conjunctival-associated lymphoid tissues (CALTs), lung airways, gut-associated lymphoid tissues (GALTs), perivascular or perhaps the skin], include three major phases of sensitization, activation and effector function (pharmacological effects or outcomes).

It is noteworthy that mast cells (MCs) that are categorized within the innate immune cells often function as effector cells for producing an effect, while B cells that are categorized as effector cells for humoral immunity within the adaptive immune cells often function as antigen presenting cells (APCs) to sensitize and activate MCs [3–10, 15–17, 38, 63–68, 72, 81, 82, 87, 89, 109, 120–124, 137, 144, 145, 159, 196].

Briefly, the three stages of sensitization, activation and effector function of immediate (type 1) hypersensitivity reactions include the following sequence of events (Figs. 2.1 and 2.4):

(a) **Tissue exposure**: Antigen, parasites or allergen inhaled, ingested or administered via lung, skin, gut or ocular tissues;
(b) **Circulating blood:** Antigen is engulfed by circulating blood phagocytes and delivered to B lymphocytes (B cells);
(c) **B cells activation and response:** B cell differentiation into plasma cells and biosynthesis of antigen-specific IgE antibodies;
(d) **Mast cells sensitization:** At low levels, IgE antibodies (Abs) circulate throughout the body without causing any reaction or harm, perhaps as part of tolerance. Upon exposure to higher levels of antigen, or repeated tissue encounter with the same antigen the circulating IgE Abs attach to the surface of mast cells (or basophils) through specific receptor binding (MCs-IgE-fcε receptors), which sensitizes MCs. Sensitization of MCs may last for weeks or years, without any severe responses. However, depending on the type of allergen or antigen, further contact of target tissue with the same antigen initiates an allergic response from the sensitized tissue (effector or pharmacological phase).
(e) **Effector phase: Mast cells activation or degranulation and pharmacological effects:** Activation of MCs occurs when IgE bound to high affinity Fc receptor (FcεR1) on the surface of sensitized MCs are cross-linked (aggregated) by allergen to trigger degranulation and release of preformed granule-derived mediators and proteases or express newly synthesized mediators. Release and expression of mediators from activated MCs include vasoactive histamine, acidic glycoproteins such as heparin, enzymes (e.g., tryptase and chymase), expression of chemotactic mediators that are released in the circulating blood to

attract and recruit other inflammatory cells (e.g., eosinophils) for additional production of toxicity at the site of injury that may cause further injury to the tissue. In occasions where IgE Abs produced against parasitic infection, helminths (e.g., Ascaris Suum or its extracts), the responses from MCs are stronger and the damage to the tissues are severe. Furthermore, while circulating IgE antibodies preferentially sensitize MCs of the susceptible host (target exposed tissue), often the circulating (homocytotropic) IgE Abs sensitize other MCs that are distant from the target. In addition, as we reported for inflammatory responses in ocular tissues (details in Chap. 4), the severity of type 1 reactions may not necessarily correlate with the circulating levels of IgE [3, 5, 81, 82, 109]. For example, repeated topical and unilateral sensitization and challenge of ocular tissues with antigen caused not only strong responses from contralateral eye (untreated eye), they occasionally produced asthma-like wheezing symptoms in immunized animals suggesting sensitization and activation of MCs in lung airways. In addition, newborn babies from repeatedly sensitized animals (guinea pigs) demonstrated severe ocular allergies upon the first or second challenge with the antigen suggesting antibody transfer maternally or paternally (genetic predisposition?) [3–5, 66–68, 81, 82, 109].

4 Molecular Mechanisms of Acute Inflammation

As noted above, the exact molecular mechanisms of activation of multiple interdependent and complex pathways that are involved in the two phases of self-terminating acute inflammation are not understood. The signals initiated/generated from the activated innate and/or adaptive immunity for the purpose of destruction of foreign elements and injured tissue during Yin (growth-arrest) responses, would simultaneously signal for induction of Yang (growth-promote) pathways to resolve, neutralize and terminate the pro-inflammatory phase-induced tissue damage and resolve inflammation [3–5, 63, 66–68, 82, 109]. Therefore, resolution of acute inflammation means returning to normal activities of all immune cells, the vasculature and the metabolic and neuronal pathways (resting status of immunity) with little or no harm to the host. The dual inherent properties of immunity during termination and resolution of acute inflammation and generation of decoy receptor molecules, in all likelihood, are inclusive of the shift in energy consumption, away from oxidative phosphorylation (in Yin) toward aerobic glycolysis (Warburg effect). Yang processes are accompanied by the scavenger roles of metabolites and antioxidants or reducing enzymes (e.g., vitamin E, ascorbate, NADPH reductase, GSH, catalase, SODs) for reducing/neutralizing the toxicities of ROS/RNS and other oxidants that are generated in host. Therefore, stimuli-induced burst of energy in immune cells and rapid production of ATP from oxidative phosphorylation causes rapid ATP hydrolysis, followed by a change (rise) in the tricarboxylic acid (TCA) cycle intermediates (e.g., succinate or citrate) that are required for lipid biosynthesis and maintenance of mitochondria energy homeostasis.

Because multiple factors are involved in inflammatory processes, the outcomes of inflammation present infinite possibilities. In general, factors influencing the outcomes of inflammation, include the nature, quantity and potency of foreign elements, frequency of inflammatory conditions, competency of immune and non immune components (individual's genetic makeup) of target tissue, route of exposure, types of target tissue (e.g., immune-privileged, immune-responsive, insulin-dependent or insulin-independent for glucose transport and/or utilization), as well as the age of individual.

5 Interrelated Cell Death Categories

The nomenclature of cell death (necrosis, accidental cell death, oncosis, pyroptosis) or apoptosis, also known as Type I, Type II or Type III, cell death are confusing and ambiguous when mechanisms of immune-independent or immune-regulated cell death are defined [3, 4, 20, 80, 63, 66–68, 109–119, 138, 197–219]. These terminologies for cell death are often used when cell death occurs principally independent of programmed cell death, without extensive involvement of immune pathways that was described for Yin and Yang of acute inflammation. Highlights of known mechanisms of cell death with limited shared features with programmed cell death include the following: (Fig. 2.5):

1. **Accidental necrosis, oncosis and pyroptosis**: Accidental tissue necrosis happens as the results of significant or sudden increases in tissue oxidative stress causing extensive depletion of adenosine triphosphate (ATP) accompanied by the loss of cytosolic components and membrane integrity. The special feature of accidental necrosis is the absence of death signaling, which is different from Yin pathways in programmed cell death. Analyses of related data suggest that accidental necrosis and programmed cell death present limited shared physiological features. Both processes occur as the result of decreased host ATP levels (or increased ATPase activity for ATP hydrolysis) followed by an increased level of intracellular sodium ions [Na^+]. These events cause opening of the ion channels that lead to membrane and cytoskeleton rupture (membrane 'leakiness'), loss of cellular membrane integrity, osmotic swelling of intracellular organelles along with disruption of nuclear components and condensation of chromatin structure, a phenomenon also called oncosis (Fig. 2.5) [20, 109–117, 197–203]. It is not clear however, what conditions (nature of stimuli or tissue type) would induce sudden drop in ATP hydrolysis and how the intrinsic inappropriate synthesis of cells (e.g., cancerous cell or viruses) or drugs contribute to the accidental cell death. Another question is whether cytotoxic T cells are able to induce accidental cell death without involvement of the programmed cell death (Fig. 2.5).

The outcomes of accidental cell necrosis are different from apoptosis in programmed cell death since in the absence of wound healing processes (Yang), necrotic bodies that accumulate in tissues need to be neutralized and/or recycled by other mechanisms. It is possible that necrotic bodies are simply digested by circulat-

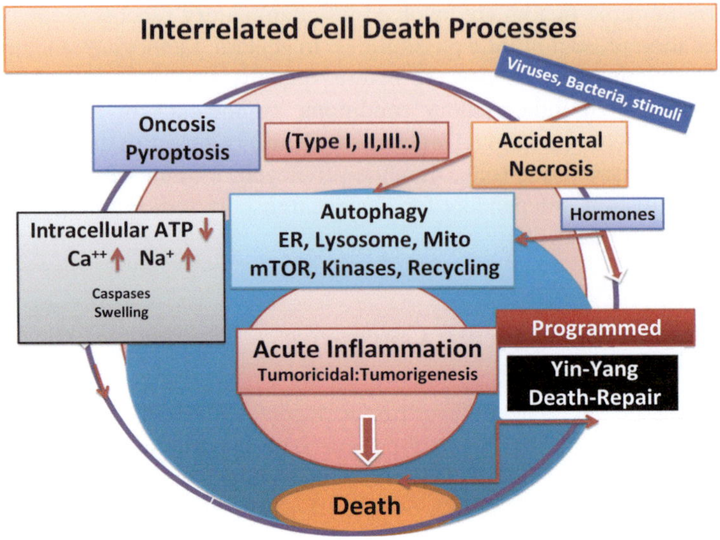

Fig. 2.5 Schematic representation of interrelated cell death. Major categories of cell death are oncosis/pyroptosis, accidental tissue necrosis and programmed cell death (Yin-Yang) of acute inflammation involving ATP hydrolysis and autophagy. See text

ing phagocytes as part of acute inflammation and/or autophagy. Accumulation of necrotic bodies from accidental necrosis may be considered as the biological byproducts in tissue; they form useless or toxic materials (antigen loads, internal stimuli) and could activate immune responses and/or autophagy. The accidental necrosis perhaps is a 'one way' cellular killing, compared with programmed cell death in 'Yin-Yang' pathways that requires complex participation of immune and non-immune pathways. However, the role of low-level activation of caspases and interleukins (e.g., IL1β), to trigger pyroptosis in non-inflammatory elimination of pathogens and maturation of dendritic cells have been demonstrated. Furthermore, activation of caspase 1 does not seem to lead to cell death (pyroptosis) in all cells such as the epithelial cells [20, 23, 26, 63, 66–68, 109–120]. These interesting observations suggest that a reason for caspase activation not leading to cell death in epithelium is that epithelium is an immune-responsive tissue and could trigger many other signals for induction of wound healing processes of acute inflammation that lead to repair and survival of the tissue.

2. **Autophagy or macroautophagy:** The term 'autophagy' derived from Latin meaning 'self' and 'eating'. Autophagy is an essential and dynamic process of tissue homeostasis, involving continuous degradation and recycling of cytosolic components, membrane formation and fusion. Autophagy has intracellular anti-viral and anti-bacterial functions and plays a role in the initiation of response processes from innate and adaptive immune system against viral and bacterial infections. In general, there are three types of autophagy, macroautophagy, microautophagy and chaperone-mediated autophagy (CMA). Briefly, the overall

processes in autophagy involve six major steps of membrane and protein assembly and degradation processes often initiated by mTOR (mammalian target of rapamycin)/PI3K/AKT signaling pathway in the induction of autophagy as the following (details in Chap. 6) [63, 109, 138, 201–219]:

(a) **Initiation of membrane isolation**. The process also called phagophore, or preautophagosome. mTOR kinase signaling initiate complex association of cell membrane and cytosolic materials [e.g., endoplasmic reticulum (ER) and related vesicles]. The process requires autophagy-related protein-enzymes complexes (e.g., DFCP1, Atgs).
(b) **Omegasome formation**. The process involves autophagy-related gene protein (Atgs) expression products, phospholipid phosphatases, ATPases, kinases complexes (e.g., Atg12-Atg5-Atg16, ULk1-Atg13-FIP200-Atg101) and components of ER and Golgi complexes, which are formed inside the ring of the omegasome.
(c) **Elongation of the isolated membranes**. This process further engulfs cytoplasmic components including mitochondria and ER. The elongation of membranes involves many negative (inhibitors) and positive (inducers) proteins and enzymes that control the extent of membrane isolation and elongation.
(d) **Autophagosome formation**. The next steps in autophagy are associated with a number of other autophagic-related proteins, enzymes and ligands (e.g., Atg5-Atg12-Atg16L), followed by membrane fusion and dissociation factors (e.g., LC3-II, LC3-PE) to form autophgosome (maturation step) that prepare the complex for degradation.
(e) **Autophagosome-lysosome fusion**. Following maturation of the autophagosome, cytoplasmic lysosome fuse with the autophagosome (autophagosome-lysosome fusion).
(f) **Degradation and recycling**. In this process, a number of lysosomal hydrolases are involved in degradation of autophagosomal contents. As the result of this process, protolysosome is elongated from autolysosome.

In brief, the essential factor or the 'core' for the above six major events involves energy-driven autophagy-related (Atg) protein kinase complexes and conjugate systems (e.g., ULK1 protein kinase, Atg9-WIPI-1, Vps34-becl in1 class III PI3-kinase, and the Atg12 and LC3), as well as PI3 binding proteins and phosphatases and Rab proteins pathways initiated through mTOR-dependent signaling. Elegant studies demonstrate that while some viruses encode virulence factors for blocking the autophagy, others utilize autophagy components for their intracellular growth or cellular budding [138, 206–220].

(g) Selective Functions of Autophagy: Mitophagy, Reticulophagy, Ribophagy and Xenophagy

In addition to the non-selective function of autophagy, the selective autophagy that includes mitophagy, a type of autophagy specific for degradation of mitochondria; reticulophagy for the recycling of endoplasmic reticulum; ribophagy for degradation/recycling of ribosomes; or piecemeal autophagy for the nucleus/chromosomal components; and xenophagy for pathogens have been identified and reported in the literature. Defects in multistep complex processes of autophagy are associated with a wide range of chronic diseases such as neurodegenerative diseases, diabetes complications, cardiomyopathy, fatty liver pathology and tumorigenesis. For example, changes in mTOR/PI3K/AKT pathways implicated in longevity, malignant transformation and growth or endocrine/hormonal control of metabolism and adipose tissue biology. Details of biological processes that are involved in non-selective or selective autophagy and degradation- assembly of cellular components for maintenance of health or induction of diseases are available in a number of recent publications (Fig. 2.5) [138, 203–229].

In summary, autophagy is a bulk process of degradation of cytoplasmic components and membrane organelles or vesicles. Autophagosomes and autolysosomes are transient structures during protein/lipid degradation and recycling in autophagy. It seems that both killing of pathogens through programmed cell death (Yin-Yang) or accidental cell death, often requires simultaneous involvement of metabolic signals that are dependent on cellular burst of energy (changes in oxido-redox potential), accompanied by increased ratios of NADP+/NADPH and hydrolysis of ATP involving ATPase and alterations in ADP/AMP levels. As noted above, accomplishing Yin-Yang events in programmed cell death of self-terminating acute inflammation, the complex apoptotic response pathways involve burst of energy from the mitochondria of activated APCs (e.g., MCs) to release mediators (e.g., Histamine) and enzymes such as tryptase or chymase, phosphatases, caspases, adenosine deaminase (ADA) and cell surface molecules (e.g., CD 73), also involving aggregation of receptor molecule (e.g., antigen-induced IgE-fcεR and MCs degranulation). These events are energy requiring and produce the required pharmacological effects. The Yin events are followed by shifting away from high energy consumption to utilization of low energy produced in glycolysis and induction of growth pathways to repair the tissue and terminate inflammation (Figs. 2.4 and 2.5).

6 Chronic Inflammation: 'Immunological Chaos' in Host Tissue and Initiation of Disease Process. Not All Immune Disruptors Created Equal!

Unresolved inflammation (oxidative stress, chronic, subclinical) was defined as the loss of balance between the two tightly regulated and biologically opposing arms of acute inflammation, Yin (growth-arrest, apoptosis or tumoricidal) and Yang (growth promote or tumorigenic) of immunity. We proposed that sustained oxidative stress could lead to exaggerated expression and co-expression of death and growth factors in susceptible host tissues. Depending on the nature of stimuli (immune disruptor) and/or the extent of expression of growth or death factors, and type and composition of host tissue (e.g., immune-responsive or immune-privileged) loss of balance in

Yin and Yang processes could determine the outcomes of tissue damage. Those immune disruptors (e.g., potent pathogens, strong carcinogens, major trauma), that manage to cause serious imbalance in the homeostasis of immunity, would take advantage of inherent dualities of dynamics of biological responses (feedback control mechanisms) to initiate serious damages in the susceptible tissues and organ systems and induction of chronic diseases [3, 4, 63, 66–68, 81, 82, 92, 109].

In 2009, Khatami proposed that unresolved inflammation was a common denominator in the genesis and progression of nearly all age-associated chronic health problems including site-specific cancers [67]. The extensive alterations or defects in the pathways of immune and non-immune networks, seem to be the principal contributors to increased risks of allergies, asthma, autoimmune and neurodegenerative diseases, hypertension, diabetes and cardiovascular complications, stroke, multiple sclerosis, Hodgkin's, lupus, Alzheimer's, and induction of soft or solid tumors, the illnesses that primarily develop in older adults [3, 4, 63, 66–68, 82]. As detailed in Chaps. 3 and 6, aging process itself induces minor or major alterations in the function of immune and non-immune systems altering the inflammatory response profiles toward new stimuli or accumulated senescent cells [3–5, 21–28, 31–34, 40, 41, 63, 66–68, 82, 92, 196, 217–237].

In brief, shifting from oxidative phosphorylation during Yin, to aerobic glycolysis and the induction of VEGF or HIF1 around neovascular tissue during Yang, are examples of inherent duality of the immune cells, assisted by non-immune systems during initiation and termination of inflammation. Oxidative stress and/or aging process could adversely influence the inherently dual capacity of immunity to generate exact amount of decoy receptors required for termination of inflammation (Yang). Retardation of immunity and expression of mismatched apoptotic or wound healing mediators accompanied by altered oxido-redox potential in tissues are perhaps essential components for immune suppression and initiation of chronic inflammatory diseases or tumorigenesis. In general, alterations in activation-induced cell death (AICD) or damage-induced cell death (DICD) of apoptosis (programmed cell death) are suggested as contributing factors in the dysfunction of immune responses during the aging process [63–68, 109, 221–232].

7 Stem Cells; Shared or Special Features in Innate and Adaptive Immune Cell Responses in Health and Age-Associated Chronic Diseases or Cancer

Antigen presenting cells (APCs), to varying degrees, possess distinct functions for regulation and control of death and survival signals that influence the effector cell function for pharmacological response. The outcomes of specific inflammatory conditions in host tissues are the results of interdependent immune responses. As schematically shown in Fig. 2.6, each immune cell that is generated by stem cells, the giant manufacturer of immune cells, has the capacity to directly or indirectly

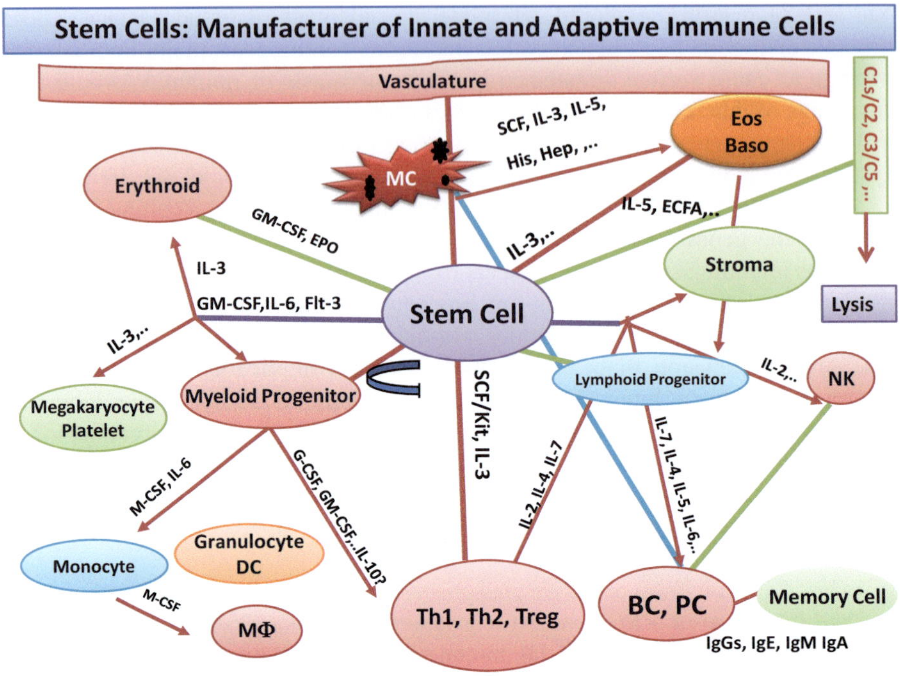

Fig. 2.6 Schematic representation of complex interdependent influence of innate and adaptive immune cells in growth and function of hematopoietic cells. Stem cells considered as the giant manufacturer of all hematopoietic cells whose growth and differentiation to specific immune cells are potentially directed by the signal transductions guided by specific tissues with special immune and non-immune compositions and/or under certain inflammatory conditions and tissue requirements. See text

influence activation, proliferation, differentiation, growth and maturation (polarization) of other immune cells. (Table 2.1) [3, 4, 63, 66, 81, 82, 109].

Depending on requirements of the target tissue and function, innate and adaptive immune cells, and their counter parts in non-immune systems are capable of diverse dual functions to change the dynamics of Yin-Yang balance (tumoricidal: tumorigenic ratio) in acute inflammation. For example, DCs, MΦs or MCs, as well as T or B lymphocytes can be induced to function as polarized cells during, development, maturation, wound healing and in response to tumorigenesis (Fig. 2.6) [3, 4, 63–65, 81, 82, 109]. Growth and maturation of immune cells include maturation and survival of self, or those of T cells subpopulation Th1, Th2 (Treg), transformation of macrophages into M1/M2 (or tumor associated TAMs) phenotypes, mast cells maturation (granulation, IgE Fcε-dependent phenotypes) and degranulation, or they can become IgEfcε-independent 'leaky' MCs or TAMCs form, transformation of dendritic cells from immature/tumoricidal (DC1) to mature/tumorigenic (DC2 or TADCs) phenotypes (Fig. 2.6, Table 2.1).

Therefore, pro- and anti-inflammatory signals regulate the levels and efficiency of inflammatory cytokine receptor coupling and amplification of effector function.

Table 2.1 Example of dual (pleiotropy) properties of immune cells and mediators in acute (AI) and chronic inflammation (CI) [3, 4, 63, 67, 109]

Mediator/Factor	Cell polarization	Major biological effects
Toll like receptors (TLRs 1–9)	DC1/DC2 (TADC); M1/M2 (TAM); MC/'leaky'(TAMC)	AI: Signal for death factor-Yin
		CI: Decoy receptor, growth promotion-Yang
Tumor necrosis factor α (TNF-α) and TNFR	DC1/DC2 (TADC); M1/M2 (TAM); MC/'leaky'(TAMC)	AI: Induction of apoptosis
		CI: Decoy receptor, growth promotion
Histamine	MC/'leaky'(TAMC)	AI: Vasoactive, apoptosis, IgE-fcε-rec-dependent, vascular hyperpermeability
		CI: Release independent of IgE- fcε-rec, growth promotion
Macrophage colony stimulating factor (M-CSF)	M1/M2/TAM	AI: Induction of apoptosis
		CI: Decoy receptor, immune suppressor, tumorigenic
Interleukins (ILs) (IL-1-α, IL-2, IL-4, IL-5, IL-6, IL-10, IL-12, IL-13,...)	Innate and adoptive immune cells	AI: Apoptosis
		CI: Decoy receptor, growth

Pro-inflammatory cytokines such as IL-1, IL-6, IL-8, TNF-α, M-CSF, GM-CSF, eotaxin, as wells as, histamine, prostaglandins (e.g., PGF1α or PGI2), leukotrienes, heparin or enzymes (e.g., chymase, tryptase) other proteases released by activated resident (local) and/or recruited inflammatory cells are capable of contributing to the progression of responses. In all likelihood, increased local concentrations of special mediators produced by resident inflammatory cells signal for expression, interactions and synergies between recruited and infiltrated cells (e.g., eosinophils, MΦs, vasculatures) are requirements of an effective immunity to accomplish a task, such as removal of an infectious agent and repair of damaged host. Details on the roles of immune cells under inflammatory conditions and carcinogenesis are provided in Chap. 6.

8 Differential Influence of Acute and Chronic Inflammation in Immune-Privileged and Immune-Responsive Tissues and Chronic Diseases

Molecular mechanisms that govern the tightly regulated processes of acute inflammation somewhat differ in immune-privileged and immune-responsive host tissues. In general, acute inflammation provides immune protection in target tissues via two mechanisms:

1. Immune surveillance in the immune-responsive tissues for killing of cancer cells, destruction of infective agents/pathogens (stimuli) and resolution of inflammation, remodeling or regeneration of host cells; and
2. Immune ignorance, immune evasiveness and tolerance in the oxidative-sensitive immune-privileged tissues.

8.1 Immune Surveillance (Protection) in Immune-Responsive Tissues

Immune-responsive tissues are generally the sites of initial contact and processing of internal or external stimuli. These tissues include squamous and glandular epithelial tissues, epithelial-associated mucosal surfaces (e.g., goblet cells), endothelial and stromal cells, fibroblasts, lymphoid tissues and vasculature.

The disease outcomes of chronic inflammation-induced immune dysfunction in immune-responsive tissues are a wide range of allergies (e.g., asthma, emphysema, food, ocular or skin allergies), chronic diseases such as hypertension, vasculitis, diabetes and cardiovascular complications, colitis, gastritis, pancreatitis, thyroiditis, esophagitis, psoriasis, lupus, prostatitis and/or cellular growth, hyperplasia, dysplasia, neoplasia/pre-cancer or cancer (e.g., prostate, lung, colorectal, uterine, breast, ovarian, stomach, pancreas, esophagus, bladder, cervix), metastasis and angiogenesis (details in Chap. 6) [3, 4, 63, 66–68, 82].

In certain chronic diseases such as diabetes complications, the hyperglycemia of diabetes is associated with glycosylation of proteins, and accumulation of advanced glycation end-products (AGE) and maillard reactions, complexes that are known to induce inflammatory reactions and interference with antigen-antibody binding [3, 4, 63, 82, 109, 238–240]. AGE, is viewed by tissues as non-self and additional risk factors for induction of not only adult on-set diabetes mellitus (DM) complications (e.g., retinopathy, cardiovascular diseases, hypertension, neuropathy, nephropathy, stroke) but they also increase the risk of several cancers (e.g., liver, pancreas, endometrium, colon, rectum, bladder, breast). The author suggested that the damaging impact of inflammatory responses toward hyperglycemia of diabetes may be different in insulin-dependent (e.g., muscle, adipocytes or liver) or insulin-independent (e.g., vasculature, retina, kidney or neuronal) tissues for glucose transport and utilization, and/or immune-privileged or immune-responsive tissues [3, 63, 109].

8.2 Immune Protection (Tolerance) in Immune-Privileged Tissues

Immunobiology of protection against pathogens, chemical or biological insults in immune-privileged tissues and neighboring cells are complex and not well understood.

Immune-privileged sites, in general, prohibit the processing and spread of pathogen-induced inflammation because these episodes can threaten delicate integrity and function of these stress-sensitive tissues. The most prominent examples of immune-privileged tissues are central nervous system (CNS), blood brain barrier (BBB), ocular tissues [e.g., cornea, neurosensory retina and retinal pigment epithelium (RPE)], hair follicles and reproductive organs (e.g., testis and uterus). Due to low capacities for self-renewal, the immune-privileged tissues are particularly vulnerable toward infections, chemical insults or injuries as even minor persistent inflammation could have long-term effects on survival of these tissues. Immune responses in these tissues either do not proceed, or proceed in a limited fashion that differs from those described for immune-responsive tissues. Induction of inflammatory processes in immune-privileged tissues is restricted by one or a combination of immunological barriers including the absence or limited presence of vasculature (e.g., avascular cornea), lymphatic channels; antigen presenting cells (APCs, Langerhans, microglial or dendritic cells/DCs) and/or immune recognition and adapter molecules (e.g., MHC class I or II, or HLA). These immunological barriers provide 'immune unresponsiveness', 'immune ignorance' or 'immune tolerance' for the immune-privileged tissues. Exposure to foreign elements often results in sequestration of antigen and avoidance of encounter with stimuli which also limits activation of lymphoid tissues for humoral and/or cell-mediated delayed hypersensitivity responses by other antigen presenting cells (Fig. 2.7, Table 2.2) [3, 4, 63, 67, 68, 109, 190, 236, 237, 241–245].

The immunological unresponsiveness in the immune-privileged tissues is termed 'immunological ignorance' or the term sometimes used for immune tolerance [3, 4, 67, 68, 109, 241–244]. In immune-privileged sites, immune protection appears to involve site-specific processes that deal with the invaders before they spread to stress-sensitive tissues. Localized immunity provided in these tissues by immune deviation or immunomodulation that includes active or passive suppression of responses from immune cells (e.g., NKs, DCs or MΦs). Preliminary studies to compare the viability of rabies virus in cultures of bovine retinal pigment epithelial (RPE) with human neuroblastoma cells suggested phagocytic/protection role for RPE cells that prevented virus's survival and propagation (Khatami, unpublished observations). Others reported the immune protection of neuroretina and cornea against pathogens [63, 67, 68, 241, 242].

Table 2.2, shows examples of immunomodulation in immune-privileged tissues, by site-specific expression of growth inhibitors, immunosuppressive cytokines, neuropeptides, limited expression of MHC I, II complex and complement regulatory proteins, as well as increased expression of selective apoptotic or death-inducing factors such as TNF-related ligands (e.g., FasL and TNF-related apoptosis-inducing ligand (TRAIL), heat shock proteins (e.g., α−β-crystalline) or

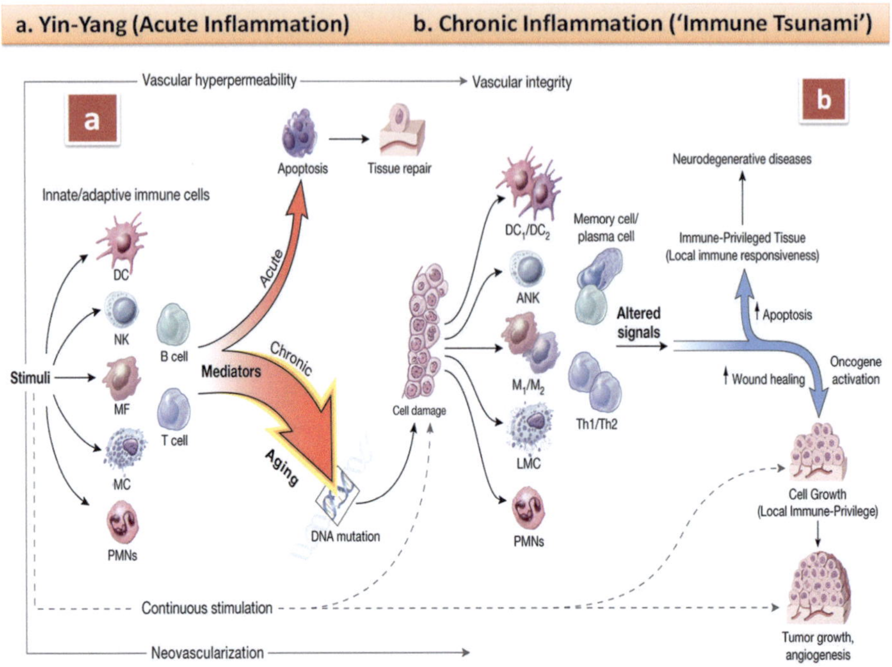

Fig. 2.7 Schematic representation of impact of acute and chronic inflammation in tissue. *Left panel* (*a*) represents self-terminating property of acute inflammation (Yin-Yang). Stimuli-induced activation of immune cell responses, facilitated by vascular hyperpermeability to defend tissues against stimuli. *Right panel* (*b*) represents oxidative stress could cause continuous activation of immune cells (e.g., DC1/DC2, M1/M2) that would lead to DNA damage and mismatched or co-expression of wound healing and apoptotic factors to differentially impact immune-privileged and immune-responsive tissues in the direction of altered architectural integrity of tissues and initiation of neurodegenerative diseases or tumorigenesis (Modified from Khatami (EXP Opin Biol Ther. Ref. [68]) with permission. All rights reserved)

proteolytic enzymes to effectively destroy inflammatory cells and limit the spread of inflammation and cell growth and minimize vascular hyperpermeability and neovascularization during exposure to stimuli or pathogenic infections (e.g., bacterial Staphylococcus aureus) [63, 67, 68]. Increased expression of selective death-inducing molecules or growth inhibitors are poised to destroy inflammatory cells that would otherwise initiates manifestation of neurodegenerative diseases and oxidative-induced damage to the brain, CNS, induction of endophthalmitis, neovascularization and infiltration of inflammatory cells within the confines of these vulnerable tissues [68].

However, the immune-privileged status of these oxidative stress-sensitive tissues does not provide complete barriers. Immune ignorance in these tissues can be breached when tissues are overwhelmed by infections or sustained oxidative stress, particularly during the aging process (Fig. 2.7). Unresolved inflammation could seriously threaten these stress-sensitive tissues, causing enhanced cell death and increased risk of neurodegenerative and autoimmune disorders such as multiple

Table 2.2 Immune tolerance and structural barriers for inflammatory mediator responses in immune-privileged tissues during acute and chronic inflammatory conditions [63, 68, 236, 237, 241–244]

Structural and response barriers	Acute inflammation	Chronic inflammation (Diseased stage)
Blood brain barrier (BBB)	Brain integrity	Loss of BBB, hemorrhage, stroke (?)
Avascular (cornea)	Limited immune response	Induction of vascular activity
Lymphatic channels NK, Langerhance, astrocytes, microglia, DCs, MΦs	Absence or limited presence- immune deviated	Induction of activity, increased presence/immune responsive
Retinal pigment epithelium/RPE	Immune deviation, informal phagocytes	Loss of phagocytic activity (?)
		Immune-responsive
Inflammatory mediators		
MHC class I,II or HLA	Limited presence	Activated
Immune suppressive cytokines	Increased activity	Reduced function (?)
FasL, (CD95L) TRAIL, complement proteins	Increased activity	Loss of activity
TGF-β	Expression of T reg (CD4-CD8)	PE (IPE, CBPE, RPE)
M-CSF	Limited expression	Increased activity
NF-kB	Limited expression	Increased activity
Thrombospondin1 (TSP-1)	Provides autoimmunity	Reduced activity (?)
CD86 (B7–2)	Expression (ocular PEs)	Reduced activity (?)
Pigment epithelial-derived factor (PEDF)	Expression (ocular PEs)	Reduced activity (?)
Cytotoxic T lymphocyte antigen-2α (CTLA-2α)	Expression (ocular PEs)	?
Heat-shock proteins (α,β crystalline)	Increased activity	Reduced function (?)
S100A (neutrophils-derived)	Increased activity (clearance)	Loss of activity (?)

sclerosis and demyelination of CNS, encephalomyelitis, stroke or Alzheimer's, ocular inflammatory complications as well as, induction of cell growth and tumorigenesis [3, 63, 67, 68, 109]. Chronic inflammation-induced expression of mediators such as GM-CSF, neuron-, or antigen-reactive lymphocytes have been demonstrated to break the immunological barriers via activation and cross-presentation of MHC class I/II to T cells (CD8 subtypes) in immune-privileged tissue causing collateral and serious damage to tissues (e.g., demyelination and axonal or cellular degeneration). Studies on pathobiology of Alzheimer's disease suggest that inflammatory cells, such as microglia, and deposition of complement proteins (e.g., C3, C4) and expression of wound healing or growth factors such as NF-kB or GM-CSF are involved in the genesis of amyloid precursor proteins (APP) plaque formation and changes of astrocyte subpopulations [26, 42, 63, 68, 197, 198, 244]. Similarly, reports on neurodegenerative diseases demonstrated that neuron- or antigen-reactive lymphocytes can escape immune tolerance and break the immunological barriers via cross-presentation of MHC class I/II to T cells (CD8 subtypes) and invade the tissues (e.g., ocular anterior chamber, retinal and neuronal tissues, CNS or brain) resulting in collateral tissue damage. The anti-inflammatory property of the intraocular environment is critical to the survival of immune-privilege ocular tissues. Induction of oxidative stress and alterations in the immune protection and clearance properties of ocular tissues are important factors in several blinding disorders, including age-associated macular degeneration, uveitis, ophthalmitis, corneal inflammatory and diabetic ocular complications (e.g., retinopathy, neuroretinopathy or retinopathy of prematurity) [63, 68, 241–243].

In certain neurodegenerative diseases such as multiple sclerosis or acute encephalomyelitis, or uveitis, it has been shown that neuron- or antigen-reactive lymphocytes can escape immune tolerance and invade the tissue (e.g., CNS) and induce significant tissue damage (e.g., demyelination and axonal degeneration) [42, 45, 63, 68, 241–244].

In summary, significant dysfunction of immune responses and progressive erosions of natural integrity in both immune-privileged and immune-responsive host tissues could be a foundation for genesis of the majority of age-associated chronic illnesses. Inflammation-induced increased expression of apoptotic factors could cause major shifts in local immune responsiveness and integrity of immune-privileged tissues that lead to neurodegenerative or autoimmune diseases. On the other hand, exaggerated co-expression of wound healing and selected apoptotic factors could induce local immune-privilege (immune tolerance, immune evasion) and loss of immune surveillance in the immune-responsive tissue, in the direction of growth promotion, neoplasia, cancer, metastasis and angiogenesis (Fig. 2.7).

We hypothesized that there are comparable mechanisms of actions in potent pathogens-induced severe acute inflammatory diseases (e.g., sepsis, or shock, meningitis or respiratory distress syndromes) with life-threatening side effects of cancer claimed 'targeted' drugs that cause cachexia, anorexia, sarcopenia and/or relapse [3, 63, 68]. Both conditions induce 'cytokine storm' or 'immune tsunami' that increase the risk of multiple organ failure (MOF) or death, due to rapid induction of immune dysfunction that otherwise occur over a longer periods of time. In acute inflammatory diseases, the prominent presence of mediators in host tissues is due to severe pathogen-driven expression of excessive amounts of apoptotic factors and toxic materials (tumoricidal) that could occur at any age. Under these conditions, it was suggested that strong pathogens would bypass orderly immunological processes by first destroying the integrity of the vasculature and gaining direct access to tissues causing induction of large amount of pro-inflammatory mediators that are toxic to host tissues [3, 55, 63, 68].

9 Clinical and Immunological Features of Immune Deficiencies

Recent studies have advanced the notion that chronic inflammation is a major risk factor underlying aging and age-related diseases. We suggested that low-grade unresolved inflammation is a common denominator in nearly all age-related pathological processes [3, 4, 63, 67, 68, 109]. Continuous (chronic) upregulation of pro-inflammatory mediators (e.g., TNF-α, IL1β, COX2, iNOS) induced during the aging process due to redox imbalance may activates many anti-inflammatory signaling pathways, including NF-kB and kinases that could inappropriately induce expression of factors in the direction of chronic illnesses such as increased allergies, atherosclerosis, arthritis, or benign or aggressive tumor growth.

The following sections describe bird's eye view on interrelated examples of inflammatory mediators, during acute and chronic inflammation in health or aging process in the direction of multistep tumorigenesis and angiogenesis. The roles that APCs play in immunity are at the center of critical decision of the immune system dynamics. That is because APCs are responsible for capturing antigens or pathogens in the periphery and migrating to the lymphoid organs and presenting the processed peptides and viral/bacterial particles to T cells for priming for either tolerance or induction of a response. The extent of expression of mediators from activated immune and non-immune cells is likely to influence the outcomes of inflammation as summarized in the following (details in Chap. 6) [3, 4, 63, 66–68, 81–100, 109]:

(a) **Angiogenesis and expression of VEGF (HIF-1)**: Formation of new capillaries is a normal process occurring in wound healing (Yang or resolution of acute inflammation), embryonic and placental development, ovulation, chronic inflammation, as well as induction of chronic diseases, tumor growth and metastasis. Angiogenesis is a key event in tumor growth and progression. The most important signal that links these different angiogenic-dependent processes is perhaps the degree of cell hypoxia. Nearly all of the components of the wound healing (Yang responses in acute inflammation, tumorigenic arm) or chronic inflammation-induced angiogenic processes have shared characteristics with the angiogenesis occurring during tumor growth and metastasis. Under oxidative stress, polarized immune cells such as macrophages produce proangiogenic, as well as antiangiogenic molecules that could cause damage to the integrity of blood vessels. For example, M-CSF-induced TAM-derived metalloelastase generates angiostatin. Irregular vascularization (neovascularization) and hypoxia are characteristics of hyperplastic and neoplastic tissues which also affect macrophage infiltration/migration, distribution and function in affected tissues [3, 4, 56, 60, 63, 66–68, 92–109, 195]. TAMs accumulate preferentially in poorly vascularized regions of tumors characterized by low oxygen tension. TAMs or skewed M2 population have altered antitumor properties; they are less mobilized or immobilized in poorly vascularized and avascular or necrotic and hypoxic areas of tumors or perhaps hyperplastic tissues. Compelling elegant studies show that hypoxic cells, particularly tumor cells, initially respond to stress by expression of vascular endothelial cytokine, originally known as hypoxia-inducible factor 1 (HIF1), or vascular endothelial growth factor (VEGF) to increase the genesis of vessel growth in an attempt to compensate for the lack of sufficient oxygen. The functional changes associated with expression of transcription factors HIF-1 HIF-2a or VEGF, bFGF and CXCL18 result in amplification of tumor angiogenesis [3, 4, 56–60, 62, 63, 66–68, 100, 109, 169, 195]. In human glioblastomas, highly expressed VEGF are identified near focal necrosis and hypoxic area where the new capillaries alongside VEGF-producing cells are localized. The extent of tumor hypoxia and angiogenesis in immune-responsive tissues likely determine the extent of tumor growth. In immune-privileged tissue, oxidative stress and induction of hypoxia could cause changes to the avascular tissues (e.g., cornea) causing local tissue immune responsiveness and vascularization, bypassing immune tolerance in these stress-sensitive tissues (Fig. 2.7, Table 2.2).

(b) **Oxidative damage: generation of ROS and RNS and physiological consequences:** The free radical theory has been primarily related to the damaging effects of reactive oxygen species (ROS) and reactive nitrogen species (RNS) and their intermediate superoxide components that are produced during inflammatory responses to destroy various toxins (Figs.2.1 and 2.2). However, generation of ROS and reactive RNS is part of normal metabolism of tissues and byproducts of oxidative metabolism. Under normal metabolism, the generation of these molecules is routinely and effectively neutralized by a wide range of cellular reducing powers and scavengers of oxidants [e.g., superoxide dismutases (SODs), NADH/NAD+, NADPH/NADP+ reductases, ascorbate-semidehydroascorbate reductase, vitamin E and glutathione recycling pathways], as well as, the presence of reducing metal ions (e.g., Zn^{2+}, Fe^{2+}, Mg^{2+}) within cellular components (e.g., Hb, albumin, mitochondria, Golgi apparatus, plasma membrane). The advanced damaging effects of enhanced state of oxidation (e.g., accumulation of free radicals and decrease in ratio of redox potentials) on biological systems toward initiation and promotion of chronic diseases such as cancer have been extensively documented [3, 4, 36, 63, 66–68, 71, 81, 82, 90, 118–124, 210, 245, 246]. Routine quantification of a panel of inflammatory mediators or the status of oxidative stress (e.g., histamine, TNF, PGs, neurotransmitters, CRP, NAD^+/NADH) to determine the status of individual health over the years, and to target for early detection of cancer, perhaps would be effective diagnostic methods of personal health. An example of dual roles that inflammatory cytokines play in carcinogenesis is tumor necrosis factor-alpha (TNF-α), a cysteine-rich family of cytokines and receptors. TNF-α is involved in maintenance of tissue homeostasis and elimination of cells with damaged DNA, pathways in apoptosis (Yin) or programmed cell death. Environmental, chemical or biological stimuli (exogenous or endogenous) can trigger the synthesis and production of TNF-α in a variety of cell types such as macrophages, T cells (Th1,Th2), MCs, or keratinocytes. The

TNF-receptors (e.g., TNFR-1, TNF-Rp55, TNF-Rp75) act as transducers of TNF by receiving and transmitting signals that trigger inflammatory responses. The TNFRs signaling is involved in mediation of a wide range of biological functions including cytotoxicity/cell death; antiviral activity; fibroblast or thymocyte proliferation, as well as induction of superoxide dismutase and NFkB activation. Accumulation of free radicals or oxidative stress will cause damage to cell components leading to inappropriate expression of decoy receptor proteins for TNF (TNFdR) or chemokines and create unresolved inflammation. Unresolved inflammation leads to damages, to varying degrees, of microstructure of tissue chromosomes or mitochondrial DNA (mutations), as well as cellular proteins or lipids and alterations in the immune system response dynamics and the function and integrity of host. An important damaging effect of oxidative stress is progressive alterations and decreases in energy output by mitochondria below the requirements of tissues that lead to hypoxia-induced growth promotion in immune-responsive tissues [63, 67, 90, 118–124, 210, 245–248] (Figs. 2.2 and 2.7, Table 2.1). In stress-sensitive immune-privileged tissues, accumulation of ROS could lead to destruction of immunity, induction of local immune-responsiveness, tissue necrosis and initiation of neurodegenerative diseases (Fig. 2.7). In brief, chronic inflammation (oxidative stress) and accumulation of ROS, RNS and superoxide radicals would increase, to varying degrees, the rate of damage to plasma and intracellular membranes and nuclear components, leading to DNA/RNA mutations and altered oxidative metabolism and bioenergetics of tissues toward the induction of hypoxia that further damage the integrity of vascular endothelial membrane structure and tissue function.

(c) **Natural Killer Cells (NKs):** NKs have critical roles in tumor immune surveillance, infections, autoimmunity and hematopoietic stem cell transplants. NKs exhibit cytotoxicity against a number of inflammatory conditions in oxidative stressed tissues by secreting a number of mediators that facilitate adaptive immune responses (Fig. 2.6). NKs share many similarities with cytotoxic T cells (CTCs) including expression of cell surface receptor molecules for perforin-dependent killing activities or NK cell-mediated lysis. However, NKs are distinct from CTCs since their inherent cytotoxicity is independent from adaptive role of MHC-related sensitization of T lymphocytes [4, 32, 49, 63, 66–68, 109, 128, 163]. While NKs cytotoxicity features have been recently considered for cancer immunotherapy, the effective use of these cells is yet to be demonstrated. As with other innate or adaptive immune cells, phenotype presence of NKs (tumor-associate NKs, TANKs) in tumor microenvironment assists immune evasion and facilitates enhanced growth requirements of tumor cells perhaps due to expression of decoy receptors or surface molecule that retards their cytotoxicity.

(d) **Macrophages (M1/M2 or TAMs):** As noted above, under oxidative stress, activated MΦs (increased M2/M1 or TAMs) could induce over-expression of monocyte-(MΦs)-colony stimulating factor-1 (MCSF-1) and/or its receptor c-fms in tissues and contribute to the tissue hyperplasia and tumorigenesis in conjunctival-associated lymphoid tissues (CALTs), vascular dysfunction, mammary glands of transgenic mice, human ovarian adenocarcinoma and other gynecological cancers and metastasis [3, 4, 37, 52, 58, 60–63, 66–68, 73–76, 87, 88, 93, 94, 109, 175, 194, 195]. Clinical features of phagocytic disorders are often found in individuals suffering from lymphadenitis, skin and visceral abscesses, cellulites, and gingivitis. Activated MΦs (TAMs or M2) and eosinophils that are recruited by tissues (e.g., conjunctiva or perhaps lung airways or gut-associated lymphoid tissues) whose principal resident immune cells are MCs and lymphocytes were suggested to play crucial synergistic roles in enhancing the growth promoting capacities of host toward tumorigenesis [3, 4, 63, 109]. Increased proliferation of neoplastic tissue is associated with increased requirements for nutrients and growth factors and induction of hypoxia. High efficiency of pro-neoplastic M2 (TAM) activity relates to their ability to accumulate and function under the oxygen-deficient regions of the tissue. In addition to over expression of MCSF, TAMs express and release an array of growth and pro-angiogenic factors that are concurrently chemotactic factors (decoy receptors) for monocytes and macrophages and act as tumorigenic or scavengers of oxidants during growth promotion and signals for abnormal growth promotion (skewed wound healing). Therefore, growth promoting factors that are normally expressed during Yang event to terminate inflammation can be excessively expressed in the hypoxic environment of accumulated TAM for expression of VEGF, bFGF, CXCL8, PDGF, EGF, and TGF-β. Factors such as PDGF promote the proliferation of neoplastic tissue and acts as a pro-angiogenic mediator for recruiting pericytes and stabilizing the newly formed vessels. Epidermal growth factor (EGF) stimulates neoplastic cells to synthesize and release M-CSF. Aside from the chemotaxis of macrophages (M2 or TAM phenotype), M-CSF1 induces differentiation and migration of peripheral monocytes that result in the enhanced infiltration of macrophages into the tumor microenvironment and enhanced expression of EGF, further influence induction of MCSF and expression of decoy receptors that would additionally facilitate macrophage-dependent intensive proliferation of neoplastic cells. MCSF-1 binding to its receptor molecule c-fms, a cell surface family of tyrosine kinase receptors, results in dimerization and phosphorylation of c-fms, the signaling requirements for macrophage proliferation to M2 phenotype to facilitate growth. We suggested that over expression of M-CSF from M2 phenotypes produces signals that are cumulative and synergistic with host mediators (e.g., low levels of histamine released into the media from 'leaky' MCs, independent of IgE-fcεR binding) causing tumor-directed expression of decoy receptors and immune suppressive factors (e.g., TNFdR, IL-5, IL-10, TGF-β, PGE2) [3, 4, 63]. Furthermore, in their role as pro-inflammatory cells, MΦs are involved in stroma remodeling releasing a slate of pro-inflammatory factors that constitute a signal of danger for immune cells. The outcomes of MΦs activities and polarization in tissue contribute to; (a), activation of cytotoxic T lymphocytes and NK cells; (b), infiltration of dendritic cells; (c), migration and differentiation of monocytes in a pro-inflammatory state (Figs. 2.2 and 2.4). M-CSF was suggested a suitable biomarker for cancer diagnosis and technology development because of its superior sensitivity and specificity, compared with conventional cancer biomarkers (e.g., CA-125, CA-19-9) (details in Chap. 6) [3, 4, 63, 109, 141].

(e) **Mast cells activation:** As discussed above, MCs activation usually occurs when IgE bound to high affinity Fcε receptor (FcεR1) on the surface of MCs cross-linked by allergen to trigger degranulation and release of preformed granule-derived mediators and proteases (effector function). Degranulation of mast cells also includes synthesis and release of newly formed lipid products (e.g., phospholipids, arachidonic acid metabolism and synthesis of prostaglandins and leukotrienes), activation of membrane enzymes (e.g., phospholipases-PLA, PLC, phosphotidylserine) and transcription of a number of cytokines that produce pharmacological effects in target tissue [3–12, 17, 38, 63, 66–68, 87, 89, 120–124, 137, 144, 159, 196, 232–234, 249, 250]. Oxidative stress-induced changes in MCs function and integrity have been associated with induction of a number of chronic allergies (e.g., asthma, emphycema, dermatitis, conjunctivitis) and cellular growth promotion and tumorigenesis, angiogenesis or cancer metastasis [3, 63, 66–68, 87, 89, 120–124, 137, 196, 249, 250].

(f) **Dendritic cells maturation**: As professional APCs, DCs are crucial for the initiation of primary immune responses. They form a network of innate or sentinel cells in the periphery to recognize, capture and transport/ferry pathogenic antigens to secondary lymphoid tissues for further processes. Immature DCs (DC0 s) in the blood can undergo polarization into immature type 1 dendritic cells, also known as DC1 (Yin response), and mature type 2 dendritic cells, known as DC2 or tumorigenic phenotype TADCs (Yang response), during migration under the influence of a variety of growth factors, cytokines/chemokines such as IL-1β, IL-10, and receptor molecules to terminate inflammation and cause immune suppression [3, 4, 42, 63, 109, 158, 166, 174, 244]. The inflammatory signals that are involved in DCs maturation and migration to lymphoid organs, simultaneously induce a chemokine receptor switch, which normally cause down-regulation of inflammatory receptors (e.g., CCR1, CCR2, CCR5) and induction of CCR7 to terminate and resolve inflammation. Concomitant exposure to lipopolysaccharide (LPS) and IL-10 blocks the chemokine receptor switch associated with DC maturation [3, 4, 29, 42, 43, 79, 158, 166, 174, 175, 244]. LPS + IL-10-treated DCs showed low expression of CCR7 and high expression of CCR1, CCR2 and CCR5 and become growth-promoting mediators. Furthermore, uncoupled receptors expressed on LPS+ IL-10-treated cells sequester and scavenge inflammatory chemokines and potentially signal for expression of imbalanced growth factors, to create unresolved inflammatory environment that scavenge the apoptotic factors and oxidants. Thus, in an inflammatory environment, it seems the mature phenotype of DCs (DC2) generates IL-10 functional decoy receptors on DCs and/or perhaps other monocytes in an attempt to terminate and resolve inflammation. Sustained oxidative stress suggested to cause a decrease in the ratios of DC1:DC2 (TADCs) leading to exaggerated expression of wound healing mediators in the direction of immune suppression and cell growth promotion. Since small numbers of DCs are sufficient to induce an immune response, DCs can act as the most potent stimulators of T cells. Furthermore, DCs are the only APCs able to present novel antigens to resting naïve T cells (T0) and initiate the primary immune response. For this reason, DCs are prime targets for immunotherapy. Owing to the highly specific and important roles of DCs in body's defense, any minor modulation in DCs function could result in significant alterations in immune responses [14, 29, 63, 78, 152, 166, 174, 175].

(g) **B cell memory function:** Analyses of data from several studies on the induction of activities and transformation of B cells into plasma cells and genesis of B memory cells, induction of tolerance and humoral immunity (HI), suggest that oxidative stress and/or aging lead to repertoire maturation of these cells to proceed at lower pace. In some instances memory B cells exhibit autoreactivity and population shifts that influence CMI such as T cell effector responses, proliferation and cyclin D2 expression and altered antibody response profiles [3–5, 7, 13, 16, 25, 30, 48, 63, 79, 82, 109, 142, 147, 149, 184, 249, 251, 252]. The minor or major changes in the ratios of Th1/Th2 (CD4+/CD8+) potentially contribute to the altered immune response dynamics of lymphoid tissues and vascularization of lymphatic channels in affected tissues. Categories in clinical features of B cell-derived immunodeficiencies relate to primary deficiencies in IgA antibodies, IgG subclass (e.g., IgG1/IgG2 or IgG3), common variable immunodeficiency (CVID), complement deficiency, and specific antibody deficiency of normal immunoglobulins. Clinical features of disorders in the function of B lymphocytes and antibody production include recurrent sinopulmonary infection, sepsis, aseptic meningitis, autoimmune diseases, dermatitis, and increased incidence of malignancies [63, 109, 235, 249, 252, 253] Deficiencies in complement cascades are often associated with pyogenic bacterial infections, neisserial meningitis, and autoimmune diseases. However, some immunodeficiencies (e.g., IgA antibodies) are clinically asymptomatic. In such cases, the inherent pleiotropic ability of immune cells, is likely to compensate and overcome the genetically defects in biological functions of such abnormalities, particularly in younger individuals. The role of dysregulated autophagy and hyperglycemia-induced glycosylation of immunoglobulins in regulation of B cells and biosynthesis of antibodies have been identified as contributing factors in B cell-related immunodeficiencies, malignancies and metabolic disorders [63, 79, 109, 239–241, 245, 248, 249].

(h) **T effector lymphocytes**. In human, T cell antigen receptors (TCRs) couple in millions of combinations that enable them complex and unique repertoires for each individual processed antigenic molecules. TCRs recognize processed foreign peptides bound to major histocompatibility complex classes (MHC I, II) proteins and lipid antigens, such as Mycobacterium tuberculosis during infections. Detailed analyses of data indicate that the antimicrobial activities of MHC class I and II and expression of inflammatory cytokines (e.g., TNFα, INF-γ) induced by T helper subclasses (e.g., Th1, Th2, Treg,Th17), and/or involvement of regulatory phenotypes (e.g,. CD4(+)CD25(+)CD127(lo) CD45RA(+) and CD4(+)CD25(+)CD127(lo)CD45RA(-)...], present highly complex polymorphic organizations in a wide range of inflammatory conditions,aging and therapies including Crohns' disease, graft vs host disease, diabetes complications, dermatitis or cancers [61, 63, 67, 109, 127, 163, 176–178, 181–184]. That is to say any given foreign protein sequence encoded by HLA-A, HLA-B, HLA-C, HLA-DP and HLA-DQ loci can bind many peptides for a response. Aging or repetitive stimulation of host cells with antigens or mitogens could retard the competency of T cells, which influence B cell production of antibodies against specific antigens that are T cell dependent (TD) and require appropriate help from CD4+ T cells in the form of cytokines and cell-cell contact. Age-induced thymic involution leads directly to a decreased production of both naïve T cells and ultimately, a decrease in repertoire diversity of T cells in the periphery [3, 4, 31, 61, 63, 67, 78, 92, 102, 109, 127, 153, 176, 177, 178, 180, 182–184, 188, 204, 222–224, 231]. However, as in the case of B-lymphocytes, the total number of circulating T cells does not appear to decrease with age, despite the decline in thymic production. These observations are suggestive of subtle changes in subpopulation distribution of T cells that result in significant accumulation of long-lived memory T cells production. Furthermore, the homeostasis of circulating T cells in older adults seems to be due to the development of extra-thymic T cell. It is reasonable to predict that age-induced increased in the presence of memory T or B cells are viewed by immune system as 'antigen overload' or oxidative stress and contributors of tardiness of immune response (immune suppression) toward new or old immune disruptors. In general, the clinical features of T cell immunodeficiency disorders often include failure to thrive, increased viral opportunistic infections (e.g., pneumonia, HIV), frequent and prolonged or severe infections, disseminated infections with unusual organisms or organisms of low virulence, chronic diarrhea, hematologic disorders, dermatitis and increased incidence of cancer malignancies (details in Chap. 6) [109, 184, 217–222, 245–246].

(i) **Cell surface markers of APCs:** Analyses of data from multiple experimental studies demonstrate that in general, long-standing chronic inflammation and aging process produce minor or major defects in the co-stimulatory activity of APCs, through surface marker regulation that contribute to the altered immune dynamics and retardation of the recognition phase of immunity. For example, specialized dendritic cells (DCs) or the follicular DCs (FDCs), have distinct function in antigen presentation to T cells through binding of immune complexes. Oxidative stress and aging cause FDCs to express considerable amount of cell surface molecules and complement receptors; but the serum levels of complement proteins seem not reflective of DCs surface molecules. This is perhaps due to the induction of immune complexes with surface molecule ligands such as CD21 (CD21L) to retard responses for B cell activation during aging or perhaps under long-standing chronic inflammatory conditions [3, 4, 46, 60, 63, 67, 102]. Oxidative stress-induced continued DCs polarization from DC1(tumoricidal) to DC2 (or TADCs, tumorigenic phenotypes) could retard the capacity of DCs to capture antigen, and present the processed antigen to T cells. This is potentially due to increased expression of surface molecule involved in chemotaxis and T cell activation of major histocompatibility complexes I and II, and costimulatory surface molecule CD-40 [3, 4, 63, 66–68, 82–87, 109, 229]. Mature DC2 also produce T cell stimulatory cytokines IL-12 and IFN-γ during wound healing processes. Under normal conditions (acute inflammatory responses), soon after antigen specific interaction with T cells occurs, mature DCs undergo apoptosis via CD40 and FAS ligation, a mechanism suggested to control unnecessary and excessive activation and expansion of T cells [63, 109, 184, 227–229, 234]. Partial activation of CD4 T cells suggests contribution to tolerance by resting B lymphocytes [184].

(j) **Antigen-induced altered prostaglandin synthesis:** Metabolism of membrane arachidonic acid and induction of activities of cyclooxygenase and lipooxygenase pathways that results in synthesis of prostaglandins (e.g., PGI2/PGF1α, PGE2) during acute and chronic inflammatory conditions have been extensively studies [3, 4, 17, 63, 66–68, 82, 109]. Increased expression of cyclooxygenase observed in LPS-stimulated macrophages, or perhaps aged DCs or during chronic inflammation would lead to enhanced production of growth promoting PGE2 and decreasing the ratios of PGI2 (PGF1α). The enhanced production of PGE2 contributes to the age-, or inflammation-induced immune suppression and inhibition of T cell function, changes in $CD4^+$:$CD8^+$ ratios, or perhaps induction of such enzymes as urokinase receptor (CD87) in tumor growth and angiogenesis [3–5, 15–17, 60, 63, 66–68, 81, 82, 109]. Analyses of data also suggest that aging and/or chronic inflammation failed the expression of phosphatidylserine in macrophages or fibroblasts that is required for recognition and ingestion of antigens and proper apoptosis. In contrast, reports on aging and oxidative stress seem to activate phosphotidylinositide-3 kinase PI3K, in MCs or other APCs leading to the induction of PGE2 and immune suppression and cell growth [63, 246, 247, 252–256].

Although it is not clear how inflammation influences the disease outcomes, one can intellectually argue that the combination of minor or major cellular/biological, genetic or immunological defects, at multi-level crosstalk of immune and non-immune systems could retard the balance between Yin (tumoricidal) and Yang (tumorigenic) of acute inflammation, particularly during the aging process. Defects in immune response pathways include one or combination of changes in the dynamics of cellular or humoral immunity (CMI, HI) and/or loss of exact biological signaling among immune and non-immune (e.g., vasculature, metabolism or neuronal) pathways that contribute to altered tissue bioenergetics and initiation of diseases. Therefore, longevity and frequent stimulation of tissues (antigen burden, oxidative stress) could induce exaggerations of the expression and co-expression of cellular and humoral response profiles to create an 'immunological chaos' and loss of balance between Yin (tumoricidal) and Yang (tumorigenic) properties of acute inflammation.

10 Challenges in Understanding Dynamics of Immune Responses and Inflammation

Maintenance of the balance between 'Yin' (tumoricidal) and 'Yang' (tumorigenic) properties of acute inflammation, is most likely a key to host defense mechanisms in preventing or delaying the onset of chronic illnesses such as neurodegenerative and autoimmune diseases, or induction of hyperplasia, neoplasia, tumor growth, cancer metastasis and angiogenesis. Strategies for promotion of the inherent ability of innate immune cells, can potentially influence proper polarization of other cells within innate and adaptive immune system including Th1 and Treg and improve the natural 'tumoricidal' versus 'tumorigenic' properties of defense mechanism [3, 4, 63, 66–68, 82, 109]. Recent approaches in immunotherapy that consider promotion of innate and adoptive immunity, through active and/or passive methods of stimulation of tumor-associated antigen or induction of monoclonal antibodies and/or enhancement of innate and adaptive immune cell defense capacity (e.g., T cells MHC complex I and II or death factors ability of DCs) are encouraging. However, there are important scientific considerations and biological gaps in conducting such studies to be effective as outlined below (details in Chaps. 5 and 6) [3, 63, 109].

Major challenges in better understanding the complexity of dynamics of immune/inflammatory responses in maintenance of health or initiation of chronic diseases or site-specific cancers include:

1. Lack of systematic studies in identification of early immune response profiles toward a wide range of immune disrupters (stimuli) that could potentially be controlled or reversed or prevented from advancing to 'mild', 'moderate' or 'severe' immune disorders.
2. Lack of understanding of the heterogeneities in immune and non-immune cell compositions of site-specific tissues, and variations of interactions and synergies between host/tissue resident immune cells and those recruited cells/factors activated and infiltrated to the host tissue. Detailed understanding of the composition and heterogeneities of immune and non-immune cell responses in site-specific tissue with host-pathogen should be the primary focus of future studies. In our studies on experimental models of acute and chronic ocular inflammatory diseases, we discovered that repeated challenges with antigen caused partially granulated mast cells (exhausted or 'leaky' MCs) to sequentially signal for recruiting other activated inflammatory cells (e.g., eosinophils and macrophages) at the site of injury contributing to the developmental phases of immune dysfunction toward tumorigenesis and angiogenesis. In the immune-responsive tissues, such as lung airways, gut-associated lymphoid tissues (GALTs) or conjunctival associated lymphoid tissues (CALTs) whose primary immune cell compositions are mast cells and lymphoid tissues, the response profiles are perhaps somewhat different from those whose primary immune cell

composition are MΦs or dendritic cells [3–5, 63, 66–68, 81, 82, 109] (details in Chaps. 4 and 6).

3. Heterogeneities in antigen clearing effects and immune response profiles (strong or weak acute inflammatory reactions) are among important challenges because the extent of antigen permeability and access to inter-epithelial and sub-epithelial cells in tissues that are immune responsive may produce significantly different outcomes. We suggested that a strong type 1 reaction could restrict the penetration/exposure of antigen to trans-epithelial surface by an outward flow of fluids (e.g., mucus secretion, tearing or copious leakage of vascular plasma from hyperpermeable vasculature) in protecting host during acute inflammation. However, whether increased or repeated exposures to stimuli and cumulative permeability of low levels antigens or low level release of histamine from exhausted MCs would predispose the epithelial tissue toward antigen penetration and tissue damage are among biological gaps that deserve further investigations. Furthermore, a weak initial type 1 response due to defects in structure or function of MCs, B/plasma cells or GCs, may result greater net promotion of antigen penetration and/or increased epithelial exposure to higher doses of antigen or environmental toxins for inducing damages to tissues [3–5, 16, 17, 63, 66–68, 81, 82, 109].
4. Poor understanding of host-pathogen interactions and extent of immune response alterations in multistep disease processes.
5. Lack of understanding in minor or major heterogeneities of immune-biological response profiles in individuals, toward potential carcinogens (external and internal stimuli) that body recognizes hazardous to its survival, particularly during aging process.
6. Major biological gaps in the role of immune protection in immune-responsive and immune-privileged tissues, as well as difference in response profiles in insulin-dependent or insulin-independent tissues, for glucose transport or metabolism, toward oxidative stress.
7. Lack of knowledge in potential differential characteristics of mitochondrial development and function for energy requirements in tissues during stages of life; fetus growth and development, after birth and adulthood and aging and disease processes. It was recently suggested that the bioenergetics of mitochondrial development and function parallel the features of high energy requirements (oxidative phosphorylation from mitochondria) for tumoricidal (Yin) and low energy requirements (from glycolysis) of tumorigenic (Yang) pathways at different stages of life (details in Chap. 6) [109].

11 Concluding Remarks

Acute inflammation is a molecular village of complex signaling and energy requiring biological events between and among immunological, neuronal, hormonal vascular, genetic and physiological responses toward intrinsic (internal) and extrinsic (external) stimuli to guard and maintain the body' health throughout life. In an effective immunity, immediate (acute) hypersensitivity reactions are initiated by a highly regulated and exquisitely precise pro- and post-inflammatory crosstalk between local and systemic immune and non-immune systems for the purpose of neutralizing and eliminating the hazardous components while repairing the damaged host tissue.

Dysfunction of immunity and development of abnormal cell growth promotion and/or tissue necrosis that often are manifested as age-associated chronic diseases, such as neurodegenerative and autoimmune diseases or benign and malignant tumors and angiogenesis are perhaps the results of slow and progressive alterations in the dynamics of biological response profiles of persistent and unresolved inflammation. The nature and extent of exposures to intrinsic and extrinsic biological hazards together with age-induced altered hormonal, metabolic and immunological changes are likely the determining factors in homeostasis of immune surveillance and the risks of chronic diseases. Identification and understanding of developmental stages of immune response dysfunction in initiation of 'mild', 'moderate' or 'severe' immune disorders that are manifested as different diseases in immune-responsive or immune-privileged tissues deserve systematic and careful studies.

With regard to cancer, a single most pointing question that needs to be addressed for future research directions is how the growth-arresting properties of acute inflammation that is the body's defense mechanism, switch to growth-promoting function under persistent inflammatory conditions in the genesis of benign or malignant tumors. Similarly, how altered immunity could lead to tissue necrosis in immune-privileged tissues and genesis of neurodegenerative or autoimmune diseases or metabolic disorders. To answer such questions systematic studies of the dynamics of inherent properties of tumoricidal vs. tumorigenic (Yin-Yang) of acute inflammation are the first steps toward understanding the complex biology of immune surveillance and the mechanisms that are involved in controlling the growth of tissue, or induction of necrosis. Focusing on the promotion of the balance between tumoricidal (Yin or apoptosis) and tumorigenic (Yang or wound healing) of acute inflammation including the differential energy requirements of the two arms of immunity could provide unique opportunities and challenges toward effective approaches to combating illnesses, developing universal vaccines for preventing diseases or treating a wide range of immune disorders including cancer for a healthier growing population around the world.

Detailed integrated studies of molecular complexes of chemical and bioenergetic signaling that fall into the biological roadmaps of factors that contribute to the maintenance of body's anabolic and catabolic molecular resources deserves careful and detailed studies. The search for answers into biology of health starts with systematically understanding of how a well orchestrated biological system can be disturbed by aging process or sustained oxidative stress.

The author's original definitions of Yin (tumoricidal) and Yang (tumorigenic) properties of effective immunity may serve larger applications for understanding the biphasic (dual) activities of system biology in sustenance of health or initiation of diseases.

Throughout this book attempts were directed to demonstrate that:

(a) Cancer is an induced disease of Twentieth century, facilitated by medical/cancer establishment for huge corporate profit;
(b) Cancer is a symptom of violations of time-controlled biological circadian rhythms with differential bioenergetics.

References

1. Ehrlich P. Uber den jetzigen Stand der Karzinomforschung. Ned Tijdschr Geneeskd. 1909;5:273–90.
2. Burnet M. Cancer; a biologic approach. I. The processes of control. Br Med J. 1957;1:779–86.
3. Khatami M. Chronic inflammation: synergistic interactions of recruiting macrophages (MFs) and eosinophils (Eos) with host mast cells (MCs) and tumorigenesis in CALTs. M-CSF, suitable biomarker for cancer diagnosis! Cancers. 2014;6:297–322.
4. Khatami M. Inflammation, aging and cancer: friend or for? In: Khatami M, editor. Inflammation, chronic diseases and cancer. Cell and molecular biology, immunology and clinical bases. Rijeka: In Tech Publishing; 2012. p. 3–30.
5. Khatami M, Donnelly JJ, John T, Rockey JH. Vernal conjunctivitis. Model studies in guinea pigs immunized topically with fluoresceinyl ovalbumin. Arch Ophthalmol. 1984;102:1683–8.
6. Baxsi A, Dharajiya N, Choudhury BK, Sur S, Boldogh I. Effects of pollen-mediated oxidative stress on immediate hypersensitivity reactions and late-phase inflammation in allergic conjunctivitis. J Allergy Clin Immunol. 2005;116:836–43.
7. Schwartz LB. The mast cell. In: Kaplan AP, editor. Allergy, vol. 1. Edingurgh: Churchil Livingston; 1985. p. 53–92.
8. Nilsson G, Blom T, Harvima I, Kusche-Gullberg M, Nilsson K, Hellman L. Stem cell factor-dependent human cord blood derived mast cells express alpha- and beta-tryptase, heparin and chondriotin sulphate. Immunology. 1996;88:308–14.
9. Galli SJ, Tsai M, Wershil BK, Tam SY, Costa JJ. Regulation of mouse and human mast cell development, survival and function by stem cell factor, the ligand for the c-kit receptor. Int Arch Allergy Immunol. 1995;107:51–3.
10. Lemura A, Tsai M, Ando A, Wershil BK, Galli SJ. The c-kit ligand, stem cell factor, promotes mast cell survival by suppressing apoptosis. Am J Pathol. 1994;144:321–8.
11. Fischetti F, Tedesco F. Cross-talk between the complement system and endothelial cells in physiologic conditions and vascular diseases. Autoimmunity. 2006;39:417–28.
12. Okayama Y. Oxidative stress in allergic and inflammatory skin diseases. Curr Drug Targets Inflamm Allergy. 2005;4:517–9.
13. Drayton DL, Liao S, Mounzer RH, Ruddle NH. Lymphoid organ development: from ontology to neogenesis. Nat Immun. 2006;7:344–53.
14. Setzu A, Lathia JD, Zhao C, Wells K, Rao MS, French-Constant C, et al. Inflammation stimulates myelination by transplanted oligodendrocyte precursor cells. Glia. 2006;54:297–303.
15. Donnelly JJ, Taylor JR, Young E, Khatami M, Lok JB, Rockey JH. Experimental ocular onchocerciasis in cynomolgus monkeys. Invest Ophthalmol Vis Sci. 1986;27:492–9.
16. Khatami M, Donnelly JJ, Haldar JP, Rockey JH. Massive follicular lymphoid hyperplasia in experimental chronic recurrent allergic conjunctivitis. Arch Ophthalmol. 1989;107:433–8.
17. Helleboid L, Khatami M, Wei Z-G, Rockey JH. Histamine and prostacyclin: primary and secondary release in allergic conjunctivitis. Invest Ophthalmol Vis Sci. 1991;32:2281–9.
18. London NR, Zhu W, Bozza FA, et al. Targeting Robo4-dependent slit signaling to survive the cytokine storm in sepsis and influenza. Sci Transl Med. 2010;17:23.

19. Anhalt GJ, Kim SC, Stanley JR, Korman NJ, Jabs DA, Kory M, et al. Paraneoplastic pemphigus. An autoimmune mucocutaneous disease associated with neoplasia. N Engl J Med. 1990;323:1729–35.
20. Fink SL, Bergsbaken T, Cookson BT. Anthrax lethal toxin and Salmonella elicit the common cell death pathway of caspase-1-dependent pyroptosis via distinct mechanisms. Proc Natl Acad Sci U S A. 2008;105:4312–7.
21. Libby P. Inflammation in atherosclerosis. Arterioscler Thromb Vasc Biol. 2012;32(9):2045–51.
22. Libby P, Ridker PM, Hansson GK. Progress and challenges in translating the biology of atherosclerosis. Nature. 2011;473:317–25.
23. Brennan MA, Cookson BT. Salmonella induces macrophage death by caspase-1-dependent necrosis. Mol Microbiol. 2000;38:31–40.
24. Gimbrone MA Jr, Garcia-Cardena G. Vascular endothelium, hemodynamics, and the pathobiology of atherosclerosis. Cardiovasc Pathol. 2013;22:9–15.
25. Moller NP. Fc-mediated immune precipitation. I. A new role of the Fc-portion of IgG. Immunology. 1979;38:631–40.
26. Culmsee C, Landshamer S. Molecular insights into mechanisms of the cell death program: role in the progression of neurodegenerative disorders. Curr Alzheimer Res. 2006;3:269–83.
27. Nguyen VT, Ndoye A, Bassler KD, Shultz LD, Shields MC, Ruben BS, et al. Classification, clinical manifestations, and immunopathological mechanisms of the epithelial variant of paraneoplastic autoimmune multiorgan syndrome: a reappraisal of paraneoplastic pemphigus. Arch Dermatol. 2001;137:193–206.
28. Issa LA. Biologic agents for inflammatory bowel disease: the current, the future and the controversy. In: Khatami M, editor. Inflammation, chronic diseases and cancer. Cell and molecular biology, immunology and clinical bases. Rijeka: InTech Publishing; 2012. p. 417–30.
29. Shortman K, Naik SH. Steady-state and inflammatory dendritic-cell development. Nat Rev Immunol. 2007;7:19–30.
30. Nishimura H, Strominger JL. Involvement of a tissue-specific autoantibody in skin disorders of murine systemic lupus erythematosus and autoinflammatory diseases. Proc Natl Acad Sci U S A. 2006;103:3292–7.
31. Asseman C, von Herrath M. Regulation of viral autoimmune responses. Novartis Found Symp. 2003;252:239–53.
32. Billet SE, Grando SA, Pittelkow MR. Paraneoplastic autoimmune multiorgan syndrome: review of the literature and support for a cytotoxic role in pathogenesis. Autoimmunity. 2006;39:617–30.
33. Aprahamian T. Autoimmunity, atherosclerosis and apoptotic cell clearance. In: Khatami M, editor. Inflammation, chronic diseases and cancer. Cell and molecular biology, immunology and clinical bases. Rijeka: InTech Publishing; 2012. p. 75–96.
34. Czernik A, Camilleri M, Pittelkow MR, Grando SA. Paraneoplastic autoimmune multiorgan syndrome: twenty years after. Int J Dermatol. 2011;50:905–14.
35. Amagai M, Klaus-Kovtun V, Stanley JR. Autoantibodies against a novel epithelial cadherin in pemphigus vulgaris, a disease of cell adhesion. Cell. 1991;67:869–77.
36. Harrois A, Huet O, Duranteau J. Alterations of mitochondrial function in sepsis and critical illness. Curr Opin Anesthesiol. 2009;22:143–9.
37. Kirma N, Luthra R, Jones J, Liu Y-G, Nair HB, Mandava U, et al. Overexpression of the colony-stimulating factor (CSF-1) and/or its receptor c-fms in mammary glands of transgenic mice results in hyperplasia and tumor formation. Cancer Res. 2004;64:4162–70.
38. D'Amato G, Salzillo A, Piccolo A, D'Amato M, Liccardi G. A review of anti-IgE monoclonal antibody (omalizumab) as add on therapy for severe allergic (IgE-mediated) asthma. Ther Clin Risk Manag. 2007;3:613–9.
39. George J, Goldstein E, Abashidze S, Deutsch V, Shmilovich H, Finkelste A, et al. Circulating endothelial progenitor cells in patients with unstable angina: association with systemic inflammation. Eur Heart J. 2004;25:1003–8.

40. Craft J, Fatenejad S. Self antigens and epitope spreading in systemic autoimmunity. Arthritis Rheum. 1997;40:1374–82.
41. Echigo T, Hasegawa M, Inaoki M, Yamazaki M, Sato S, Takehara K. Antiphospholipid antibodies in patients with autoimmune blistering disease. J Am Acad Dermatol. 2007;57:397–400.
42. Karni A, Abraham M, Monosonego A, Guifang C, Freeman GJ, Hafler D, et al. Innate immunity in multiple sclerosis: myeloid dendritic cells in secondary progressive multiple sclerosis are activated and drive a proinflammatory immune response. J Immunol. 2006;177:4196–202.
43. Desvignes L, Ernst JD. Interferon-γ-responsive nonhematopoietic cells regulate the immune response to mycobacterium tuberculosis. Immunity. 2009;31:974–85.
44. Aggarwal BB, Kunnumakkara AB, Harikumar KB, Gupta SR, Tharakan ST, Koca C, et al. Signal transducer and activator of transcription-3, inflammation, and cancer: how intimate is the relationship? Ann N Y Acad Sci. 2009;1171:59–76.
45. Cavaletti G. Current status and future prospective of immunointervention in multiple sclerosis. Curr Med Chem. 2006;13:2329–43.
46. Rothe G, Gabriel H, Kovacs E, et al. Peripheral blood mononuclear phagocyte subpopulations as cellular markers in hypercholesterolemia. Arterioscler Thromb Vasc Biol. 1996;16(12):1437–47.
47. Hotamisisligil GS. Inflammation and metabolic disorders. Nature. 2006;444:860–7.
48. Heinz C, Fanihagh F, Steuhl KP. Squamous cell carcinoma of the conjunctiva in patients with atopic eczema. Cornea. 2003;22:135–7.
49. Hoglund P, Klein E. Natural killer cells in cancer. Semin Cancer Biol. 2006;16:331–2.
50. Khatami M. Induction of conjunctival-associated lymphoid hyperplasia by antigen and tumor promoting agents: targeting mediators of inflammatory responses as biomarkers for early detection of tumor/cancer. Special Conference Proceedings: The Biology and Genetics of Early Detection and Chemoprevention of Cancer, Am Assoc Cancer Research, Bal Harbour, FL, USA, 6–10 October 1999.
51. Dvorak HF. Tumors: wounds that do not heal. Similarities between tumor stroma generation and wound healing. N Engl J Med. 1986;315:1650–9.
52. Weitzman SA, Gordon LI. Inflammation and cancer: role of phagocytic-generated oxidants in carcinogenesis. Blood. 1990;76(4):655–63.
53. Vesterinen E, Oukkala E, Timonen T, Aromaa A. Cancer incident among 78000 asmatic patients. Int J Epidemiol. 1993;22:976–82.
54. Huovinen E, Kapiro J, Vesterinen E, Koshenvuo M. Mortality of adults with asthma: a prospective cohort study. Thorax. 1997;52:49–54.
55. Khatami M. Unresolved inflammation and cancer: loss of natural immune surveillance as the correct "target" for therapy! Seeing the "elephant" in the light of logic. Cell Biochem Biophys. 2012;62:501–9.
56. Folkman J, Watson K, Ingber D, Hanahan D. Induction of angiogenesis during the transition from hyperplasia to neoplasia. Nature. 1989;339:58–61.
57. Hanahan D, Folkman J. Patterns and emerging mechanisms of the angiogenic switch during tumorgenesis. Cell. 1996;86:353–64.
58. Montovani A, Ming WJ, Balotta C, Abdeljalil B, Bottazzi B. Origin and regulation of tumor-associated macrophages: the role of tumor-derived chemotactic factor. Biochim Biophys Acta. 1986;865:59–67.
59. Vartanian RK, Weidner N. Correlation of intratumoral endothelial cell proliferation with microvessel density (tumor angiogenesis) and tumor cell proliferation in breast carcinoma. Am J Pathol. 1994;144:1188–94.
60. Hildenbrand R, Wolf G, Böhme B, Bleyl U, Steinborn A. Urokinase plasminogen activator receptor (CD87) expression of tumor-associated macrophages in ductal carcinoma in situ, breast cancer, and resident macrophages of normal breast tissue. J Leukoc Biol. 1999;66:40–9.
61. Luboshits G, Shina S, Kaplan O, et al. Elevated expression of the CC chemokine regulated on activation, normal T cell expressed and secreted (RANTES) in advanced breast carcinoma. Cancer Res. 1999;59:4681–7.

62. Al-Sarireh B, Eremin O. Tumour-associated macrophages (TAMs): disordered function, immune suppression and progressive tumour growth. J R Coll Surg Edinb. 2000;45:1–16.
63. Khatami M (2016) In: Cancer research and therapy: scam of century–promote immunity [Yin-Yang]. ISBN-10:153043100X; ISBN-13: 978–1530431007; Amazon-Createspace. p 1–166.https://www.createspace.com/6123573
64. Khatami M. Safety concerns and hidden agenda behind HPV vaccines: another generation of drug-dependent society? Clin Transl Med. 2016;5(1):46. Epub 2016 Dec 5
65. Khatami M. Book review on cancer research and therapy: Safety concerns for HPV vaccination of young generation, paid by Obamacare and V.P. Biden Moonshot initiative. Global Vaccines and Immunol, 2016. ISSN: 2397-575X https://oatext.com/pdf/GVI-1-118.pdf
66. Khatami M. Yin and Yang in inflammation: duality in innate immune cell function and tumorigenesis. Exp Opin Biol Ther. 2008;8:1461–72.
67. Khatami M. Inflammation, aging and cancer: Tumoricidal vs tumorigenesis of immunity: a common denominator mapping chronic diseases. Cell Biochem Biophys. 2009;55:55–79.
68. Khatami M. Unresolved inflammation: 'immune tsunami' or erosion of integrity in immune-privileged and immune-responsive tissues and acute and chronic inflammatory diseases or cancer. Exp Opin Biol Ther. 2011;11:1419–32.
69. Amiri-Kordestani L, Fojo T. Why do phase III clinical trials in oncology fail so often? J Natl Cancer Inst. 2012;104:568–9.
70. Zou W. Immunosuppressive networks in the tumour environment and their therapeutic relevance. Nat Rev Cancer. 2005;5:263–74.
71. Farrow B, Sugiyama Y, Chen A, Uffort E, Nealon W, Evers BM. Inflammatory mechanisms contributing to pancreatic cancer development. Ann Surg. 2004;239:763–71.
72. Kondo K, Muramatsu M, Okamoto Y, Jin D, Takai S, Tanigawa N, et al. Expression of chymase-positive cells in gastric cancer and its correlation with the angiogenesis. J Surg Oncol. 2006;93:36–43.
73. DiCarlo E, Forni G, Lollini PL, Colombo MP, Modesti A, Musiani P. The intriguing role of polymorphonuclear neutrophils in antitumor reactions. Blood. 2001;97:339–45.
74. Lamagna C, Aurrand-Lions M, Imhof BA. Dual role of macrophages in tumor growth and angiogenesis. J Leukoc Biol. 2006;80(4):705–13.
75. Lin EY, Nguyen AV, Russell RG, Pollard JW. Colony-stimulating factor 1 promotes progression of mammary tumors to malignancy. J Exp Med. 2001;193:727–39.
76. Ingman WV, Wyckoff J, Gouon-Evans V, Condeelis J, Pollard JW. Macrophages promote collagen fibrillogenesis around terminal end buds of the developing mammary gland. Dev Dyn. 2006;235:3222–9.
77. Yu H, Pardoll D, Jove R. STATs in cancer inflammation and immunity: a leading role for STAT3. Nat Rev Cancer. 2009;9:798–809.
78. Gounaris E, Blatner NR, Dennis K, Mahnusso F, et al. T-regulatory cells shift from a protective anti-inflammatory to a cancer-promoting proinflammatory phenotype in polyposis. Cancer Res. 2009;69:5490–7.
79. Stoecker MM, Wang E. Histiocytic/dendritic cell transformation of B-cell neoplasms: pathologic evidence of lineage conversion in differentiated hematolymphoid malignancies. Arch Pathol Lab Med. 2013;137:865–70.
80. Ballaz S, Mulshine JL. The potential contributions of chronic inflammation to lung carcinogenesis. Clin Lung Cancer. 2003;5:46–62.
81. Khatami M. Cyclooxygenase inhibitor Ketorolac or mast cell stabilizers: immunological challenges in cancer therapy. Letters to the editor. Clin Cancer Res. 2005;11:1350–2.
82. Khatami M. Developmental phases of inflammation-induced massive lymphoid hyperplasia and extensive changes in epithelium in an experimental model of allergy. Implications for a direct link between inflammation and tumorigenesis. Am J Ther. 2005;12:117–26.
83. Rodriguez PC, Ernstoff MS, Hernandez C, Atkins M, Zabaleta J, Sierra R, Ochoa AC. Arginase I-producing myeloid-derived suppressor cells in renal cell carcinoma are a subpopulation of activated granulocytes. Cancer Res. 2009;69:1553–60.

84. Fridlender ZG, Sun J, Kim S, Kapoor V, Cheng G, Ling L, Worthen GS, Albelda SM. Polarization of tumor-associated neutrophil phenotype by TGF-β: "N1" versus "N2" TAN. Cancer Cell. 2009;16:183–94.
85. Ding T, Xu J, Wang F, et al. High tumor-infiltrating macrophage density predicts poor prognosis in patients with primary hepatocellular carcinoma after resection. Hum Pathol. 2009;40(3):381–9.
86. Ilkovitch D, Lopez DM. The liver is a site for tumor-induced myeloid-derived suppressor cell accumulation and immunosuppression. Cancer Res. 2009;69:5514–21.
87. Tataroğlu C, Kargi A, Ozkal S, Eşrefoğlu N, Akkoçlu A. Association of macrophages, mast cells and eosinophil leukocytes with angiogenesis and tumor stage in non-small cell lung carcinomas (NSCLC). Lung Cancer. 2004;43(1):47–54.
88. Wang R, Ma Z, Wang Y, Cheng Z, Xu H, Li W, et al. The interaction of coagulation factor XII and monocyte/macrophages mediating peritoneal metastasis of epithelial ovarian cancer. Gynecol Oncol. 2010;117:460–6.
89. Tomita M, Matsuzaki Y, Edagawa M, Shimizu T, Hara M, Onitsuka T. Distribution of mast cells in mediastinal lymph nodes from lung cancer patients. World J Surg Oncol. 2003;1:25.
90. Ardies CM. Inflammation as cause for scar cancers of the lung. Integr Cancer Ther. 2003;2:238–46.
91. Muller AJ, DuHadaway JB, Donover PS, Sutanto-Ward E, Prendergast GC. Inhibition of indoleamine 2,3-dioxygenase, an immunoregulatory target of the cancer suppression gene Bin1, potentiates cancer chemotherapy. Nat Med. 2005;11:312–9.
92. Hakim FT, Flomerfelt FA, Boyiadzis M, Gress RE. Aging, immunity and cancer. Curr Opin Immunol. 2004;18:151–8.
93. Itzkowitz SH, Yio X. Inflammation and cancer IV. Colorectal cancer in inflammatory bowel disease: the role of inflammation. Am J Physiol Gastrointest Liver Physiol. 2004;287:G7–17.
94. Teranishi A, Akada S, Saito S, Hatake K, Morikawa H. Macrophage colony-stimulating factor restored chemotherapy-induced granulocyte dysfunctions: role of Il-8 production by monocytes. Int Immunopharmacol. 2002;2:83–94.
95. Fisher-Wilson J. Angiogenesis therapy moves beyond cancer. Ann Intern Med. 2004;141:165–8.
96. Kido S, Kitadai Y, Hattori N, et al. Interleukin 8 and vascular endothelial growth factor—prognostic factors in human gastric carcinomas? Eur J Cancer. 2001;37(12):1482–7.
97. Gasser S, Raulet D. The DNA damage response, immunity and cancer. Semin Cancer Biol. 2006;16:344–7.
98. Ohno S, Inagawa H, Dhar DK, et al. The degree of macrophage infiltration into the cancer cell nest is a significant predictor of survival in gastric cancer patients. Anticancer Res. 2003;23(6):5015–22.
99. Leek RD, Lewis CE, Whitehouse R, Greenall M, Clarke J, Harris AL. Association of macrophage infiltration with angiogenesis and prognosis in invasive breast carcinoma. Cancer Res. 1996;56(20):4625–9.
100. Pestell RG, Li Z. Antisense to cyclin D1 inhibits VEGF-stimulated growth of vascular endothelial cells: implication of tumor vascularization. Clin Cancer Res. 2006;12:4459–62.
101. Mumberg D, Wick M, Schreiber H. Unique tumor antigens redefined as mutant tumor-specific antigens. Semin Immunol. 1998;8:289–93.
102. Nishikawa H, Kato T, Tawara I, Ikeda H, Kuribayashi K, Allen PM, et al. IFN-gamma controls the generation/activation of CD+CD25+ regulatory T cells in antitumor immune response. J Immunol. 2005;175:4433–40.
103. Schramm H. Comparison of the impact of pro-and anti-inflammatory immune processes at the two immune-deviated sites, eye and solid tumor and possible consequences for the antitumoral therapy with fever inducers. Forsch Komplementarmed Klass Naturheilkd. 2005;12:37–46.
104. Nash MA, Ferrandina G, Gordinier M, Loercher A, Freedman RS. The role of cytokines in both the normal and malignant ovary. Endocr Relat Cancer. 1999;6:93–107.

105. Barbul A, Lazarou SA, Efron G. Arginine enhances wound healing and lymphocyte immune responses in humans. Surgery. 1990;108:331.
106. Ledford H. Translational research: 4 ways to fix the clinical trial. Nature. 2011;477:526–8.
107. Amiri-Kordestani L, Basseville A, Kurziel K, Fojo AT, Bates SE. Targeting MDR in breast and lung cancer: discriminating its potential importance from the failure of drug resistance reversal studies. Drug Resist Updat. 2012;15:50–61.
108. U.S. FDA. Silver Spring (MD) U.S. FDA. Proposal to withdraw approval for the breast cancer indication for bevacizumab (avastin). FDA Public Hearing. June 29, 2011. http://www.fda.gov/downloads/NewsEvents/MeetingsConferencesWorkshops/UCM261697.pdf
109. Khatami M. Is cancer a severe delayed hypersensivitity reaction and histamine a blueprint? Clin Transl Med. 2016;5:35. doi:10.1186/s40169-016-0108-3.
110. Kroemer G, Galluzzi L, Vandenabeele P, Abrams J, Alnemri ES, Baehrecke EH, et al. Classification of cell death: recommendations of the nomenclature committee on cell death. Cell Death Differ. 2009;16:3–11.
111. Lockshin RA, Williams CM. Programmed cell death II. Endocrine potentiation of the breakdown of the intersegmental muscles of silkmoths. J Insect Physiol. 1964;10:643–9.
112. Schweichel JU, Merker HJ. The morphology of various types of cell death in prenatal tissues. Teratology. 1973;7:253–66.
113. Galluzzi L, Maiuri MC, Vitale I, Zischka H, Castedo M, Zitvogel L, et al. Cell death modalities: classification and pathophysiological implications. Cell Death Differ. 2007;14:1237–43.
114. Grando SA, Bystryn JC, Chernyavsky AI, Frusic-Zlotkin M, Gniadecki R, Lotti R, et al. Apoptolysis: a novel mechanism of skin blistering in pemphigus vulgaris linking the apoptotic pathways to basal cell shrinkage and suprabasal acantholysis. Exp Dermatol. 2009;18:764–70.
115. Kinnally KW, Peixoto PM, Ryu SY, Dejean LM. Is mPTP the gatekeeper for necrosis, apoptosis, or both? Biochim Biophys Acta. 2011;1813:616–22.
116. Rasola A, Bernardi P. Mitochondrial permeability transition in ca(2+)-dependent apoptosis and necrosis. Cell Calcium. 2011;50:222–33.
117. Frisch SM, Francis H. Disruption of epithelial cell–matrix interactions induces apoptosis. J Cell Biol. 1994;124:619–26.
118. Erwig LP, Henson PM. Immunological consequences of apoptotic cell phagocytosis. Am J Pathol. 2007;171:2–8.
119. Hirie RA, Reczek E, Horner JS, Khachatrian L, Sage J, Jacks T, et al. Perp is a mediator of p53-dependent apoptosis in diverse cell types. Curr Biol. 2003;13:1985–90.
120. Hundley TR, Giffillan AM, Tkaczyk C, Andrade MV, Metcalf DD, Beaven MA. Kit and FCeR1 mediate unique and convergent signals for release of inflammatory mediators from human mast cells. Blood. 2004;104:2410–7.
121. Hauswirth AW, Florian S, Schernthaner GH, Krauth MT, Sonneck K, Sperr WR, et al. Expression of cell surface antigens on mast cells: mast cell phenotyping. Methods Mol Biol. 2006;315:77–90.
122. Valent P, Schernthaner GH, Sperr WR, Fritsch G, Agis H, Willheim M, et al. Variable expression of activation-linked surface antigens on human mast cells in health and disease. Immunol Rev. 2001;179:74–81.
123. Ishizuka T, Chayama K, Takeda K, Hamelmann E, Terada N, Keller GM, et al. Mitogen-activated protein kinase activation through fc epsilon receptor 1 and stem cell factor receptor is differentially regulated by phosphatidyinositol 3-kinase and calcineurin in mouse bone marrow-derived mast cells. J Immunol. 1999;15:2087–94.
124. Ishizuka T, Kawasome H, Terada N, Takeda K, Gerwins P, Keller GM, et al. Stem cell factor augments Fc epsilon RI-mediated TNF-alpha production and stimulates MAP kinases via a different pathway in MC/9 mast cells. J Immunol. 1998;161:3624–30.
125. Thompson PA, Khatami M, Baglole CJ, Sun J, Harris SA, Moon EY, et al. Environmental immune disruptors, inflammation and cancer risk. Carcinogenesis. 2015;36(Suppl 1):S232–53. doi:10.1093/carcin/bgv038.

126. Freeman JD, Warren RL, Webb JR, Nelson BH, Holt RA. Profiling the T-cell receptor β-chain repertoire by massively parallel sequencing. Genome Res. 2009;19:1817–24.
127. Hermansson A, et al. Inhibition of T cell response to native low-density lipoprotein reduces atherosclerosis. J Exp Med. 2010;207:1081–93.
128. Kobayashi M, Fitz L, Ryan M, Hewick RM, Clark SC, Chan S, et al. Identification and purification of natural killer cell stimulatory factor (NKSF), a cytokine with multiple biologic effects on human lymphocytes. J Exp Med. 1989;170:827–45.
129. Bawa AS, Anilakumar KR. Genetically modified foods: safety, risks and public concerns-a review. J Food Sci Technol. 2013;50:1035–46. Epub 2012 Dec 19
130. Poulsen LK. Allergy assessment of foods or ingredients derived from biotechnology, gene-modified organisms, or novel foods. Mol Nutr Food Res. 2004;48(6):413–23.
131. Pedersen MH, Hansen TK, Sten E, Seguro K, Ohtsuka T, Morita A, et al. Evaluation of the potential allergenicity of the enzyme microbial transglutaminase using the 2001 FAO/WHO decision tree. Mol Nutr Food Res. 2004;48:434–40.
132. Spök A, Gaugitsch H, Laffer S, Pauli G, Saito H, Sampson H, et al. Suggestions for the assessment of the allergenic potential of genetically modified organisms. Int Arch Allergy Immunol. 2005;137(2):167–80.
133. Metcalfe DD. Introduction: what are the issues in addressing the allergenic potential of genetically modified foods? Environ Health Perspect. 2003;111:1110–3.
134. Scheideler SE, Rice D, Smith B, et al. Evaluation of nutritional equivalency of corn grain from DAS-Ø15Ø7–1 (Herculex I) in the diets of laying hens. J Appl Poult Res. 2008;17:383–9.
135. Kruger TE, Smith LR, Harbour DV, Blalock JE. Thyrotropin: an endogenous regulator of the in vitro immune response. J Immunol. 1989;142:744.
136. Coutelier J-P, Kehrl JH, Bellur SS, Kohn LD, Notkins AL, Prabhakar BS. Binding and functional effects of thyroid stimulating hormone on human immune cells. J Clin Immunol. 1990;10:204.
137. Valent P, Bettelheim P. Cell surface structures on human basophils and mast cells: biochemical and functional characterization. Adv Immunol. 1992;52:333–423.
138. Lee YS, Kang YS, Lee JS, Nicolova S, Kim JA. Involvement of NADPH oxidase-mediated generation of reactive oxygen species in the apoptotic cell death by capsaicin in Hep G2 human hepatoma cells. Free Radic Res. 2004;38:405–12.
139. Shahabuddin S, Ponath P, Schleimer RP. Migration of eosinophils across endothelial cell monolayers: interactions among IL-5, endothelial-activating cytokines, and C-C chemokines. J Immunol. 2000;164:3847–54.
140. Carow B, Rottenberg ME. Suppressor of cytokine signalling: molecules in infection and inflammation. In: Khatami M, editor. Inflammation, chronic diseases and cancer. cell and molecular biology, immunology and clinical bases. Rijeka: In Tech Publishing; 2012. p. 279–306.
141. Khatami M. Standardizing cancer biomarkers criteria: data elements as a foundation for a database. Inflammatory mediator/M-CSF as model marker, Cell Biochem Biophy. 2007; 47:187–198.
142. Monteseirin J, Chacon P, Vega A, El Bekay R, Alvarez M, Alba G, et al. Human neutrophils synthesize IL-8 in an IgE-mediated activation. J Leukoc Biol. 2004;76:692–700.
143. Bernstein C, Bernstein H, Payne CM, Garewal H. DNA repair/pro-apoptotic dual-role proteins in five major DNA repair pathways: fail-safe protection against carcinogenesis. Mutat Res. 2002;511(2):145–78.
144. Theoharides TC, Alysandratos KD, Angelidou A, Delivanis DA, Sismanopoulos N, Zhang B, et al. Mast cells and inflammation. Biochim Biophys Acta. 1822;2012:21–33.
145. Theoharides TC. Mast cell: a neuroimmunoendocrine master player. Int J Tissue React. 1996;18:1–21.
146. Geissmann F, Gordon S, Hume DA, Mowat AM, Randolph GJ. Unravelling mononuclear phagocyte heterogeneity. Nat Rev Immunol. 2010;10:453–60.
147. Mebius RE. Organogenesis of lymphoid tissues. Nat Rev Immunol. 2003;3:292–303.

148. Kabelitz D, Medzhitov R. Innate immunity-cross-talk with adaptive immunity through pattern recognition receptors and cytokines. Curr Opin Immunol. 2006;19:1–3.
149. Oliver G. Lymphatic vasculature development. Nat Rev Immunol. 2004;4:35–45.
150. Klebanoff SJ, Vadas MA, Harlan JM, Sparks LH, Gamble JR, Agosti JM, et al. Stimulation of neutrophils by tumor necrosis factor. J Immunol. 1986;136:4220–5.
151. Dolan S, Field LC, Nolan AM. The role of nitric oxide and prostaglandin signaling pathways in spinal nociceptive processing in chronic inflammation. Pain. 2000;86:311–20.
152. Naik SH, Sathe P, Park HY, Metcalf D, Proietto AI, Dakic A, et al. Development of plasmacytoid and conventional dendritic cell subtypes from single precursor cells derived *in vitro* and *in vivo*. Nat Immunol. 2007;8:1217–26.
153. Schumacher TN, Gerlach C, van Heijst JW. Mapping the life histories of T cells. Nat Rev Immunol. 2010;10:621–31.
154. Dong C. Genetic controls of Th17 cell differentiation and plasticity. Exp Mol Med. 2011;43:1–6.
155. Pober JS. Interleukin-17 and atherosclerotic vascular disease. Arterioscler Thromb Vasc Biol. 2011;31:1465–6.
156. Trinchieri G. Interleukin-12 and the regulation of innate resistance and adaptive immunity. Nat Rev Immunol. 2003;3:133–46.
157. Venturi V, Price DA, Douek DC, Davenport MP. The molecular basis for public T-cell responses? Nat Rev Immunol. 2008;8:231–8.
158. Fukao T, Matsuda S, Koyasu S. Synergistic effects of IL-4 and IL-18 on IL-12- dependent IFN-γ production by dendritic cells. J Immunol. 2000;164:64–71.
159. Tam SY, Tsai M, Yamaguchi M, Yano K, Butterfield JH, Galli SJ. Expression of functional TrkA receptor tyrosine kinase in the HMC-1 human mast cell line and in human mast cells. Blood. 1997;90:1807–20.
160. Putnam CD, Arvai AS, Bourne Y. Active and inhibited human catalase structures: ligand and NADPH binding and catalytic mechanism. J Mol Biol. 2000;296:295–309.
161. Sander LE, Sackett SD, Dierssen U, Beraza N, Linke RP, Müller M, et al. Hepatic acute-phase proteins control innate immune responses during infection by promoting myeloid-derived suppressor cell function. J Exp Med. 2010;207:1453–64.
162. Delgado M, Munoz-Elias EJ, Kan Y, Gozes I, Fridkin M, Brenneman DE, et al. Vasoactive intestinal peptide and pituitary adenylate cyclase-activating polypeptide inhibit tumor necrosis factor α transcriptional activation by regulating nuclear factor-κB and cAMP response element-binding protein/c-Jun. J Biol Chem. 1998;273(47):31427–36.
163. Provinciali M, Di Stefano G, Fabris N. Improvement in the proliferative capacity and natural killer cell activity of murine spleen lymphocytes by thyrotropin. Int J Immunopharmacol. 1992;14:865–70.
164. Klein JR. Hormone regulation of immune homeostasis: local or long distance? Biochem Pharmacol. 1998;56:1–5.
165. Sansonetti PJ. War and peace at mucosal surfaces. Nat Rev Immunol. 2004;4:953–64.
166. Wilson NS, Villadangos JA. Lymphoid organ dendritic cells: beyond the Langerhans cells paradigm. Immunol Cell Biolo. 2004;82:91–8.
167. de St F, Groth B. The evolution of self-tolerance: a new cell arises to meet the challenge of self-reactivity. Immunol Today. 1998;19:448–54.
168. Friedberg EC. DNA damage and repair. Nature. 2003;421(6921):436–40.
169. Gordon S, Taylor PR. Monocyte and macrophage heterogeneity. Nat Rev Immunol. 2005;5:953–64.
170. Robinson SC, Scott KA, Balkwill FR. Chemokine stimulation of monocyte matrix metalloproteinase-9 requires endogenous TNF-alpha. Eur J Immunol. 2002;32:404–12.
171. Locati M, Deuschle U, Massardi ML, et al. Analysis of the gene expression profile activated by the CC chemokine ligand 5/RANTES and by lipopolysaccharide in human monocytes. J Immunol. 2002;168(7):3557–62.

172. Ivanov II, et al. Induction of intestinal Th17 cells by segmented filamentous bacteria. Cell. 2009;139:485–98.
173. Gool CJ, Thijs C, Dagnelie PC, Henquet CJ, Van Houwelingen AC, Schrander J, et al. Determinants of neonatal IgE level: parity, maternal age, birth season and perinatal essential fatty acid status in infants of atopic mothers. Allergy. 2004;59(9):961–8.
174. De Wilde V, Van Rompaey N, Hill M, Lebrun JF, Lemaitre P, Lhomme F, et al. Endotoxin-induced myeloid-derived suppressor cells inhibit alloimmune responses via heme oxygenase-1. Am J Transplant. 2009;9:2034–47.
175. Kaiser F, Cook D, Papoutsopoulou S, Rajsbaum R, Wu X, Yang HT, et al. TPL-2 negatively regulates interferon-β production in macrophages and myeloid dendritic cells. J Exp Med. 2009;206:1863–71.
176. Goronzy JJ, Wevand CM. T cell development and receptor diversity during aging. Curr Opin Immunol. 2005;17:468–75.
177. Fabris N, Mocchegiani E, Mariotti S, Pacini F, Pinchera A. Thyroid-thymus interactions during development and aging. Horm Res. 1989;31:85–9.
178. Berthiaume F, Aparicio CL, Eungdamrong J, Yarmush ML. Age- and disease-related decline in immune function: an opportunity for "thymus-boosting" therapies. Tissue Eng. 1999;5(6):499–514.
179. Palsson-Mcdermott EM, O'Neill AJ. The Warburg effect then and now. From cancer to inflammatory diseases. Bioassays. 2013;35:965–73.
180. Wang J, Klein JR. Thymus-neuroendocrine interactions in extrathymic T cells development. Science. 1994;265:1860–962.
181. Wang J, Klein JR. Hormone regulation of extrathymic gut T cell development: involvement of thyroid stimulating hormone. Cell Immunol. 1995;161:299–302.
182. Wang J, Klein JR. Hormone regulation of murine T cells: potent tissue-specific immunosuppressive effects of thyroxine targeted to gut T *cells*. Int Immunol. 1996;8:231–5.
183. Wang J, Whetsell M, Klein JR. Local hormone networks and intestinal T cells homeostasis. Science. 1997;275:1937–9.
184. Croft M, Joseph SB, Miner KT. Partial activation of naive CD4 T cells and tolerance induction in response to peptide presented by resting B cells. J Immunol. 1997;159:3257–65.
185. Litvinenko GI, Shurlygina AV, Dergacheva TI, Mel'nikova EV, Trufakin VA. Chrono- and Immunocorrection of inflammatory disorders of internal reproductive organs in women of reproductive age. Bull Exp Biol Med. 2015;159(1):62–5. doi:10.1007/s10517-015-2890-0. Epub 2015 Jun 3
186. Pierpaoli W, Kopp HG, Muller J, Keller M. Interdependence between neuroendocrine programming and the generation of immune recognition in ontogeny. Cell Immunol. 1977;29:16–27.
187. Beisel WR, Rapoport MI. Inter-relations between adrenocortical functions and infectious illness. N Engl J Med. 1969;280:596–604.
188. Mellor AL, Munn DH. Physiologic control of the functional status of Foxp3^{+} regulatory T cells. J Immunol. 2011;186:4535–40.
189. Rollins DA, Coppo M, Rogatsky I. Nuclear Receptor Coregulators of the p160 family: Insights into Inflammation and Metabolism. Mol Endocrinol. 2015 Feb 3:me20151005. [Epub ahead of print].
190. Wang Y, Li M, Tang J, Song M, Xu X, Xiong J, et al. Glucocorticoids facilitate astrocytic amyloid-*β*peptide deposition by increased expression of APP and BACE1 and decreasing the expression of amyloid-*β*-degrading proteases. Endocrinology. 2011;152:2704–15. doi:10.1210/en.2011-0145.
191. Caratti G, Matthews L, Poolman T, Kershaw S, Baxter M, Ray D. Glucocorticoid receptor function in health and disease. Clin Endocrinol (Oxf). 2015 Jan 27. doi: 10.1111/cen.12728. [Epub ahead of print].
192. Grant RW, Dixit VD. Adipose tissue as an immunological organ. Obesity (Silver Spring). 2015 Jan 22. doi: 10.1002/oby.21003.. [Epub ahead of print].

193. Mauer J, Denson JL, Brüning JC. Versatile functions for IL-6 in metabolism and cancer. Trends Immunol. pii: S1471–4906(14)00233–6. doi: 10.1016/j.it.2014.12.008. [Epub ahead of print], 2015.
194. Mauer J, Chaurasia B, Goldau J, Vogt MC, Ruud J, Nguyen KD, et al. Signaling by IL-6 promotes alternative activation of macrophages to limit endotoxemia and obesity-associated resistance to insulin. Nat Immunol. 2014;15:423–30. doi:10.1038/ni.2865. Epub 2014.
195. Kiriakidis S, Andreakos E, Monaco C, Foxwell B, Feldmann M, Paleolog E. VEGF expression in human macrophages is NF-κB-dependent: studies using adenoviruses expressing the endogenous NF-κB inhibitor IκBα and a kinase-defective form of the IκB kinase 2. J Cell Sci. 2003;116:665–74.
196. Galli SJ. Biology of disease: new insights into 'the riddle of mast cells'; microenvironmental regulation of mast cell development and phenotypic heterogeneity. Lab Investig. 1990;62:5–33.
197. Stovkova A. Cachexia: the interplay between the immune system, brain control and metabolism. In: Khatami M, editor. Inflammatory diseases: immunopathology, clinical and pharmacological bases. Rijeka: In Tech Publishing; 2012. p. 27–56.
198. Nakanishi H. Involvement of microglial cathepsin B in pro-interleukin-1b processing and persistent pain. In: Khatami M, editor. Inflammation, chronic diseases and cancer: cell and molecular biology, immunology and clinical bases. Rijeka: In Tech Publishing; 2012. p. 265–72.
199. Fink SL, Cookson BT. Apoptosis, pyroptosis, and necrosis: mechanistic description of dead and dying eukaryotic cells. Infect Immun. 2005;73:1907–16.
200. Fink SL, Cookson BT. Pyroptosis and host cell death responses during salmonella infection. Cell Microbiol. 2007;9:2562–70.
201. Bergsbaken T, Fink SL, Cookson BT. Pyroptosis: host cell death and inflammation. Nat Rev Microbiol. 2009;7:99–109.
202. Yu SW, Andrabi SA, Wang H, Kim NS, Poirier GG, Dawson TM, et al. Apoptosis-inducing factor mediates poly(ADP-ribose) (PAR) polymer-induced cell death. Proc Natl Acad Sci U S A. 2006;103:18314–9.
203. Cho YS, Challa S, Moquin D, Genga R, Ray TD, Guildford M, et al. Phosphorylation-driven assembly of the RIP1–RIP3 complex regulates programmed necrosis and virus-induced inflammation. Cell. 2009;137:1112–23.
204. Akbar AN, Salmon M. Cellular environments and apoptosis: tissue microenvironments control activated T-cell death. Immunol Today. 1997;18:72–6.
205. Frisch SM, Screaton RA. Anoikis mechanisms. Curr Opin Cell Biol. 2001;13:555–62.
206. Tanida I, Ueno T, Kominami E. LC3 conjugation system in mammalian autophagy. Int J Biochem Cell Biol. 2004;36:2503–18.
207. Zhang K. Integration of ER stress, oxidative stress and the inflammatory response in health and disease. Int J Clin Exp Med. 2010;3:33–40.
208. Ohsumi Y. Historical landmarks of autophagy research. Cell Res. 2014;24:9–23. doi:10.1038/cr.2013.169.
209. Nakatogawa H, Suzuki K, Kamada Y, Ohsumi Y. Dynamics and diversity in autophagy mechanisms: lessons from yeast. Nat Rev Mol Cell Biol. 2009;10:458–67.
210. Rambold AS, Kostelecky B, Lippincott-Schwartz J. Together we are stronger: fusion protects mitochondria from autophagosomal degradation. Autophagy. 2011;7:1568–9.
211. Andrabi SA, Kim NS, Yu SW, Wang H, Koh DW, Sasaki M, et al. Poly(ADP-ribose) (PAR) polymer is a death signal. Proc Natl Acad Sci U S A. 2006;103:18308–13.
212. Albert ML. Death-defying immunity: do apoptotic cells influence antigen processing and presentation? Nat Rev Immunol. 2004;4:223–31.
213. Yang Z, Klionsky DJ. An overview of the molecular mechanism of autophagy. Curr Top Microbiol Immunol. 2009;335:1–32.
214. Itakura E, Mizushima N. Characterization of autophagosome formation site by a hierarchical analysis of mammalian Atg proteins. Autophagy. 2010;6:764–76.

215. Vergne I, Roberts E, Elmaoued RA, Tosch V, Delgado MA, Proikas-Cezanne T, et al. Control of autophagy initiation by phosphoinositide 3-phosphatase jumpy. EMBO J. 2009;28:2244–58.
216. Mailleux AA, Overholtzer M, Schmelzle T, Bouillet P, Strasser A, Brugge JS. BIM regulates apoptosis during mammary ductal morphogenesis, and its absence reveals alternative cell death mechanisms. Dev Cell. 2007;12:221–34.
217. Mabuchi S, Kuroda H, Takahashi R, Sasano T. The PI3K/AKT/mTOR pathway as a therapeutic target in ovarian cancer. Gynecol Oncol. 2015 Feb 10. pii: S0090-8258(15)00606-X.
218. Matarrese P, Ciarlo L, Tinari A, Piacentini M, Malorni W. Xeno-cannibalism as an exacerbation of self-cannibalism: a possible fruitful survival strategy for cancer cells. Curr Pharm Des. 2008;14:245–52.
219. Lamming DW. Diminished mTOR signaling: a common mode of action for endocrine longevity factors. Spring. 2014 Dec 15;3:735. doi: 10.1186/2193-1801-3-735. eCollection 2014.
220. Hodes RJ, Sierra F, Austad SN, Epel E, Neigh GN, Kristine M, Erlandson KM, et al. Disease drivers of aging Ann N Y Acad Sci. Author manuscript; available in PMC 2017 Mar 30. Published in final edited form as: Ann N Y Acad Sci. 2016;1386(1):45–68. doi: 10.1111/nyas.13299.
221. Bar-Peled L, Sabatini DM. Regulation of mTORC1 by amino acids. Trends Cell Biol. 2014;24:400–6.
222. Ginaldi L, De Martinis M, Monti D, Franceschi C. The immune system in the elderly: activation-induced and damage-induced apoptosis. Immunol Res. 2004;30:81–94.
223. Ginaldi L, De Martinis M, D'Ostilio A, Marini L, Loreto MF, Corsi MP, et al. Cell proliferation and apoptosis in the immune system in the elderly. Immunol Res. 2000;21(1):31–8.
224. Ginaldi L, De Martinis M, D'Ostilio A, Marini L, Quaglino D. Changes in antigen expression on B lymphocytes during HIV infection. Pathobiology. 1998;66:17–23.
225. Cargnello M, Tcherkezian J, Roux PP. The expanding role of mTOR in cancer cell growth and proliferation. Mutagenesis. 2015;30:169–76.
226. Gupta S. Molecular steps of cell suicide: an insight into immune senescence. J Clin Immunol. 2000;20:229–39.
227. De Martinis M, Franceschi C, Monti D, Ginaldi L. Apoptosis remodeling in immunosenescence: implications for strategies to delay ageing. Curr Med Chem. 2007;14(13):1389–97.
228. De Martinis M, Modesti M, Ginaldi L. Phenotypic and functional changes of circulating monocytes and polymorphonuclear leucocytes from elderly persons. Immunol Cell Biol. 2004;82:415–20.
229. Ciccarelli F, De Martinis M, Ginaldi L. An update on autoinflammatory diseases. Curr Med Chem. 2013;21:261–9.
230. Domey J, Bergemann C, Bremer-Streck S, Krumbein I, Reichenbach JR, Teichgräber U, Hilger I. Long-term prevalence of NIRF-labeled magnetic nanoparticles for the diagnostic and intraoperative imaging of inflammation. Nanotoxicology, Early Online: 1–12! Informa UK Ltd. doi: 10.3109/17435390.2014.1000413. 2015.
231. Bouchlaka MN, Sckisel GD, Chen M, et al. Aging predisposes to acute inflammatory induced pathology after tumor immunotherapy. J Exp Med. 2013;210:2223–37.
232. Fang KC, Raymond WW, Lazarus SC, et al. Dog mastcytoma cell secrete a 92-kDa gelatinase activated extracellularly by mast cell chymase. J Clin Invest. 1996;97:1589–96.
233. Romagnolo DF, Papoutsis AJ, Selmin O. Nutritional targeting of cyclooxygenase-2 for colon cancer prevention. Inflamm Allergy Drug Targets. 2010;9:181–91.
234. Rafi A, Castle SC, Uyemura K, Makinodan T. Immune dysfunction in the elderly and its reversal by antihistamines. Biomed Pharmacol. 2003;57:246–50.
235. Kuhn HG, Biebl M, Wilhelm D, Li M, Friedlander RM, Winkler J. Increased generation of granule cells in adult Bcl-2-overexpressing mice: a role for cell death during continued hippocampal neurogenesis. Eur J Neurosci. 2005;22(8):1907–15.
236. Lee HO, Herndon JM, Barreiro R, Ferguson TA. TRAIL: a mechanism of tumor surveillance in an immune privileged site. J Immunol. 2002;169:4739–47.
237. Naito M, Itoh M. Patterns of infiltration of lymphocytes into the testis under normal and pathological conditions in mice. Am J Reprod Immunol. 2008;59:55–61.

238. Valcourt U, Merle B, Gineyts E, Viguet-Carrin S, Delmas PD, Garnero P. Non-enzymatic glycation of bone collagen modifies osteoclastic activity and differentiation. J Biol Chem. 2007;282:5691–703.
239. Dunn EJ, Philippou H, Ariëns RA, Grant PJ. Molecular mechanisms involved in the resistance of fibrin to clot lysis by plasmin in subjects with type 2 diabetes mellitus. Diabetologia. 2006;49:1071–80.
240. Kennedy DM, Skillen AW, Self CH. Glycation of monoclonal antibodies impairs their ability to bind antigen. Clin Exp Immunol. 1994;98:245–51.
241. Niederkorn JY. See no evil, hear no evil, do no evil: the lessons of immune privilege. Nat Immunol. 2006;7:354–9.
242. Hamrah P, Huq SO, Liu Y, Zhang Q, Dana MR. Corneal immunity is mediated by heterogeneous population of antigen-presenting cells. J Leukoc Biol. 2003;74:172–8.
243. Streilein JW, Masli S, Takeuchi M, Kezuka T. The eye's view of antigen presentation. Hum Immunol. 2002;63:435–43.
244. Fischer HG, Reichmann G. Brain dendritic cells and macrophages/microglia in central nervous system inflammation. J Immunol. 2001;166:2717–26.
245. Hart AB, Samuels DC, Hulgan T. The other genome: a systematic review of studies of mitochondrial DNA haplogroups and outcomes of HIV infection and antiretroviral therapy. AIDS Rev. 2013;15:213–20.
246. Ng Kee Kwong F, Nicholson AG, Harrison CL, Hansbro PM, Adcock IM, Chung KF. Is mitochondrial dysfunction a driving mechanism linking COPD to nonsmall cell lung carcinoma? Eur Respir Rev. 2017 Oct 25;26(146). pii: 170040. doi: 10.1183/16000617.0040-2017. Print 2017 Dec 31.
247. Ochs HD, Hagin D. Primary immunodeficiency disorders: general classification, new molecular insights, and practical approach to diagnosis and treatment. Ann Allergy Asthma Immunol. 2014;112:489–95.
248. Ridker PM, Danielson E, Fonesca FA, Genest J, Gotto AM Jr, Kastelein JJ, et al. Rosuvastatin to prevent vascular events in men and women with elevated C-reactive protein. N Engl J Med. 2008;359:2195–207.
249. Liadaki K, Sun J, Hammarström L, Pan-Hammarström Q. New facets of antibody deficiencies. Curr Opin Immunol. 2013;25:629–38.
250. Dardenne M, Savino W, Bach J-F. Modulation of thymic endocrine function by thyroid and steroid hormones. Int J Neurosci. 1988;39:325–34.
251. Xu X. ALK-negative anaplastic large cell lymphoma primarily involving the bronchus: a case report and literature. Int J Clin Exp Pathol. 2014;7:460–3.
252. Bork P, Holm L, Sander C. The immunoglobulin fold. Structural classification, sequence patterns and common core. J Mol Biol. 1994;242:309–20.
253. Slack EC, Robinson MJ, Hernanz-Falcon P, Brown GD, Williams DL, Schweighoffer E, et al. Syk-dependent ERK activation regulates IL-2 and IL-10 production by DC stimulated with zymosan. Eur J Immunol. 2007;37:1600–12.
254. Saraiva M, Christensen JR, Veldhoen M, Murphy TL, Murphy KM, O'Garra A. Interleukin-10 production by Th1 cells requires interleukin-12-induced STAT4 transcription factor and ERK MAP kinase activation by high antigen dose. Immunity. 2009;31:209–19.
255. Redford PS, Murray PJ, O'Garra A. The role of IL-10 in immune regulation during *M. tuberculosis* infection. Mucosal Immunol. 2011;4:261–70.
256. Esser-von Bieren J. Immune-regulation and -functions of eicosanoid lipid mediators. Biol Chem. 2017;398(11):1177–91. https://doi.org/10.1515/hsz-2017-0146.

Chapter 3
Theories of Aging and Chronic Diseases: Chronic Inflammation an Interdependent 'Roadmap' to Age-Associated Illnesses

We have confused illness with the process of aging, which can be thoroughly healthy. Illness is not a necessary part of aging!

Dr. Charles Eugster, 94-year-old World Master Rowing Champion.

Abstract

Cancer is a symptom of violations of controlled biological circadian rhythms.

Living long is a biological process characterized by progressive alterations in tissue/organ function, often associated with increased risk of chronic diseases. Among major theories of aging are retardation of immune response dynamics, increased free radicals (oxido-redox imbalance) and increased genetic mutations. These age-associated biological changes cause minor or major readjustments of organs systems known as biological senescent and immunosenescent. In this chapter, the focus will be to discuss that these changes are interdependent processes and persistent or unresolved inflammation (oxidative stress) is a common denominator in increasing the risk of nearly all age-associated chronic illnesses and site-specific cancers. Attempts were made to demonstrate the interrelationships between unresolved inflammation and the induction of immune response shifts in immune-responsive and immune-privileged tissues in initiation and progression of major chronic illnesses. Evaluation of scattered data on aging process suggests that in general, longevity is a biologically intrinsic process characterized by steady and progressive declines in the integrity and function of organs/tissues. However, the rate of susceptibility and severity to illnesses vary among individuals due to complex combination of interactions and heterogeneities between intrinsic and extrinsic factors that would determine the biology of aging. Strategies for reducing oxidative stress or correcting the balance between Yin and Yang response profiles of acute inflammation may prove to be important targets for delaying or preventing the onset of disabling illnesses and reducing the cost of sick-care.

M. Khatami, *Inflammation, Aging and Cancer*,
https://doi.org/10.1007/978-3-319-66475-0_3

Keywords Aging theories • American health status • Alopecia • Antioxidants • Antigenic-load • Aspirin • Atrophy • Biological clocks • Bioenergetics • Biological wear and tear • Caloric restriction • C-elegans • DCs maturation • Genomic theory • Redox imbalance theory • Hematopoietic cells • Hormones • Hypoxia • Immune competency • Immunosenescence theory • Immune compromised • Inflammatory mediators • 'Leaky' MCs • Mitochondrial theory • Polarization • Reactive oxygen species • Respiration • Stem cell attrition • Super oxide dismutases • T cell immunity • Thymus involution • Amifostine • Mercaptoethanol • N-acethylcysteine • Captopril • Werner syndrome • Cokayne syndrome • Trichothiodystrophy • Dyskeratosis congenital • Ataxia-telangiectasia • Skewed cytotoxicity • Yin-Yang

1 Introduction

Aging seems to be the only way to live longer!

Fascination with studying the biology of aging process has intensified only in the mid-twentieth century, as the growth of population of older adults is rapidly rising around the world and the economic cost of healthcare for elderly with chronic illnesses is becoming a significant national burden. With advanced aging, the likelihood of development of one or more significant medical illnesses in the elderly increases. However, the increased rate of population among healthy older individuals around the globe suggests that the aging process is not necessarily associated with illnesses. Older people can lead a healthy, active and productive life well beyond the standard age of retirement of 65–70 years.

Several clinical reports demonstrate that the risks for older adults to develop community-acquired pneumonia (CAP) or hospital-acquired pneumonia (HAP) rise when various illnesses such as swallowing disorders, recurrent aspiration, cognitive impairment, malnutrition, alcoholism, obstructive lung disease, congestive heart failure, diabetes, renal disease or immunosuppressive therapy are also present [1–8]. Published guidelines by various health organizations have limitations for diagnosis and treatment of these aging health conditions. The issues are often complicated by patient's capacity to make decision when professionals require to observe practices on mental capacity of the patients, consent issues, criteria for safe discharge of patients from different health centers and related variables [8–17]. The principal clinical options recommended for management of patients that are exposed to specific pathogens (e.g., staphylococcus aureus, gram-positive cocci, bacteria) include steroid administration (e.g., glucocorticosteroid), antibiotic intervention, gas exchange and airway pressure control. Such clinical practices present limitations of frequencies, duration or combination therapies, to be effective for all older individuals in different settings [5, 9, 14–17]. Furthermore, prevention strategies including vaccination (e.g., flu, meningitis) or life style recommendations and management advice with alternative or complementary treatment procedures (e.g., saline nebulizer, granulocyte-colony stimulating factor, fluid intake, physiotherapy, nutrition) or palliative care often produce complications such as the follow-up after discharge from hospital for microbiological tests in patients with moderate or severe CAP [12–17].

Biologically, defects in in cellular immunity (T cell) and cytokine production (e.g., IFN-γ) are considered risk factors for the increased morbidity in older adults (mean age 75 years) that are exposed to infective viruses such as respiratory syncytial virus (RSV), when compared with younger (mean age 31 years) adults [16, 17]. It should also be noted that even the older individuals who have no evidence of any clinical diseases may be at greater risk for developing pneumonia due to skewed immune dynamics and alterations of microbial clearance associated with advancing in age [1–6, 12–18].

As noted in Chap. 1, according to a 2014 report by Mirror, Mirror [18], comparing health status and performance of general population of Americans with 11 other developed nations (Australia, Canada, France, Germany, Netherlands, New Zealand, Norway, Sweden, Switzerland, the United Kingdom), ***"The United States health care system is the most expensive in the world"***, but consistently shows that U.S.A ranks last and underperforms [18]. The reported health performance dimensions that USA consistently rated last included:

(a) **Health Quality:** The indicators were effective care, safe care, coordinated care, and patient-centered care. "While there has been some improvement in recent years, lower scores on safe and coordinated care pull the overall U.S. quality score down".
(b) **Health Access:** Due to the absence of universal coverage, while patients 'in the U.S. have rapid access to specialized health care services, … they are less likely to report rapid access to primary care than people in leading countries in the study.
(c) **Health Efficiency:** On health performance, USA measures last on expenditures and administrative costs, as well as on administrative hassles and avoidable emergency room use and duplicative medical testing compared with other developed nations.
(d) **Health Equity:** "Americans with below-average incomes were much more likely than their counterparts in other countries to report not visiting a physician when sick; not getting a recommended test, treatment, or follow-up care; or not filling a prescription or skipping doses when needed because of costs."
(e) **Healthy Living:** The Americans rank last overall with poor scores on all three indicators of healthy living …"mortality amenable to medical care, infant mortality, and healthy life expectancy at age 60. The U.S. and U.K. had much higher death rates in 2007 from conditions amenable to medical care than some of the other countries…"

Economic burden to the society, particularly with regard to cost of cancer care and therapy is becoming unsustainable in USA and other developed countries such as Japan and England [18, 19]. As detailed in Chaps. 5 and 6, cancer therapy and cost of care for patients in USA is the reason for almost half of the home foreclosures, while, the outcomes of claimed cancer 'targeted' therapies, 'personalized' or 'precision' medicine produced 90% (±5) failure rates for solid tumors [19–22].

In this chapter, the author attempted to extend her recently published hypotheses that the different health conditions, which increase the reported risks of community-acquired pneumonia (CAP) in older adults or other age-associated health conditions have shared biological features; and that oxidative stress (unresolved, sub-clinical or chronic inflammation) is the hallmark of nearly all chronic diseases including site-specific cancers.

In this effort, outlined analyses of major interrelated biological features including important knowledge gaps in understanding the age-associated illnesses, as well as, problems in managing the care for the elderly are provided in the following [21–55]:

(a) Older adults are immune compromised to varying degrees;
(b) The differently known age-associated illnesses have oxidative stress as interdependent common links that are manifested in vulnerable-susceptible tissue/organ systems as distinct diseases;
(c) Oxidative stress or unresolved (sub-clinical, chronic) inflammation differentially influences the tissue-specific features (e.g., immune-responsive and immune-privileged tissues, insulin-dependent and insulin-independent tissues for glucose transport and metabolism) that lead to the induction and manifestation of different diseases;
(d) Special or shared biological features (complications) of full-blown disease that generally determine the outcomes of nearly all chronic diseases fall into three major interdependent categories, tissue necrosis, vascular complications and tissue growth;
(e) Effective immunity (immune surveillance) that is 'friend' for protecting the body against all harmful elements becomes 'foe' during aging and chronic inflammation (oxidative stress) and utilizes same molecular tools of inherent duality of immune and non-immune systems in favor of initiation and progression of chronic conditions in vulnerable tissues;
(f) The majority of age-associated chronic illnesses are very likely preventable or correctable, if the scientific understanding of the biology of aging was focused on the maintenance of effective immunity (balancing the inherent tumoricidal vs tumorigenic properties of immune surveillance), and caring for the elderly in hospital settings were significantly improved;

Detailed discussion of clinical or basic research on the individual chronic diseases is out of the scope of this book. Attempts were made to demonstrate that longevity and oxidative stress (unresolved, subclinical, persistent or chronic inflammation) are co-morbidity and co-mortality risk factors in the induction of nearly all age-associated chronic diseases such as neurodegenerative and autoimmune diseases, diabetes and cardiovascular complications, stroke, hypertension, Alzheimer's, Parkinson's, lupus, colitis, as well as, site-specific tissue growth, neoplasia, hyperplasia, cancer metastasis and angiogenesis.

2 Principals in Biology of Aging Process

Until a few decades ago and despite the development of numerous modern technologies for detection of hundreds and thousands of isolated molecular entities in the fields of OMICS (e.g., proteomics, genomics, lipidomics, metabolomics, glycomics), little serious scientific efforts were invested for systematic understanding of the aging process, the immunosenescence and the initiation of age-associated chronic diseases. Numerous risk factors have been identified that predispose the elderly to several chronic diseases such as neurodegenerative and autoimmune diseases, asthma/emphysema and lower respiratory tract infections, Alzheimer's, adult on-set diabetes and cardiovascular complications, Parkinson's, osteoporosis and many site-specific cancers [21–55]. However, the molecular or cellular bases of these health problems are yet to be integrated or understood sufficiently enough to achieve better outcomes for improving public health. Admittedly, a biological reason for the lack of progress in studying the interdependent events during the induction of age-associated health problems is the combined and complex extrinsic and intrinsic heterogeneities that are involved in the pathobiology of common illnesses.

To appreciate the complexity of the biology of aging and age-associated chronic diseases, the core principals that govern biological activities in eukaryotic cells are outlined in the following. It is important to note that from birth to death, the multicellular organism of the human body is subject to continued energy-requiring wear and tear processes to accommodate repairing and adaptation that are required for maintenance of health. Aging and weakened status and eventual loss of controlled wear and tear processes (regeneration, degeneration and recycling) are likely the bases for initiation and progression of diseases as well as death (details in Chap. 6) (Fig. 3.1) [56–80]:

(i) The body is a dynamic system of complex and highly interactive multiple organs, whose function continually evolves, from the conception and fetal growth all the way through life including the aging process.

(ii) The proper functioning of organ systems involves a wide range of well-orchestrated and energy-dependent physical, mechanical, molecular and chemical signal transduction mechanisms involving genetic/epigenetic, enzymatic, metabolic and neuronal activities for the purpose of regeneration, degradation and turnover processes and survival. The highly regulated crosstalks occur continuously between and among organs, glands, tissues and cells of the skin, liver, kidney, lung, heart, stomach, eyes, bones, muscles, thymus, immune cells, vasculature, neuronal, and gastrointestinal tract.

(iii) Among critical steps in sustenance of normal living cells are the proton pumping across the membrane and generation of differential acidity between cellular membrane and cytoplasm. Continued proton pumping and generated electricity is required for numerous routine cell activities such as lysosomal digestion and protein recycling, ion/solute transport, degradation of pathogen's structural proteins/lipids/genes for immune recognition/activation, as well as cellular proliferation. The extent of proton pumping provided through vascular and other cell membrane ATPases alter, to varying degrees, from the time of fetal growth and after birth, as well as during aging or disease processes including carcinogenesis. Agents that are foreign to the body as well as aging process and diseases can temporarily or permanently disturb the membrane effective potential of cell environmental pH causing skewed signal transduction and crosstalk between and among cells/tissues for achieving and controlling the required activities of the cells.

(iv) Interactions and signal transductions between immune and non-immune tissue components (e.g., cells, organelles, proteins/enzymes, lipids, DNA/RNA) are amazingly successful complexes of turnover and regeneration processes with durations lasting from a fraction of seconds to several minutes; few days or months and even years. To achieve various crosstalks all types of cells and organ systems must follow biological rules of rhythmicity at different and precise levels. The links among physio-immune-neuronal-hormonal or pathological features of nearly all tissue/organ systems follow the control mechanisms of circadian rhythms (positive-negative response cycles). The circadian system is defined as a principal pacemaker in the suprachiasmatic nucleus circadian (SNC) in coordination with a number of peripheral circadian oscillators. Pathophysiological features of chronic diseases such as metabolic syndrome, site-specific cancers, diabetes and cardiovascular complications are very likely associated with disruptive conditions of certain components of the circadian cycle. The insufficient circadian rhythms could be the results of mutations of the clock genes, circadian control genes, or physiological and perhaps immunological deficiencies that lead to altered synchronization between SCN and other peripheral dual features of biological oscillators.

(v) The various synchronization properties are defined as the natural positive and negative duality (oscillations) or biphasic events that are required for maintenance of health. In general, approximate duration of biological rhythms (collectively labeled as 'effective acquisition time') are classified into three major categories:

(a) Ultradian, lasting seconds to several hours (e.g., neuronal and visual signal transduction, ion fluxes, hormonal release, enzymatic reactions, transporter activities, biosynthesis of receptor molecules, chromosomal repair activities, type 1 or immediate hypersensitivity responses),
(b) Circadian, lasting approximately 24 h (e.g., skin turnover, melatonin, cellular and extracellular membrane component biosynthesis),
(c) Infradian, also known as tidal or annual pathways, lasting more than a few days (e.g., biosynthesis and turnover of hemoglobin, mast cell sensitization and responses). Regeneration of complex organ systems (e.g., liver, lung or kidneys) may take a few years to be completed,

(vi) Aging process itself is a dynamic phenomenon of biological regeneration and degeneration characteristic of all multicellular organisms with minor or major declines skewed/retarded in the biological switches. For example, aging pro-

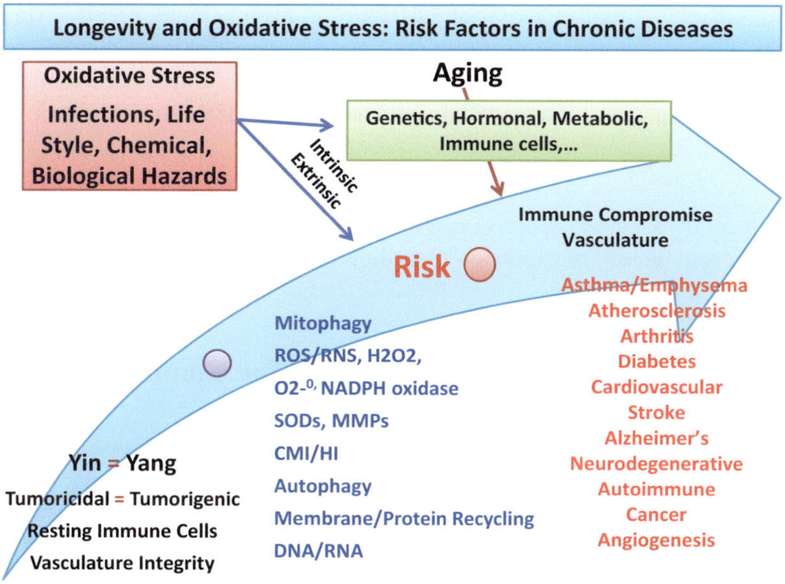

Fig. 3.1 Schematic representation of maintenance of Yin-Yang (tumoricidal vs tumorigenic) of acute inflammation in health (*left panel*) and induction of oxidative stress in alterations of intrinsic and extrinsic factors toward increased risk of chronic diseases during aging process (*right panel*). It represents that aging and oxidative stress increase risk of chronic diseases. Alterations or loss of mitochondrial function (mitophagy), ribosomal activities (autophagy), accumulation of oxidants (ROS/RNS), increased mutated genes (DNA/RNA) and immune suppression (changes in CMI/HI) lead to increased risk of asthma/emphysema, diabetes and cardiovascular diseases, stroke, Alzheimer's, neurodegenerative or autoimmune diseases or cancer and angiogenesis) (Reproduced from Khatami Clin Trans Med 2016 [80]. All rights reserved)

cess and altered hormonal and related activities lead to declines or accelerations (skewed) of physiological activities (biological rearrangements) in organs/tissues (biological senescence). Aging process also induces minor or major changes in immune response dynamics within organ systems (immunosenescence). The age-induced altered natural biological and immunological activities, in general, lead to altered effectiveness of immune surveillance or the balance between tumoricidal vs. tumorigenic properties of immune system, weakening the body to effectively challenge toxicity of components that potentially threaten the body's survival.

It is hypothesized that the overall control switches of the stimulating and inhibitory processes that follow the above rhythmic rules are larger version of the original definitions that the author proposed [30] for effective immunity, possessing 2 highly regulated and biologically opposing arms (biphasic or Yin and Yang) mechanisms provided through acute inflammation (immune surveillance) for maintenance of health.

In summary, maintenance of health depends on the inherently precise expression and regulations of energy-requiring positive and negative biological control switches (biological rhythms or clocks) between the local (host) and distant immune and non-immune (e.g., vasculature, metabolism neuroendocrine or neuro-physiological) systems [80].

The recently accepted adaptive origin of life is somewhat in contrast with the evolutionary theory of exclusion as traditionally known.

3 Biological Theories of Aging: Search for Common Link

In the last few decades, numerous biological theories of aging have been proposed to explain the mechanisms of aging process. To date, among the popular theories of aging are the genetic program theory, wear-and-tear theory, telomere theory, endocrine/hormonal theory, melatonin theory, DNA damage hypothesis, error catastrophe theory, the rate of living theory, mitochondrial theory, the nitric oxide hypothesis, the free radical and/or the oxidative stress theory, mitochondrial and immune/inflammation theory (reviewed in [45, 56, 61–63, 65–90]). These reports address and argue some of the challenges on the validity and pitfalls of documented theories that include isolated efforts to prevent diseases or slow down aging and prolong life, by means of food and nutrition intake, exercise and diet restrictions [47, 49, 58, 71–120].

As discussed in the following sections, the various aging theories, in all likelihood, are interdependent and the oxidative stress is the major influence on the intrinsic and extrinsic biological systems affecting the immune surveillance (immunity) that Burnet theorized over six decades ago [28]. Support for interdependence of the known theories of aging comes from the observations that age-induced alterations of hormonal, immunological, genomic functions are co-morbidity and co-mortality risk factors whose declines are accelerated by oxidative stress and accumulation of free radicals in tissues in the direction of initiation of nearly all age-associated chronic diseases (Figs. 3.1 and 3.2) [21–26, 80].

The following outlines the analyses of data on major interdependent biological dynamics in aging process based on reported theories with emphasis on the role of oxidative stress. The mechanisms of actions of immune disruptors and induction of chronic/unresolved inflammation are suggested as common links in the genesis of nearly all chronic illnesses and site-specific cancers [reviewed in 21–26, 31–36, 50, 80–150]:

(a) Aging accompanies the atrophy or shrinkage of thymus followed by shortage of biosynthesis of stem cells, the giant manufacturer of immune cells. The shortage of stem cells often leads to altered/inefficient synthesis and response dynamics of innate and adaptive immune cells. The effects of aging on the immune system are widespread and extend from altered functions of the hematopoietic stem cells and lymphoid progenitors in the bone marrow and thymus to mature lymphocytes in secondary lymphoid organs. The combined

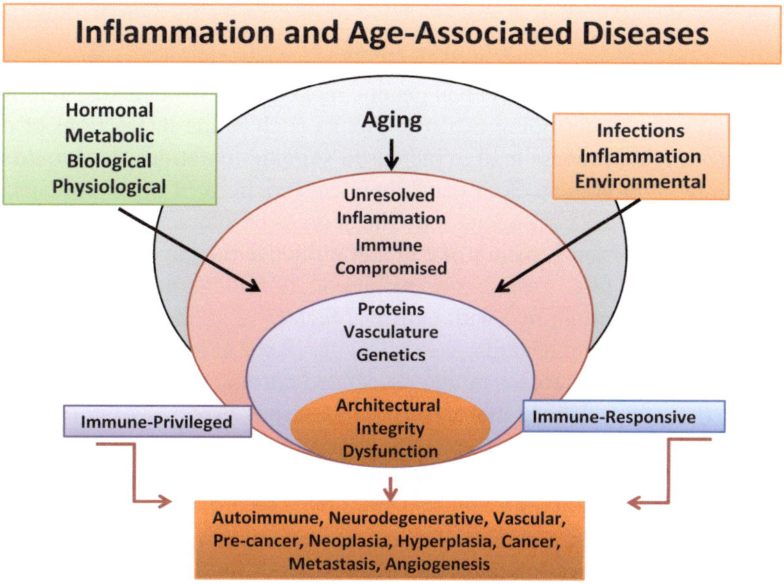

Fig. 3.2 Schematic representation that longevity and oxidative stress are co-morbidity and co-mortality risk factors that would increase the risk of chronic illnesses. As depicted in the figure, chronic inflammation differentially influences the tissues that are immune-responsive or immune-privileged leading to a wide range of illnesses that are potentially interrelated. See text

changes result in a diminution of immune responsiveness in the elderly (immunosenescence);

(b) The endocrine system and the function or levels of hormones (e.g., estrogen, insulin, testosterone, DHA) that play important roles in modulation of oxidative stress, metabolism and physiology of tissues alter in aging. Endocrine deficiencies impact the dynamics of immune responses;

(c) Oxidative stress-induced altered chromosomal components and increased mutations of the genetics and epigenetics materials that damage the DNA/RNA and expression profiles and functions of proteins/enzymes, hormones, cytokines/chemokines or lipids influence tissue physiology and function;

(d) Aging can cause impaired or insufficient transport properties of metabolites (e.g., glucose, myo-inositol, pyridoxine/pyridoxal phosphate, vitamin C), their receptors and cell surface molecules and loss of effectiveness in homeostasis of oxido-redox potential and bioenergetics in tissues (e.g., nuclear and membrane phosphorylation and dephosphorylation by kinases and phosphatases);

(e) Accumulation of senescence cells and loss of effectiveness in protein/lipid recycling pathways involving intracellular organelles such as lysosomes, ER, Golgi apparatus and mitochondria and induction of pathological status in autophagy and mitophagy;

(f) Promotion of telomere attrition is an important contributing factor in aging;

(g) Free radicals accumulation and induction of impaired circadian rhythmicity and cardiac output are among important factors in aging process;

While the importance of individual genetic makeup (intrinsic factor) in longevity is logical, how the confounding extrinsic factors such as the interactions of oxidative stress and aging process lead to increased somatic mutations that would affect the regulations of biological clocks and chemical functions of organ systems in the direction of diseases are not understood. The degrees of interactions between intrinsic (innate) factors or the genetic makeup that influence the physiological behaviors of the organs/tissues (e.g., vasculature, metabolic, hormonal, neuronal and immune response pathways), combined with extrinsic factors (e.g., exposures to chemical, environmental, biological hazards, life styles) are likely to impose major impacts in aging process and the outcomes of age-associated chronic conditions (Fig. 3.2).

In 2008, the author defined that acute inflammation possesses 2 tightly regulated and biologically opposing arms (biphasic), termed Yin (tumoricidal, apoptosis) and Yang (tumorigenic, wound healing) properties of immunity. Yin and Yang control an elaborate and precise crosstalk between immune and non-immune (e.g., vasculature, neuroendocrine and metabolic pathways) systems to protect the body against all foreign elements that threatens the body's survival [30, 80]. It was further hypothesized that chronic inflammation is a major risk factor underlying aging and age-related diseases [23–27, 30, 80]. Since 1998 at the National Cancer Institute (NCI) a major goal of the author has been to promote the important roles that inflammation play in cancer biology. In the last decade, heavily funded projects and significant number of publications are devoted to fragmented proposed hypotheses on the role of inflammation in cancer research, immunotherapy and related network and conferences around the world. However, except for our 'accidental' discoveries that were established in 1980's, little efforts have been invested to systematically understand the early events that occur between tissues and immune disruptors that alter immune dynamics in tissue toward multistep carcinogenesis ([21–27, 30, 31, 50–60, 80], submitted documents to NCI/NIH since 1998).

4 Free Radical Concept and Oxidative Stress Theory of Aging: Role of Mitochondria

Half a century ago, Harman [65] originally postulated that the free-radical theory of aging is the accumulation of the molecular damage in tissue caused by byproducts of the normal oxidative metabolism, called reactive oxygen species (ROS). Harman further extended his theory and explained the role of mitochondria in aging process since mitochondria is the main source of generation of ROS and SODs [65, 66]. Since then, other studies following the discovery of detoxifying enzymes such as the superoxide dismutases (SODs), within cellular components and organelles (e.g., cytosol, mitochondria) that neutralize the superoxide anions; catalases and detection of the hydrogen peroxide (H_2O_2) provided credibility and support for the free-radical theory of aging [80–118]. Understanding of the signaling pathways in aging that involve free radical theory largely comes from the investigations on the nematode *Caenorhabditis elegans* (*C-elegans*) organism [99–116]. Analyses of reported data using this model address how reactive oxygen species (ROS) influence the aging process. Data demonstrate that over time ROS and/or oxidative stress accumulate some types of damage in specific targets such as the proteins, lipids, or nucleic acids contributing to the aging process. However, further analyses of such data on the oxidative biology of *C. elegans* show debates and controversies that ROS are not the toxic byproducts of the oxidative metabolism, since using antioxidant interventional therapies to alter the effects of accumulation of ROS remain inconclusive. It has been suggested that the overall rise in oxidative damage is not a major factor determining lifespan, due to duality of oxido-redux or rhythmic biology in organ systems that are capable of neutralizing the impact of ROS or other oxidants through effective function of anti-oxidants in healthy aging body. Furthermore, the notion that a general increase in oxidative stress does not limit lifespan in this model organism suggests that under stressful conditions, resistant to oxidative stress might be important to normal lifespan and reproduction in *C-elegans*, or other experimental model systems and human subjects.

In the last few decades many oxidants and enzymes have been identified that are not free radicals but, if not properly neutralized and removed by antioxidants and growth factors, they produce oxidative damage to tissues, perhaps participating in the loss of balance between the Yin and Yang (tumoricidal and tumorigenic) properties of acute inflammation [21–27, 30–36, 80, 117–165]. Several studies demonstrate that the normal byproducts of cellular metabolism including the intermediates of mitochondrial respiration or the activities of oxidative enzymes (e.g., cytochrome P-450, NADPH oxidase, myeloperoxidases, NO synthase, glutathione peroxidase, or xanthine oxidases), generate highly reactive molecules with unpaired electrons or free radicals (e.g., ROS, RNS, superanions-HO^-, peroxynitrile, H2O2, NADP+). The generation of oxidants are routinely neutralized by cellular antioxidants and scavengers of free radicals, agents that possess reductive capacity and protect tissue components from oxidative damage and maintenance of the oxido-reductive status of cells. Generation of normal amounts of ROS is required for routine regulation of cell functions, including apoptosis and proliferation that influence intracellular signaling pathways, gene expression, fragmentation of DNA, membrane lipid peroxidation and increased vulnerability of extracellular matrix to proteases. For example, hydroxyl ions (HO^-) or $O2^-$ can interact and oxidize free iron (Fe^+2, reduced form) or copper (Cu^+) ions, or NO to their oxidized forms (e.g., Fe^{3+}, Cu^{2+}, or $ONOO^-$) and thereby modify and regulate the function of specialized carrier proteins (e.g., ferritin) or availability of NO [21, 23, 25, 30–38, 46–50, 80, 86, 150–180]. Related information supports that oxidative stress induces activation of enzymes [e.g., NADPH oxidase, peroxisome proliferators-activated receptors (PPARs), pro-inflammatory mediators (e.g., IL-6, IL-10, TNF-α, PGs] and alters redox state of binding proteins (e.g., Fos, c-jun, c-myc, beta actin), altered activities of genomic, chromosomal or epigenetic component, DNA/RNA/mRNA or telomere and telomerase activities that would lead to early abnormal genetic responses and hematopoietic activation [170–255]. These changes are known to contribute to the induction of numerous mild or severe conditions such as, asthma, atheroma, emphysema, atherosclerosis, autoimmune and neurodegenerative diseases, hypertension, stroke, multiple sclerosis, arthritis, neurodegenerative diseases, diabetes or Alzheimer's or carcinogenesis and angiogenesis. Furthermore, the extent of presence of energy-consuming peroxidation-induced extracellular membrane damage (e.g., activities of MMPs and expression of type IV collagenase or lipid peroxidation) may determine the extent of immune response profiles and chromosomal/genomic damage in tissues and the fate of tumor growth, metastasis and angiogenesis in susceptible tissues such as squamous and epithelial tissues in lung, prostate, colorectal, stomach or ovary [80, 163–270].

An overall review of data provide compelling evidence that the aging process is centrally regulated by a complex energy-requiring metabolic activity, cellular proliferation and differentiation, immune response crosstalk and autophagy for protein/lipid recycling events. Among several energy-driven pathways, the major complex processes involve 2 distinct forms of mammalian target of rapamycin (mTORC1 and mTORC2), an evolutionary conserved family of serine/threonine kinase and member of the family of phosphoinositide-3 kinase (PI3K) related kinases (PIKK). The role of mTORC1 has been shown to engage with complexes such as NAD+ -dependent deacetylase enzymes, SIRT1 pathways and include mediation by ROS-induced activation of S6 kinase and H2O2 production for signal transduction and regulation of cell growth and proliferation involving the immune response crosstalk. Abnormal function of TOR contributes to the tissue hypertrophy and hyperactivity toward cellular damage and age-related health conditions. Furthermore, activation of TOR-dependent pathways seems to limit lifespan by accelerating age-related diseases even before the accumulation of ROS induces death (details in Chap. 6).

Several age-associated diseases (e.g., atherosclerosis, stroke, cardiovascular complications, adult diabetes, neurodegenerative diseases or site-specific cancers) clearly are affected by increased oxidative stress. Oxidative stress inactivates or alters functions of critical enzymes (e.g., superoxide dismutases, catalase, glutathione peroxidase and glutathione reductase), intrinsic metabolites (e.g., uric acid, bilirubin, SH-proteins, glutathione), extrinsic reducing agents (e.g., vitamins C, D, E, carotenoids, flavonoids) or other antioxidants, and metal chelating proteins that prevent Fenton and Haber-Weiss chemistry have been identified as potential contributors of age-associated diseases. The reported loss of numerous natural protective mechanisms that prevent cellular damages associated with chronic diseases strongly support that the oxidative damage theory play a key role in aging [21–27, 30, 80, 111–146, 183–285].

The classic free radical theory of aging includes mitochondria-related specific processes of senescence. Age-associated generation of free radicals and accumulation of ROS are toxins to the mitochondrial function including induction of numerous mitochondrial DNA mutations and progressive reduction in energy output that are significantly below the required levels of body's function. The reduced output energy from mitochondria implicated in a number of age-associated health conditions such as the loss of memory, hearing, vision, stamina and tumorigenesis.

Increased damage by free radicals is linked to the impairments of mitochondrial function, which further alters inflammatory processes required for routine immune or tissue remodeling. The release of pro-inflammatory cytokines from DNA-damaged cells and dysfunctional mitochondria (mitophagy or mitotically arrested DNA) that exhibit the senescence-associated secretory phenotype (SASP) present several adverse effects including mutations of stem cells that reduce the capacity of tissue regeneration processes and induction of cancer stem cells and abnormal tissue growth. Senescence-associated secretory phenotype also could potentially be involved in antigen-load and chronic inflammation that would lead to necrosis and neurodegenerative diseases in immune-privileged tissues [21, 23, 26, 27, 30–38, 80, 100, 142–216].

Review of several excellent reports suggest that in the mitochondrial concept (mitohormesis theory) under normal metabolism, the production of ROS seems an important molecular signal that induce 'hormetic' effect by triggering stress resistance and longevity and induction of specific antioxidants in response to ROS. Combined aging process and cumulative effects of ROS are important factors in the impaired mitochondrial metabolism, oxidative phosphorylation and differential bioenergetics in cell that participate in altered dynamics of immunity and induction of chronic diseases processes. Among important known factors that are involved in the ROS-induced dysfunction of mitochondria (mitophagy) are mutations of certain genes (mit mutants) such as clk-1, isp-1 or neu-6, involved in expression of enzymes (e.g., increased SOD and catalase activities, or hypoxia-inducible transcription factor-HIF-1), perhaps biological attempts to offset the damaging effects of a rise in tissue ROS levels. Furthermore, inhibition of mitochondrial respiration leads to altered mitochondrial protein folding response (e.g., UPR^{mito} and increased hsp-6 expression). The uncoupling of respiration could disturb the integrity of mitochondrial architectural integrity, causing abnormalities in membrane composition (e.g., cardiolipin), effective bioenergetics and signals for production of anti-oxidants and expression of enzymes (e.g., SOD) that are required for effective metabolism and immunity of organ systems and life span (see Sect. 7 below).

The natural antioxidants within organ systems include several enzymes [e.g., superoxide dismutases (SODs), $NADP^+$ reductase or catalase], hydrophilic agents [e.g., glutathione (GSH), vitamin C, uric acid], lipophilic compounds (e.g., vitamin E, carotenoids, and bilirubin), mitochondrial thioredoxin and metal ions with electron transfer capacity such as $Fe2^+$, Cu^+. These antioxidants are ubiquitously distributed within cytoplasm, mitochondria and/or extracellular tissue compartments throughout the body. Antioxidant enzymes such as SODs prevent formation of highly reactive free radicals such as ROS by readily accepting and scavenging the unpaired electrons and transferring or converting the oxidants to other electron accepting molecules. For example, SODs convert superoxide anion (free radical $O2^-$) to the less aggressive oxidant H2O2, which is further removed by other antioxidant enzymes such as GSH peroxidase or catalase, involving other reducing metabolites such as GSH, NADPH, vitamins E or C (ascorbate, semidehydroascorbate) recycling pathways [21–27, 30, 40–65, 80, 101–124, 144, 155–165]. It is likely that neutralization of ROS by natural antioxidants would reduce/regulate activation of mTOR and related kinase pathways that are associated with tissue hypertrophy and growth.

Thus far, the recommended caloric restriction is the only known strategy tested to increase the life span in rodents and may also applies to primates, and presumably humans [95–98, 127, 128, 158]. However, potential health benefits of a number of antioxidants, vitamins (e.g., vit D, E, C), anti-inflammatory agents, or sulfhydryl-containing agents (e.g., asprin, Amifostine, isothiocyanate, mercaptoethanol, N-acethylcysteine or captopril) and precursors of reduced glutathione on cellular redox-sensitive transcription factors (e.g., NF-kB), leukocyte adherence or ACE or mast cell stabilizers (e.g., Na-cromolyn) could also be important in delaying or preventing age-associated diseases including cancer ([21–27, 30, 51, 78–80, 91, 96, 101, 116, 130–132, 148] Khatami submitted documents to NCI/NIH, since 1998).

In brief, the 'oxidative stress' theory, also known as the 'free radical' theory seems to have stood the test of time, as this biological phenomenon has been the most broadly investigated topic in biology of aging. The tightly controlled concentrations of ROS and fluctuations/oscillations (negative-positive switches) of the tissue redox potentials are important mediators of signaling processes for inflammatory responses and metabolism in tissues. The ongoing controversies to the oxidative damage theory of aging using the experimental models of aging are, most likely, due to the enormous knowledge gaps and lack of systematic understanding of the age-associated altered molecular dynamics of oxidative stress during the progressive deterioration of feedback controls of the immunity; the giant umbrella of the immune cells, the neuro-endocrine and the metabolic networks that lead to increased somatic mutations in the genesis of molecular catastrophic errors and initiation of site-specific diseases [24–30, 33–36, 50, 80, 112–124, 148]. Insights into the mechanisms of accumulation of ROS and the redox status of tissue compartments and response dynamic contributions in aging require detailed bioenergetic studies that would enable scientists to accurately detect the initial interrelated biological processes. In all likelihood, the functional loss of neutralizing ROS factors is the result of a progressive pro-oxidizing shift in the redox state of the cells during aging. This would lead to over-oxidation of the redox-sensitive proteins and consequently the disruption of redox-regulated signaling mechanisms.

5 Genomic Theory of Aging

Biological aging and tendency to decay the ordered systems into general disorder applies to all body's cellular and molecular networks, including DNA and chromosomal damage [e.g., depurination and depyrimidation at normal acidity or temperature] that often lead to injury by water nucleophillic properties that could alter structural integrity and function of genetic, epigenetic and influence expression of proteins/enzymes as well as recycling pathways. Several elegant studies demonstrate that normal tissue metabolism including mitochondrial oxidative phosphorylation are associated with DNA mutations at the rate of about 10,000 bases/cell/day (for depurination or depyrimidation), or an average of 100 bases/cell/day (for cytosine deamination) that involve hydroxyl radical-mediated oxidative damage and altered immune response crosstalk among organ/tissues [168–237]. Normal aging process causes changes in the features of chromosomal function, including the shortening of telomere and expression of related proteins and enzymes that are required for maintenance of regeneration as well as degeneration pathways for nearly all activities of tissue components [30, 80, 172–197].

To maintain health and effective immunity throughout life, correction of generation of genetic errors and mismatches, require routine and simultaneous molecular repair pathways involving biological and immunological pathways of protein expression and recycling/regeneration processes or replication/repair of DNA/RNA molecules and nuclear components [80, 175–229]. The DNA repair mechanisms by AP Pol β base replacement (base excision repair BER) and related repair enzymes occasionally lead to base pair excision or modifications and rearrangements of one strand of DNA (mismatch repair) while the second strand remains as template for zip or fork replication. The process of fork replication on one strand seems to provide temporary vulnerability causing potential increased damage to DNA before the natural double-stranded DNA is repaired. The accumulation of mismatched or modified and unprocessed DNA bases would induce altered molecular signals for repair mechanisms including protein kinase signaling pathways leading to destabilization of recombination pathways during the loss of multi-potency of mesenchymal stromal cells and dysregulation of crosstalk in immune and non-immune pathways that could lead to the multistep chronic diseases such as epilepsy, bone and pulmonary diseases and cancer [30, 80, 168–191, 205–207, 213–229, 231–237]. It is suggested that accumulation of senescent cells with features of inactive/suppressed DNA/RNA or chromosomal activities present additional burden (antigen-load) to organ systems for clearance and recycling pathways as potential contributing factors in aging.

Among the many factors involved in chromosomal and DNA damage, in the course of normal cellular metabolism, are oxidative damage to DNA during mitochondrial respiration, immune cell maturation and responses toward stimuli and exogenous factors (e.g., exposure to UV radiation or perhaps carcinogens), as well as cellular DNA synthesis during cell cycle transit [30, 80, 150–215, 228, 229]. During cellular DNA synthesis the damaged DNA is often magnified through slow process of replacement of an excised base and base pairing excision in the G1 phase (nicks) that may cause collapsed forks preventing correct replication forks into DNA double strand, leading to further large deletions and chromosomal damage and deficiencies in cell cycle progression and checkpoints (ATR protein kinase) and fork stability. Therefore, the normal DNA replication processes, over time, create sufficient damage to DNA to cause stem and progenitor cell attrition and deplete tissue regeneration capacity leading to accelerated or premature decline in tissues renewal capacity of stem and progenitor cell fates that influence senescence and apoptosis and increased risks for onset of age-associated chronic diseases. It is also important to note that as is the case for immune response activities, nucleotide biosynthesis and related DNA/RNA repair pathways are ATP-dependent and require efficient mitochondrial integrity [30, 80, 159, 167, 171–178, 206, 207, 210–225, 228, 232].

Deficiencies in genome maintenance are associated with various aspects of premature aging in genetically modified animal models and in humans. Human specific genetic diseases featured by Werner syndrome, Cockayne syndrome, trichothiodystrophy, dyskeratosis congenital, and ataxia-telangiectasia, as well as age-associated conditions such as graying hair, alopecia, hyphosis, osteoporosis, and impaired tissue regeneration, have been reported in mouse models of aging in which targeted mutations have been generated in DNA damage response (DDR) regulators caused by mutation of genes involved in the efficient repair of DNA damage or the cell cycle regulatory response molecular patterns [165–175, 204]. Loss of stem and progenitor cells attrition and tissue homeostasis including impaired genome regenerative capacity in adult stem cells have been proposed as the general organismal decline in aging [30, 80, 172–187, 206, 207, 214, 219–222].

It is noteworthy, that only in the last decade, the decision makers in the cancer community have come to accept and appreciate that inflammation is a precancerous state of cells that initiates adaptive changes in epigenetic structures resulting in accumulation of genetic errors and impairments of regulation of gene expression in multistep carcinogenesis [25, 26, 159, 166–172, 200–229]. Epigenetics and post-mitotic modification events of gene expression pathways (e.g., DNA methylation, methylated DNA binding proteins, histone modification-related enzymes, microRNAs) or telomere-telomerase pathways are sensitive to immune dysfunction and oxidative stress [21–27, 30, 38–44, 48, 50–56, 73, 80, 135–137, 143, 171, 178, 255, 280, 282].

5.1 *Role of Hyperactivation of Suppressor Gene Pathways in Aging*

As described above, the process of restarting DNA replication forks and preventing collapse require 50 different genes during the complex multistage processes of DNA homologous recombination such as double-strand break recognition, strand invasion and space-'holiday' junction resolution. Defects in any steps of these molecular sequences could influence mutagenic types of repair processes and accumulation of DNA damage at bridge-breakage fusion cycles during the chromosomal translocations.

Analyses of relevant data demonstrate that aging and oxidative stress, to varying degrees, increase the genetic mutations at multiple locations leading to inactivation or defective function of suppressor gene molecules (e.g., p25, p35, p38, or p53) and increased instabilities in somatic maintenance and repair, proliferative control of gene expression as well as misguided expression of apoptosis or wound healing mediators [172–229]. The increased genetic mutations could also damage chromosomal contents and alter DNA methylation (hypo-, and hypermethylation) causing defects in cell contact inhibition and cell cycle regulation such as cyclin-dependent kinases (e.g., ser-thr kinases-cdks), telomere dysfunction or shortening as well as epigenetic and posttranslational events. A specific example of the role of suppressor genes mutations in senescence is the role of p38 pathways. The inactivation or mutation of P38 mitogen-activated protein kinase (MAPK) that are involved in regulation of extracellular-signal regulated kinase (ERK), c-Jun N-terminal kinase (JNK) could lead to enhanced cellular transformation and disruption in the induction of senescence that follows tumor growth. Furthermore, impaired DNA methylation of CpG islands, important molecular checkpoints in gene expression pathways influence carcinogenesis, inflammation and viral infection [21, 31, 92, 170, 178, 180, 181, 201, 202, 212–226, 237].

6 Immunosenescence Theory: Connecting the Dots with Oxidative Stress and Skewed Dynamics of Immunity in Aging

Immunoscenescence is the results of age-induced readjustment and/or remodeling of the immune cell dynamics, combined with age-associated physiological rearrangements and altered hormonal and metabolic changes (biological senescence). Immunoscencence-induced remodeling of immune system includes minor or major alterations in innate and adaptive immune cells and bone changes in the activities of bone morphogenesis and remodeling and initiation of disease processes [21–30, 33–36, 38–45, 48, 50–56, 80, 239–259, 284, 308–310].

A clinical feature of immunosenescence is the development of hyper-, or hyposensitivity reactions toward new antigen challenges and/or self-antigens and the observed increased allergies or autoimmune diseases in older adults. The immune dysfunction results from cumulative impairments in the complex network of cellular and humoral interactions of the critical cells in the immune system, including the dendritic, natural killer and mast cells, macrophages, B and T cell subpopulations (e.g., Th1/Th2 cells or B memory cell). Aging response to inflammation is cell and humoral mediated pathways (CMI, HI), with active participation of nearly all other components of organ systems (e.g., vascular, metabolic, neuronal and hormonal pathways). Furthermore, the protective roles of immune responses (immune surveillance) depend on the ability of immune cells to generate and retain 'memory cells' to recognize and respond in an accelerated defensive manner to pathogen exposures. The aging body generally retains immunity against previously encountered pathogens. However, components of immunologic memory show skewed responses toward new stimuli (pathogens or carcinogens) [21–27, 30, 41, 50, 80, 241–283, 311–355].

In general, aging causes minor or major alterations in the response ability of APCs to present antigen to the resting/naïve T cells (T0). The changes are likely due to the proposed altered balance between tumoricidal vs tumorigenic (Yin-Yang) properties of immune response dynamics, or the loss of homeostasis of oxido-redox potential of immune and non-immune cells. Depending on the tissue immune cell composition and vulnerability toward oxidative stress, the loss of Yin-Yang balance could result in untimely maturation or polarity of APCs such as changes in DCs (DC1/DC2 ratios), granulation and degranulation of MCs (MCs-'leaky' or TAMC) and/or macrophage (M1/M2 or TAM) phenotype population. The altered response dynamics of APCs, could further contribute to the impaired inflammatory signals in maturation, migration or recruitment and infiltration of other inflammatory cells and/or defects in communications with adaptive T or B cells. Data on aging provide evidence that the dysfunction of humoral response profiles associated with changes in expression of antibody profiles (e.g., IgG, IgE, IgM, IgA and isotypes) are, in part, due to decreases in Th1 (tumoricidal) response ability to provide appropriate crosstalk through co-stimulatory molecules, expression of cytokines and/or effective production of immunoglobulins. Aging is also associated with defects in T cell responses to viral infections. As detailed below, defects in cellular and humoral immunity (CMI, HI) could likely result in increased morbidity in older adults when exposed to infective viruses (e.g., respiratory syncytial virus, RSV) or increased chronic allergies (e.g., asthma, emphysema).

6.1 Immune Competency in Aging: Role of Antigen Presenting Cells (APCs) in Immunosenescence

In general, advance aging appears to cause decreases in both non-immune and immune defenses, although many aspects of immunity remain robust in centenarians. A growing body of evidence supports the notion that aging- and oxidative stress-induced impaired function of antigen presenting cells (APCs) could alter response profiles of adoptive immunity, which collectively cause retardation of the dynamics of crosstalk in non-immune (e.g., vasculature, neuronal, hormonal and metabolic) pathways in the direction of initiation and manifestation of chronic health problems. For example, APCs are responsible for recognition, uptake, processing and presentation of processed/digested antigens/pathogens to the antigen-specific receptor molecules (epitopes) of major histocompatibility complexes (MHC, MHC I and II) on T cells [21, 30, 80, 205–207, 221–345].

The intrinsic processes of T cell activation (adaptive or adoptive immunity) require interactions between T cells and APCs. In an acute inflammation, APCs and the expression of specific cytokines and mediators initiate and determine the outcomes of effector T cell responses (pharmacological effects) and the maintenance of balance in dual properties of Th1/Th2 and cytokine expression profiles [21–27, 30, 50, 80, 217, 336, 348–369].

In general, innate immune cells express invariant receptors, as opposed to adaptive immune cells, which express rearranged receptors for a wide range of processed antigens presented by APCs. Among major antigen presenting cells are the dendritic cells (DCs, the most professional APCs), and macrophages (MΦs, also professional phagocytes/monocytes). Activation of inflammatory cells (e.g., DCs, MΦs, MCs, eosinophils/Eos) and the production of diverse pro-inflammatory signals, cytokines and chemokines initiate crosstalk between innate and acquired immune response systems for generation of memory B cells and humoral response mechanisms. The APCs play key roles in protection of epithelium and mucosal surfaces through specific receptors that recognize, capture and ferry specific moieties of pathogens such as bacteria, viruses or other microorganisms such as mannose-rich glycoproteins or lipopolysaccharides (LPS). APCs are able to produce specific anti-bacterial peptides/cytokines or reactive oxygen species and neurotoxins that kill/destroy the infective pathogens or tumor cells. As a result, APCs generate various pro-inflammatory (apoptotic or tumoricidal) mediators that interact with and upregulate their counterparts in adaptive immune cells for acquired immune responses and activation or recruitment of other inflammatory cells [21, 80, 217, 265–285, 336, 348–369] (see Chap. 6).

With advancing age, naïve T cell population gradually decline while memory cells become predominant and tend to cause skewed (hypo-, or hyper-) responsiveness toward stimuli as bases for the increased prevalence of age-associated conditions such as asthma, emphysema, ocular and skin allergies, arthritis or neuro-degenerative and autoimmune diseases or cell growth [21, 80, 280–297, 370–388]. Older adults often demonstrate higher allergen sensitization as evaluated by total IgE levels. Furthermore, age-related T cell immune deficiency is preceded by intrinsic changes within bone marrow stem cells and the involution of the thymus. Bone marrow stem cells show decreased affinity for the thymic stroma. Atrophy of the thymus is associated with loss of thymic hormone and alterations in T cell function as well as changes in metabolic activities of the tissues as integrated factors in diseases processes [21, 80, 81, 289–294, 370–390] (see Chap. 6).

It is noteworthy that the collective alterations in anti-inflammatory and bioenergetics of aging (e.g., changes in hormonal, metabolic, physiological and mitochondrial activities) accompanied by sustained oxidative stress could induce expression or co-expression of mismatched growth and apoptotic factors in susceptible tissues. The extra caloric intake may additionally disturb the feedback controls of metabolism in tissues in the direction of growth promotion and induction of site-specific cancers. Suggestions that caloric restriction and exercise would delay the age-related declines of physiological function and chronic illnesses and promote healthy aging are biologically logical as obesity and extra caloric intake may additionally impair the oxido-redox balance in tissue in favor of growth promotion (see below) [21–64, 78–80, 97–138, 155, 158, 176, 247–252].

6.2 *Multipotent Hematopoietic Stem Cells*

Cells of the immune system are constantly renewed and supplied by the giant manufacturer of hematopoietic multipotent stem cells. Well documented data demonstrate that with aging the thymus involutes and the supply of naïve T cells gradually falls causing a reduction in the overall renewal capacity of stem cell. The critical deficits that occur in stem cells, particularly changes in T cells, are termed immunosenescence. The inefficiency of immune system to defend against new pathogens or cancerous cells and the increased incidence of autoimmune, inflammatory and infectious diseases during the aging process is recognized in the last few decades (Fig. 3.3) [21–27, 30–56, 178, 193–200, 221, 243–345]. For example, the proliferative activity of bone marrow peaks in middle age and then gradually decreases in older individuals, a phenomenon perhaps associated with increased apoptosis in aging. Consistent with these observations, CD 34+ stem cells mobilize less effectively in the elderly when compared to younger donors. Moreover, thymic involution, decreased lymphopoiesis along with reduction in the ability of marrow stroma to support lymphopoiesis have been reported in aging. Aging also causes cumulative expansion of memory cells and increased expression/ co-expression of apoptotic (Yin) and wound healing (Yang) mediators. These changes alter CMI and HI immune competence in aging [21, 24, 30, 31, 80, 178, 193, 199, 200, 219, 288–337, 459, 489].

The changes in multipotent hematopoietic stem cell population originate from alterations of bone marrow remodeling and regenerative processes as well as thymic and spleen T-lineage committed to stem cell biosynthesis and function. The features of immunosenescence are the following three primary changes in hematopoietic (innate and adaptive) immune cells that result in skewed immune response dynamics of CMI and HI accompanied by altered vasculature, metabolic and physiological activities in organs/tissues [21–50, 80, 186, 200, 226, 244–254, 264–522]:

(a) A decline in the number of naïve cells due to diminished thymopoiesis;
(b) An increase in the number of memory cells resulting in abnormal expression of cytokines/chemokines, other mediators or antibodies and mucosal secretion activities;
(c) Dysfunctional accumulation of activated effector cells, limited mutations of activated effector cells and limited T cell repertoire occupying T cell space.

Upon infection, adoptive immunity provides protection through three basic phases of recognition, activation/effector and memory. The age-induced immune dysfunction may occur at any of these phases, particularly in the recognition phase where the immune response alterations are attributed to intrinsic B cell numerous molecular defects including skewed antigen presentation, mucosal secretion, reduced co-stimulation, antibody profiles, repertoire constrictions, or a combination of colonotypic immune responses as features of immunosenescence [21–27, 30, 37–50, 80, 186, 200, 226, 266–463].

As schematically represented in Fig. 3.3, myeloid cells, originated from megakaryocytes express a number of cytokines and receptor molecules with various functions in the genesis of monocytes (MΦs) or granulocytes. There are at least 24 different immune cell types with distinct genetic profiling (at least 155 reported genes). They include innate and adaptive subpopulations/phenotypes, present in resting/normal (unstimulated) status or present distinct activities under a wide range of acute or chronic inflammatory responses or immunosenescence. Different immune cell phenotypes including platelets, innate and adaptive cells inherit expression of many cytokines and chemokines and receptor molecules with shared, over-

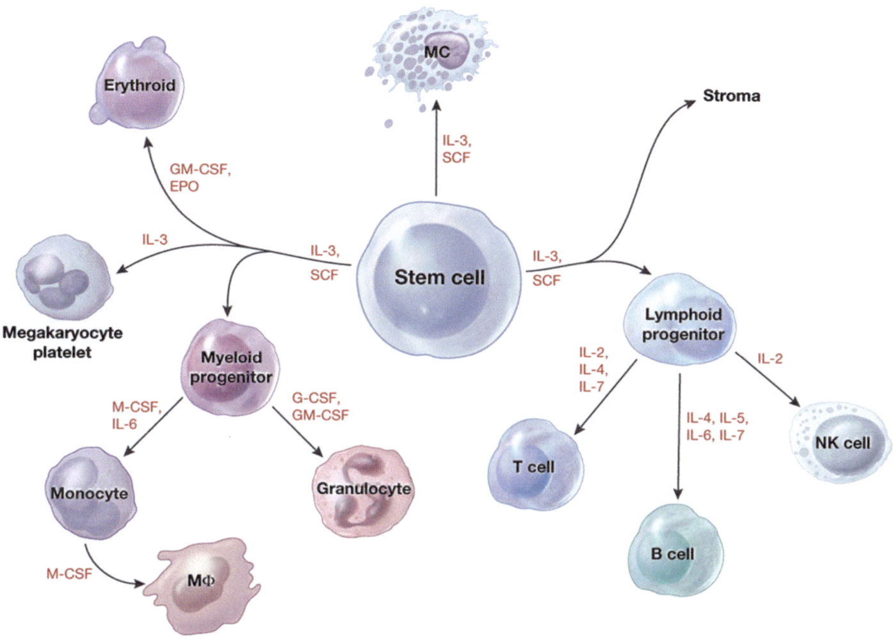

Fig. 3.3 Schematic representation of stem cells as the giant manufacturer (pluripotent cells) of hematopoietic immune cells. As depicted, growth and differentiation of each immune cell is regulated by induction of expression of special or shared mediators, cytokines, chemokines and growth factors. See text

lapping/compensating or distinct features under specific conditions to main the body's health [21–24, 31, 80, 147–155]. During antigen processing, the major functions of APCs are outlined below:

(d) Expression of receptor/ligands and surface molecules, such as toll-like receptors (TLRs, IL types), surface molecules (over 100 proteins, such as CD40/CD40L, CD22, CD73), cytokines such as tumor necrosis factor superfamily (22 molecular expression entities), complement cascade (at least 12 reported genetic profiles). The expression of these factors requires them to recognize and bind pathogens or pathogen-processed structures for presentation to other immune cells or responses from non-immune cells;
(e) Expression of innate cell-like (invariant) receptors (e.g., from platelets) for ingestion and destruction of microbiomes and prevention (termination) of pathogenicity;
(f) Release of molecular signals to communicate with other immune or non-immune cells in the tissue microenvironment or at distance to facilitate inflammatory conditions;
(g) Contribution to signaling molecular responses, facilitating polarization, differentiation and growth of other cells during apoptosis or wound healing or tissue repair and remodeling;

Therefore, the proper function of stem cells seems to be a key to healthy aging for making the body resistance to oxidative stress and delayed on-set of chronic diseases. However, longevity and the rate of functional capacities of organ systems and susceptibility to disabling diseases vary in individuals, perhaps due to a combination of genetics, immunological or biological factors as well as the frequency of exposure to diverse environmental hazards.

6.3 Cytokine/Chemokine Dynamics: Role of Decoy Receptors in Control of Acute or Chronic Inflammation in Health and Diseases

Pro- and anti-inflammatory signals from activated immune and non-immune cells regulate the levels and efficiency of inflammatory cytokine receptor coupling in a variety of inflammatory conditions to maintain the balance between Yin and Yang of immune surveillance or the control of immunity.

A major feature in the biology of immune system in aging is upregulation of inflammatory responses that seems detrimental to longevity. Data on age-dependent increased expression of several cytokines such as IL-2, IFN-γ, TNF-α (identified as Type 1), or IL-4, IL-6, IL-10 (identified as Type 2) that influence T cells, particularly CD8+ subset of effector/cytotoxic and memory cells in chronic inflammatory state and inability to fight viral infections in aging are not understood and often confusing [21–41, 80, 134–138, 203–207, 238–264]. Detailed analyses of several reports, however, support the author's recent hypotheses that loss of balance between Yin (pro-inflammatory) and Yang (anti-inflammatory) processes of acute inflammation is the major force in the induction of chronic state of unresolved inflammation. In all likelihood, oxidative stress and aging process lay a foundation for persistent viral infections by EBV and CMV or the induction of other illnesses such as hypertension, neurological diseases, cardiovascular problems as well as site-specific cancers. In other words, aging and persistent viral infection induce chronic antigenic stimulation status (antigen-load, oxidative stress) and generate modifications of CD8+ subsets and inability to clear/resolve antigen-(infection)-induced activation of immune dynamics. Furthermore, age-dependent expansions of CD-8 + CD28- T cells, and co-expression of pro-inflammatory cytokines including CMV-epitope specific cells, underline the importance of chronic antigenic stimulation in the pathogenesis of immunological alterations that could favor the appearance of pathologies (e.g., arteriosclerosis, dementia, osteoporosis, cardiovascular complications, cancer), all of which share aspects of inflammatory components [21–55, 68, 80, 266–286].

Further analyses of data demonstrate that stimuli-induced expression of pro-inflammatory cytokines and enzymes (e.g., IL-1, IL-6, IL-8, TNF−α, M−CSF, GM-CSF, eotaxin, histamine, PGs, LTs, heparin, chymase, tryptase) from activated resident (local) and/or recruited inflammatory cells, contribute to the amplification and progression of responses. The required signals to destroy the pathogens are often generated in part, by increasing the local concentrations of pro-inflammatory mediators produced by resident inflammatory cells or by producing additional cytokines or mediators (e.g., ROS/RNS, TGF-β) from infiltrated macrophages, platelets or complement activation to accomplish a function (e.g., removal of an irritant or lysing of an infectious agent).

It appears that the major bases for age-associated persistent (chronic/unresolved) inflammatory status in the induction of chronic health conditions fall into two principal categories:

1. Loss of vascular integrity and function (vascular toning), further facilitated by skewed metabolic responses and impaired immune signals- resulting in increased vascular permeability and changes in the balance between angiogeneic and anti-angiogenic factors;
2. Impaired balance in the oxido-redox potentials or bioenergetic features in tissues/organ systems, as the principal loss of protective mechanisms of body's health;

During an inflammatory response, the decoy receptors seem to function as control switches or checkpoints (feedback mechanisms) that simultaneously initiate the termination processes (Yang, wound healing) following the Yin events (Fig. 3.4).

Decoy receptor molecules are agonist-binding proteins that sequester inflammatory cytokines and signaling receptor components during termination or control of self-terminating acute inflammation. The cytokine receptor dual function (decoy behavior) was originally formulated for IL-1 and IL II receptors. Decoy receptors are structurally incapable of participating in signaling receptor complexes. However, they are able to sequester ligands that have subsequently been identified for IL-8, a member of the IL-1 family, and the TNFR superfamily (e.g., osteoprotegerin) [19–30, 80, 227, 250–266, 286–288, 297, 298, 303–311]. An example of extensively studied cytokine and decoy receptor function that is involved in the multistep carcinogenesis is tumor necrosis factor-alpha (TNF-α), a cysteine- rich cytokine and its receptor molecules (TNFR-1, TNF-Rp55, TNF-Rp75). The TNFRs act as transponders of TNF by receiving and transmitting signals that trigger inflammatory responses. The TNFR signaling mediates several biologically different functions during Yin and Yang of acute inflammation (programmed cell death) for maintenance of tissue homeostasis and elimination of host cells with damaged DNA. Environmental or chemical stimuli (exogenous or endogenous) can trigger the synthesis and production of TNF-α and its receptor molecules in a variety of cell types [e.g., MΦs, T cells (Th1, Th2), DCs, MCs or keratinocytes]. TNFR also has proliferative capabilities for growth of fibroblasts or thymocytes and induction of expression of superoxide dismutases to terminate acute inflammation (Yang), likely through expression of decoy receptor molecules (e.g., TNFdr). Other decoy receptors that participate in termination event of inflammation (Yang response) or proliferation of other immune or non-immune cells and cancer growth and angiogenesis, include receptor molecules for MCSF, iNO, PGE2 and/or histamine (released from 'leaky MCs into tissue microenvironment, independent from IgE-fcεR binding) [21–27, 80, 200, 227, 265–270, 287–293] (see Chap. 6).

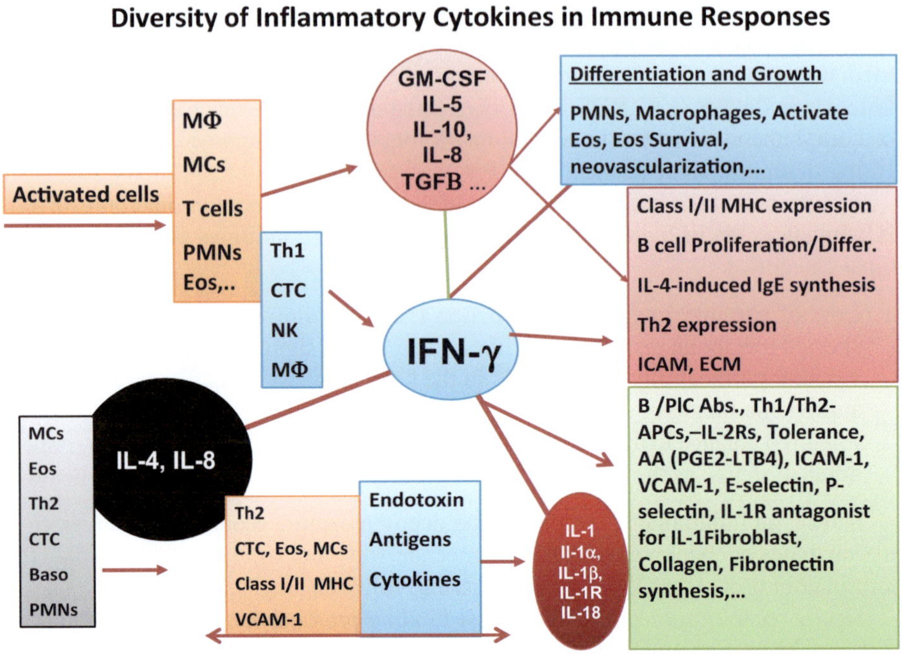

Fig. 3.4 Schematic representation of interdependent roles of inflammatory cytokines during tissue stimulation in acute or chronic inflammatory conditions. See text

In brief, the expression of apoptotic or pro-inflammatory mediators (Yin events) has two distinct features:

(a) Activation-induced cell death (AICD), which is a specific but 'peculiar' complex immune response dynamics for eliminating useless/excess lymphocytes that are produced during clonal expansion as a response to tissue antigenic stimulation;
(b) Damaged-induced cell death (DICD), which is a more generalized immune response to a variety of cellular insults, particularly oxidative metabolism, biological byproducts and autophagy/mitophagy function in tissues;

Antigenic-load and the presence of pro-inflammatory status in aging process are associated with subtle remodeling on the functions of apoptotic processes in AICD and DICD. Other minor or major changes in immune cell function (e.g., changes in DCs and MΦs, MCs, NKs functions, or T- and B- cell response profiles) including induction of decoy receptor molecules, are likely to contribute to the unresolved inflammation and age-induced immunosenescence and initiation of chronic diseases [21–44, 50–60, 80, 226, 240–298].

Accumulation of free radicals (e.g., ROS, RNS, ROO^-) signals that the status of oxidative-reductive potentials in tissue is imbalanced. Since stimuli-induced acute inflammatory responses are initiated through expression of danger molecules or the signaling receptors (e.g., TLRs, TNFR), long-standing inflammatory conditions (oxidative stress) or the loss of effective defense could also be through altered signals of decoy receptor molecules to control acute inflammation. Under-, or over-expression of decoy receptor signaling could influence the activities of tissue components, such as vasculature integrity; shifts in the ratios of tissue oxidative-reductive status and altered synthesis of cell phenotypes (e.g., changes in M1/M2/TAM or DC1/DC2) that would lead to tissue growth-arrest or growth-promotion, or altered tumoricidal vs. tumorigenic ratios of immune cells (Figs. 3.3 and 3.4).

6.4 *Role of Natural Killer Cells in Aging: Skewed Cytotoxicity*

Natural killer (NKs) cells have important and diverse functions within innate immunity as first line of defense. Recent studies demonstrate critical roles for NKs in reproduction and the most abundant cells (50–70%) at the maternal/fetal interface for induction of angiogenesis through specific MHC molecules. They also participate in control of adaptive immune cells and memory responses [21, 305, 312–328]. While the absolute number of NK cells, and the IFN-γ production and phagocytosis are increased in aging individuals, the NK-cell cytotoxicity on a 'per-cell' basis and the response to IL-2 is impaired. Age-associated increases in NK cells and in T cells expressing NK receptors was suggested to play a beneficiary role in immunosenescence and these effectors might blunt the growth of neoplastic cells in older individuals.

In the innate immune system, the levels of cytotoxic activities of natural killer (NK) cells has been shown to play critical roles in inhibiting tumor growth and metastasis in a number of studies. However, whether the inherent dual roles NKs (mature vs immature phenotypes) of immune surveillance is skewed during aging or carcinogenesis and metastasis are not well understood. Analyses of recent data suggest that cytotoxicity of human NKs and the presence of CD56 for lysing infected cells or oncogenically transformed cells may be altered by growth factors and membrane proteins such as human aspartyl-β-hydroxylase (HAAH), a member of the α-ketoglutarate-dependent 2,3 dioxygenase family that hydroxylates epidermal growth factor (EGF)-like domain in transformation-associated proteins [21, 305, 312–328].

Under certain inflammatory conditions, NKs may be considered as humoral as well as, cellular elements of the immune system for initiating crosstalk between innate and acquired/adoptive immunity through activation of vascular components. Some of the critical deficits in immunosenescence occur in stem cells and NKs, particularly, causing changes in T cell subpopulations that underlie the functional deficits of aging and extractable recovery from therapy [21, 80, 305, 312–328].

A number of reports show there are three primary changes in NKs-T cell function in aging:

(a) Decline in the number of naïve cells due to diminished thymopoiesis;
(b) Increased number of memory cells resulting in increased cytokine production;
(c) Dysfunctional accumulation of activated effector cells of limited T cell mutation and skewed T cell repertoire.

As noted above, while the absolute number of NK cells and the IFN-γ production and phagocytosis increases in older individuals, the NK-cell cytotoxicity on a 'per-cell' basis and the response to IL-2 is impaired. Age-associated increases in NK cells and in T cells expressing NK receptors was suggested to contribute and benefit immunosenescence that might blunt the growth of neoplastic cells in older individuals [21, 80, 305, 312–328].

6.5 *T Cell Immunity in Aging*

T cell dysfunction is associated with reduced thymic generation of naïve T cells, virus-induced expansion of terminal effectors and increased levels of memory cells producing skewed pro-and anti-apoptotic responses. One of the most critical components of the immune system during aging process is alterations in T cell immunity. The mechanisms that alter the normal homeostatic balance of T cell subpopulations during the aging process and stimulation of pro-inflammatory cytokine production and perpetuating large oligoclonal populations of immune dysfunctional cells are the topics of intense investigations [21, 22, 132, 133, 188, 232, 238–241, 243–246, 329–345]. The diminished diversity of the T cell receptor repertoire in aging, in all likelihood, is primarily due to two interdependent conditions:

(a) Elevation of pro-inflammatory cytokine milieu present in the elderly;
(b) Persistent oxidative stress-induced additional changes in the ratios of immune cells in the direction of Th2 and Treg expression;

A crucial event during an innate immune response is the process of antigen recognition and presentation by antigen presenting cells (APCs), to specific immune T cells for destruction. Both DCs and macrophages have been demonstrated to possess diverse functions depending on their microenvironments. Age-induced declines in T cell repertoire and accumulation of memory effector cells and genesis of oligoclonal complexes (megaclones) cause a condition of 'antigen-load' that could changes the dynamics of effective immunity in defending the vulnerable tissue against ubiquitous infectious agents or new antigen challenges. Age-associated changes in T cells include shifts in the population of subtypes of naïve and memory T cells which changes the cytokine profiles and T cell proliferative and cytotoxic responses. However, despite the extensive research on characterizing the alterations (decreases) in T cell immunity in elderly, little is known about correlation between immunological changes and clinically relevant decline in health outcomes. It is therefore essential to understand the details of alterations in T cell immunity, the potential relationships with vascular function as well as oxidative-reductive status so that the future of clinical interventions can be designed according to the extent of such changes to better manipulate and restore these fundamental systems for the aging population [30, 31, 309–342].

Overall analyses of data on the role of T cells in the induction of chronic diseases demonstrate that the formation of oligoclonal complexes results from accumulation of combined defects in one or more interdependent immune regulatory events including:

(i) Changes in immune response dynamics due to modifications of T cell MHC-binding regions (epitopes);
(ii) Alterations in antigen processing components that influence accumulation of terminally differentiated effector T cells;
(iii) Increased accumulation of genetic errors, leading to exaggerated or mismatched expression and synthesis of apoptotic and wound healing mediators (creating sustained inflammation);
(iv) Skewed expression of Th1/Th2 and Treg in response to infective agents;
(v) Skewed lymphocytes clonal expansion or polyclonal complexes and inability of immune and non-immune systems to properly respond to new challenges (e.g., viral, bacterial, neoplastic cells or vaccines);
(vi) Release of histamine, a vasoactive component from activated ('leaky') MCs, into microenvironment of vulnerable tissue;
(vii) Minor or major damages in mitochondrial oxidative phosphorylation and energy status of tissue, contributing to frailty;
(viii) Enhanced vulnerability of aging body toward new antigens and infective agents in the induction of chronic illnesses or cancer (Figs. 3.3–3.5).

The changes (decreased) in the ratios of Th1: Th2 responses are likely important contributing factors in age-associated immune dysfunction and multistep carcinogenesis. Release of histamine, an important vasoactive pro-inflammatory mediator (alkaline) from activated MCs, not only promotes a Th2 response, but it also induces polarization of DCs into Th2 cell-promoting effector DCs or DC2 s via interaction with the Th2 receptor, leading to immune suppression and carcinogenesis. Inhibition of histamine-receptor (H2) to reverse the polarization of activated DCs back to Th1 response and improve immune function in the frail elderly has been postulated [21, 46, 80, 344, 392, 395, 399–422].

The intrinsic process of T cell activation requires interaction between the T cell and antigen presenting cells (APCs). APCs are responsible for the uptake, processing and presentation of antigen in association with distinct major histocompatibility complexes (MHC) epitopes to antigen receptors on T cells [80, 337, 344, 392, 395, 399–422]. APCs work along with cytokines to initiate and determine the outcome of effector T cell responses.

Given the predominance of the Th2 and Treg response in the elderly, vaccine strategies may need to focus on mechanisms where humoral immunity predominates. In addition, nutritional supplements such as vitamin E, minerals, Cox-2 inhibitors that have shown initial promise for immunomodulation require further systematic investigation to ascertain their role in manipulating the immune system [21, 47, 80, 97–99, 327, 331, 337, 345, 399–422].

The T cell population displays an age-dependent decline of the absolute number of total T cells (CD3+), involving both CD4+ and CD8+ subsets, accompanied by an increase of NK cells with well preserved cytotoxic function and by a reduction of B cells. As noted above, one of the main characteristics of the immune system during aging is a progressive, age-dependent decline of the virgin T cells (CD95-), which is particularly profound at the level of the CD8+ subpopulation of the oldest old subjects. The progressive exhaustion of this important T cell subpopulation dedicated primarily to the defense against new antigenic challenges (viral neoplastic, bacteria or pathogen-specific vaccines), could be a consequence of both the thymic involution and the lifelong chronic antigenic stimulation. The immune function of the elderly, therefore, is weakened by the exhaustion of CD95- virgin cells (TH^0) that are replaced by large clonal expansion of CD28- T-cells. The origin of CD28- cells has not been completely clarified but it is assumed that they present cells in the phase of replicative senescence characterized by shortening telomeres and reduced proliferative capacity [329–337, 339–350].

In brief, upon maturation, T cells polarize into either T helper 1 (Th1) or Th2 cells, based on their cytokine profile.Th1 and Th2 cells represent two polarized forms of T helper cells. T cells which express patterns of both Th1 and Th2 cells are designated Th0 cells and they mediate intermediate effects that depend on the ratio of cytokines produced and the nature of responding cells. Th1 cells are involved in coordination or mediation of inflammatory or immune responses against bacterial, viral, and parasitic infections as well as other allergens or pathogens. The major cytokines associated with Th1 responses are interferon gamma (IFN-γ), tumor necrosis factor-β (TNF-β), interleukin-2 (IL-2) and IL-12. Impairments of Th1 responses have been associated with the pathogenesis of organ-specific autoimmune disorders, such as Crohn's disease, sarcoidosis, and unexplained recurrent abortions.

Th2 cells produce cytokines such as IL-4, IL-5, IL-6, IL-9 and IL-10. These cytokines are associated with humoral immunity and evoke a strong antibody response in certain diseases such as in accelerated progression from HIV infection, and AIDS, various atopic and inflammatory disorders, parasitic infections and allograft tolerance [21, 285, 329–337, 339–350].

Better understanding of the roles of Th1 and Th2 cells is of paramount importance for comprehending the mechanisms of protection against infectious agents and the pathogenesis of immunopathologic disorders as well as for the future directions for development of novel therapeutic strategies.

6.6 B Cells and Lymphoid Organ Function in Aging

The lymph nodes (LNs) and spleen have highly organized structural features that would allow interaction between T and B cells and the antigen-presenting dendritic cells (DCs) on a matrix made up by stromal cells. The optimal structure of the LNs and spleen require formation of tertiary lymphoid organs (TLOs) at the sites of infection or chronic immune stimulation and genesis of germinal centers. The knowledge gaps and controversies on the molecular mechanisms of TLOs formation and functions of these structures under a wide range of inflammatory conditions such as infections, transplantation, autoimmunity, humoral immunity (HI), as well as, aging processes, make it difficult to better appreciate the important roles that these immune-responsive systems play in health or diseases [21, 24, 30, 31, 336, 344–349].

The reported decreases in circulating memory B cells and germinal center formation in the elderly are suggestive of altered function of follicular dendritic-cells that also skew T cell responses and virus-induced expansion of terminal effectors and increased tissue levels of memory cells. The observed loss of response dynamics in innate immune cells and T and B cell subpopulation (cell-mediated immunity-CMI and humoral immunity-HI) in aging suggests their significant contributions in the increased risk of many infections, autoimmune diseases and other chronic health problems such as cancer in older adults. In addition, the response to vaccination that requires CMI-induced humoral response is significantly decreased in the elderly. Although memory lymphocytes can proliferate fairly rapidly upon stimulation with specific antigens; in general, the generation of such responses in the lung is not necessary unless components of innate immunity are overwhelmed by pathogen challenges that cannot be contained primarily by the innate immune system [21, 329–336, 339, 364].

Oxidative stress-induced skewed clearance ability of immune system and generation of dysfunctional lymphocytes could be viewed as additional foreign elements (self antigens), adding to the 'pool' of antigen-load and potentiating inappropriate immune responses and the induction of hyper- or hypo-sensitivity reactions or cross-reactivity, toward a wide range of stimuli that are not normally considered antigenic.

Several studies demonstrate the interactions between thymic epithelial tissues and thymocytes in experimental models of aging [21, 23, 131, 132, 133, 238, 239, 244–246, 249, 262, 363, 364]. The analyses of data illuminated many of the fundamental signaling pathways that are involved in regulation of thymopoiesis and the critical control points that potentially could reverse the age-associated thymic involution or immune reconstitution. For example, increased in thymopoiesis was shown in animal models of age-induced thymic involution after marrow transplant, by treatment with IL-7, growth hormone (GH) and Keratinocyte growth factor (KGF). GH therapy was shown to also enhance bone marrow cellularity and multi-lineage hematopoiesis, although improvement in follicular dendritic cells or B cells has not been established [21, 32, 244, 249, 363, 364].

The extension of these studies and applications of growth hormones or other cytokines involved in thymopoiesis and related marrow transplant for human should await a better understanding of the fundamental immunobiological heterogeneities that are unique to humans, particularly when therapeutic approaches are considered for site-specific cancers.

6.7 Germinal Center Dynamics: Antibody-Forming and Memory Cells

During germinal center (GC) reaction, B cells receive signals to produce high–affinity, isotype-switched antibodies as well as differentiate to memory cells or antibody-forming cells (AFCs). Therefore, changes in the GC reaction can dramatically affect humoral immunity. In aged animals, GCs are fewer in number and smaller. Antibodies from aged individuals exhibit less somatic mutation and are of less affinity [21, 41, 137, 356, 363, 364]. In an analysis on heavy genes and lineage trees of post-GC B cells, the mechanisms of somatic hypermutation was found to be intact in aged mice, and the changes in mutations observed in antibodies from aged animals were thought to be due to founder cells effects and/or the process of selection [342–346]. Additionally, striking tissue-specific differences were seen. Many of these observations of diminished germinal center responses can be attributed to poor APC (FDC) and Th cell function. During GC reaction, some B cells are triggered to enter the memory cell pathway. It is clear then, that a poor GC response in the elderly can attribute not only to the inability to clear an existing infection, but also the inability to protect against future infections. Defects in B cell memory are reported at all stages, from generation of memory cells in the GC to poor maintenance of the memory cells due to defective iccosomes, to ineffective reactivation of low-affinity, non-isotype-switched clones [41, 137, 138, 356, 363, 364]. B cell themselves may be defective in generating memory. GC reaction was suggested to be intact in aged mice, but its function merely delayed for B cell antibody production as demonstrated in a number of studies. Using murine model of aging it was shown that aged B cells were able to produce high affinity, isotype-switched antibodies in response to TD antigen, when provided with an appropriate environment. Another plasma cell population, the long-lived bone marrow plasma cells are decreased in number and have fewer germline mutations than AFCs in young animals [138, 356, 363, 364]. These studies suggest that B cell responses in aged animals are not defective but may merely have slower kinetics or decreased specificity.

6.8 Role of Neutrophils in Remodeling Extracellular Matrix and Angiogenesis

Polymorphonuclear cells (PMNs) are not a major constituent of the leukocyte infiltrate, but they might have a key role in triggering and sustaining the inflammatory cascade. Analyses of several reported data suggest that neutrophils participate in acute inflammatory processes, particularly during termination of inflammation (Yang or wound healing) and/or induction of tumorigenesis [21, 31, 365, 366, 367, 369, 393]. Briefly, during termination of an acute inflammation (Yang), neutrophils respond to signals of IL-8, expressed from activated innate immune cells, and release a series of enzymes that are involved in remodeling of the extracellular matrix (ECM) and neovascularization of target tissue. Activated neutrophils initially adhere to vascular endothelium and then potent binding occurs during this reaction. Adhesion molecules expressed on granulocytes such as CD11a, CD11b, CD18 are involved in these phenomena. After the initial reactions, granulocytes migrate out of blood vessels via LFA-1 (CD11a.CD18) and Mac-1 (CD11b/CD18) to exert bactericidal effects [21, 31, 365–367, 369, 393, 492–497]. Neutrophils-induced ECM remodeling involve activation of enzymes, such as matrix metalloproteinases (MMPs) including MMP-9 (gelatinase B), a family of Zn^{2+}-dependent extracellular proteases, to initially digest extracellular components (acting initially in the apoptotic arm of Yin process?). Following their actions, these enzymes are inhibited or inactivated by the tissue inhibitors of metalloproteinases (TIMPs). Neutrophils activation by IL-8 signaling and ECM remodeling processes also involve release of specific sulfatase and heparanase and growth factors (e.g., bFGF, chemoattractants) expressed from activated vascular endothelial cells and lymphocytes. The ECM remodeling events would allow activation and migration of neutrophils and expedite the recruitment of other immune cells responding the inflammatory cascade established by IL-8 release. It is suggested that the action of enzymes and growth factors that are involved in remodeling of the extracellular matrix provide less resistance or temporary loss of matrix integrity during termination of inflammation. Under oxidative stress or during carcinogenesis, lack of ECM resistance could provide an opportunity to facilitate influx of clumps of tumor cells and take advantage of the diminished cell-cell interactions in favor of tumor infiltrations and subsequent metastasis in secondary organ systems. Therefore, the presence of growth or wound healing factors could facilitate tumor angiogenesis and create an environment to further use wound healing signals such as IL-8 to attract neutrophils for remodeling in favor of tumor angiogenesis. Indirect support for the suggestion comes from analyses of related data that show another cytokine such as M-CSF induces cytokine production by monocytes (e.g., MΦs) and secondarily enhances expression of cell adhesion molecule (CAM) and superoxide anion production by granulocytes. In this process, IL-8 was reported to accelerate granulocyte chemotaxis and expression of adhesion molecules such as Mac-1 (CD11b/CD18), as well as synthesis of superoxide anion production by granulocytes [21–23, 31, 32, 80, 171, 276, 368, 497]. Teranishi et al. [368] showed that IL-8 production by monocytes from ovarian cancer patients, at day 14 after chemotherapy, dose-dependently increased with M-CSF, while the levels of GM-CSF and G-CSF secretion were not influenced. In general, the biological systems involved in IL-8 production by monocytes seem to have important roles in activation and expression of other cytokines such as the M-CSF and potential improvement of granulocyte functions. They also could secondarily enhance neutrophils chemotaxis that are further influenced by IL-8 expression of monocytes.

6.9 *Mast Cells: Innate Immune Cells Possessing Effector Cell Properties*

In mammalians, including humans, mast cells (MCs) as other immune cells originate from the hematopoietic lineage. MCs complete their differentiation in various peripheral tissues, and ubiquitously present in organs throughout the body. Originating from CD34+ progenitor cells in the bone marrow, mast cells circulate as undifferentiated mononuclear cells in the peripheral circulation and express c-kit (CD117), the receptor for stem cell factor [21–26, 30, 50, 51, 80, 367, 373–382]. MCs have tendency to localize around blood vessels, nerves, glandular duct as well as inflammatory neoplastic foci (Figs. 3.4 and 3.5). All MCs possess common characteristics of cytoplasmic granules storing biogenic amines (e.g., vasoactive histamine) and acidic proteoglycans (e.g., heparin), expression of plasma membrane receptors binding for IgE antibodies, cytokines and neutral proteases. However, MC populations are heterogeneous and show marked differences in their phenotypic expression of different proteases in their granules in distinct anatomical sites. Mast cell containing tryptase (MCT), also known as immune cell associated MCs, are predominantly located in the respiratory and intestinal mucosa, where they co-localize around T lymphocytes. MCs containing both tryptase and chymase (MCTC) are predominantly found in connective tissue areas of the skin, conjunctiva and synovium. MCs stain metachromatically, because of the presence of sulphated glycosaminoglycan heparin. In many organs and under physiological conditions, MCs are numerous and close to the capillaries. Maintenance of MCs growth is facilitated by dermal endothelial cells expressing growth mediators and chemotactic stem cell factor (SCF) [21–26, 30, 50, 51, 80, 367, 373–382, 386, 397–403, 405–418].

Possessing and expressing a wide range of biologically active mediators within their granules and cellular membranes, mast cells are considered multipotent effector cells of the immune system. Mast cells express a number of functionally important cell surface antigens and growth factors, such as stem cell factor receptor (SCFR also called kit ligand or CD117) as well as immunoglobulin E receptor (IgER, FC high affinity epsilon receptor). Tryptases (alpha and beta) are selectively and abundantly produced by mast cell degranulation and the levels of tryptase in the circulation provide a precise indicator of mast cell activation [e.g., during anaphylaxis]. Systemic anaphylaxis arises when mast cells, possibly along with other cell types, are provoked to secrete mediators that evoke a systemic response including vascular hyperpermeability reactions. Generally, in anaphylaxis elevations of histamine levels in circulation have been detected. However, suggestions of involvement of other innate immune cells such as basophiles and release of additional histamine in genetically modified food allergy-induced conditions such as asthma, utricaria, angioderma, atopic dermatitis, conjunctivitis, shock and cardiac arrhythmias deserve further studied (see Chaps. 5 and 6) [21].

Upon activation, MCs can induce or promote degranulation, migration, and/or cytokine production through respective ligand binding. Interactions and communication of external and internal molecules of activated mast cells can mediate surface molecule adhesion and also cell aggregation. The extent of mast cell activation and physiological responses e.g., expression of critical molecules on the surface of mast cells, depends not only on the extent of signal on the effected tissue/organ environment, but also on the stage of cell maturation. Under a variety of conditions mast cells express variable amount of activated surface antigen proteins such as CD25, CD63, CD69, CD88; cell recognition molecules, such as CD2, CD11, CD18, CD 50, CD54 or cytokine receptors [21, 80, 367, 373–382, 386, 397–403, 405–418].

MCs are recognized as the key cells in immediate or type 1 hypersensitivity reactions. However, their distribution throughout serosal and mucosal tissues and their close proximity to blood vessels have suggested their involvement in several other diseases. The number of MCs, primarily non-functional MCs, rise in pathological conditions often during oxidative stress involving increased angiogenic activity, such as psoriasis, atherosclerosis, rheumatoid arthritis, haemangioma and other neoplasms and tumorigenesis [21, 80, 367, 373–382, 386, 397–403]. We suggested that the rise in number of MCs, was due to oxidative-stress-induced production of unscheduled (not fully granulated) or increased in number of 'leaky' mast cells [21–26, 50, 80]. The extent of mast cell granulation and degranulations, or "leakiness" could determine the tumoricidal vs tumorigenesis function of MCs and contributions in cell growth. It was further hypothesized that the release of low-level histamine (independent from antigen-specific IgE-fc binding receptor aggregation), from 'leaky' or exhausted MCs in the microenvironment of tissue could signal for induction of angiogenesis and tumorigenesis (Fig. 3.5). Similar to allergic rhinitis, the atopic dermatitis, asthma, or conjunctivitis are often accompanied by increased circulating IgE. However, the circulating levels of IgE may not always correlate with the extent of clinical reactions as we reported for conjunctival-associated lymphoid tissues (details in Chaps. 4 and 6) [21, 23, 50]. In acute (immediate) inflammatory responses or hypersensitivity (type1) reactions, activation of MCs leads to

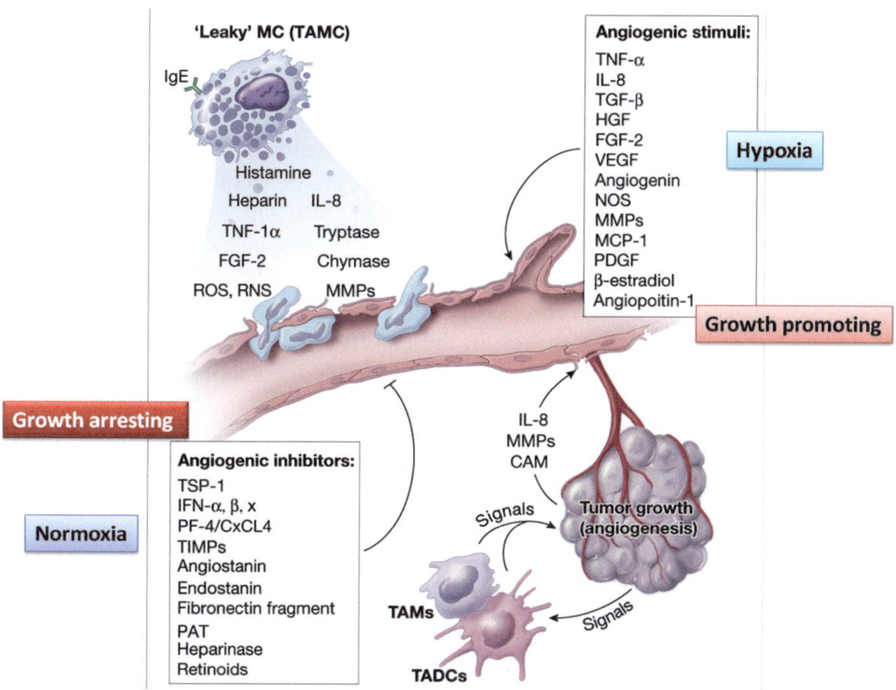

Fig. 3.5 Schematic representation of mast cells activities in chronic inflammation and the induction of angiogenesis and tumorigenesis. Modified from Khatami [30] Exp.Opin. Biol. Ther. 2008. See text.

crosslinking of receptor molecules Fcε RI-IgE and release of preformed vasoactive mediators such as histamine, synthesis of prostaglandins and leukotrienes, and the transcription of several other inflammatory cytokines, oxidants and neurotransmitters (Fig. 3.4) [21, 80, 367, 373–382, 386, 397–403]. The inflammatory mediators rapidly induce mucosal edema and mucus secretion, constriction of smooth muscle and hyperpermeability of vasculature to facilitate inflammatory cell infiltration.

Histamine, a potent vasoactive mediator of mast cell degranulation, exerts its effects via at least three receptors, H1, H2 and H3 expressed on vascular endothelial and lymphoid cells and the neuronal systems including the brain [21, 22, 50, 51, 80, 386, 397–403]. Histamine is a regulator of inflammatory responses and promotes allergic reactions, gastric acid secretion, and tumorigenesis. Studies using antibody titers and delayed type hypersensitivity reactions in rats demonstrated H2 selective antihistamines improved responses in HI and CMI. Analyses of data on using histamine H2 antagonists demonstrated boost of the proliferative response of T cells to IL-2 and improved healing of Herpes Zoster as well as increased survival of patients with gastric and colorectal cancers. The overall analyses of data on these and related studies on inhibition of histamine receptors seem to support the author's hypothesis that using mast cell stabilizers may be immunologically effective in preventing multistep pathways of tumorigenesis in mast-cell dependent tissue growth stimulation (details in Chap. 6) [21, 50, 80]. Among several mediators affected by continuous release of histamine into the target tissue are inhibition of apoptotic cytokines (e.g., IL-12, involved in Th1 responses or Yin), stimulation of IL-10 (mediated by H2 receptor during Th2 response and immunosuppressive or Yang) [21, 22, 50, 51, 80, 284, 285, 306, 307, 340, 360, 386, 397–403]. It was suggested that continuous release of histamine signals for shifts (decrease) in the dynamics of adaptive immune cells (Th1/Th2 ratios), similar to, or contributing to the response shifts occurring in favor of Th2 response immune compromise, and the observed increased allergic reactions in frail elderly (details in Chap. 6) [21, 80]. The hypothesis is further supported by an increased severity of inflammatory responses and inappropriate feedback control loop observed in atopic disorders and increased asthma in aging. The evidence also supports the use of H2 antihistamines to restore the Th2/Th1 and/or downregulate Th2 responses seen in the elderly. If the Th2 response could be restored to a level that is seen in the healthy individuals, a more normal Th1/Th2 ratio would result in improvement of immune function.

Through H1 and H2 receptor molecules, histamine also polarizes human immature DCs (DC1) into Th2 cell-promoting effector DCs (DC2 or TADCs) that would contribute to the immune suppression [21–27, 80, 308, 419, 420, 424]. As previously suggested, in acute inflammation, histamine initially signals for Th2 polarization and expression of growth factors for termination of inflammation. However, prolonged release of histamine (independent of IgE-binding to receptor occurs by 'leaky' MCs) is likely an attempt to induce termination of inflammation by induction of Th2 polarization (Yang). Overexpression of the CSF-1 and/or its receptor c-fms in mammary glands of transgenic mice results in hyperplasia and tumor formation [226]. Binding of CSF-1 to its receptor c-fms, which is a cell surface receptor belonging to a family of tyrosine kinase receptors, results in the dimerization and phosphorylation of c-fms, leading to macrophage proliferation via signal transduction pathways. Studies involving certain hematopoietic growth factors, such as CSF-1, have demonstrated that these substrates also affect normal and malignant cells of nonhematopoietic origin. Involvement of MCs and/or high expression of CSF-1 has been associated with a variety of disorders such as stroke, conjunctivitis, gynecological cancers (ovarian adenocarcinoma), non-Hodgkin lymphoma and hyperplasia, neoplasia and other cancers [21, 22, 23, 80, 226, 384, 389].

It is suggested that the release of low-level histamine, a negatively charged vasoactive agent, produced non-specifically in the microenvironment of tumor associated MCs (TAMC) or 'leaky' MCs is an immune suppressor, similar to production of arginine (also a negatively charged/alkaline amino acid) release from activated MΦs (TAMs or M2 phenotype) in the direction of tumor growth promotion (Figs. 3.4. and 3.5) [21, 22, 23, 80].

Mast cells have been shown to directly and indirectly influence growth and cellular functions of eosinophils, macrophages and T cells. The mediators involved, include T cell-derived IL-5, granulocyte-macrophage colony-stimulating factor (GM-CSF). These mediators also play a role in eosinophil activation, chemotaxis, and macrophage growth promoting activity. Mast cells also induce the release of factors/cytokines for program cell death, tumor necrosis factor-α (TNF-α) that interacts with eosinphil chemotaxic during apoptosis and cell growth arrest. Furthermore, synthesis and release of factors, such as mast cell/stem cell factor (SCF)-c-kit and its receptors regulates the function of mast cells. The level and nature of cytokines and chemokines present in the tissue would perhaps produce signals that regulate the activation or suppression of oncogene pathways such as Ras-MAPK through c-fos gene expression and induction of cancers or other systemic diseases (Figs. 3.4 and 3.5) [21–26, 50, 80, 375–382].

6.10 Function of Dendritic Cells in Immunity and Aging

Dendritic cells (DCs), originate in the bone marrow and found in peripheral sites of antigen uptake (skin, spleen, thymus, colon and synovia) as well as the blood. They are routinely responsible for initiation, activation and outcome of effector T cells (Th1 or Th2) resulting in immune responses. Resting immature DCs, also called DC0s, are derived from monocytes and are highly efficient for capturing foreign antigens. DCs form a network of sentinel cells in the periphery to capture and transport/ferry pathogenic antigens to secondary lymphoid tissues. Therefore, DCs are crucial for the initiation of primary immune responses [21, 52, 80, 308, 335, 419–422, 424–431, 439].

At least two classes of dendritic cells are considered as highly specialized APCs. However, other phenotypes of DCs have been identified in site-specific tissues under a wide range of inflammatory conditions and experimental model studies.

The following outlines the origins and basic function of dendritic cells in immunity:

(a) **Class 1 DCs – induction of tolerance.** Derived from bone marrow, DCs present the processed antigen to T cells and act as ferry for delivery/presentation of processed antigens to the naïve and memory T cells resulting in CD4+ and CD8+ immunity and tolerance. These cells do not synthesize antibodies or many cytokines and are not normally involved in phagocytic or antimicrobial activities.
(b) **Class 2 DCs-follicular dendritic cells (FDCs)**: FDCs are involved in presentation of native antigens as immune complexes to B cells to develop antibody memory-affinity maturation and immunity. The origins of FDCs are not clear but they may also arise from bone marrow.

Immature DCs (DC0 s, resting cells) are thought to undergo step maturation or transition (polarization) from type 1 (tumoricidal) dendritic cells (DC1) and type 2 (tumorigenic) dendritic cell phenotypes (DC2) during stimuli-induced migration and under the influence of growth factors/cytokines such as IL-1β [419–422, 424–431, 439, 452]. The inflammatory signals, that are involved in DCs maturation and migration to lymphoid organs, also induce a chemokine receptor switch, which normally cause down-regulation of inflammatory receptors (such as CCR1, CCR2, CCR5) and induction of CCR7, perhaps as contributing signals for termination of an acute inflammation (Yin-Yang). For example, as noted above, concomitant tissue exposure to lipopolysaccharide (LPS, stimuli) and IL-10, blocks the chemokine receptor switch associated with DC maturation. LPS + IL-10-treated DCs showed low expression of CCR7 (signal for apoptosis Yin arm?) and high expression of CCR1, CCR2 and CCR5. These chemokines receptors were unable to elicit migration. Relevant data showed that uncoupled receptors expressed on mixture of LPS+ IL-10-treated cells sequester and scavenge inflammatory chemokines. Similar results were obtained for monocytes exposed to activating signals and IL-10. Thus, in an inflammatory environment, it is likely that IL-10 generates functional decoy receptors on DC and monocytes, which act as molecular sinks and scavengers for inflammatory chemokines, to regulate and terminate (resolve) inflammation [21–27, 419–422, 424–431, 439, 452].

Again, since small numbers of DC are sufficient to induce an immune response, DCs are the most potent stimulator cells of T cells. Analyses of related data suggest that in addition to their roles for presentation of processed antigen to T cells during the induction of tolerance, DCs seem to be the only APCs capable of presenting novel antigens, to resting naïve T cells to initiate the primary immune response. This important feature of DCs has currently become the focus of considering DCs as prime targets for immunotherapy. Therefore, due to the highly importance of the DCs, any minor modulation in DCs function could result in significant alterations in immune responses. As recent data suggested, methods could be developed in the near future to provide elderly individuals with protection through enhanced route of administration, such as repeated vaccination (details in Chaps. 5 and 6) [422, 424–431, 439, 452].

Major or minor alterations in the number or function of DCs are associated with immune dysfunction, in chronic/persistent inflammation and the aging process [21–27, 80, 422, 424–431, 439, 452]. These changes include:

(a) Oxidative stress-induced DCs polarization to DC2 phenotypes (perhaps on both classes of DCs) and maturation processes resulting in the loss of capacity to capture antigen, increased capacity to present processed antigens to T cell due to increased expression of surface molecule involved in chemotaxis and T cell activation of major histocompatibility complexes I and II and costimulatory molecules (e.g., (CD-40) or potential loss of tolerance to antigens that ordinarily do not stimulate responses from T cells.
(b) Mature DC2 also produce T cell stimulatory cytokines IL-12 and IFN-γ. Soon after antigen specific interaction with T cells, mature DC undergo apoptosis via CD40 and FAS ligation, a mechanism thought to regulate unnecessary and excessive T cell or perhaps natural killer cells activation and expansion.

While, the current approaches to modulate the activities of DCs for, immunotherapeutic vaccination methods against infectious diseases in frail older adults are attractive, applications of such strategies require detailed understanding of the potential interactions and synergies between DCs and other APCs in site-specific tissues for effectiveness of such approaches as we recently demonstrated in conjunctival-associated lymphoid tissues [22, 80] (details in Chaps. 4 and 6).

6.11 Role of Macrophages in Acute and Chronic Inflammation and Aging

Macrophages are terminally differentiated cells of bone marrow derived from peripheral monocytes and reside in tissues (Fig. 3.3). In general, activation of monocytes by pathogens/microbial or their fragments, cause expression of pro-inflammatory death signals and mediators leading to migration into tissues and differentiation to pro-inflammatory cells or MI (tumoricidal), which are involved in the destruction of microorganisms and neoplastic cells. M1 function includes activation of other innate and adaptive immune cells and non-immune (vasculature, metabolism and neuronal) responses that facilitate enhanced synthesis and release of pro-inflammatory cytokines such as TNF-*α*, IL-1, IL-6, IL-12, and IL-23 and expression of chemokines such as CCL5, CCL8, CXCL2, and CXCL4 (Figs. 3.3 and 3.6) [21–26, 80, 260, 308, 337, 367, 368, 384, 393, 435–451, 504].

Macrophages occupy distinct regions of lymphoid tissues in the gut and mucosa. MΦs are influenced and activated by signals from intracellular microbial cell walls and by cytokines (e.g., TNF or IFN-γ), to produce numerous cytokines, enzymes, reactive oxygen species/ROS, reactive nitrogen species/RNS to kill intracellular microbes and to clear antigens, from the B cells and/or follicules of the lymphoid organs, the mucosal surface of the gut and the circulation. In addition, B cell proliferation and induction of plasma cell for specific antibody production are influenced

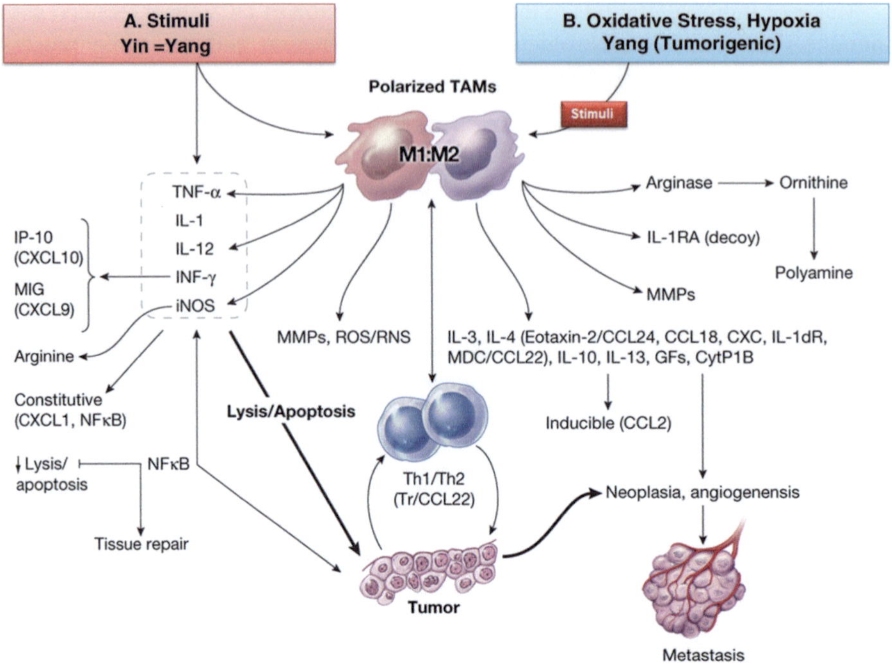

Fig. 3.6 Schematic representation of pleiotropic properties (duality) of macrophages (MΦs) in acute and chronic inflammation. Self-termination acute inflammation induces generation of a wide range of precise signals for apoptotic and wound healing from activated MΦs in their M1 and M2 (tumoricidal vs tumorigenic) phenotypes (**A**, *left panel*, Yin = Yang). The mediators include tumor necrosis factor alpha (TNFα), interleukins (ILs, IL-1, IL-12), interferon gamma (INF-γ), chemokines (e.g., IP-10 or CXCL10 or MIG- CXCL9), inducible nitric oxide synthase (iNOS) for arginine (Arg) metabolism, matrix metalloproteases (e.g., MMP-2, 7, 8, 9), reactive oxygen species (ROSs), reactive nitrogen species (RNs) other chemokines (e.g., CXCL 1) as well as expression of NF-kB and wound healing pathways. The outcomes are destruction (lysis) of viruses, defective tumor cells and infected host tissue as well as termination of inflammation and tissue repair. The **B** (*right panel*) oxidative stress-induced hypoxia favors polarization of MΦs in M2 (TAMs) phenotypes and expression of tumorigenic factors including activation of arginase and ornithine pathways toward polyamine biosynthesis, generation of decoy receptors in IL-1 RA (IL-1dR), MMPs (MMP-2, 9, 10, 11) or ILs (IL-3, IL-4, IL-10, IL-13), chemonkines such as CCL24 (Eotaxin-2), CCL18, CXC, MDC/CCL22, Cytp1B, which influence tumor growth, neoplasia, angiogenesis, and metastasis. Alterations in the ratios of M1/M2 impact cell-mediated immunity (CMI), Th1/Th2 ratios including regulatory T cells (Tr/ CCL22) leading to immune suppression and tumorigenesis (Modified from Ref. [23] with permission, All right reserved)

by signals from surface Ig receptor proteins of immune cells or lymphocyte-derived cytokines (lymphokines) such as IL-2, IL-4, IL-5, under inflammatory conditions, and could influence the dynamics of immune responses [balance between tumoricidal (Yin) and tumorigenic (Yang) properties] in the direction of tissue necrosis or growth and induction of chronic diseases (Figs. 3.5 and 3.6).

Macrophages have major roles in tissue remodeling and repair in inflammatory conditions and ontogenesis in adult life. Macrophage heterogeneity, possessing at least two types of cells (M1 and M2) perhaps reflects the plasticity and versatility of these cells in response to exposure to diverse microenvironmental signals. The immunoregulatory roles of these cells are increasing being recognized [21–23, 80, 260, 308, 337, 367, 368, 435–451, 504]. Differential cytokine production (pro- and anti-inflammatory mediators) is a key feature of polarized macrophages. The classically activated M1 macrophages are potent effector cells that kill microorganisms and lyse the tumor cells by producing copious amount of proinflammatory cytokines. In contrast, TAMs or M2 phenotypes produce a host of growth factors that affect tumor-cell proliferation, angiogenesis and the deposition and dissociation of connective tissues. By expressing cytokines from M2 (TAMs) phenotypes, MΦs participate in circuits that regulate tumor growth and progression, adaptive/acquired immune dysregulation, stroma formation and angiogenesis. Inflammatory conditions, causing dynamic shifts in immune responses include alterations in the ratios of polarized APCs, infiltrating macrophages, changes in the T cell subpopulation (e.g., decreases in Th1:Th2) that could promote tumor progression and metastasis in a cascade of events (Fig. 3.6).

The progressive immune dysfunction raises the possibility that systematic monitoring of molecular and cellular profiles involved at identifiable phases of inflammation-induced tumorigenesis might represent novel and valuable therapeutic targets. For instance, arginine metabolism is characterized by high levels of inducible nitric oxide synthase (iNOS) in M1 cells, whereas the arginase pathways predominates in the M2 cells with generation of ornithine and polyamines (Fig. 3.6) [21–26, 80, 367, 368, 384, 393, 435–451, 504]. Others have shown that inhibition of polyamine synthesis has been used in preclinical studies for cancer chemoprevention. Whether inhibition of polyamine synthesis restores antitumor properties of macrophages, e.g., shifting the ratios of M1: M2 polarities and favoring their tumoricidal effects, are yet to be understood. CCL8, for example, is a highly inducible chemokine that is clearly responsible for the elicitation of neutrophils as part of an innate response to a wide variety of challenges. In contrast, CCL19 and CCL20 chemokines are expressed constitutively and are intimately involved in the basal migration patterns of T cell and the formation of secondary lymphoid organs involved in adaptive response [21, 435–440].

As schematically demonstrated in Fig. 3.6, the maintenance of body homeostasis requires maintaining a proper ratio of both M1 (tumoricidal):M2 (tumorigenic or TAM) phenotype of macrophages. This balance is disturbed during altered immune response dynamics and unresolved inflammation in aging. Tumor associated macrophages (TAM) and the M2 phenotypes demonstrated similar functions in immune suppression and promotion of cell growth. M2 and TAMs phenotypes are poor APCs and express little apoptotic factors (IL-12) or toxins such as NO, but express high levels of mannose receptors (MR) and IL-10 primarily involved in growth promotion. Therefore, polarization of macrophage (and other innate immune cells) is a simplified model for conceptual framework of feedback control mechanisms describing how the Yin and Yang of acute inflammation may continue diverse operation of immune responses in health and diseases [21–23, 80, 260, 368, 384, 393, 435–451, 504].

In brief, the sequence of events and diverse biological activities of macrophages (professional APCs), under a wide range of acute (simultaneous Yin-Yang events) or chronic inflammatory conditions that may lead to tumorigenesis includes, but not limited to, the following (Fig. 3.6):

(a) Polarization/activation (M1) for recognition of antigen, induction of TLR molecules;
(b) Cytotoxicity and phagocytosis, burst of energy (ATP) from mitochondrial oxidative phosphorylation for antigen processing involving secretion of biologically active molecules, generation of toxins and oxidants (e.g., TNF-a, IL-1, caspases, NO) and related receptor molecules;
(c) Activation of cytotoxic T lymphocytes, NK cells and vasculature and generation of signaling molecules and receptors (e.g., MHC class I or II, CAMs, platelets activation) to facilitate apoptosis;
(d) High capacity for presentation of antigen to antigen-naive T lymphocytes;
(e) Activation, migration and differentiation of monocytes such as DCs in the direction of pro-inflammatory process for additional required oxidants and toxins for destruction of pathogens and target tissue;
(f) Immune response towards Th1 and/or Th17;
(g) Control/regulation of inflammatory process through induction of M2 (tumorigenic or TAM) phenotype during termination phase of acute inflammation (Yang);
(h) Termination of inflammation occurs by induction of decoy receptor molecules (e.g., IL-1 dR, TNFdR or IRAK-M), activation of arginase, induction of suppression of adaptive immune cells through expression of factors [e.g., NFkB, PGE2, IL-10, CCR2/CCL2, CCL17 and CCL22, MMP-2 and MMP-9, urokinase-type plasminogen activator (uPA)]. Expression of these wound healing mediators of M2 also facilitates tumor invasion and influence induction of Th2 phenotype, influx of T regulatory cells (Treg) and altered TCR during tumor growth promotion;
(i) Activation of B and plasma cells and induction of higher expression of certain membrane/surface receptors, including type 2 Fc receptor for IgG (Fc-R2, CD23), mannose receptor (MR), and receptor for LPS (CD14);
(j) Suppression of adaptive immunity, remodeling and repair of damaged target tissue and termination of inflammation;
(k) Persistent oxidative stress or aging could induce infiltrations, interactions and synergies of TAMs to the site of injury by activated host immune cells in the direction of immune suppression and tumorigenesis;
(l) Induction of hypoxia and expression of mismatched apoptotic and growth factors (immune chaos or immune tsunami) facilitate enhanced growth requirements of cancer cells with oncogenic features could lead to immune suppression and opportunities for tumor cells to evade immune surveillance;

Furthermore, maintenance of macrophages in TAM phenotype is assisted by T cells infiltrating human tumors in Th2 phenotype, with a predominance of $CD8^{+}$ in conditions such as Kaposi's sarcoma, perhaps gastric malignancies or colorectal cancer. Presence of TAM further induce expression of growth promoting mediators such as IL-4, IL-13, IL-10 or PGE2, which facilitate skewing of macrophage polarization in tumor environment. However, infiltration of TAM at site-specific tumors may not correlate with cancer patients' survival, as the presence of M1 in tissue have been shown to have cytotoxic and apoptotic activities that compensate for growth promoting activities of TAM in improving survival. As recently suggested, promotion of Yin and Yang activities of immune cells such as enhancing anti-tumoricidal properties of M1 in certain regions of neoplastic tissue may improve survival [21–27, 30, 50, 80]. As noted above, TAM are capable of modifying subunit of T cell receptor (TCR-ζ) or T-helper lymphocytes, which play a role in the activation of Th2 leading to induction of energy and apoptosis of T lymphocyte (Th1). Therefore, as with other immune cells, the duality or immunoregulatory roles of macrophages might contribute to the fate of tissue repair, growth promotion or necrosis under a wide range of inflammatory conditions [21–27, 30, 50, 80, 431, 303, 337, 434–451].

As schematically represented in Fig. 3.6, chemokines expressed from MΦs present both growth-arresting (Yin) and growth-promoting activities in vitro and in vivo depending on the conditions that they exert their effects. In general, in acute inflammation inducible chemokines are involved in attracting leukocytes (e.g., DCs, MΦs) to the tissue site of inflammation while constitutive chemokines control the basal trafficking of T lymphocytes for termination/resolution of acute inflammation. For example, monocyte chemoattractant protein-1 (MCP-1), also known as macrophage chemoattractant protein (CCL2), fits the role of inducible chemokine. At basal (resting), MCP-1 is rarely expressed but under inflammatory conditions, it can be rapidly induced [21–27, 30, 80].

Oxidative stress-induced expression of chemokines (e.g., CCL2, CCL22, CCL18) from activated MΦs (M2/TAMs phenotypes) are involved in amplification and regulation of the polarized immune cells such as T cell responses and often lead to changes in the Th1 to Th2 ratios influencing immune suppression and tissue growth in the direction of tumorigenesis or cancer. Reports on the formation of fibrous tissue in tumor stoma are major features in human tumors. Fibrous tissue formation, known to encapsulate parasites (or perhaps their substructures) could induce oxidative stress and continuous activation of M2 (TAMs) that signal for expression of chemokines or growth factors (e.g., CCL2 and IL-13, or TGF-β) and the induction of Th2 responses and suppression of apoptosis. It should be noted that nearly all tumor cells produce and/or induce abundant quantities of several chemokines (e.g., CCL2, M-CSF, TGF-β), in the direction of growth survival by either changing the receptor function (expression of decoy receptors) or by altering the chemokine response function that result in "hijacking" and satisfying their enhanced growth requirements (Fig. 3.6) [21–27, 30, 50, 80, 303, 337, 434–451].

6.12 Inefficiency of Immune System to Overcome New Challenges in Aging. A Cycle of Skewed Response Dynamics in Immune and Non-immune Systems

Immunosenescence is the result of minor and major skewed responses of immunity, including altered functions of vasculature and metabolic response dynamics that affects the immune-responsive and immune-privileged tissues as the bases for the genesis and progression of a wide range of age-associated chronic diseases. Numerous reports clearly indicate that the activity, availability and function of immune, vascular, hormonal and neuroendocrine systems change or deteriorate with aging. For instance, as the organisms age, changes in the activities, architectural and function of immune and non-immune systems influence reproductive, morphological, behavioral and biochemical properties in the organs/tissues. Age-related increased oxidative damage in a variety of cell types (e.g., T and B cell, APCs, mucus-secreting goblet cells, epithelial or endothelial cells) or cellular components (mitochondria, ER, lysosome, Golgi apparatus) and molecules (e.g., DNA/RNA, proteins and lipids) or transport systems in organisms, invertebrates or humans have been demonstrated [21–45, 80, 196, 197, 300–369]. Analyses of relevant data suggest that immunosenescence is not accompanied by progressive deterioration of the immune function, but it is rather the result of immune system remodeling where some functions are reduced, others remain unchanged or even increased. It appears that the ancestral/innate compartment of the immune system is relatively preserved during aging in comparison with the more acquired sophisticated adaptive compartment that exhibit profound modifications. Furthermore, data on biology of aging strongly suggests that continuous (chronic) up-regulation of pro-inflammatory mediators (e.g., TNF-α, IL1-b, COX-2, iNOS) that are expressed in aging are due to redox imbalance that activates many pro-inflammatory signaling pathways, including NF-kB signaling pathway [21–31, 186, 303, 335, 337, 380–562].

7 Cytobiology of Vasculature, Platelets and Complement in Acute or Chronic Inflammatory Diseases

Vasculogenesis is the earliest event in the fetal growth development. Activation of vasculature, neovascularization and angiogenesis are also normal required physiological events for growth and development, and facilitation of acute inflammatory conditions.

At resting, the homeostasis of vascular function (toning) and integrity is maintained by basal expression of vascular-derived angiognenic and anti-angiogenic factors. Mediators of activated vascular components participate in both apoptosis and wound healing processes. During inflammation, activation of vascular tissue components is necessary for increased vascular permeability (hyperpermeability) and infiltration of inflammatory cells to the target tissue. Stimuli induce vascular tissues to express mediators such as cell adhesion molecules (CAMs), vascular endothelial growth factor (VEGF), endostatin, epidermal growth factor (EGF), heparin and histamine receptors, membrane metaloproteases-MMPs. Other events such as activation of histaminase, heparinase or inhibitors of prostaglandin synthesis or NOS also participate during vascular tissue activation and inflammatory processes. These events are required for regulation of vascular permeability and passage of blood components (e.g., inflammatory cells, plasma proteins or complements), differentiation and migration of cells at the site of injury during both apoptosis and wound healing processes and for termination of inflammation (Figs. 3.5 and 3.6) [21–27, 30, 50, 80, 338, 452–454, 456–477].

Considered the tree of life, vasculature plays key roles in health and diseases with three principal functions:

(a) Delivery of nutrients and oxygen to tissues/organ systems and removal of gases and waste products from the tissues throughout the body;
(b) Gate-keeper of immune cells; involved in proliferation, differentiation and infiltration of inflammatory cells into stimulated (infected or injured) targeted tissues, facilitate both apoptosis (Yin) and wound healing (Yang) processes;
(c) Maintenance of crosstalk between neuronal-immune systems and organs/ tissues;

Being the gatekeepers for leukocyte trafficking, vasculature was suggested to play a most crucial role during both arms of Yin (apoptosis) and Yang (wound healing) responses with active participation of neuronal pathways and induction of mediators such as cortisol, epinephrine or norepinephrine [21–27, 30, 50, 80]. Upon tissue stimulation, vascular responses include leukocyte activation; differentiation and migration to the target/injured tissue; appropriate expression of cytokines and chemokines and receptor molecules as well as vascular-derived neuronal/hormonal components (epinephrine, norepinephrine, cortisol) during tumoricidal (growth-arresting) and tumorigenic (growth-promoting) responses. In an acute inflammation, activation, infiltration and trafficking of leukocytes to target tissue often involve vascular hyperpermeability reactions and crosstalk between mediators of immune inflammatory cells (e.g., TLR, TNF-α, ILs) and vascular components (e.g., CAMs, VEGF, FGF, PDGF), extracellular matrix and membrane proteases (e.g., ECMs, MMPs), responses from neuroendocine system (e.g., cortisol or epinephrine). A wide range of nutrients, metabolites and gases (e.g., adenosine, glucose, arginine, NO, CO/CO2), hormones (e.g., insulin), vasoactive components (e.g., histamine) and their respective receptors or surface molecules, also influence blood flow regulation and growth, B and T cell activities that initiate from fetal growth and undergo minor or major changes in aging [21–27, 30, 37, 47, 48, 58, 87, 117, 452–473]. It should also be noted that under oxidative stress, vascular permeability, function and integrity differentially impact tissues that are immune-privileged or immune-responsive leading to manifestation of site-specific diseases such as neurodegenerative and autoimmune diseases, diabetes and cardiovascular complications or neoplasia and cancer (Figs. 3.5 and 3.6) [21–27, 30, 50, 80, 224, 338, 399, 408, 452–497].

Outlined examples of major biological properties of angiogenesis in health and chronic diseases and cancer are provided below (Figs. 3.5 and 3.6).

1. Angiogenesis is part of the complex networks of immunity that functions within the highly regulated mechanisms of Yin and Yang of self-terminating properties of effective defense mechanism provided through acute inflammation.
2. Under acute inflammatory conditions, vasculature expresses required angiogenic and anti-angiogenic factors to facilitate both arms of Yin (pro-inflammatory) and Yang (anti-inflammatory) responses for maintaining body's protection against harmful foreign elements.
3. Maintenance of vascular quiescence (integrity) normally is achieved by the homeostasis of endogenous inhibitors of angiogenesis (anti-angiogenic) that are balanced by the pro-angiogenic factors.
4. Aging and oxidative stress alter, to varying degrees, the vascular toning or integrity leading to expression or co-expression of anti-, and pro-angiogenic factors and induction of molecular deposition of complexes and micro coagulation (unresolved inflammation) products such as oxidized lipids, proteins, metabolites (e.g., glucose, uric acid or creatinine), and immune cell complexes of under-, or over-expressed mediators that create an antigen-load. The complexes (antigen-load) could further signal for mismatched responses from immune and metabolic pathways leading to additional aggregated complexes at the vascular bed and initiation and progression of organ-specific health problems.
5. Generation of adenosine and receptor molecules (ARs) involves expression of vascular and immune cells ectonucleotidases and surface molecules (e.g., CD39, CD73) that are involved in regulation of blood flow and B and T cell dynamics (e.g., CD4+ and subset of NKT, Treg) during acute or chronic inflammatory conditions. Adenosine involvement in blood flow and immune cell dynamics is particularly important in solid organ transplantation-induced ischemia and promotion of immunogenicity of donor organ that could increase the risk of organ rejection [64, 295, 302, 390, 477, 478–481, 497, 515].
6. Tumor angiogenesis is associated with a more serious shift in the equilibrium between positive (angiogenic) and negative (anti-angiogenic) regulators of vasculature function that benefit tumor growth.

Several reports present compelling evidence that aging and unresolved inflammation induces minor or major changes in vascular biology and function, involving a wide range of chronic diseases such as adult-onset diabetes complications (e.g., retinopathy, neuropathy, angiopathy, nephropathy), impotence, neurodegenerative and autoimmune diseases, rheumatoid arthritis, stroke, epilepsy, cardiovascular complications, neoplasia/hyperplasia and cancer metastasis. Among the most important reported biological features of vascular dysfunction are neovascularizati on/angiogenesis, induction of hypoxia, loss of balance between pericytes and endothelial cells, association and deposition of molecular complexes [64, 295, 302, 390,

477, 478–481, 497, 507, 510–520]. Similar to the duality of the immune cells, under physiological conditions, angiogenesis is regulated by maintenance of balance between positive and negative factors and modulators requiring expression of angiogenic and anti-angiogenic factors, involving extracellular matrix proteins, adhesion molecules and receptors, growth factors and proteolytic enzymes. There are distinct gene expression patterns of angiogenic endothelial cells that are characterized by control switches of cell proteolytic balance towards an invasive phenotype as well as by the expression of specific adhesion molecules.

As part of the inflammatory response, the localization of leukocytes depends on cytokine-induced expression of vascular cell adhesion molecule-1 (VCAM-1) on endothelial cells (EC). Several reports demonstrate that VCAM-1 expression is induced on human umbilical vein EC (HUVEC) by both TNF-α, and IL-1α, in contrast to human dermal microvascular EC (HDMEC) that only TNF-α leads to expression of VCAM-1. To explore molecular mechanisms responsible for these contrasting patterns of VCAM-1 transcriptional activation, contrast studies with VCAM-1, and in vitro binding assays using two adjacent NF-kappa B binding sequences of the VCAM-1 promoter as a DNA probes, suggested requirements of the NF-kB motifs for VCAM-1 transcription and related pathways [492–497]. Furthermore, it was shown that the gene regulatory region of VCAM-1 is distinct from the NF-kappa B sites and potentially function as IL-1α -mediated transcriptional repressor within human dermal microvascular endothelial cell. It was concluded that the repressor region conveys IL-1α−dependent, but not TNF α−dependent, inhibition of transcription driven by a heterologous cytokine response on promoter gene [21, 64, 80, 470, 494–497, 507, 511–514].

Among pro-angiogenic factors, vascular endothelial growth factor (VEGF) plays crucial roles in biology of neovascularization and neoplasm growth. In acute inflammation, expression of VEGF is receptor-dependent, interacting with VEGF-R1 (pro-inflammatory for chemotaxis, activation of peripheral monocytes and MMP-9 and vascular hyperpermeability) and VEGF-R2 (anti-inflammatory and inhibition of vascular permeability) processes (Yin-Yang), respectively. The serum concentration of VEGF in patients is often higher than the plasma level, potentially due to the secretory activity of thrombocytes, which release high amounts of VEGF during blood coagulation. Analyses of relevant data on the role of VEGF in neoplasm growth suggest that VEGF acts through several interdependent pathways involving gelatinase A, decreased in tissue inhibition of endothelial metalloproteases (e.g., MMP 9), altered cell adhesion molecules and selective alterations in IL-1, as well as enhanced expression of NFkB that would lead to alterations of integrity of extracellular matrix and growth of neoplasm. It is possible that the continued expression of MMP-9 that normally signals for wound healing (Yang or termination) of acute inflammation, is viewed by neoplastic tissues as extended signals for wound healing and continued expression of VEGF-R2. The increased activity of VEGF-R2 receptor leads to an enhanced permeability of blood vessels ('leaky' vessels) and promotion of neovascularization processes within the neoplastic tissue resulting in proliferation of vascular endothelial cells and decreased ratios of pericytes:

endothelial cells. Furthermore, abnormal proliferation of endothelial cells are associated with inhibition of dendritic cell maturation and altered/decreased ratios of DC1/DC2 (TADCs), induction of NO, expression of CAMs, or perhaps altered ratios of M1/M2 (TAM), events that contribute to immune suppression, chronic inflammatory diseases, carcinogenesis and hypoxia-induced angiogenesis [21, 80, 478–481, 496, 497, 507, 510–520].

Other mediators, chemokines or pro-angiogenic factors whose altered activities are known to contribute to age-associated chronic diseases include (Figs. 3.4, 3.5, and 3.6):

(a) Basic fibroblast growth factor (bFGF) interacting through receptor molecules (e.g., FGF-R and FGF-R2);
(b) Epidermal growth factor and its receptor (EGFR);
(c) Interleukin-8 (IL-8), a chemokine acting through receptor molecules (A/CXCR1 and B/CXCR2) inducing migration of monocytes to neoplastic tissues. IL-8 directly correlates with vascularization of proliferating tissue, poor prognosis and advanced growth of cancers such as gastric cancer cells.

7.1 Platelets Contributions in Immunity: Shared Features with Innate Immune Cells

Until recently, platelets were considered as non-immune cell moieties with some immune functions. However, compelling data demonstrate that blood platelets display a number of functions and are special facilitators of acute inflammation contributing effectively in Yin (apoptosis), and Yang (wound healing) crosstalks. Platelets originate from myeloid cells and belong to the megakaryocytes (Fig. 3.3). During acute inflammatory processes, platelets play crucial roles in repairing (Yang, anti-inflammatory) the damaged vascular endothelium and stop bleeding and behave as innate immune cells, primarily through expression of PDGF and other wound healing mediators. They also participate in apoptotic events when they recognize a variety of danger signals from infectious agents, including pathogen-(bacteria)-induced acute inflammatory conditions such as sepsis. At least 1000 proteins/factors are reported in platelets activities, many are membrane-bound proteins and actively participate in immune response dynamics such as blood hemostasis, surface molecular shedding as well as pathobiology of diseases [21, 80, 462–468, 476, 505, 532–536]. For example, platelet-activating factor (PAF) is a potent phospholipid mediator and expressed in response to diverse immunologic and non-immunologic stimuli. In vivo and in vitro studies using PAF receptor antagonists demonstrated PAF involvement in a number of cardiac disorders such as ischemia, infarction and sudden cardiac death. PAF directly affects cardiac tissue by modification of chronotropic and inotropic activity; or indirectly causing coronary artery constriction, modulation of myocardial contractility and induction of arrhythmias by activation of membrane arachidonic acid pathways (e.g., cyclooxygenase-COX, lipooxygenase-LO) and the synthesis of eicosanoids such as thromboxane A2 (TXA2), leukotrienes (LTs) as well as expression of pro-inflammatory cytokines such as TNF-α [21, 80, 476, 505, 532–536].

An overall analyses of data demonstrate that platelets express several receptors with diverse (dual or pleiotropy) functions as other immune cells. The major known functions of platelets that closely resemble the duality of innate immune responses include (details in Chap. 6):

(a) Expression of non-mutated ligands (naïve proteins?) and toll-like receptors (TLRs), through pattern recognition receptor for binding to pathogens or pathogen-derived components (e.g., lipopolysaccharides) using distinct lipid A moiety that are different from classical receptor molecules (e.g., CRs or FcRs) of innate immune cells.
(b) Expression of innate/invariant receptors for the ingestion of a variety of microorganisms through different mechanism of actions for the purpose of destruction or inhibition of pathogenicity;
(c) Release a variety of molecular signals for crosstalk with other cells in the tissue microenvironment and/or to influence recruiting cells during an inflammatory process;
(d) Polarize and respond to activate cellular machinery upon receiving danger signals to repair tissue damage and wound healing processes;
(e) Expression of infection-induced TLRs possesses efficient functions for pathogen-specific production of receptors for antibodies and complement factors and interactions with innate immunity. The roles that CD40-CD40L (ligand) and adhesion molecules play in crosstalk between immune and non-immune cells, under inflammatory conditions, particularly during damage to vascular endothelium and disorders are under extensive studies [476, 505, 532–536].

7.2 *Nitric Oxide in Inflammation and Aging*

Nitric oxide (NO) is synthesized by vascular endothelial, immune and neuronal cells via NO synthases (NOS). The role of mediator is ubiquitous in controlling the function of almost every, if not all, organ systems in the body. Bacterial or viral products such as lipopolysaccharides (LPS) induce massive amount of inducible NOS (iNOS) from activated host cells that is toxic to the invading pathogens and inactivation of constituent enzymes, leading to target cell death. Actions of all NO (constituent and inducible) are mediated by the free radical oxidant properties of this soluble gas, as well as by activation of guanylase cyclase (GC), leading to the production of cyclic guanosine monophosphate (cGMP) for immune cell activation (e.g., induction of M2 or TAM) that mediate numerous physiological actions in health and a wide range of chronic diseases and cancer [21, 47, 84–90, 491, 492,

503, 506, 509, 511, 515–530]. For example, NO activates cyclooxygenase and lipoxygenase enzymes leading to the production of physiologically relevant quantities of PGE2 and leukotrienes as well as induction of IRAK-M for tolerance or growth (details in Chap. 6). In the case of iNOS, the massive release of NO, PGE2 and leukotrienes produce toxic effects [85, 491, 492, 503, 506, 509, 511, 515, 516–530]. Systemic injection of LPS causes induction of expression of IL-1 β mRNA followed by IL-β synthesis and by induction of iNOS mRNA in a time-course delay of 2 h and 4 h, respectively. The LPS-induced synthesis of NO affects the anterior pituitary and pineal glands, meninges and choroids plexus, regions outside the blood-brain barrier, and shortly thereafter, in hypothalamic regions, such as the temperature-regulating centers, paraventricular nucleus containing releasing and inhibitory hormone neurons, and the arcuate nucleus, a region containing these neurons and axons bound for the median eminence [85–88, 509, 516–530]. The question has been raised whether LPS similarly activates production of inflammatory cytokines and iNOS in the cardiovascular system and the gonads. It has been suggested that recurrent infections over the life span play a significant role in producing aging changes in all systems outside the BBB via release of toxic quantities of NO [85, 509–534]. NO may be a major factor in the development of coronary heart disease (CHD). Accumulating data indicate a role for the infections in the induction of CHD and indeed patients treated with a tetracycline derivative has 10 times less complications of CHD than their controls [47, 85, 503, 506, 509–530]. Inflammatory conditions induced by infection have been shown to cause activation of iNOS in rats that lead to progression of coronary arteriosclerosis and coronary occlusion. In aging, infections and activation of iNOS may play a role in the decreased secretion of the pituitary and pineal hormones (e.g., melatonin) in anterior pituitary and pineal gland as well as the temperature-regulating centers and the observed loss of thermosensitive neurons [85, 509–512]. Furthermore, aging and recurrent infection-induced iNOS in the paraventricular nucleus may cause the decreased nocturnal secretion of growth hormone (GH) and prolactin, leading to the destruction of luteinizing hormone-releasing hormone (LHRH), neurons that follow decreased genesis of gonadotropins. Persistent infections (unresolved inflammation) may play a role in the observed increases in the numbers of brain astrocytes expressing IL-1β in older patients [85, 509–538]. Published data also suggest that IL-1 and products of NO activity accumulate around the plaques in Alzheimers' patients. During World War I, a role for activation of iNOS was suggested in early onset of Parkinson's disease, coupled with aging process, damaging the survival of cells adjacent to substantia nigra dopaminergic neurons as the result of flu-induced encephalitis. It should be noted that the pathology of the central nervous system (CNS) in patients with AIDS bears striking resemblance to aging biological changes, and may also be largely caused by the action of iNOS. Antioxidants, such as melanin, vitamins C, D, E, probably play important acute and chronic roles in reducing or eliminating the oxidant damage produced by NO [47, 85, 503, 506, 509–530].

8 Autophagy and Mitophagy in Inflammation and Aging

Among numerous biological alterations that occur under oxidative stress and aging, the body's 'self eating' processes provided through cellular lysosome, mitochondria and Golgi membrane recycling pathways for degradation and regeneration of proteins and lipids, termed autophagy (macroautophagy) and mitohormesis play crucial roles in maintenance of immunity, physiology and metabolism of tissues and during immunosenescence and chronic diseases. Mitochondrial dysfunction (mitophagy) has been linked to a number of age-associated or chronic health conditions, including migraine, cardiovascular and neurodegenerative diseases, sarcopenia, cancer, infertility, kidney and liver diseases, drug toxicities and related illnesses [21, 23, 30, 66, 75, 80, 91, 100, 102, 110–120, 148, 149, 154–167, 275–277, 510, 511, 542–584]. Relevant data indicate that the key biochemical functions of mitochondria are beyond its physiological roles as the energy power plant of the body's tissues and cells. In recent decades, the biology of mitochondria has been the focus of active basic research and clinical studies and as potential target for drug development and prevention for a number of pathological and chronic conditions including aging process and cancer (details in Chaps. 2 and 6) (Fig. 3.7) [21, 23, 30, 66, 75, 80, 91, 100, 102, 110–120, 156, 159, 160, 164, 165, 275–277, 510, 511, 543–548].

Observations on the association of defects in energy metabolism in cancer cells in relationship with respiration (oxidative phosphorylation) and the abnormal rates of aerobic glycolysis for ATP synthesis that originally reported by Otto Warburg, led to mitochondrial injury (mitophagy) concept [557–562]. Since these important observations research in metabolism of cancer cells and the role that mitochondria

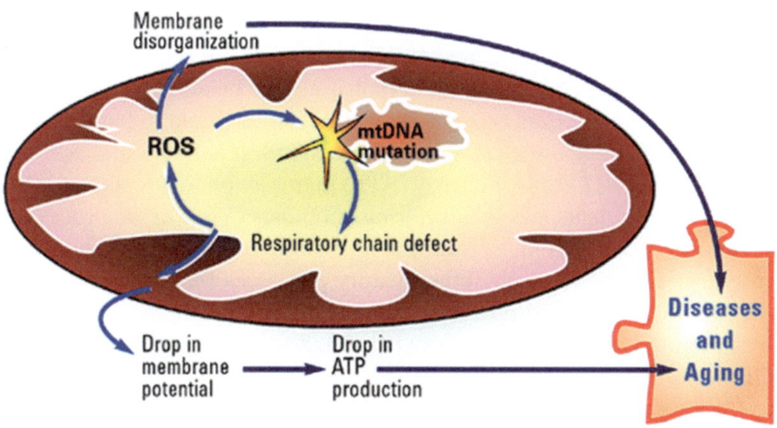

Fig. 3.7 Proposed mechanisms of mitochondria dysfunction. (*1*) Mitochondrial DNA (mDNA) mutation caused by free radical damage; (*2*) Kreb's cycle decreased efficiency due to inadequate Kreb's cycle intermediates; (*3*) Respiratory chain defect due to enzyme and substrate alteration; and (*4*) Membrane Disorganization and loss of fluidity (Reproduced from Rustin et al. 'Defective mitochondria, free radicals, cell death-Reality or myth-ochondria'. Mech Age Develop, Ref. [75])

play in cancer growth extended to the presentation of two well-known hypotheses of 'Crabtree effect' and the 'Pasteur effect' that may be defined as the following interdependent (cause and effect) biological events that would satisfy tumor growth [21, 80, 561, 565, 569, 578–582]:

(a) **Crabtree Effect:** the tumor cells trigger the competitive inhibition of oxidative phosphorylation (respiration) for phosphate groups (Pi) and ADP, by glycolysis for their enhanced growth requirements;
(b) **Pasteur Effect:** the tumor cells induce inhibition of glycolysis by elevated oxygen concentration.

These concepts argue that cancer cells have higher rates of consumption for either oxygen or glucose, when concentration of the either nutrient is reduced in the microenvironment of cancerous tissue. The concepts suggest the survival adaptability of cancer cell metabolism in adjusting to their microenvironment under the following conditions that are toxic to normal cell survival:

(a) Increased mutations or alterations and damage in mitochondrial DNA;
(b) Elevation of hexokinase production;
(c) Lysis or loss of mitochondrial cristae structures and altered mitochondrial protein and lipid content;
(d) Potential utilization of mitochondrial cardiolipin as additional sources of energy;

Furthermore, as analyses of recent data suggest cancer cell mutations and dysregulation of pathways for expression of PI3K/Akt and the altered balance in the activity of c-MYC, HIF, or p53 alter glucose and amino acids transport and metabolism [21, 80, 177, 438, 483, 544–547, 561, 565, 569–577, 582]. The content and composition of cardiolipin, a key mitochondrial lipid located in the inner membrane of mitochondria, necessary for efficient cellular oxidative phosphorylation (respiration) or maintenance of chemiosmosis demonstrated to be abnormal in cancer cells. While details of reported data on the role of mitochondria and inflammation in diseases of aging are debatable and not well understood, it is likely that acute inflammation initially causes a burst of energy (ATP) in mitochondria of activated immune cells, to generate oxidants and toxins during apoptosis (Yin). In the process cardiolipin molecules oscillates/moves from the inner to outer mitochondrial membrane, apparently to facilitate the acute inflammatory processes for termination or wound healing (Yang) events and to prevent further oxidative metabolism, contributing to the protective mechanisms of immunity [21, 23, 80].

Validation of the above integrated concepts awaits systematic studies of the relationships between bioenergetics of mitochondria during acute and chronic inflammatory processes, and better understanding of the bases for dysregulated protein recycling pathways (autophagy) and the roles that genetics and epigenetics play in health or disease processes to be beneficiary for prevention or treatment of chronic diseases.

9 Hormonal, Metabolic and Lipid Adaptations-Rearrangements in Aging

Multiple and diverse roles of important hormones (e.g., estrogen, progesterone, insulin, glucagons, androgen, andosterone, testosterone, thyroxine, glucocorticoids, mineralcorticoids, dehydroepiandosterone-DHEA) and hormone-like growth factors (e. g., IGF-1, FGF, EGF, VEGF) on the regeneration and function of organ systems and tissue physiology, development and metabolism in health and age-associated diseases have been extensively documented [21–27, 30, 50, 58, 64, 77, 80, 102, 103, 111, 128, 176, 247, 271, 540, 547, 587–634]. The influence of these important hormones and growth factors in the biology of aging tissues (e.g., neurogenesis, myelination, cognition, bone, immunity, metabolism) in the induction of chronic diseases (e.g., diabetes, vascular complications, cardiovascular diseases, atherosclerosis, osteoporosis, Alzheimer's and site-specific cancers) also have been the focus of many recent studies (Figs. 3.1 and 3.2). For example, the age-associated hormonal alterations on thymic atrophy and associated declines in the genesis of subsets of T cells, particularly peripheral T cells have been linked to immune dysfunction, cell death and immunosenescence [23, 25, 131–134].

In general, hormones including gonadal and sex steroids (e.g., estrogen, androgens, testosterone, progerstrone), DHA/DHEA, insulin or parathyroid hormones (e.g., 1–25 dihydroxy vitamin D, and calcitonin) play crucial roles in the regulations of a wide range of physiological functions in the body such as reproductive systems, organogenesis, fluid homeostasis, bone structure, membrane and intracellular signaling pathways, metabolic and immune responses to stress. The roles that these hormones play, to varying degrees on the physiology, function and remodeling of bone, neuronal function, myelination and neurogeneration of brain and CNS and/or membrane-associated fatty acid metabolism have been extensively studied in experimental models of diseases and in human subjects [21, 23, 58, 80, 590–599, 602–622]. Details on the role of the hormones in health and diseases are beyond the scope of this book. A brief overview of some of the known function of hormones under the influence of oxidative stress and age-associated diseases should help understand the common links in the biology of aging. For example, changes in estrogen or testosterone are associated with increased production of pro-inflammatory cytokines; alterations in bone resorption and remodeling, and changes in essential fatty acid metabolism as contributing factors in osteoporosis and other age-associated illnesses such as atherosclerosis or cancer. Furthermore, insulin deficiency and glucose toxicity (hyperglycemia), or insulin-induced expression of inflammatory mediators such as NF-kB and Ikappa B kinase (IKK-beta, encoded by IKbKb), or surface proteins (e.g., CD40L) in platelets', adhesion molecules (e.g., VCAM-1) on hepatocytes, endothelial or myeloid cells have been reported. Details of the role that insulin deficiencies play in insulin-dependent (e.g., muscle, liver, adipocytes) or insulin-independent tissues (e.g., vasculature, kidney, nerves, retina,

RPE, lens) as well as, the influence of increased non-enzymatic glycosylation of proteins in alterations of functions of important proteins or metabolites has been extensively studied [21, 23, 58, 64, 77, 102, 111, 271, 540, 547, 548, 598]. A closer examination of the available data on a variety of cytokines (e.g., TNF-α, ILs, VEGF) and receptor molecules on the endogenous hormones and hormone-like factors such as cortisol, epinephrine, neurotransmitters (e.g., norepinephrine) or melatonin, which also contribute to the growth and immune responses, suggest that aging process elevates the circadian rhythm of these factors and the observed pathophysiological responses. The overall responses are suggestive of compensatory sympathetic outflow increases, that elevate norepinephrine levels, via activation of adrenoceptors (α & β)-stimulation of the heart, vasculature, kidney and significant changes in the heart rate that influence cardiac output, peripheral vascular resistance, renal blood flow or urine output. In addition, the effect of age on response to dexamethasone treatment among the control group supports the hypotheses that the sensitivity of glucocorticoids negative feedbacks decrease with age [21, 70, 80, 251, 589]. Whether these effects reflect the stress-induced down-regulation of pituitary corticotrophin releasing factor (CRF) receptors and/or accumulation of mismatched inflammatory mediators and changes in the circadian nature of body's biology (positive and negative feedback control mechanisms or Yin and Yang of immunity) remain to be understood. Other biological systems with important potential pleiotropic roles are the suppressor molecule, silence signal regulating factor 1 (SIRT1, sitruin 1, also known as silent information regulator 1) and melatonin-related processes as clock proteins in facilitating cellular and metabolic dynamics of sensing and controlling the induction of senescence and carcinogenesis [21, 74, 122, 526, 619, 620].

9.1 Inflammation-Induced Sarcopenia or Cachexia in Aging

Sarcopenia or muscle loss (waste) in aging has multifactorial origins, involving activities of neuronal, immunological and physiological pathways [21, 23, 80, 146, 199, 291, 346, 347, 551–553, 575, 628]. Analyses of related data including cancer targeted drug-induced cachexia or sarcopenia suggest that sarcopenia is a smoldering inflammatory dynamics, driven by mismatched expression and co-expression of mediators and accelerated rate of unresolved inflammation (immune tsunami or immunological chaos) similar to other diseases of aging including arthritis or cancer affecting different organ systems. The severe conditions resemble the life-threatening effects of cancer 'targeted' drugs and induction of cachexia or aneroxia (details in Chap. 6) [21, 23, 80]. The overall contributing factors in the complications of age-associated sarcopenia or cachexia include:

(a) Changes in the anabolic hormones such as DHA, glucocorticoids, thyroxine, insulin, estrogen, testosterone and related receptor proteins;
(b) Loss of alpha-motor neuron input, decreased intake of dietary protein, and decline in physical activity;

(c) Associated changes in glucocorticoid negative feedback inhibition of hypothalamic corticotropin-releasing factor (CRF) and pituitary ACTH;
(d) Elevated levels of interleukin-6 and C-reactive protein;
(e) Sarcopenic obesity often displays inflammatory burden due to continued activation of adipocytes and associated expression of adipokines.

There are debates whether sarcopenia is a distinct feature of a disease or it is a milder and evolving form of cachexia or anorexia observed in older adults. Furthermore, the beneficiary roles of hormones such as dehydroepiandrosterone (DHEA) and its sulfate ester (DHEAS, a reservoir for DHEA) which are antioxidants and weak androgens and primarily produced by adrenal gland, have been reported in treatment of such metabolic disorders (e.g., diabetes or hepatic injury) or longevity and prevention of cancer. Potential recommended interventions for sarcopenia include nutritional supplements, physical activity/resistance exercise, caloric restriction, anabolic hormones, anti-inflammatory agents, vitamin E and other antioxidants [21, 23, 80, 97–99, 139, 346, 551, 553].

9.2 *Fatty Acid (Lipid) Biology in Inflammation and Aging*

Long-chain polyunsaturated fatty acids (essential fatty acids-FAs) including membrane arachidonic acid (AA) metabolites such as prostaglandins (e.g., PGI2/PGF-1α, PGD, PGE2), leukotrienes (e.g., LT4, LTC), phosphatidylinositol (PI), phosphatidylserine (PS) together with their respective receptors and enzymes (e.g., COX, LO, phospholipases A, B and C, leukotriene synthases) play crucial roles in regulation, metabolism and function of tissues. For example, membrane fatty acids are involved in a wide range of signal transduction mechanisms and crosstalk during immune and hormonal responses, vasculogenesis and vascular toning, bone remodeling and function in health and diseases of aging [21–27, 80, 87, 157, 153, 287, 370, 420, 441, 450, 505, 544, 589, 621]. Aging-associated thymus involution along with oxidative stress and certain life styles (e.g., smoking, heavy alcohol consumption) are factors associated with increased levels of pro-inflammatory mediators (e.g., IL-1, TNF-σα, IL-6) and decreased body's capacity to metabolize and convert precursor of FAs into polyunsaturated FAs that could lead to physiological changes such as decreased in bone mass, resorption and remodeling and impaired calcium balance, alterations of osteoblastogenesis, osteoclastogenesis, and functions of osteoblast and osteoclast during menopause, as well as rheumatoid arthritis. Bone and vascular remodeling and function are controlled by activation of a sophisticated membrane-lipid complex interactions involving intracellular soluble form of ligands and inflammatory mediators [e.g., receptor-activator of nuclear-kappa B (RANK) and ligand binding (RANKL), decoy receptor proteins and bone-specific osteoprotegrin (OPG)] that are essential for differentiation and activation of osteoclasts [192, 283, 408, 417, 434, 493, 575, 602].

10 Concluding Remarks

The increased rate of population among healthy older individuals around the globe suggests that the aging process is not necessarily associated with illnesses. Older people can lead a healthy, active and productive life well beyond the current standard age of retirement that is set at 65–70 years. However, longevity and extensive inflammatory response alterations in the pathways of immune and non-immune networks, particularly the vascular system, seem to be the principal common links in many age-associated chronic health problems such as asthma, hypertension, autoimmune and neurodegenerative diseases, diabetes and cardiovascular complications, stroke, neuronal dysfunctions, Alzheimer's, Parkinson's and site-specific cancers. Aging process itself cause minor or major alterations in the function of immune and non-immune systems that are the bases for altered inflammatory responses to various old and new stimuli. It should be emphasized that the loss of effective immunity is the combined changes of the balance between the biphasic response profiles (two biologically opposing arms) of acute inflammation, initiated by activation of immune cells and facilitated by negative and positive factors of vasculature (angiogenic and antiangiogenic mediators), oxido-redox potentials (oxidants and anti-oxidants), as well as, dysregulated dual capacities of metabolic and neuronal pathways.

The second laws of thermodynamics and physics may apply to the body's growth dynamics from fetus development to the aging process. Here we assume that in a normal healthy adult effective immunity conducts orchestration of a fascinating successful and orderly network of positive and negative chemical/biological signals (biological control switches) that constitutes the Yin-Yang of self-terminating acute inflammation for protecting the body against exposures to all potential hazards throughout life. However, biological and immunological rearrangements that occur in organ systems during normal aging are associated with decays or retardation, to varying degrees, of the ordered duality of Yin-Yang that would create general biological chaos. Recently, we hypothesized a concept specifically related to the role that chronic inflammation-(oxidative stress)-induced 'immunological chaos' or 'immune tsunami' damages to the architectural integrity and function of tissues toward retardation or altered dynamics of immunity in the direction of tissue necrosis or neoplasia [21–27, 80]. It is likely that the type and extent of vulnerability of an organ or tissue toward the drifts in the three fundamental systems of genomic stability, immune cells and oxidative stress determine the outcomes of a particular disease process. For example, loss of immunity and altered vascular integrity, including changes in oxido-redox balance in tissues that are immune-privileged (e.g., blood brain barrier or CNS) could result in diverse manifestations of neurodegenerative diseases such as the stroke, Alzheimer's, Parkinson's or even brain tumors. This takes into consideration of the anatomical barriers loss in brain (BBB) and biological differences of the brain architectural structure (e.g., vasculature, glial and neuronal tissue) and function within the oxidative-sensitive tissues of the brain, compared with those tissues that are classically known as immune-responsive (e.g., epithelial, endothelial, vasculature).

Experimental manipulations that slow down aging, such as dietary restriction and result in promotion of immunity are proposed to increase oxidative stress resistance and longevity. Strategies for maintaining the pleiotropic roles of antigen presenting cells (APCs) are highly desirable targets as these cells are responsible for enhancing and preserving the T cell responses during the aging process. It is noteworthy that modulations of T cell differentiation have limited capacity after puberty. Therefore, stabilizing the duality of innate (APCs) immune cell responses at APC-T cell interface could prove to be a key in reversing impaired immune function.

Significant improvement of health, particularly for the older population ultimately comes from better understanding of the complex molecular and cellular processes that are collectively involved in declines of immunity during aging. The future directions for systematic studies of the heterogeneities of the biological systems would require constructing a useful 'roadmap' that identifies the interrelationships between inflammation and a wide range of biological events that are considered co-morbidity and co-mortality risk factors in increasing the genesis and progression of chronic illnesses. Developing a 'roadmap' to identify the key biological control mechanisms that govern the biology of aging process is a timely, challenging and important undertaking for the scientific community toward improving the health of growing population around the world.

11 Author's Personal Note

The current combination of economic burden of sick-care to the society and the increased population of older adults around the globe require making conscience decisions that the public deserves; that is the need for switching to a culture of healthcare for a more productive society, particularly in the USA. As reflected throughout this book, a personal goal of the author is to continue these challenging scientific and professional attempts for making professionals and public to appreciate that the mission of public health should not be maintenance of costly 'sick-care' that only benefit the medical/cancer establishment and associates in big pharma and food industry.

Again, there is a need to switch this wasteful culture of 'sick care' to the culture of 'health care' where prevention of diseases outweighs the therapeutic approaches.

Immunity in Health and Disease
Effective immunity is crosstalk between the molecular village of negative and positive (Yin-Yang) signals that guard the body for maintaining health. However, a few bugs or aging process can disturb this amazingly orchestrated and secretively successful molecular operation to make us sick!

References

1. Komiya K, Ishii H, Kadota J. Healthcare-associated pneumonia and aspiration pneumonia. Aging Dis. 2014;6:27–37.
2. Hedlund J. Community-acquired pneumonia requiring hospitalisation. Factors of importance for the short-and long term prognosis. Scand J Infect Dis. 1995;97(Suppl):1–60.
3. Swenson CE, Sadikot RT. Achromobacter respiratory infections. Ann Am Thorac Soc. 2015;12:252–8.
4. Komiya K, Ishii H, Kushima H, Sato S, Kimura H, et al. Physicians' attitudes toward the definition of "death from age-related physical debility" in deceased elderly with aspiration pneumonia. Geriatr Gerontol Int. 2013;13:586–90.
5. Bruce AM, Spencer JM. Prevalence of community-acquired methicillin-resistant Staphylococcus Aureus in a private dermatology office. J Drugs Dermatol. 2008;7:751–5.
6. Mpenge MA, MacGowan AP. Ceftaroline in the management of complicated skin and soft tissue infections and community acquired pneumonia. Ther Clin Risk Manag. 2015;11:565–79. doi:10.2147/TCRM.S75412. eCollection 2015
7. Ewig S, Welte T, Chastre J, Torres A. Rethinking the concepts of community-acquired and health-care-associated pneumonia. Lancet Infect Dis. 2010;10:279–87.
8. Health Protection Agency Surveillance of Healthcare Associated Infections Report. 2008. [Accessed April 29, 2014]. Available from: http://www.hpa.org.uk/webc/HPAwebFile/HPAweb_C/1216193833496.
9. Torok E, Moran E, Cooke F. Oxford handbook of infectious diseases and microbiology. Oxford: Oxford University Press; 2009.
10. Attridge RT, Frei CR. Health care-associated pneumonia: an evidence-based review. Am J Med. 2011;124:689–97.
11. Chalmers JD, Taylor JK, Singanayagam A, Fleming GB, Akram AR, et al. Epidemiology, antibiotic therapy, and clinical outcomes in health care-associated pneumonia: a UK cohort study. Clin Infect Dis. 2011;53:107–13.
12. DHHS. DHHS report: Health United States with special feature on prescription drugs. Washington, DC: DHHS; 2013.
13. Riquelme R, Torres A, El-Ebiary M, de la Bellacasa JP, Estruch R, Mensa J, Fernández-Solá J, Hernández C, Rodriguez-Roisin R. Community-acquired pneumonia in the elderly: a multivariate analysis of risk and prognostic factors. Am J Respir Crit Care Med. 1996;154:1450–5.
14. Sader HS, Farrell DJ, Jones RN. Antimicrobial susceptibility of gram-positive cocci isolated from skin and skin-structure infections in European medical centres. Int J Antimicrob Agents. 2010;36:28–32.
15. Terracciano A, Löckenhoff CE, Zonderman AB, Ferrucci L, Costa PT. Personality predictors of longevity: activity, emotional stability, and conscientiousness. Psychosom Med. 2008;70:621–7.
16. Boucher H, Miller LG, Razonable RR. Serious infections caused by methicillin-resistant Staphylococcus aureus. Clin Infect Dis. 2010;51(Suppl 2):S183–97.
17. Baik I, Curhan GC, Rimm EB, Bendich A, Willett WC, Fawzi WW. A prospective study of age and lifestyle factors in relation to community-acquired pneumonia in US men and women. Arch Intern Med. 2000;160:3082–8.
18. Davis K, Stremikis K, Schoen C, Squires D. Mirror, Mirror on the Wall, 2014 Update: How the U.S. Health Care System Compares Internationally, The Commonwealth Fund, June 2014.
19. McNulty J, Khera N. Financial hardship-an unwanted consequence of cancer treatment. Curr Hematol Malig Rep. 2015;26:205–12. [Epub ahead of print]
20. Janssen I, Shepard DS, Katzmarzyk PT, Roubenoff R. The healthcare costs of sarcopenia in the United States. J Am Geriatr Soc. 2004;52:80–5.

21. Khatami M. Cancer research and therapy: scam of century – promote immunity [Yin-Yang], 2016; ISBN-10:153043100X;ISBN-13:978–1530431007; Amazon-Createspace p1–166, http://www.createspace.com/6123573.
22. Khatami M. Chronic inflammation: synergistic interactions of recruiting macrophages (TAMs) eosinophils (Eos) with host mast cells (MCs) and tumorigenesis un CALTs. MCSF, suitable biomarker for cancer diagnosis! Cancers (Basel). 2014;6:297–322.
23. Khatami M. Inflammation, aging, and cancer: tumoricidal versus tumorigenesis of immunity: a common denominator mapping chronic diseases. Cell Biochem Biophys. 2009;55:55–79.
24. Khatami M. Unresolved inflammation and cancer: loss of natural immune surveillance as the correct 'target' for therapy! Seeing the 'elephant' in the light of logic. Cell Biochem Biophys. 2012;62:501–9.
25. Khatami M. Inflammation, aging and cancer: Friend or foe? In: Khatami M, editor. Inflammation, Chronic Diseases and Cancer-Cell and Molecular Biology, Immunology and Clinical Bases. Rejeka, Croatia: InTech Publishing., [ISBN 978-953-51-0102; 2012. p. 3–30.
26. Khatami M. Unresolved inflammation: 'immune tsunami' or erosion of integrity in immune-privileged and immune-responsive tissues and acute and chronic inflammatory diseases or cancer. Expert Opin Biol Ther. 2011;11:1419–32.
27. Williams GC. Pleiotropy, natural selection and the evolution of senescence. Evolution. 1957;11:398–411.
28. Burnet M: Cancer: a biological approach. The processes of control. Br Med J.. 1957.
29. Lee RD. Rethinking the evolutionary theory of aging: transfers, not births, shape senescence in social species. Proc Natl Acad Sci (USA). 2003;100:9637–42.
30. Khatami M. 'Yin and Yang' in inflammation: duality in innate immune cell function and tumorigenesis. Expert Opin Biol Ther. 2008;8:1461–71.
31. Hakim FT, Flomerfelt FA, Boyiadzis M, Gress RE. Aging, immunity and cancer. Current Opin Immunol. 2004;18:151–8.
32. Knight JA. The biochemistry of aging. Adv Clin Chem. 2000;35:1–62.
33. Fleg JL, Morrell CH, Bos AG, Brant LJ, Talbot LA, Wright JG, et al. Accelerated longitudinal decline of aerobic capacity in healthy older adults. Circulation. 2005;112:674–82.
34. Franceschi C, Bonafè M, Valensin S. Human immunosenescence: the prevailing of innate immunity, the failing of clonotypic immunity, and the filling of immunological space. Vaccine. 2000;18:1717–20.
35. Franceschi C, Bonafè M, Valensin S, Olivieri F, De Luca M, Ottaviani E, De Benedictis G. Inflamm-aging. An evolutionary perspective on immunosenescence. Ann N Y Acad Sci. 2000;908:244–54.
36. Baggio G, Donazzan S, Monti D, Mari D, Martini S, Gabelli C, Dalla Vestra M, Previato L, Guido M, Pigozzo S, Cortella I, Crepaldi G, Franceschi C. Lipoprotein(a) and lipoprotein profile in healthy centenarians: a reappraisal of vascular risk factors. FASEB J. 1998;12:433–7.
37. Kipling D, Davis T, Ostler EJ, Faragher RG. What can progeroid syndromes tell about human aging? Science. 2004;305:1426–31.
38. Brod SA. Unregulated inflammation shortens human functional longevity. Inflamm Res. 2000;49:561–70.
39. Bruunsgaard H. The clinical impact of systemic low-level inflammation in elderly populations. With special reference to cardiovascular disease, dementia and mortality. Dan Med Bull. 2006;53:285–309.
40. Quaglino D, Ginaldi L, Furia N, De Martinis M. The effect of age on hemopoiesis. Aging (Milano). 1996;8:1–12.
41. McGlauchlen KS, Vogel LA. Ineffective humoral immunity in the elderly. Microbes Infect. 2003;5:1279–84.
42. Hansson GK, Libby P. The immune response in atherosclerosis: a double-edged sword. Nat Rev Immunol. 2006;6:508–19.
43. Meyer KC. Lung infection and aging. Ageing Res Rev. 2004;3:55–67.

44. Croce K, Libby P. Intertwining of thrombosis and inflammation in atherosclerosis. Curr Opin Hematol. 2007;14:55–61.
45. Blagosklonny MV. Aging and immortality: quasi-programmed senescence and its pharmacologic inhibition. Cell Cycle. 2006;5:2087–102.
46. Rafi A, Castle SC, Uyemura K, Makinodan T. Immune dysfunction in the elderly and its reversal by antihistamines. Biomedicine & Pharmacology. 2003;57:246–50.
47. Ignarro LJ, Balestrieri ML, Napoli C. Nutrition, physical activity, and cardiovascular disease: an update. Cardiovasc Res. 2007;73:326–40.
48. Chung HY, Cesari M, Anton S, Marzetti E, Giovannini S, Seo AY, Carter C, Yu BP, Leeuwenburgh C. Molecular inflammation: Underpinning of aging and age-related diseases. Ageing Res Rev. 2008;8:18–30.
49. Arking R. The Biology of Aging: Observarion and principles. 2nd ed. Sunderland, MA, USA: Sinauer Associates Inc.; 1998. p. 153–250.
50. Khatami M. Developmental phases of inflammation-induced massive lymphoid hyperplasia and extensive changes in epithelium in an experimental model of allergy: implications for a direct link between inflammation and carcinogenesis. Am J Ther. 2005;12:117–26.
51. Culmsee C, Landshamer S. Molecular insights into mechanisms of the cell death program: role in the progression of neurodegenerative disorders. Curr Alzheimer Res. 2006;3:269–83.
52. Sansoni P, Vescovini R, Fagnoni F, Biasini C, Zanni F, Zanlari L, Telera A, Lucchini G, Passeri G, Monti D, Franceschi C, Passeri M. The immune system in extreme longevity. Exp Gerontol. 2008;43:61–5.
53. Ginaldi L, DiBenedetto MC, DeMartinis M. Osteoporosis inflammation and ageing. Immun Ageing. 2005;2:14. doi:10.1186/1742-4933-2-14.
54. Keibel A, Singh V, Sharma MC. Inflammation, microenvironment, and the immune system in cancer progression. Curr Pharm Des. 2009;15:1949–55.
55. Davalos AR, Coppe JP, Campisi J, Desprez PY. Senescent cells as a source of inflammatory factors for tumor progression. Cancer Metastasis Rev. 2010;29:273–83.
56. Sohal RS, Orr WC. The redox stress hypothesis of aging. Free Radic Biol Med. 2012;52:539–55.
57. Huppertz B, Ghosh D, Sengupta J. An integrative view on the physiology of human early placental villi. Prog Biophys Mol Biol. 2014;114:33–48.
58. Dunlop K, Cedrone M, Staples JF, Regnault TR. Altered fetal skeletal muscle nutrient metabolism following an adverse in utero environment and the modulation of later life insulin sensitivity. Forum Nutr. 2015;7:1202–16.
59. Moreno E, Rhiner C. Darwin's multicellularity: from neurotrophic theories and cell competition to fitness fingerprints. Curr Opin Cell Biol. 2014;31:16–22.
60. Moreno E, Basler K. Morata G: cells compete for decapentaplegic survival factor to prevent apoptosis in *Drosophila* wing development. Nature. 2002;416:755–9.
61. Virchow R. Cellular pathology. London: Churchill; 1860.
62. De Loof A, De Haes W, Boerjan B, Schoofs L. The fading electricity theory of aging: the missing biophysical principal? Aging Res Rev. 2013;12:58–66.
63. Lucia U. The Gouy-Stodola theorem in bioenergetic analysis of living systems (irreversibility in bioenergetics of living systems). Energies. 2014;7:5717–39.
64. Guzmán-Gutiérrez E, Arroyo P, Salsoso R, Fuenzalida B, Sáez T, Leiva A, Pardo F, Sobrevia L. Role of insulin and adenosine in the human placenta microvascular and macrovascular endothelial cell dysfunction in gestational diabetes mellitus. Microcirculation. 2014;21:26–37.
65. Harman D. Aging: a theory based on free radical and radiation chemistry. J Gerontol. 1956;11:298–300.
66. Harman D. The biologic clock: the mitochondria? J Am Geriatr Soc. 1972;20:145–7.
67. Mittledorf JJ. Adaptive aging in the context of evolutionary theory. Biochemistry (Mosc). 2012;77:716–25.
68. Weinert BT, Timiras PS. Invited review: theories of aging. J Appl Physiol. 2003;95:1706–16.

69. Arellanes-Licea E, Caldelas I, De Ita-Pérez D, Díaz-Muñoz M. The circadian timing system: a recent addition in the physiological mechanisms underlying pathological and aging processes. Aging Dis. 2014;5:406–18. doi:10.14336/AD.2014.0500406. eCollection 2014
70. Nader N, Chrousos GP, Kino T. Circadian rhythm transcription factor CLOCK regulates the transcriptional activity of the glucocorticoid receptor by acetylating its hinge region lysine cluster: potential physiological implications. FASEB J. 2009;23:1572–83.
71. Vielhaber E, Eide E, Rivers A, Gao ZH, Virshup DM. Nuclear entry of the circadian regulator mPER1 is controlled by mammalian casein kinase I epsilon. Mol Cell Biol. 2000;13:4888–99.
72. Jones DP. Redox theory of aging. Redox Biol. 2015;5:71–8.
73. Chung HY, Kim HJ, Kim KW, Choi JS, Yu BP. Molecular inflammation hypothesis of aging based on the anti-aging mechanism of calorie restriction. Microsc Res Tech. 2002;59:264–72.
74. Hardeland R. Melatonin and the theories of aging: a critical appraisal of melatonin's role in antiaging mechanisms. J Pineal Res. 2013;55:325–56.
75. Rustin P, von Kleist-Retzow JC, Vajo Z, Rotig A, Munnich A. Detective mitochondria, free radicals, cell death-reality or myth-ochrondria. Mech Age Develop. 2000;114:201–6. http://www.britannica.com/EBchecked/topic/271624/Horace
76. Muller FL, Lustgarten MS, Jang Y, Richardson A, Van Remmen H. Trends in oxidative aging theories. Free Radic Biol Med. 2007;43:477–503.
77. Tatar M, Bartke A, Antebi A. The endocrine regulation of aging by insulin-like signals. Science. 2003;299:1346–51.
78. Lapointe J, Hekimi S. When a theory of aging ages badly. Cell Mol Life Sci. 2010;67:1–8.
79. Vitale G, Salvioli S, Franceschi C. Oxidative stress and the ageing endocrine system. Nat Rev Endocrinol. 2013;9:228–40.
80. Khatami M. Is cancer a severe delayed hypersensitivity reaction and histamine a blueprint? Perspective. Clin Trans Med. 2016;5:35. doi:10.1186/s40169-016-0108-3. Epub 2016 Aug 23
81. Khalyavkin AV, Krut'ko VN. Early thymus involution--manifestation of an aging program or a program of Development? Biochemistry (Mosc). 2015 Dec;80(12):1622–5. doi:10.1134/S0006297915120111.
82. Beckman KB, Ames BN. The free radical theory of aging matures. Physiol Rev. 1998;78:547–81.
83. Margulis L. Symbiosis and evolution. Sci Am. 1971;225:48–57.
84. Beckman JS, Koppenol WH. Nitric oxide, superoxide and peroxynitrite: The good, the bad, and the ugly. Am. J. Physiol. (Cell Physiol.). 1996;271:C1424–37.
85. McCann SM, Mastronardi C, de Laurentiis A, Rettori V. The nitric oxide theory of aging revisited. Ann N Y Acad Sci. 2005;1057:64–84.
86. Halliwell B, Gutteridge JMC. Free radicals in biology and medicine. 4th ed. Oxford: Oxford University Press; 2007.
87. Liu X, Miller MJS, Joshi MS, Thomas DD, Lancaster JR Jr. Accelerated reaction of nitric oxide with O_2 within the hydrophobic interior of biological membranes. Proc Natl Acad Sci U S A. 1998;95:2175–9.
88. Madej E, Folkes LK, Wardman P, Czapski G, Goldstein S. Thiyl radicals react with nitric oxide to form S-nitrosothiols with rate constants near the diffusion-controlled limit. Free Radic Biol Med. 2008;44:2013–8.
89. Eiserich JP, Butler J, Van Der Vliet A, Cross CE, Halliwell B. Nitric oxide rapidly scavenges tyrosine and tryptophan radicals. Biochem J. 1995;310:745–9.
90. Huie RE, Padmaja S. The reaction of NO with superoxide. Free Radic Res Commun. 1993;18:195–9.
91. Zorov DB, Plotnikov EY, Silachev DN, Zorova LD, Pevzner IB, Zorov SD, Babenko VA, Jankauskas SS, Popkov VA, Savina PS. Microbiota and mitobiota. Putting an equal sign between mitochondria and bacteria. Biochemistry (Mosc). 2014;79:1017–31.
92. Klass M, Nguyen PN, Dechavigny A. Age-correlated changes in the DNA template in the nematode *Caenorhabditis elegans*. Mech Ageing Dev. 1983;22:253–63.

93. Gems D, Doonan R. Antioxidant defense and aging in *C. elegans*: is the oxidative damage theory of aging wrong? Cell Cycle. 2009;8:1681–7.
94. Sekirov I, Russell SL, Antunes LC, Finlay BB. Gut microbiota in health and disease. Physiol. Rev. 2010;90:859–904.
95. Yamaza H, Chiba T, Higami Y, Shimokawa I. Lifespan extension by caloric restriction: an aspect of energy metabolism. Microsc Res Tech. 2002;59:325–30.
96. Ames BN, Shigenaga MK, Hagen TM. Oxidants, antioxidants, and the degenerative diseases of aging. Proc Natl Acad Sci U S A. 1993;90:7915–22.
97. Kim CI. Treatment: nutrition alimentotherapy. Geriatrics. Seoul: Seoul National University Press; 1997. p. 122–31.
98. DeBoer S, Olson FK, Schultz C, Starkson S, Wiitanen EM. Geriatric nutrition. In: Nelson JK, Mozness KE, Jensen MD, Gastineau CF, editors. Diet manual. 7th ed. St. Louis: Mosby; 1994. p. 58–70.
99. Harrington LA, Harley CB. Effect of vitamin E on lifespan and reproduction in *Caenorhabditis elegans*. Mech Ageing Dev. 1988;43:71–8.
100. Feng J, Bussière F, Hekimi S. Mitochondrial electron transport is a key determinant of life span in *Caenorhabditis elegans*. Dev Cell. 2001;1:633–44.
101. Doonan R, McElwee JJ, Matthijssens F, et al. Against the oxidative damage theory of aging: superoxide dismutases protect against oxidative stress but have little or no effect on life span in *Caenorhabditis elegans*. Genes Dev. 2008;22:3236–41.
102. Brys K, Castelein N, Matthijssens F, Vanfleteren JR, Braeckman BP. Disruption of insulin signalling preserves bioenergetic competence of mitochondria in ageing *Caenorhabditis elegans*. BMC Biol. 2010;8:91. doi:10.1186/1741-7007-8-91.
103. Yasuda K, Adachi H, Fujiwara Y, Ishii N. Protein carbonyl accumulation in aging dauer formation-defective (*daf*) mutants of *Caenorhabditis elegans*. J Gerontol A. 1999;54:B47–51.
104. Minniti AN, Cataldo R, Trigo C, et al. Methionine sulfoxide reductase a expression is regulated by the DAF-16/FOXO pathway in *Caenorhabditis elegans*. Aging Cell. 2009;8:690–705.
105. Honda Y, Honda S. The *daf-2* gene network for longevity regulates oxidative stress resistance and Mn-superoxide dismutase gene expression in *Caenorhabditis elegans*. FASEB J. 1999;13:1385–93.
106. Petriv OI, Rachubinski RA. Lack of peroxisomal catalase causes a progeric phenotype in *Caenorhabditis elegans*. J Biol Chem. 2004;279:19996–20001.
107. Back P, Braeckman BP, Matthijssens F. ROS in aging *Caenorhabditis elegans*: damage or signaling? Oxidative Med Cell Longev. 2012;608478:2012. doi:10.1155/2012/608478. Epub 2012 Aug 15.
108. Jee C, Vanoaica L, Lee J, Park BJ, Ahnn J. Thioredoxin is related to life span regulation and oxidative stress response in *Caenorhabditis elegans*. Genes Cells. 2005;10(12):1203–10.
109. Hernández-García D, Wood CD, Castro-Obregón S, Covarrubias L. Reactive oxygen species: a radical role in development? Free Radic Biol Med. 2010;49:130–43.
110. Melov S, Lithgow GJ, Fischer DR, Tedesco PM, Johnson TE. Increased frequency of deletions in the mitochondrial genome with age of *Caenorhabditis elegans*. Nucleic Acids Res. 1995;23:1419–25.
111. Honda Y, Tanaka M, Honda S. Modulation of longevity and diapause by redox regulation mechanisms under the insulin-like signaling control in *Caenorhabditis elegans*. Exp Gerontol. 2008;43:520–9.
112. Bokov A, Chaudhuri A, Richardson A. The role of oxidative damage and stress in aging. Mech Ageing Dev. 2004;125:811–26.
113. Matthijssens F, Back P, Braeckman BP, Vanfleteren JR. Prooxidant activity of the superoxide dismutase (SOD)-mimetic EUK-8 in proliferating and growth-arrested *Escherichia coli* cells. Free Radic Biol Med. 2008;45:708–15.
114. Hebert DN, Molinari M. In and out of the ER: protein folding, quality control, degradation, and related human diseases. Physiol Rev. 2007;87:1377–408.

115. Taub J, Lau JF, Ma C, et al. A cytosolic catalase is needed to extend adult lifespan in *C. elegans* daf-C and clk-1 mutants. Nature. 1999;399:162–6.
116. Van Raamsdonk JM, Hekimi S. Reactive oxygen species and aging in *Caenorhabditis elegans*: causal or casual relationship? Antioxid Redox Signal. 2010;13:1911–53.
117. Toldo S, Seropian IM, Mezzaroma E, Van Tassell BW, Salloum FN, Lewis EC, et al. Alpha-1 antitrypsin inhibits caspase-1 and protects from acute myocardial ischemia-reperfusion injury. J Mol Cell Cardiol. 2011;51:244–51.
118. Orrenius S, Gogvadze V, Zhivotovsky B. Calcium and mitochondria in the regulation of cell death. Biochem Biophys Res Commun. 2015;460:72–81.
119. Orrenius S. Reactive oxygen species in mitochondria-mediated cell death. Drug Metab Rev. 2007;39:443–55.
120. Ott M, Gogvadze V, Orrenius S, Zhivotovsky B. Mitochondria, oxidative stress and cell death. Apoptosis. 2007;12:913–22.
121. Apel K, Hirt H. Reactive oxygen species: metabolism, oxidative stress, and signal transduction. Annu Rev Plant Biol. 2004;55:373–99.
122. Cetrullo S, D'Adamo S, Tantini B, Borzi RM, Flamigni F. mTOR, AMPK, and Sirt1: key players in metabolic stress management. Crit Rev Eukaryot Gene Expr. 2015;25:59–75.
123. Wataya-Kaneda M. Mammalian target of rapamycin and tuberous sclerosis complex. J Dermatol Sci. 2015;S0923-1811(15):00154–1.
124. Corradetti MN, Guan KL. Upstream of the mammalian target of rapamycin: do all roads pass through mTOR? Oncogene. 2006;25:6347–60.
125. Albert V, Hall MN. mTOR signaling in cellular and organismal energetics. Curr Opin Cell Biol. 2014;33C:55–66.
126. Sengupta S, Peterson TR, Sabatini DM. Regulation of the mTOR complex 1 pathway by nutrients, growth factors, and stress. Mol Cell. 2010;40:310–22.
127. Lakowski B, Hekimi S. The genetics of caloric restriction in *Caenorhabditis elegans*. Proc Natl Acad Sci USA. 1998;95(22):13091–6.
128. Bishop NA, Guarente L. Two neurons mediate diet-restriction-induced longevity in *C. elegans*. Nature. 2007;447(7144):545–9.
129. Miller RA. The aging immune system: primer and prospectus. Science. 1996;273:70–4.
130. Michaud M, Balardy L, Moulis G, Gaudin C, Peyrot C, Vellas B, Cesari M, Nourhashemi F. Proinflammatory cytokines, aging, and age-related diseases. J Am Med Dir Assoc. 2013;14:877–82.
131. Makinodan T, Kay MM. Age influence on the immune system. Adv Immunol. 1980;29:287–330.
132. Qi Q, Zhang DW, Weyand CM, Goronzy JJ. Mechanisms shaping the naïve T cell repertoire in the elderly thymic involution or peripheral homeostatic proliferation? Exp Gerontol. 2014;54:71–4.
133. Appay V, Sauce D. Naive T cells: the crux of cellular immune aging? Exp Gerontol. 2014;54:90–3.
134. Ghia P, Melchers F, Rolink AG. Age-dependent changes in B lymphocyte development in man and mouse. Exp Gerontol. 2000;35:159–65.
135. Chen H, Zheng X, Zheng Y. Lamin-B in systemic inflammation, tissue homeostasis, and aging. Nucleus. 2015;15:1–4.
136. Fulop T, Larbi A, Kotb R, de Angelis F, Pawelec G. Aging, immunity, and cancer. Discov Med. 2011;61:537–50.
137. Blaseser A, McGlauchlen K, Vogel LA. Aged B lymphocytes retain their ability to express surface markers but are dysfunctional in their proliferative capacity during early activation event. Immun Ageing. 2008;5:5–15. doi:10.1186/1742-4933-5-15.
138. Powers DC, Belshe RB. Effect of age on cytotoxic T lymphocyte memory as well as serum and local antibody responses elicited by inactivated influenza virus vaccine. J Infect Dis. 1993;167:584–92.
139. Allain TJ, Dhesi J. Hypovitaminosis D in older adults. Gerontology. 2003;49:273–8.

140. Sawyer DT. Oxygen chemistry. New York: Oxford University Press; 1991.
141. Borel P, Caillaud D, Cano NJ. Vitamin d bioavailability: state of the art. Crit Rev Food Sci Nutr. 2015;55:1193–205.
142. Thompson P, Khatami M, Baglole CJ, Sun J, Harris SA, Moon EY, et al. Environmental immune disruptors, inflammation and cancer risk. Carcinogenesis. 2015;36(Suppl 1):S232–53. doi:10.1093/carcin/bgv038.
143. Inoue H, Hisamoto N, An JH, et al. The *C. elegans* p38 MAPK pathway regulates nuclear localization of the transcription factor SKN-1 in oxidative stress response. Gene Dev. 2005;19:2278–83.
144. Cross AR, Segal AW. The NADPH oxidase of professional phagocytes—prototype of the NOX electron transport chain systems. Biochim Biophys Acta. 2004;1657:1–22.
145. Cochemé HM, Quin C, McQuaker SJ, et al. Measurement of H_2O_2 within living *Drosophila* during aging using a ratiometric mass spectrometry probe targeted to the mitochondrial matrix. Cell Metab. 2011;13:340–50.
146. Mishina NM, Tyurin-Kuzmin PA, Markvicheva KN, et al. Does cellular hydrogen peroxide diffuse or act locally? Antioxid Redox Signal. 2011;14:1–7.
147. Kim SG, Buel GR, Blenis J. Nutrient regulation of the mTOR complex 1 signaling pathway. Mol Cells. 2013;35:463–73.
148. Edeas M. Strategies to target mitochondria and oxidative stress by antioxidants: key points and perspectives. Pharm Res. 2011;28:2771–9.
149. Degenhardt K, Mathew R, Beaudoin B, Bray K, Anderson D, Chen G, Mukherjee C, Shi Y, Gelinas C, Fan Y, Nelson DA, Jin S, White E. Autophagy promotes tumor cell survival and restricts necrosis, inflammation, and tumorigenesis. Cancer Cell. 2006;10:51–64.
150. Krtolica A, Campisi J. Cancer and aging: a model for the cancer promoting effects of the aging stroma. Int J Biochem Cell Biol. 2002;34:1401–14.
151. Reuter S, Gupta SC, Chaturvedi MM, Aggarwal BB. Oxidative stress, inflammation, and cancer: how are they linked? Free Radic Biol Med. 2010;49:1603–16.
152. McCord JM, Edeas MA. SOD, oxidative stress and human pathologies: a brief history and a future vision. Biomed Pharmacother. 2005;59:139–42.
153. Stone JR, Yang S. Hydrogen Peroxide: a signaling messenger. Antiox Redox Signaling. 2006;8:243–70.
154. Ungvari Z, Labinskyy N, Mukhopadhyay P, et al. Resveratrol attenuates mitochondrial oxidative stress in coronary arterial endothelial cells. Am J Physiol. 2009;297:H1876–81.
155. Emerit J, Edeas M, Bricaire F. Neurodegenerative diseases and oxidative stress. Biomed Pharmacother. 2004;58:39–46.
156. Kroemer G. Autophagy: a druggable process that is deregulated in aging and human disease. J Clin Invest. 2015;125:1–4. doi:10.1172/JCI78652. Epub 2015 Jan 2
157. Galluzzi L, Zamzami N, de La Motte RT, Lemaire C, Brenner C, Kroemer G. Methods for the assessment of mitochondrial membrane permeabilization in apoptosis. Apoptosis. 2007;12:803–13.
158. Sohal RS, Weindruch R. Oxidative stress, caloric restriction, and aging. Science. 1996;273(5271):59–63.
159. Galluzzi L, Morselli E, Kepp O, Vitale I, Rigoni A, Vacchelli E, Michaud M, Zischka H, Castedo M, Kroemer G. Mitochondrial gateways to cancer. Mol Asp Med. 2010;31:1–20.
160. Pedersen PL. Tumor mitochondria and the bioenergetics of cancer cells. Prog Exp Tumor Res. 1978;22:190–274.
161. Kiebish MA, Han X, Cheng H, Chuang JH, Seyfried TN. Cardiolipin and electron transport chain abnormalities in mouse brain tumor mitochondria: lipidomic evidence supporting the Warburg theory of cancer. J Lipid Res. 2008;49:2545–456.
162. Cloonan SM, Choi AMK. Mitochondria: commanders of innate immunity and disease? Curr Opin Immunol. 2012;24:32–40.

163. Takahashi E, Sato M. Anaerobic respiration sustains mitochondrial membrane potential in a prolyl hydroxylase pathway-activated cancer cell line in a hypoxic microenvironment. Am J Physiol Cell Physiol. 2014;306:C334–42.
164. Bonnet S, Archer SL, Allalunis-Turner J, Haromy A, Beaulieu C, Thompson R, Lee CT, Lopaschuk GD, Puttagunta L, Bonnet S, Harry G, Hasimoto K, Porter CJ, Andrade MA, Thebaud B, Michelakis ED. A mitochondria-K+ channel axis is suppressed in cancer and its normalization promotes apoptosis and inhibits cancer growth. Cancer Cell. 2007;11:37–51.
165. Frezza C, Gottlieb E. Mitochondria in cancer: not just innocent bystanders. Sem Cancer Bio. 2009;119:4–11.
166. Zhang XV, Martin ST. Driving parts of Krebs Cycle in reverse through mineral photochemistry. J Am Chem Soc. 2006;128:16032–3.
167. Poyton RO, Ball KA, Castello PR. Mitochondrial generation of free radicals and hypoxic signaling. Trends Endocrinol Metab. 2009;20:332–40.
168. Sharma G, Sharma AR, Seo EM, Nam JS. Genetic polymorphism in extracellular regulators of Wnt signaling pathway. Biomed Res Int. 2015;2015:847529.
169. Lovering RC, Camon EB, Blake JA, Diehl AD. Access to immunology through the gene ontology. Immunology. 2008;125:154–60.
170. Collins LV, Hajizadeh S, Holme E, Jonsson I-M, Tarkowski A. Endogenously oxidized mitochondrial DNA induces in vivo and in vitro inflammatory responses. J Leukoc Biol. 2004;75:995–1000. doi:10.1189/jlb.0703328.
171. Landis GN, Tower J. Superoxide dismutase evolution and life span regulation. Mech Ageing Dev. 2005;126:365–79.
172. De Magalhaes JP, Wuttke D, Wood SH, Plank M, Vora C. Genome-environment interactions that modulate aging: powerful targets for drug discovery. Pharmacol Rev. 2012;64:88–101.
173. Vijg J, Hasty P. Aging and p53: getting it straight. A commentary on a recent paper by Gentry and Venkatachalam. Aging Cell. 2005;4:335–8.
174. Vogelstein B, Kinzler KW. Cancer genes and the pathways they control. Nat Med. 2004;10:789–99.
175. Fukada S, Morikawa D, Yamamoto Y, Yoshida T, Sumie N, Yamaguchi M, et al. Genetic background affects properties of satellite cells and mdx phenotypes. Am J Pathol. 2010;176:2414–24.
176. Rudolph KL, Chang S, Lee HW, Blasco M, Gottlieb GJ, Greider C, DePinho RA. Longevity, stress response, and cancer in aging telomerase-deficient mice. Cell. 1999;96:701–12.
177. Chin L, Artandi SE, Shen Q, Tam A, Lee SL, Gottlieb GJ, Greider CW, DePinho RA. p53 deficiency rescues the adverse effects of telomere loss and cooperates with telomere dysfunction to accelerate carcinogenesis. Cell. 1999;97:527–638.
178. Nijnik A, Woodbine L, Marchetti C, Dawson S, Lambe T, Liu C, et al. DNA repair is limiting for haematopoietic stem cells during ageing. Nature. 2007;447:686–90.
179. Nagata S, Suda T. Fas and Fas ligand: lpr and gld mutations. Immunol Today. 1995;16:39–43.
180. Alves H, Munoz-Najar U, De Wit J, Renard AJ, Hoeijmakers JH, Sedivy JM, et al. A link between the accumulation of DNA damage and loss of multi-potency of human mesenchymal stromal cells. J Cell Mol Med. 2010;14:2729–38.
181. Heyn H, Li N, Ferreira HJ, et al. Distinct DNA methylomes of newborns and centenarians. Proc Natl Acad Sci U S A. 2012;109:10522–7.
182. Jinnah HA, de Gregorio L, Harris JC, Nyhan WL, O'Neill JP. The spectrum of inherited mutations causing HPRT deficiency: 75 new cases and a review of 196 previously reported cases. Mutat Res. 2000;463:309–26.
183. Harley CB, Futcher AB, Greider CW. Telomeres shorten during ageing of human fibroblasts. Nature. 1990;345:458–60.
184. Slagboom PE, Droog S, Boomsma DI. Genetic determination of telomere size in humans: a twin study of three age groups. Am J Hum Genet. 1994;55:876–82.
185. Armanios M. Syndromes of telomere shortening. Ann Rev Genomics HumGenet. 2009;10:45–61.

186. Noebels J. Pathway-driven discovery of epilepsy genes. Nat Neurosci. 2015;18:344–50.
187. Greider CW. Telomeres and senescence: the history, the experiment, the future. Curr Biol. 1998;8:R178–81.
188. Savage SA, Bertuch AA. The genetics and clinical manifestations of telomere biology disorders. Genet Med. 2010;12:753–64.
189. Calado RT, Young NS. Telomere diseases. N Engl J Med. 2009;361:2353–65.
190. Diaz de LA, Cronkhite JT, Katzenstein AL, Godwin JD, Raghu G, Glazer CS, Rosenblatt RL, Girod CE, Garrity ER, Xing C, Garcia CK. Telomere lengths, pulmonary fibrosis and telomerase (TERT) mutations. PLoS One. 2010;5:e10680.
191. Son NH, Murray S, Yanovski J, Hodes RJ, Weng N. Lineage-specific telomere shortening and unaltered capacity for telomerase expression in human T and B lymphocytes with age. J Immunol. 2000;165:1191–6.
192. Gadalla SM, Cawthon R, Giri N, Alter BP, Savage SA. Telomere length in blood, buccal cells, and fibroblasts from patients with inherited bone marrow failure syndromes. Aging (Albany, NY). 2010;2:867–74.
193. Hiyama E, Hiyama K. Telomere and telomerase in stem cells. Br J Cancer. 2007;96:1020–4.
194. Blackburn EH, Greider CW, Szostak JW. Telomeres and telomerase: the path from maize, Tetrahymena and yeast to human cancer and aging. Nat Med. 2006;12:1133–8.
195. Weng NP. Telomeres and immune competency. Curr Opin Immunol. 2012;24:470–5.
196. Weng NP, Levine BL, June CH, Hodes RJ. Human naive and memory T lymphocytes differ in telomeric length and replicative potential. Proc Natl Acad Sci U S A. 1995;92:11091–4.
197. Chou JP, Effros RB. Tcell replicative senescence in human aging. Curr Pharm Des. 2013;19(9):1680–98.
198. Wong JM, Collins K. Telomere maintenance and disease. Lancet. 2003;362:983–8.
199. Bjornson CR, Cheung TH, Liu L, Tripathi PV, Steeper KM, Rando TA. Notch signaling is necessary to maintain quiescence in adult muscle stem cells. Stem Cells. 2012;30:232–42.
200. Sharpless NE, DePinho RA. Telomeres, stem cells senescence and cancer. J Clin Invest. 2004;113:160–8.
201. Bohr VA, Anson RM. DNA damage, mutation and fine structure DNA repair in aging. Mutat Res. 1995;338:25–34.
202. Medová M, Aebersold DM, Zimmer Y. The molecular crosstalk between the MET receptor tyrosine kinase and the DNA damage response-biological and clinical aspects. Cancers. 2014;6:1–27.
203. Obokata H, Wakayama T, Sasai Y, Kojima K, Vacanti MP, Niwa H, Yamato M, Vacanti CA. Stimulus-triggered fate conversion of somatic cells into pluripotency. Nature. 2014;505:641–7.
204. Huang Q, Lan F, Wang X, Yu Y, Quyang X, Zheng F, et al. IL-1beta-induced activation of p38 promotes metastasis in gastric adenocarcinoma via upregulation of AP-1/c-fos, MMP2 and MMP9. Mol Cancer. 2014;13:18. doi:10.1186/1476-4598-13-18.
205. Ebert MP, Fei G, Kahmann S, et al. Increased beta-catenin mRNA levels and mutational alterations of the APC and beta-catenin gene are present in intestinal-type gastric cancer. Carcinogenesis. 2002;23:87–91.
206. Resende C, Ristimaki A, Machado JC. Genetic and epigenetic alteration in gastric carcinogenesis. Helicobacter. 2010;15:34–9.
207. Vogiatzi P, Vindigni C, Roviello F, Renieri A, Giordano A. Deciphering the underlying genetic and epigenetic events leading to gastric carcinogenesis. J Cell Physiol. 2007;211:287–95.
208. Marimuthu A, Jacob HK, Jakharia A, et al. Gene expression profiling of gastric cancer. J Proteomics Bioinform. 2011;4:74–82.
209. Pasini FS, Zilberstein B, Snitcovsky I, et al. A gene expression profile related to immune dampening in the tumor microenvironment is associated with poor prognosis in gastric adenocarcinoma. J Gastroenterol. 2013;49(11):1453–66.
210. Liu N, Liu X, Zhou N, Wu Q, Zhou L, Li Q. Gene expression profiling and bioinformatics analysis of gastric carcinoma. Exp Mol Pathol. 2014;96(3):361–6.

211. Subramanian A, Tamayo P, Mootha VK, et al. Gene set enrichment analysis: a knowledge-based approach for interpreting genome-wide expression profiles. Proc Natl Acad Sci U S A. 2005;102:15545–50.
212. Jinawath N, Furukawa Y, Hasegawa S, et al. Comparison of gene-expression profiles between diffuse- and intestinal-type gastric cancers using a genome-wide cDNA microarray. Oncogene. 2004;23:6830–44.
213. Hasegawa S, Furukawa Y, Li M, et al. Genome-wide analysis of gene expression in intestinal-type gastric cancers using a complementary DNA microarray representing 23, 040 genes. Cancer Res. 2002;62:7012–7.
214. Dallaire A, Garand C, Paquel ER, et al. Down regulation of miR-124 in both Werner syndrome DNA helicase mutant mice and mutant *Caenorhabditis elegans*wrn-1 reveals the importance of this microRNA in accelerated aging. Aging (Albany NY). 2012;4:636–47.
215. Honeywell DR, Cabrita MA, Zhao H, Dimitroulakos J, Addison CL. miR-105 inhibits prostate tumour growth by suppressing CDK6 levels. PLoS One. 2013;8:e70515.
216. Yanaihara N, Caplen N, Bowman E, et al. Unique microRNA molecular profiles in lung cancer diagnosis and prognosis. Cancer Cell. 2006;9:189–98.
217. Hsu SD, Lin FM, Wu WY, et al. miRTarBase: a database curates experimentally validated microRNA-target interactions. Nucleic Acids Res. 2011;39(Database issue):D163–9.
218. Zahn JM, Poosala S, Owen AB, et al. AGEMAP: a gene expression database for aging in mice. PLoS Genet. 2007;3:e201.
219. Card DA, Hebbar PB, Li L, et al. Oct4/Sox2-regulated miR-302 targets cyclin D1 in human embryonic stem cells. Mol Cell Biol. 2008;28(20):6426–38.
220. Sirotkin AV, Laukova M, Ovcharenko D, Brenaut P, Mlyncek M. Identification of microRNAs controlling human ovarian cell proliferation and apoptosis. J Cell Physiol. 2010;223:49–56.
221. Gaur A, Jewell DA, Liang Y, et al. Characterization of microRNA expression levels and their biological correlates in human cancer cell lines. Cancer Res. 2007;67:2456–68.
222. Huang da W, Sherman BT, Lempicki RA. Systematic and integrative analysis of large gene lists using DAVID bioinformatics resources. Nat Protoc. 2009;4:44–57.
223. Li CP, Huang TS, Chao Y, Chang FY, Whang-Peng J, Lee SD. Advantages of assaying telomerase activity in ascites for diagnosis of digestive tract malignancies. World J Gastroenterol. 2004;10:2468–71.
224. Malumbres M, Barbacid M. RAS oncogenes: the first 30 years. Nat Rev Cancer. 2003;3:459–65.
225. Hingorani SR, Tuveson DA. Ras redux: rethinking how and where Ras acts. Curr Opin Genet Dev. 2003;13:6–13.
226. Kirma N, Luthra R, Jones J, Liu Y-G, Nair HB, Mandava U, Tekmal RR. Overexpression of the colony-stimulating factor (CSF-1) and/or its receptor c-fms in mammary glands of transgenic mice results in hyperplasia and tumor formation. Cancer Res. 2004;64:4162–70.
227. Campbell SL, Khosravi-Far R, Rossman KL, Clark GJ, Der CJ. Increasing complexity of Ras signaling. Oncogene. 1998;17:1395–413.
228. Vaziri H, Benchimol S. From telomere loss to p53 induction and activation of a DNA-damage pathway at senescence: the telomere loss/DNA damage model of cell aging. Exp Gerontol. 1996;31:295–301.
229. Schmitt CA, Fridman JS, Yang M, Lee S, Baranov E, Hoffman RM, Lowe SW. A senescence program controlled by p53 and p16INK4a contributes to the outcome of cancer therapy. Cell. 2002;109:335–46.
230. Thomson JM, Gaucher EA, Burgan MF, De Kee DW, Li T, Aris JP, Benner SA. Resurrecting ancestral alcohol dehydrogenases from yeast. Nat Genet. 2005;37:630–5.
231. Feldmann J, Prieur AM, Quartier P, Berquin P, Certain S, Cortis E. Chronic infantile neurological cutaneous and articular syndrome is caused by mutations in CIAS1 a gene highly expressed in polymorphonuclear cells and chondrocytes. Am J Hum Genet. 2002;71:198–203.
232. Croce CM. Causes and consequences of microRNA dysregulation in cancer. Nat Rev Genetics. 2009;10:704–14.

233. Otero M, Plumb DA, Tsuchimochi K, et al. E74-like factor 3 (ELF3) impacts on matrix metalloproteinase 13 (MMP13) transcriptional control in articular chondrocytes under proinflammatory stress. J Biol Chem. 2012;287:3559–72.
234. Gayen JR, Zhang K, RamachandraRao SP, et al. Role of reactive oxygen species in hyperadrenergic hypertension: biochemical, physiological, and pharmacological evidence from targeted ablation of the chromogranin a (Chga) gene. Circ Cardiovasc Genet. 2010;3:414–25.
235. Xiao F, Zuo Z, Cai G, Kang S, Gao X. Li T: miRecords: an integrated resource for microRNA-target interactions. Nucleic Acids Res. 2009;37(Database issue):D105–10.
236. Wang D, Yan L, Hu Q, et al. IMA: an R package for high-throughput analysis of Illumina's 450K Infinium methylation data. Bioinformatics. 2012;28:729–30.
237. Saeed AI, Sharov V, White J, et al. TM4: a free, open-source system for microarray data management and analysis. BioTechniques. 2003;34:374–8.
238. Engwerda CR, Handwerger BS, Fox BS. Aged T cells are hyporesponsive to costimulation mediated by CD28. J Immunol. 1994;152:3740–7.
239. Linton PJ, Haynes L, Klinman NR, Swain SL. Antigen-independent changes in naïve $CD4^+$ T cells with aging. J Exp Med. 1996;184:1891–900.
240. Haynes L, Eaton SM, Burns EM, Rincon M, Swain SL. Inflammatory cytokines overcome age-related defects in $CD4^+$ T cell responses in vivo. J Immunol. 2004;172:5194–9.
241. McElhaney JE, Xie D, Hager WD, Barry MB, Wang Y, Kleppinger A, Ewen C, Kane KP, Bleackley RC. T cell responses are better correlates of vaccine protection in the elderly. J Immunol. 2006;176:6333–9.
242. Simi A, Ibáñez CF. Assembly and activation of neurotrophic factor receptor complexes. Dev Neurobiol. 2010;70:323–31.
243. Deng Y, Jing Y, Campbell AE, Gravenstein S. Age-related impaired type 1 T cell responses to influenza: reduced activation ex vivo, decreased expansion in CTL culture in vitro, and blunted response to influenza vaccination in vivo in the elderly. J Immunol. 2004;172:3437–46.
244. Vissinga C, Hertogh-Huijbregts A, Rozing J, Nagelkerken L. Analysis of the age-related decline in alloreactivity of $CD4^+$ and $CD8^+$ T cells in CBA/RIJ mice. Mech Ageing Dev. 1990;51:179–94.
245. Schmucker DL, Daniels CK, Wang RK, Smith K. Mucosal immune response to cholera toxin in ageing rats. I Antibody and antibody-containing cell response. Immunology. 1988;64:691–5.
246. Jones SC, Clise-Dwyer K, Huston G, Dibble J, Eaton S, Haynes L, Swain SL. Impact of post-thymic cellular longevity on the development of age-associated CD4+ T cell defects. J Immunol. 2008;180:4465–75.
247. Blaeser A, Panwar A, Vogel LA. Humoral immunity and aging: intrinsic B cell defects. Curr Trends Immunol. 2007;8:61–7.
248. Johnson KM, Owen K, Witte PL. Aging and developmental transitions in the B cell lineage. Int Immunol. 2002;14:1313–23.
249. Zheng B, Han S, Takahashi Y, Kelsoe G. Immunosenescence and germinal center reaction. Immunol Rev. 1997;160:63–77.
250. Ruffolo RR Jr. Fundamentals of receptor theory: basics for shock research. Circ Shock. 1992;37:176–84.
251. Hibberd C, Yau JL, Seckl JR. Glucocorticoids and the ageing hippocampus. J Anat. 2000;197(Pt 4):553–62.
252. Barzilai N, Huffman DM, Muzumdar RH, Bartke A. The critical role of metabolic pathways in aging. Diabetes. 2012;61:1315–22.
253. Martin FM, Bydlon G, Friedman JS. SOD2-deficiency sideroblastic anemia and red blood cell oxidative stress. Antioxid Redox Signal. 2006;8:1217–25.
254. Vaishnaw AK, Toubi E, Ohsako S, Drappa J, Buys S, Estrada J, Sitarz A, Zemel L, Chu JL, Elkon KB. The spectrum of apoptotic defects and clinical manifestations, including systemic lupus erythematosus, in humans with CD95 (Fas/APO-1) mutations. Arthritis Rheum. 1999;42:1833–42.

255. Chung HY, Lee EK, Choi YJ, et al. Molecular inflammation as an underlying mechanism of the aging process and age-related diseases. J Dent Res. 2011;90:830–40.
256. Ryan KA, Smith MF Jr, Sanders MK, Ernst PB. Reactive oxygen and nitrogen species differentially regulate toll-like receptor 4-mediated activation of NF-kappa B and interleukin-8 expression. Infect Immun. 2004;72(4):2123–30.
257. Schwab L, Goroncy L, Palaniyandi S, Gautam S, Triantafyllopoulou A, Mocsai A, et al. Neutrophil granulocytes recruited upon translocation of intestinal bacteria enhance graft-versus-host disease via tissue damage. Nat Med. 2014;20:648–54. doi:10.1038/nm.3517.
258. Pérez VI, Bokov A, Van Remmen H, et al. Is the oxidative stress theory of aging dead? Biochim Biophys Acta. 2009;1790:1005–14.
259. Kuhns DB, Nelson EL, Alvord WG, Gallin JI. Fibrinogen induces IL-8 synthesis in human neutrophils stimulated with formyl-methionyl-leucyl-phenylalanine or leukotriene B(4). J Immunol. 2001;167:2869–78. doi:10.4049/jimmunol.167.5.2869.
260. Smiley ST, King JA, Hancock WW. Fibrinogen stimulates macrophage chemokine secretion through toll-like receptor 4. J Immunol. 2001;167:2887–94. doi:10.4049/jimmunol.167.5.2887.
261. Dostert C, Pétrilli V, van Bruggen R, Steele C, Mossman BT, Tschopp J. Innate immune activation through Nalp3 inflammasome sensing of asbestos and silica. Science. 2008;320:674–7.
262. Song H, Price PW, Cerny J. Age-related changes in antibody repertoire: contribution from T cells. Immunol Rev. 1997;160:55–62.
263. Hitchler MJ, Domann FE. An epigenetic perspective on the free radical theory of development. Free Radic Biol Med. 2007;43:1023–36.
264. Kim C, Kang D, Lee EK, Lee JS. Long noncoding RNAs and RNA-binding proteins in oxidative stress, cellular senescence, and age-related diseases. Oxidative Med Cell Longev. 2017;2017:2062384. https://doi.org/10.1155/2017/2062384. Epub 2017 July 25.
265. Marshak-Rothstein A, Rifkin IR. Immunologically active autoantigens: the role of toll-like receptors in the development of chronic inflammatory disease. Annu Rev Immunol. 2007;25:419–41. doi:10.1146/annurev.immunol.22.012703.104514.
266. Blagosklonny MV. Aging: ROS or TOR. Cell Cycle. 2008;7:3344–54.
267. Levine RL, Stadtman ER. Oxidative modification of proteins during aging. Exper Gerontol. 2001;36:1495–502.
268. Hawkins S, Wiswell R. Rate and mechanism of maximal oxygen consumption decline with aging: implications for exercise training. Sports Med. 2003;33:877–88.
269. Campisi J, Andersen JK, Kapahi P, Melov S. Cellular senescence: a link between cancer and age-related degenerative disease? Sem Cancer Biol. 2011;21:354–9.
270. Tower J. Programmed cell death in aging. Ageing Res Rev. 2015;23:90–100. doi:10.1016/j.arr.2015.04.002. Epub 2015 Apr 8
271. Goldstein BJ, Mahadev K, Wu X. Redox paradox: insulin action is facilitated by insulin-stimulated reactive oxygen species with multiple potential signaling targets. Diabetes. 2005;54:311–21.
272. Remillard CV, Yuan JX. Activation of K+ channels: an essential pathway in programmed cell death. Am J Physiol Lung Cell Mol Physiol. 2004;286:L49–67.
273. Schafer FQ, Buettner GR. Redox environment of the cell as viewed through the redox state of the glutathione disulfide/glutathione couple. Free Radic Biol Med. 2001;30:1191–212.
274. Elchuri S, Oberley TD, Qi W, et al. CuZnSOD deficiency leads to persistent and widespread oxidative damage and hepatocarcinogenesis later in life. Oncogene. 2005;24:367–80.
275. Croteau DL, Bohr VA. Repair of oxidative damage to nuclear and mitochondrial DNA in mammalian cells. J Biol Chem. 1997;272:25409–12.
276. Melov S, Ravenscroft J, Malik S, et al. Extension of life-span with superoxide dismutase/catalase mimetics. Science. 2000;289:1567–9.
277. Gehrke N, Mertens C, Zillinger T, Wenzel J, Bald T, Zahn S, et al. Oxidative damage of DNA confers resistance to cytosolic nuclease TREX1 degradation and potentiates STING-dependent immune sensing. Immunity. 2013;39:482–95. doi:10.1016/j.immuni.2013.08.004.

278. Gutscher M, Sobotta MC, Wabnitz GH, et al. Proximity-based protein thiol oxidation by H_2O_2-scavenging peroxidases. J Biol Chem. 2009;284(46):31532–40.
279. Bulcao C, Ferreira SR, Giuffrida FM, Ribeiro-Filho FF. The new adipose tissue and adipocytokines. Curr Diabetes Rev. 2006;2:19–28.
280. Jabaut J, Ckless K. Inflammation, immunity and redox signaling. In: Khatami M, editor. Inflammation, chronic diseases and cancer. Cell and molecular biology, immunology and clinical bases. Rijeka: InTech; 2012. p. 145–60.
281. Fischetti F, Tedesco F. Cross-talk between the complement system and endothelial cells in physiologic conditions and vascular diseases. Autoimmunity. 2006;39:417–28. doi:10.1080/08916930600739712.
282. Aprahamian T. Autoimmunity, atherosclerosis and apoptic cell clearance. In: Khatami M, editor. Inflammation, chronic diseases and cancer. Cell and molecular biology, immunology and clinical bases. Rijeka: InTech; 2012. p. 75–96.
283. Meur YL, Tesch GH, Hill PA, Mu W, Foti R, Nikolic-Paterson DJ, Atkins RC. Monocyte proliferation outside the bone marrow has also been demonstrated in vitro studies using monocytes extracted from peripheral blood and glomeruli. J Leukocyte Biology. 2002;72:530–7.
284. Barnes PJ, Chung KF, Page CP. Inflammatory mediators of asthma: an update. Pharmacol Rev. 1998;50:515–96.
285. Finkelman FD, Shea-Donohue T, Morris SC, Gildea L, Strait R, Madden KB, Schopf L, Urban JF Jr. Interleukin-4- and interleukin-13-mediated host protection against intestinal nematode parasites. Immunol Rev. 2004;201:139–55.
286. Balkwill F. Cancer and the chemokine network. Nat Rev Cancer. 2004;4:540–50.
287. Machado ER, Ueta MT, Lourenço EV, Anibal FF, Sorgi CA, Soares EG, et al. Leukotrienes play a role in the control of parasite burden in murine strongyloidiasis. J Immunol. 2005;175:3892–9.
288. Rossi DJ, Jamieson CH, Weissman IL. Stem cells and the pathways to aging and cancer. Cell. 2008;132:681–96.
289. Krishnamurthy J, Sharpless NE. Stem cells and the rate of living. Cell Stem Cell. 2007;1:9–11.
290. Van Zant G, Liang Y. The role of stem cells in aging. Exp Hematol. 2003;31:659–72.
291. Collins CA, Zammit PS, Ruiz AP, Morgan JE, Partridge TA. A population of myogenic stem cells that survives skeletal muscle aging. Stem Cells. 2007;25:885–94.
292. Fukada S, Ma Y, Uezumi A. Adult stem cell and mesenchymal progenitor theories of aging. Front Cell Dev Biol. 2014;2:10. doi:10.3389/fcell. 2014.00010. eCollection 2014
293. Caplan AI, Dennis JE. Mesenchymal stem cells as trophic mediators. J Cell Biochem. 2006;98:1076–84.
294. Hartman M, Piliponsky AM, Temkin V, Levischaffer F. Human peripheral blood eosinophils express stem cell factor. Blood. 2001;97:1086–91.
295. Lama VN, Smith L, Badri L, Flint A, Andrei AC, Murray S, et al. Evidence for tissue-resident mesenchymal stem cells in human adult lung from studies of transplanted allografts. J Clin Invest. 2007;117:989–96.
296. Biteau B, Jasper H. EGF signaling regulates the proliferation of intestinal stem cells in Drosophila. Development. 2011;138:1045–55.
297. Cheung TH, Rando TA. Molecular regulation of stem cell quiescence. Nat Rev Mol Cell Biol. 2013;14:329–40.
298. Yuzankina Y, Asare A, Brown EJ. Replicative stress, stem cells and aging. Mech Aging Dev. 2008;129:460–6.
299. Nishimura EK. Melanocyte stem cells: a melanocyte reservoir in hair follicles for hair and skin pigmentation. Pigment Cell Melanoma Res. 2011;24:401–10.
300. Nishimura EK, Granter SR, Fisher DE. Mechanisms of hair graying: incomplete melanocyte stem cell maintenance in the niche. Science. 2005;307:720–4.
301. Morikawa S, Mabuchi Y, Niibe K, Suzuki S, Nagoshi N, Sunabori T, et al. Development of mesenchymal stem cells partially originate from the neural crest. Biochem Biophys Res Commun. 2009;379:1114–9.

302. Brennan TV, Lin L, Huang X, Cardona DM, Li Z, Dredge K, et al. Heparan sulfate, an endogenous TLR4 agonist, promotes acute GVHD following allogeneic stem cell transplantation. Blood. 2012;120:2899–908. doi:10.1182/blood-2011-07-368720.
303. Nowarski R, Gagliani N, Huber S, Flavell RA. Innate immune cells in inflammation and cancer. Cancer Immunol Res. 2013;1:77–84. doi:10.1158/2326-6066.CIR-13-0081.
304. DiCarlo E, Forni G, Lollini PL, Colombo MP, Modesti A, Musiani P. The intriguing role of polymorphonuclear neutrophils in antitumor reactions. Blood. 2001;97:339–45.
305. Sigal LJ, Crotty S, Andino R, Rock KL. Cytotoxic T-cell immunity to virus-infected non-haematopoietic cells requires presentation of exogenous antigen. Nature. 1999;398:77–80.
306. D'Amico G, Frascaroli G, Bianchi G, Transidico P, Doni A, Vecchi A, Sozzani S, Allavena P, Mantovani A. Uncoupling of inflammatory chemokine receptors by IL-10: generation of functional decoys. Nat Immunol. 2000;1:387–91.
307. Lloyd CM, Hawrylowicz CM. Regulatory T cells in asthma. Immunity. 2009;31:438–49.
308. Werling D, Hope JC, Howard CJ, Jungi TW. Differential production of cytokines, reactive oxygen and nitrogen by bovine macrophages and dendritic cells stimulated with toll-like receptor agonists. Immunology. 2004;111:41–52.
309. Daly C, Dube C, Rollins BJ. Chemokine influences on adaptive immunity and malignancies of the immune system. Emst Schering Res Found Workshop. 2004;45:11–30.
310. Hadler-Olsen E, Winberg JO, Uhlin-Hansen L. Matrix metalloproteinases in cancer: their value as diagnostic and prognostic markers and therapeutic targets. Tumour Biol. 2013;34:2041–51.
311. Mendelsohn J, Baselga J. Epidermal growth factor receptor targeting in cancer. Semin Oncol. 2006;33:369–85.
312. Cooper MA, Fehniger TA, Caligiuri MA. The biology of human natural killer-cell subsets. Trends Immunol. 2001;22:633–40.
313. Rajagopalan S. HLA-G-mediated NK cell senescence promotes vascular remodeling: implications for reproduction. Cell Mol Immunol. 2014;11:460–6. doi:10.1038/cmi.2014.53. Epub 2014 Jul 7
314. Cooper MA, Fehniger TA, Fuchs A, Colonna M, Caligiuri MA. NK cell and DC interactions. Trends Immunol. 2004;25:47–52.
315. Robertson MJ, Ritz J. Biology and clinical relevance of human natural killer cells. Blood. 1990;76:2421–38.
316. Lanier LL, Le AM, Civin CI, Loken MR, Phillips JH. The relationship of CD16 (Leu-11) and Leu-19 (NKH-1) antigen expression on human peripheral blood NK cells and cytotoxic T lymphocytes. J Immunol. 1986;136:4480–6.
317. Grubeck-Loebenstein B, Della Bella S, Iorio AM, Michel JP, Pawelec G, Solana R. Immunosenescence and vaccine failure in the elderly. Aging Clin Exp Res. 2009;21:201–9.
318. Lanier LL. NK cell recognition. Annu Rev Immunol. 2005;23:225–74.
319. Caligiuri MA, Zmuidzinas A, Manley TJ, Levine H, Smith KA, Ritz J. Functional consequences of interleukin 2 receptor expression on resting human lymphocytes: identification of a novel natural killer cell subset with high affinity receptors. J Exp Med. 1990;171:1509–26.
320. Smyth MJ, Cretney E, Kelly JM, Westwood JA, Street SE, Yagita H, et al. Activation of NK cell cytotoxicity. Mol Immunol. 2005;42:501–10.
321. Zwirner NW, Fuertes MB, Girart MV, Domaica CI, Rossi LE. Cytokine-driven regulation of NK cell functions in tumor immunity: role of the MICA-NKG2D system. Cytokine Growth Factor Rev. 2007;18:159–70.
322. Pende D, Parolini S, Pessino A, Sivori S, Augugliaro R, Morelli L, et al. Identification and molecular characterization of NKp30, a novel triggering receptor involved in natural cytotoxicity mediated by human natural killer cells. J Exp Med. 1999;190:1505–16.
323. Balch CM, Tilden AB, Dougherty PA, Cloud GA, Abo T. Depressed levels of granular lymphocytes with natural killer (NK) cell function in 247 cancer patients. Am Surg. 1983;198:192–9.
324. DiPenta JM, Johnson JG, Murphy RJ. Natural killer cells and exercise training in the elderly: a review. Can J Appl Physiol. 2004;29:419–43.

325. Shephard RJ, Shek PN. Cancer, immune function, and physical activity. Can J Appl Physiol. 1995;20:1–25.
326. Haaland DA, Sabljic TF, Baribeau DA, Mukovozov IM, Hart LE. Is regular exercise a friend or foe of the aging immune system? A systematic review. Clin J Sport Med. 2008;18:539–48. doi:10.1097/JSM.0b013e3181865eec.
327. Albers R, Antoine JM, Bourdet-Sicard R, Calder PC, Gleeson M, Lesourd B, Samartín S, Sanderson IR, Van Loo J, Vas Dias FW, Watzl B. Markers to measure immunomodulation in human nutrition intervention studies. Br J Nutr. 2005;94:452–81.
328. Ince N, de la Monte SM, Wands JR. Overexpression of human aspartyl (asparaginyl) beta-hydroxylase is associated with malignant transformation. Cancer Res. 2000;60:1261–6.
329. Perica K, Varela JC, Oelke M, Schneck J. Adoptive T cell immunotherapy for cancer. Rambam Maimonides Med J. 2015;6:e0004. doi:10.5041/RMMJ.10179. eCollection 2015
330. Gaber T, Strehl C, Sawitzki B, Hoff P, Buttgereit F. Cellular energy metabolism in T-lymphocytes. Intl Rev of Immunol. 2015;34:34–49. doi:10.3109/08830185.2014.956358.
331. Fulop T Jr, Larbi A, Dupuis G, Pawelec G. Ageing, autoimmunity and arthritis: perturbations of TCR signal transduction pathways with ageing- a biochemical paradigm for the ageing immune system. Arthritis Res Ther. 2003;5:290–302.
332. Aspinall R. Age-related changes in the function of T cells. Microsc Res Tech. 2003;62:508–13.
333. Ait-Oufella H, Salomon BL, Potteaux S, Robertson A-KL, Gourdy P, Zoll J, Merval R, Esposito B, Cohen JL, Fisson S, et al. Natural regulatory T cells control the development of atherosclerosis in mice. Nat Med. 2006;12:178–80.
334. Zhou X, Nicoletti A, Elhage R, Hansson GK. Transfer of CD4(+) T cells aggravates atherosclerosis in immunodeficient apolipoprotein E knockout mice. Circulation. 2000;102:2919–22.
335. Hammad H, Plantinga M, Deswarte K, Pouliot P, Willart MA, Kool M, Muskens F, Lambrecht BN. Inflammatory dendritic cells–not basophils–are necessary and sufficient for induction of Th2 immunity to inhaled house dust mite allergen. J Exp Med. 2010;207:2097–111.
336. Linton PJ, Dorshkind K. Age-related changes in lymphocyte development and function. Nat Immunol. 2004;5:133–9.
337. Herrero C, Sebastian C, Marques L, Comalada M, Xaus J, Valledor AF, Lioberas J, Celada A. Immunosenescence of macrophages: reduced MHC class II gene expression. Exp Gerontol. 2002;37:389–94.
338. Galkina E, Kadl A, Sanders J, Varughese D, Sarembock IJ, Ley K. Lymphocyte recruitment into the aortic wall before and during development of atherosclerosis is partially L-selectin dependent. J Exp Med. 2006;203:1273–82.
339. Mckinnon JG, Hoover SK, Inge TH, Bear HD. Activation and expansion of cytotoxic T lymphocytes from tumor-draining lymph nodes. Cancer Immunol Immunother. 1990;32:38–44.
340. Gu L, Tseng S, Horner RM, Tam C, Loda M, Rollins BJ. Control of TH2 polarization by the chemokine monocyte chemoattractant protein-1. Nature. 2000;404:407–11.
341. Hsieh FH, Lam BK, Penrose JF, Austen KF, Boyce JA. T helper cell type 2 cytokines coordinately regulate immunoglobulin E-dependent cysteinyl leukotriene production by human cord blood-derived mast cell: profound induction of leukotriene C(4) synthase expression by interleukin 4. J Exp Med. 2001;193:123–33.
342. Serelli-Lee V, Ling KL, Ho C, et al. Persistent *Helicobacter pylori* specific Th17 responses in patients with past H. pylori infection are associated with elevated gastric mucosal IL-1beta. PLoS One. 2012;7(6):e39199.
343. Fu TM, Ulmer JB, Caulfield MJ, Deck RR, Friedman A, Wang S, Liu X, Donnelly JJ, Liu MA. Priming of cytotoxic T lymphocytes by DNA vaccines: requirement for professional antigen presenting cells and evidence for antigen transfer from myocytes. Mol Med. 1997;3:362–71.
344. Rafi A, Castle SC, Uyemura K, Makinodan T. Immune dysfunction in the elderly and its reversal by antihistamines. Biomed Pharmacoth. 2003;57:246–50.
345. Yang K, Chi H. AMPK helps T cell survive nutrient starvation. Immunity. 2015;42:4–6.

346. Khor SC, Abdul Karim N, Ngah WZ, Yusof YA, Makpol S. Vitamin E in sarcopenia: current evidences on its role in prevention and treatment. Oxidative Med Cell Longev. 2014;2014:914853. doi:10.1155/2014/914853. Epub 2014 Jul 6
347. Kim J, Wilson JM, Lee S. Dietary implications on mechanisms of sarcopenia: roles of protein, amino acids and antioxidants. J Nutrit Biochem. 2010;21:1–13.
348. Gashev AA, Chatterjee V. Aged lymphatic contractility: recent answers and new questions. Lymphat Res Biol. 2013;11:2–13.
349. Choi YS, Baumgarth N. Dual role for B-1a cells in immunity to influenza virus infection. J Exp Med. 2008;205:3053–64.
350. Matsumura Y, Abe M, Makimura K. Commensal fungi are involved in antigen-specific antibody production in the elderly. Brit J Med Medical Res. 2015;5:1562–70. Article no.BJMMR.2015.176–ISSN: 2231-0614
351. Perry HM, Bender TP, McNamara CA. B cell subsets in atherosclerosis. Front Immunol. 2012;3:373.
352. Vidarsson G, Dekkers G, Rispens T. IgG subclasses and allotypes: from structure to effector functions. Front Immunol. 2014;5:520. doi:10.3389/fimmu.2014.00520.
353. Abraham E, Wunderink R, Silverman H, Perl TM, Nasraway S, Levy H, Bone R, Wenzel RP, Balk R, Allred R, Pennington JE, Wherry JC. Efficacy and safety of monoclonal antibody to human tumor necrosis factor alpha in patients with sepsis syndrome. JAMA. 1995;273:934–41.
354. Schroeder HW Jr. The evolution and development of the antibody repertoire. Front Immunol. 2015; doi:10.3389/fimmu.2015.00033.
355. Daugherty A, Puré E, Delfel-Butteiger D, Chen S, Leferovich J, Roselaar SE, Rader DJ. The effects of total lymphocyte deficiency on the extent of atherosclerosis in apolipoprotein E−/− mice. J Clin Invest. 1997;100:1575–80.
356. Blaeser A, McGlauchlen K, Vogel LA. Aged-B lymphocytes retain their ability to express surface markers but are dysfunctional in their proliferative capability during early activation events. Immun Ageing. 2008;5:15. doi:10.1186/1742-4933-5-15.
357. Iwasaki A, Medzhitov R. Regulation of adaptive immunity by the innate immune system. Science. 2010;327:291–5. doi:10.1126/science.1183021.
358. Major AS, Fazio S, Linton MF. B-lymphocyte deficiency increases atherosclerosis in LDL receptor-null mice. Arterioscler Thromb Vasc Biol. 2002;22:1892–8.
359. Tsiantoulas D, Diehl CJ, Witztum JL, Christoph J. Binder B cells and humoral immunity in atherosclerosis. Circ Res. 2014;114:1743–56.
360. Howard WA, Gibson KL, Dunn-Walters DK. Antibody quality in old age. Rejuvenation Res. 2006;9:117–25.
361. Dailey RW, Eun SY, Russell CE, Vogel LA. B cells of aged mice show decreased expansion in response to antigen, but are normal in effector function. Cell Immunol. 2001;214:99–109.
362. Neyt K, Perros F, Geurtsvan-Kessel CH, Hammad H, Lambrecht BN. Tertiary lymphoid organs in infection and autoimmunity. Trends Immunol. 2012;33:297–305.
363. Linterman MA. How T follicular helper cells and the germinal centre response change with age. Immunol Cell Biol. 2014;92:72–9.
364. Good-Jacobson KL, Shlomchik MJ. Plasticity and heterogeneity in the generation of memory B cells and long-lived plasma cells: the influence of germinal center interactions and dynamics. J Immunol. 2010;185:3117–25. doi:10.4049/jimmunol.1001155.
365. Tseng CW, Liu GY. Expanding roles of neutrophils in aging hosts. Curr Opin Immunol. 2014;29:43–8.
366. De Larco JE, Wuertz BRK, Furcht LT. The potential role of neutrophils in promoting the metastatic phenotype of tumor releasing interleukin -8. Clin Cancer Res. 2004;10:4895–900.
367. Jackaman C, Nelson DJ. Are macrophages, myeloid derived suppressor cells and neutrophils mediators of local suppression in healthy and cancerous tissues in aging hosts. Exp Gerontol. 2014;54:53–7.

368. Teranishi A, Akada S, Saito S, Hatake K, Morikawa H. Macrophage cology-stimulating factor restored chemotherapy-induced granulocyte dysfunction: role of IL-8 production by monocytes. Int Immunopharmacol. 2002;2:83–94.
369. Rijken F, Bruijzeel-Koomen CA. Photoaged skin: the role of neutrophils, preventive measures and potential pharmacological targets. Clin Pharmacol Ther. 2010;89:120–4.
370. Gomez-Cambronero J, Kantonen S. A river runs through it: how autophagy, senescence, and phagocytosis could be linked to phospholipase D by Wnt signaling. J Leukoc Biol. 2014;96:779–84.
371. Ohbayashi H, Shimokata K. Matrix metalloproteinase-9 and airway remodeling in asthma. Curr Drug Targets Inflamm Allergy. 2005;4:177–81.
372. Ibusuki K, Sakiyama T, Kanmura S, Maeda T, Iwashita Y, Nasu Y, Sasaki F, Taguchi H, Hashimoto S, Numata M, Uto H, Tsubouchi H, Ido A. Human neutrophil peptides induce interleukin-8 in intestinal epithelial cells through the P2 receptor and ERK1/2 signaling pathways. Int J Mol Med. 2015;35:1603–9. doi:10.3892/ijmm.2015.2156. Epub 2015 Mar 26
373. Ribatti D, Crivellato E. Mast cell ontology: an historical overview. Immunol Lett. 2014;159:11–4. doi:10.1016/j.imlet.2014.02.003. Epub 2014 Feb 14
374. Shakoory B, Fitzgerald SM, Lee SA, Chi DS, Krishnawamy G. The role of human mast cell-derived cytokines in eosinophil biology. J Interferon Cytokine Res. 2004;24:271–81.
375. Theoharides TC, Alysandratos KD, Angelidou A, Delivanis DA, Sismanopoulos N, Zhang B, Asadi S, Vasiadi M, Weng Z, Miniati A, Kalogeromitros D. Mast cells and inflammation. Biochim Biophys Acta. 2012;1822:21–33. doi:10.1016/j.bbadis.2010.12.014.
376. Valent P, Bettelheim P. Cell surface structures on human basophils and mast cells: biochemical and functional characterization. Adv Immunol. 1992;52:333–423.
377. Valent P, Schernthaner GH, Sperr WR, Fritsch G, Agis H, Willheim M, Buhring HJ, Orfao A, Escribano L. Variable expression of activation-linked surface antigens on human mast cells in health and disease. Immunol Rev. 2001;179:74–81.
378. Schwartz LB. The mast cell. In: Kaplan AP, editor. Allergy, vol. 1. Edingurgh: Churchil Livingston; 1985. p. 53–92.
379. Tomita M, Matsuzaki Y, Onitsuka T. Correlation between mast cells and survival rates in patients with pulmonary adenocarcinoma. Lung Cancer. 1999;26:103–8.
380. Brightling CE, Bradding P, Pavord ID, Wardlaw AJ. New insights into the role of the mast cell in asthma. Clin Exp Allergy. 2003;33:550–6.
381. Renauld J-C. New insights into the role of cytokines in asthma. J Clin Pathol. 2001;54:577–89.
382. Kelley JL, Chi DS, Abou-Auda W, Smith JK, Krishnaswamy G. The molecular role of mast cells in atherosclerotic cardiovascular disease. Mol Med Today. 2000;6:304–8.
383. Barcante JMP, Barcante TA, Peconick AP, Pereira LJ, Lima WS. Parasitic infections and inflammatory diseases. In: Khatami M, editor. Inflammation, chronic diseases and cancer. Cell and molecular biology, immunology and clinical bases. Rijeka: InTech; 2012. p. 205–18.
384. Le Meur Y, Tesch GH, Hill PA, Mu W, Foti R, Nikolic-Paterson DJ, Atkins RC. Macrophage accumulation at a site of renal inflammation is dependent on the M-CSF/c-fms pathway. J Leukocyte Biol. 2002;72:530–7.
385. Lambrecht BN, Hammad H. Death at the airway epithelium in asthma. Cell Res. 2013;23:588–9.
386. Khatami M, Donnelly JJ, John T, Rockey JH. Vernal conjunctivitis. Model studies in guinea pigs immunized topically with fluoresceinyl ovalbumin. Arch Ophthalmol. 1984;102:1683–8.
387. Khatami M, Donnelly JJ, Rockey JH. Induction and down-regulation of conjunctival type-1 hypersensitivity reactions in guinea pigs sensitized topically with fluoresceinyl ovalbumin. Ophthalmic Res. 1985;17:139–47.
388. El-Malky M, Maruyama H, Hirabayashi Y, Shimada S, Yoshida A, Amano T, et al. Intraepithelial infiltration of eosinophils and their contribution to the elimination of adult intestinal nematode, *Strongyloides venezuelensis* in mice. Parasitol Int. 2003;52:71–910.
389. Austen KF, Boyce JA. Mast cell lineage development and phenotypic regulation. Leuk Res. 2001;25:511–8.

390. Tobin MJ. Chronic obstructive disease, pollution, pulmonary vascular disease, transplantation, pleural disease, and lung cancer. Am J Respir Crit Care Med. 2000;164:1789.
391. Galli SJ, Maurer M, Lantz CS. Mast cells as sentinels of innate immunity. Curr Opin Immunol. 1999;11:53–9.
392. Galli SJ. Biology of disease: new insights into 'the riddle of mast cells'; microenvironmental regulation of mast cell development and phenotypic heterogeneity. Lab Investig. 1990;62:5–33.
393. Galli SJ, Borregaard N, Wynn TA. Phenotypic and functional plasticity of cells of innate immunity: macrophages, mast cells and neutrophils. Nat Immunol. 2011;12:1035–44.
394. Walls AF, Roberts JA, Godfrey RC, Church MK, Holgate ST. Histochemical heterogeneity of human mast cells: disease-related differences in mast cell subsets recovered by bronchoalveolar lavage. Intl Arch Allergy Appl Immunol. 1990;92:233–41.
395. Burnet FM. The probable relationship of some or all mast cells to the T-cell system. Cell Immunol. 1977;30:358–60.
396. Palomares O. The role of regulatory T cells in IgE-mediated food allergy. J Investig Allergol Clin Immunol. 2013;23(6):371–82.
397. Helleboid L, Khatami M, Wei Z-G, Rockey JH. Histamine and prostacyclin: primary and secondary release in allergic conjunctivitis. Invest Ophthalmol Vis Sci. 1991;32:2281–9.
398. Rockey JH, Donnelly JJ, John T, Khatami M, Schwartzman RM, Stromberg BE, Bianco AE, Soulsby EJL. IgE antibodies in ocular immunopathology. In: O'Conner GR, Chandler JW, editors. Advances in immunology and immunopathology of the eye. New York: Masson; 1985. p. 199–202.
399. Ribatti D, Nico B, Ranieri G, Specchia G, Vacca A. The role of angiogenesis in human non-hodgkin lymphomas. Neoplasia. 2013;15:231–8.
400. Ribati D. The crucial role of mast cells in blood-brain barrier alterations. Exp Cell Res. 2015; doi:10.1016/j.yexcr.2015.05.013. pii: S0014–4827(15)00193–7. [Epub ahead of print]
401. Ribatti D. Mast cells as therapeutic target in cancer. Eur J Pharmacol. 2015; doi:10.1016/j.ejphar.2015.02.056. pii: S0014-2999(15)00356-8. [Epub ahead of print]
402. Ribatti D, Ranieri G. Tryptase, a novel angiogenic factor stored in mast cell graules. Exp Cell Res. 2015;332:157–62. doi:10.1016/j.yexcr.2014.11.014. Epub 2014 Dec 3
403. Vesterinen E, Oukkala E, Timonen T, Aromaa A. Cancer incident among 78000 asmatic patients. Intl J Epidemiol. 1993;22:976–82.
404. Huovinen E, Kapiro J, Vesterinen E, Koshenvuo M. Mortality of adults with asthma: a prospective cohort study. Thorax. 1997;52:49–54.
405. Tomita M, Matsuzaki Y, Edagawa M, Shimizu T, Hara M, Onitsuka T. Distribution of mast cells in mediastinal lymph nodes from lung cancer patients. World J Surg Oncol. 2003;1:25.
406. Khatami M. Cyclooxygenase inhibitor ketorolac or mast cell stabilizers: immunological challenges in cancer therapy. Clin Cancer Res. 2005;11:1349–51.
407. Medhurst SJ, Collins SD, Billinton A, Bingham S, Dalziel RG, Brass A, Roberts JC, Medhurst AD, Chessell IP. Novel histamine H3 receptor antagonists GSK189254 and GSK334429 are efficacious in surgically-induced and virally-induced rat models of neuropathic pain. Pain. 2008;138:61–9. doi:10.1016/j.pain.2007.11.006. Epub 2007 Dec 31
408. Ammendola M, Marech I, Sammarco G, Zuccalà V, Luposella M, Zizzo N, et al. Infiltrating mast cells correlate with angiogenesis in bone metastases from gastric cancer patients. Int J Mol Sci. 2015;16(2):3237–50. doi:10.3390/ijms160232372015.
409. Baylin SB, Abeloff MD, Wieman KC, Tomford JW, Ettinger DS. Elevated histaminase (diaminase) activity in small-cell carcinoma of the lung. N Engl J Med. 1975;293:1286–90.
410. Dvorak A, Seder R, Paul W, Morgan E, Galli S. Effects of interleukin-3 with or without the c-kit ligand, stem cell factor, on the survival and cytoplasmic granule formation of mouse basophils and mast cells in vitro. Am J Pathol. 1994;11:160–70.
411. Bijanzadeh M, Ramachandra NB, Mahesh PA, Savitha MR, Vijayakumar GS, Kumar P, et al. Soluble intercellular adhesion molecule-1 and E-selectin in patients with asthma exacerbation. Lung. 2009;187:315–20.

412. Bot I, de Jager SC, Zernecke A, Lindstedt KA, van Berkel TJ, Weber C, Biessen EA. Perivascular mast cells promote atherogenesis and induce plaque destabilization in apolipoprotein E-deficient mice. Circulation. 2007;115:2516–25.
413. Chatterjee V, Gashev AA. Aging-associated shifts in functional status of mast cells located by adult and aged mesenteric lymphatic vessels. Am J Physiol Heart Circ Physiol. 2012;303:H693–702.
414. Grimbaldeston MA, Metz M, Yu M, Tsai M, Galli SJ. Effector and potential immunoregulatory roles of mast cells in IgE-associated acquired immune responses. Curr Opinion Immunol. 2006;18:751–60.
415. Gunin AG, Kornilov NK, Vasilieva OV, Petrov VV. Age-related changes in proliferation, the numbers of mast cells, eosinophils, and cd45-positive cells in human dermis. J Gerontol Biol Sci Med Sci. 2011;66:385–92.
416. Okayama Y, Benyon RC, Rees PH, Lowman MA, Hillier K, Church MK. Inhibition profiles of sodium cromoglycate and nedocromil sodium on mediator release from mast cells of human skin, lung, tonsil, adenoid and intestine. Clin Exp Allergy. 1992;22:401–9.
417. Gong J, Yang NS, Croft M, Weng IC, Sun L, Liu FT, Chen SS. The antigen presentation function of bone marrow-derived mast cells is spatiotemporally restricted to a subset expressing high levels of cell surface FcepsilonRI and MHC II. BMC Immunol. 2010;11:34. doi:10.1186/1471-2172-11-34.
418. Cundell DR, Mickle KE. Developing the perfect antihistamine for use in allergic conditions: a voyage in H1 selectivity. eBook, Frontiers in Clinical Drug Research-Anti Allergy Agents. 2016.
419. Agrawal A, Agrawal S, Gupta S. Dendritic cells in human aging. Exp Gerontol. 2007;42:421–6.
420. Gosset P, Bureau F, Angeli V, Pichavant M, Faveeuw C, Tonnel AB, Trottein F. Prostaglandin D2 affects the maturation of human monocyte-derived dendritic cells: consequence on the polarization of naive Th cells. J Immunol. 2003;170:4943–52.
421. Inaba K, Turley S, Yamaide F, Iyoda T, Mahnke K, Inaba M, et al. Efficient presentation of phagocytosed cellular fragments on the major histocompatibility complex class II products of dendritic cells. J Exp Med. 1998;188:2163–73.
422. Spies B, Hochrein H, Vabulas M, Huster K, Busch DH, Schmitz F, Heit A, Wagner H. Vaccination with plasmid DNA activates dendritic cells via toll-like receptor 9 (TLR9) but functions in TLR9-deficient mice. J Immunol. 2003;171:5908–12.
423. Khatami M. Safety concerns and hidden agenda behind HPV vaccines: another generation of drug-dependent society? Clin Trans Med. 2016;5(1):46. Epub 2016 Dec 5
424. Lambrecht BN, Hammad H. Lung dendritic cells in respiratory viral infection and asthma: from protection to immunopathology. Annu Rev Immunol. 2012;30:243–70.
425. Bobryshev YV. Dendritic cells and their role in atherogenesis. Lab Investig. 2010;90:970–84.
426. Trombetta ES, Ebersold M, Garrett W, Pypaert M, Mellman I. Activation of lysosomal function during dendritic cell maturation. Science. 2003;299:1400–3.
427. Uyemura K, Castle SC, Makinodan T. The frail elderly: role of dendritic cells in the susceptibility of infection. Mech Ageing Dev. 2002;123:955–62.
428. Romagnoli G, Nisini R, Chiani P, Mariotti S, Teloni R, Cassone A, Torosantucci A. The interaction of human dendritic cells with yeast and germ-tube forms of Candida Albicans leads to efficient fungal processing, dendritic cell maturation, and acquisition of a Th1 response-promoting function. J Leukoc Biol. 2004;75:117–26. Epub 2003 Oct 2
429. Reid SD, Penna G, Adorini L. The control of T cell responses by dendritic cell subsets. Curr Opin Immunol. 2000;12:114–21.
430. Gerosa F, Baldani-Guerra B, Nisii C, Marchesini V, Carra G, Trinchieri G. Reciprocal activating interaction between natural killer cells and dendritic cells. J Exp Med. 2002;195:327–33.
431. Jonuleit H, Schmitt E, Steinbrink K, Henk AH. Dendritic cells as a tool to induce anergic and regulatory T cells. Trends Immunol. 2001;22:394–400.
432. Paschen A, Dittmar KE, Grenningloh R, Rohde M, Schadendorf D, Domann E, Chakraborty T, Weiss S. Human dendritic cells infected by *Listeria monocytogenes*: induction of matu-

ration, requirements for phagolysosomal escape and antigen presentation capacity Eur. J Immunol. 2000;30:3447–56.
433. Dieu MC, Vanbervliet B, Vicari A, Bridon JM, Oldham E, Ait-Yhia S, Briere F, Zlotni A, Lebecque S, Caux C. Selective recruitment of immature and mature dendritic cells by distinct chemokines expressed in different anatomic sites. J Exp Med. 1998;188:373–86.
434. Hirsch S, Austyn JM, Gordon S. Expression of the macrophage-specific antigen F4/80 during differentiation of mouse bone marrow cells in culture. J Exp Med. 1981;11:713–25. doi:10.1084/jem.154.3.713.
435. Sanghera JS, Weinstein SL, Aluwalia M, Girn J, Pelech SL. Activation of multiple proline-directed kinases by bacterial lipopolysaccharide in murine macrophages. J Immunol. 1996;156:4457–65.
436. Montovani A, Ming WJ, Balotta C, Abdeljalil B, Bottazzi B. Origin and regulation of tumor-associated macrophages: the role of tumor-derived chemotactic factor. Biochim Biophys Acta. 1986;865:59–67.
437. Gordon S. Alternative activation of macrophages. Nat Rev Immunol. 2005;5:953–64. doi:10.1038/nri1733.
438. Bae YS, Lee JH, Choi SH, Kim S, Almazan F, Witztum JL, Miller YI. Macrophages generate reactive oxygen species in response to minimally oxidized low-density lipoprotein: toll-like receptor 4- and spleen tyrosine kinase-dependent activation of NADPH oxidase 2. Circ Res. 2009;104:210–8.
439. Mantovani A, Schioppa T, Biswas SK, Marchesi F, Allavena P, Sica A. Tumor-associated macrophages and dendritic cells as prototypic type II polarized myeloid populations. Tumori. 2003;89(5):459–68.
440. Mantovani A, Sozzani S, Locati M, Allavena P, Sica A. Macrophage polarization: tumor-associated macrophages as a paradigm for polarized M2 mononuclear phagocytes. Trends Immunol. 2002;23(11):549–55.
441. Fadok VA, de Cathelineau A, Daleke DL, Henson PM, Bratton DL. Loss of phospholipids asymmetry and surface exposure of phosphatidylserine is required for phagocytosis of apoptotic cell by macrophages and fibroblasts. J Biol Chem. 2001;276:1071–7.
442. Al-Sarireh B, Eremin O. Tumour-associated macrophages (TAMs): disordered function, immune suppression and progressive tumour growth. J R Coll Surg Edinb. 2000;45:1–16.
443. Stranks AJ, Hansen AL, Panse I, Mortensen M, Ferguson DJP, Puleston DJ, Shenderov K, Watson AS, Veldhoen M, Phadwal K, Cerundolo V, Simon AK. Autophagy controls acquisition of aging features in macrophages. J Innate Immun. 2015;7:375–91. doi:10.1159/000370112.
444. Weitzman SA, Gordon LI. Inflammation and cancer: role of phagocytic-generated oxidants in carcinogenesis. Blood. 1990;76:655–63.
445. Srivastava P. Interaction of heat shock proteins with peptides and antigen presenting cells: chaperoning of the innate and adaptive immune responses. Annu Rev Immunol. 2002;20:395–425.
446. Zhu L, Zhao Q, Yang T, Ding W, Zhao Y. Cellular metabolism and macrophage functional polarization. Int Rev Immunol. 2015;34:82–100.
447. Herbeuval JP, Lelievre E, Lambert C, Dy M, Genin C. Recruitment of STAT3 for production of IL-10 by colon carcinoma cells induced by macrophage-derived IL-6. J Immunol. 2004;172(7):4630–6.
448. Clinton SK, Underwood R, Hayes L, Sherman ML, Kufe DW, Libby P. Macrophage colony-stimulating factor gene expression in vascular cells and in experimental and human atherosclerosis. Am J Pathol. 1992;140:301–16.
449. Barton GM. A calculated response: control of inflammation by the innate immune system. J Clin Invest. 2008;118:413–20.
450. Schumann J. The impact of macrophage membrane lipid composition on innate immune response mechanisms. In: Khatami M, editor. Inflammation, chronic diseases and cancer; cell and molecular biology, immunology and clinical bases. Rijeka: Intech Publishing; 2012. p. 31–52.

451. Guilliams M, Lambrecht BN, Hammad H. Division of labor between lung dendritic cells and macrophages in the defense against pulmonary infections. Mucosal Immunol. 2013;6:464–73.
452. Folkman J. Angiogenesis. Ann Rev Med. 2006;57:1–18.
453. Wagner DD, Frenette PS. The vessel wall and its interactions. Blood. 2008;111:5271–81.
454. Saghiri MA, Asatourian A, Orangi J, Sorenson CM, Sheibani N. Functional role of inorganic trace elements in angiogenesis-Part I: N, Fe, Se, P, Au, and Ca. Crit Rev Oncol Hematol. 2015; doi:10.1016/j.critrevonc.2015.05.010. pii: S1040-8428(15)00099-2. [Epub ahead of print]
455. Benito-Martin A, Di Giannatale A, Ceder S, Peinado H. The new deal: a potential role for secreted vesicles in innate immunity and tumor progression. Front Immunol. 2015;24 doi:10.3389/fimmu.2015.00066.
456. Oliver G. Lymphatic vasculature development. Nat Rev Immunol. 2004;4:35–45.
457. Ozerdem U, Stallcup WB. Early contribution of pericytes to angiogenic sprouting and tube formation. Angiogenesis. 2003;6:241–9. doi:10.1023/b:agen.0000021401.58039.a9.
458. Jackson SP. The growing complexity of platelet aggregation. Blood. 2007;109:5087–95.
459. Williamson K, Stringer SE, Alexander MY. Endothelial progenitor cells enter the aging arena. Front Physiol. 2012;3:30. doi:10.3389/fphys.2012.00030.
460. Ribeiro AL, Okamoto OK. Combined effects of pericytes in the tumor microenvironment. Stem Cells Int. 2015;2015:868475.
461. Liao D, Johnson RS. Hypoxia: a key regulator of angiogenesis in cancer. Cancer Metastasis Rev. 2007;26:281–90.
462. Nurden AT, Nurden P, Sanchez M, Andia I, Anitua E. Platelets and wound healing. Front Biosci. 2008;13:3532–48.
463. Feuerstein G, Rabinovici R, Leor J, Winkler JD, Vonhof S. Platelet-activating factor and cardiac diseases: therapeutic potential for PAF inhibitors. J Lipid Mediat Cell Signal. 1997;15:255–84.
464. Cognasse F, Hamzeh H, Chavarin P, Acquart S, Genin C, Garraud O. Evidence of toll-like receptor molecules on human platelets. Immunol Cell Biol. 2005;83:196–8.
465. Andonegui G, Kerfoot SM, YK MN, Ebbert KV, Patel KD, Kubes P. Platelets express functional toll-like receptor-4. Blood. 2005;106:2417–23.
466. Fong KP, Barry C, Tran AN, Traxler EA, Wannemacher KM, Tang HY, Speicher KD, Blair IA, Speicher DW, Grosser T, Brass LF. Deciphering the human platelet sheddome. Blood. 2011;117:e15.
467. Anitua E, Andia I, Ardanza B, Nurden P, Nurden AT. Autologous platelets as a source of proteins for healing and tissue regeneration. Thromb Haemost. 2004;91:4–15.
468. Garraud O, Hamzeh-Cognasse H, Cognasse F. Platelets and cytokines: how and why? Transfus Clin Biol. 2012;19:104–8.
469. Shahabuddin S, Ponath P, Schleimer RP. Migration of eosinophils across endothelial cell monolayers: interactions among IL-5, endothelial-activating cytokines, and C-C chemokines. J Immunol. 2000;164:3847–54.
470. Dvorak HF, Brown LF, Detmar M, Dvorak AM. Vascular permeability factor/vascular endothelial growth factor, microvascular hyperpermeability, and angiogenesis. Am J Pathol. 1995;146:1029–39.
471. Mabeta P, Pepper MS. Hemangiomas – current therapeutic strategies. Int J Dev Biol. 2011;55(4–5):431–7. doi:10.1387/ijdb.103221pm.
472. Naito AT, Sumida T, Nomura S, Liu ML, Higo T, Nakagawa A, et al. Complement C1q activates canonical Wnt signaling and promotes aging-related phenotypes. Cell. 2012;149:1298–313.
473. Pathak AP, Hochfeld WE, Goodman SL, Pepper MS. Circulating and imaging markers for angiogenesis. 2008;11:321–35.
474. Wilson JF. Angiogenesis therapy moves beyond cancer: Ann Intern Med. 2004;141:165–8.
475. D'Alessio P. Aging and the endothelium. Exp Gerontol. 2004;39:165–71.

476. Garraud O, Hamzeh-Cognasse H, Pozzetto B, Cavaillon J-M, Cognasse F. Bench-to-bedside review: platelets and active immune functions – new clues for immunopathology? Critical Care. 2013;17:–236. doi:10.1186/cc12716.
477. Saze Z, Schuler PJ, Hong C-S, Cheng D, Jackson EK, Whiteside TL. Adenosine production by human B cells and B cell-mediated suppression of activated T cells. Blood. 2013;122:9–18.
478. Deaglio S, Dwyer K, Gao W, Friedman D, Usheva A, Erat A, et al. Adenosine generation catalyzed by CD39 and CD73 expressed on regulatory T cells mediates immune suppression. J Exp Med. 2007;204:1257–65.
479. Eltzschig HK, Thompson LF, Karhausen J, Cotta RJ, Ibla JC, Robson SC, et al. Endogenous adenosine produced during hypoxia attenuates neutrophil accumulation: coordination by extracellular nucleotide metabolism. Blood. 2004;104:3986–92.
480. Eltzschig HK. Adenosine: an old drug newly discovered. Anesthesiology. 2009;111:904–1510.
481. Roberts V, Stagg J, Dwyer KM. The role of ectonucleotidases CD39 and CD73 and adenosine signaling in solid organ transplantation. Front Immunol. 2014;5:64. eCollection 2014
482. Karshovska E, Weber C, Von Hundelshausen P. Platelet chemokines in health and disease. Thromb Haemost. 2013;110:894–902.
483. Kamath BM, Spinner NB, Emerick KM, Chudley AE, Booth C, Piccoli DA, Krantz ID. Vascular anomalies in Alagille syndrome: a significant cause of morbidity and mortality. Circulation. 2004;109:1354–8.
484. Hiratsuka S, Maru Y, Okada A, Seiki M, Noda T, Shibuya M. Involvement of Flt-1 tyrosine kinase (vascular endothelial growth factor receptor-1) in pathological angiogenesis. Cancer Res. 2001;61:1207–13.
485. Ferrara N. Role of vascular endothelial growth factor in regulation of physiological angiogenesis. Am J Physiol Cell Physiol. 2001;280:C1358–66.
486. Veale DJ, Maple C. Cell adhesion molecules in rheumatoid arthritis. Drugs Aging. 1996;9:87–92.
487. Hansson GK, Hermansson A. The immune system in atherosclerosis. Nat Immunol. 2011;12:204–12.
488. Semenza GL, Roth PH, Fang HM, Wang GL. Transcriptional regulation of genes encoding glycolytic enzymes by hypoxia-inducible factor 1. J Biol Chem. 1994;269:23757–63.
489. George J, Goldstein E, Abashidze S, Deutsch V, Shmilovich H, Finkelste A, Herz I, Miller H, Keren G. Circulating endothelial progenitor cells in patients with unstable angina: association with systemic inflammation. Eur Heart J. 2004;25:1003–8.
490. Harris AL, Zhang H, Moghaddam A, Fox S, Scott P, Pattison A, Gatter K, Stratford L, Bicknell R. Breast cancer angiogenesis- new approaches to therapy via antiangiogenesis, hypoxic activated drugs, and vascular targeting. Breast Cancer Res. 1996;38:97–108.
491. Napoli C, Ignarro LJ. Nitric oxide and pathogenic mechanisms involved in the development of vascular diseases. Arch Pharm Res. 2009;32:1103–8. doi:10.1007/s12272-009-1801-1. Epub 2009.
492. Napoli C, Hayashi T, Cacciatore F, Casamassimi A, Casini C, Al-Omran M, Ignarro LJ. Endothelial progenitor cells as therapeutic agents in the microcirculation: an update. Atherosclerosis. 2011;215:9–22.
493. Arnett TR, Gibbons DC, Utting JC, Orriss IR, Hoebertz A, Rosendaal M, Meghji S. Hypoxia is a major stimulator of osteoclast formation and bone resorption. J Cell Physiol. 2003;196:2–8.
494. Lamoreaux WJ, Fitzgerald ME, Reiner A, Hasty KA, Charles ST. Vascular endothelial growth factor increases release of gelatinase a and decreases release of tissue inhibitor of metalloproteinases by microvascular endothelial cells in vitro. Microvasc Res. 1998;55:29–42.
495. Meldrum DR. Tumor necrosis factor in the heart. Am J Phys. 1998;274:R577–95.
496. Gille J, Swerlick RA, Lawley TJ, Caughman SW. Differential regulation of vascular cell adhesion molecule-1 gene transcription by tumor necrosis factor alpha and interleukin-1 alpha in dermal microvascular endothelial cells. Blood. 1996;87:211–7.

497. Lee KH, Lawley TJ, Xu YL, Swerlick RA. VCAM-1-, ELAM-1-, and ICAM-1-independent adhesion of melanoma cells to cultured human dermal microvascular endothelial cells. J Invest Dermatol. 1992;98:79–85.
498. Zdrojewicz Z, Pachura E, Pachura P. The thymus: a forgotten, but very important organ. Adv Clin Exp Med. 2016;25(2):369–75. doi:10.17219/acem/58802.
499. Chaudhry MS, Velardi E, Dudakov JA, van den Brink MR. Thymus: the next (re)generation. Immunol Rev. 2016;271(1):56–71. doi:10.1111/imr.12418.
500. Sepp NT, Gille J, Li LJ, Caughman SW, Lawley TJ, Swerlick RA. A factor in human plasma permits persistent expression of E-selectin by human endothelial cells. J Invest Dermatol. 1994;102:445–50.
501. Rutkowski MJ, Sughrue ME, Kane AJ, Ahn BJ, Fang S, Parsa AT. The complement cascade as a mediator of tissue growth and regeneration. Inflamm Res. 2010;59:897–905.
502. LaRocca TJ, Stivison EA, Hod EA, Spitalnik SL, Cowan PJ, Randis TM, Ratner AJ. Human-specific bacterial pore-forming toxins induce programmed necrosis in erythrocytes. MBio. 2014;5:e01251–14.
503. del Fresno C, Gomez-Garcia L, Caveda L, et al. Nitric oxide activates the expression of IRAK-M via the release of TNF-alpha in human monocytes. Nitric Oxide. 2004;10:213–20.
504. Weinstein SL, Gold MR, DeFranco AL. Bacterial lipopolysaccharide stimulates protein tyrosine phosphorylation in macrophages. Proc Natl Acad Sci. 1991;88:4148–52.
505. Hawiger J, Hawiger A, Timmons S. Endotoxin-sensitive membrane component of human platelets. Nature. 1975;256:125–7.
506. Keaney JF, Hare JM, Balligand JL, Loscalzo J, Smith TW, Colucci WS. Inhibition of nitric oxide synthase augments myocardial contractile responses to beta-adrenergic stimulation. Am J Physiol. 1996;271(Heart Circ. Physiol. 40):H2646–52.
507. Chen ZS, Pohl J, Lawley TJ, Swerlick RA. Human microvascular endothelial cells adhere to thrombospondin-1 via an RGD/CSVTCG domain independent mechanism. J Invest Dermatol. 1996;106:215–20.
508. Swerlick RA, Lawley TJ. Role of microvascular endothelial cells in inflammation. J Invest Dermatol. 1993;100:111S–5S.
509. Olsen KR, Donald JA. Nervous control of circulation: the role of gasotransmitters, NO, CO and H_2S. Acta Histochem. 2009;111:244–56.
510. Giulivi C, Kato K, Cooper CE. Nitric oxide regulation of mitochondrial oxygen consumption I: cellular physiology. Am J Physiol Cell Physiol. 2006;291:C1225–31.
511. Taylor CT, Moncada S. Nitric oxide, cytochrome c oxidase, and the cellular response to hypoxia. Arterioscler Thromb Vasc Biol. 2010;30:643–7.
512. Siddiq A, Aminova LR, Ratan RR. Hypoxia inducible factor prolyl 4-hydroxylase enzymes: center stage in the battle against hypoxia, metabolic compromise and oxidative stress. Neurochem Res. 2007;32:931–46.
513. Semenza GL. Regulation of oxygen homeostasis by hypoxia-inducible factor 1. Physiology. 2009;24:97–106.
514. Inoue Y, Hatta Y, Takeuchi J, Kosugi S, Miura I. Successful treatment of refractory acute GVHD complicated by severe intestinal transplant-associated thrombotic microangiopathy using recombinant thrombomodulin. Thromb Res. 2011;127:603–4.
515. Metzen E, Zhou J, Jelkmann W, Fandrey J, Brune B. Nitric oxide impairs normoxic degradation of HIF-1α by inhibition of prolyl hydroxylases. Mol Biol Cell. 2003;14:3470–81.
516. Li F, Sonveaux P, Rabbani ZN, Liu S, Yan B, Huang Q, Vujaskovic Z, Dewhirst MW, Li C-Y. Regulation of HIF-1α stability through S-nitrosylation. Mol Cell. 2007;26:63–74.
517. Kim-Shapiro DB, Gladwin MT, Patel RP, Hogg N. The reaction between nitrite and hemoglobin: the role of nitrite in hemoglobin-mediated hypoxic vasodilation. J Inorg Biochem. 2005;99:237–46.
518. Pierucci M, Galati S, Valentino M, Di Matteo V, Benigno A, Pitruzzella A, Muscat R, Di Giovanni G. Nitric oxide modulation of the basal ganglia circuitry: therapeutic implica-

tion for Parkinson's disease and other motor disorders. CNS Neurol Disord Drug Targets. 2011;10:777–91.

519. Amento EP, Ehsani N, Palmer H, Libby P. Cytokines and growth factors positively and negatively regulate interstitial collagen gene expression in human vascular smooth muscle cells. Arterioscler Thromb Vasc Biol. 1991;11:1223–30.
520. Li L, Moore PK. An overview of the biological significance of endogenous gases: new roles for old molecules. Biochem Soc Trans. 2007;35:1138–41.
521. Moncada S, Palmer RMJ, Higgs EA. Nitric oxide: physiology, pathophysiology and pharmacology. Pharmacol Rev. 1991;43:109–41.
522. Meldrum DR, Gambone JC, Morris MA, Esposito K, Giugliano D, Ignarro LJ. Lifestyle and metabolic approaches to maximizing erectile and vascular health. Int J Impot Res. 2012;24:61–8. doi:10.1038/ijir.2011.51. Epub 2011 Nov 10
523. Fukuto JM, Ignarro LJ. In vivo aspects of nitric oxide (NO) chemistry: does peroxynitrite ($^{-}$OONO) play a major role in cytotoxicity? Acc Chem Res. 1997;30:149–52.
524. Pryor WA, Houk KN, Foote CS, Fukuto JM, Ignarro LJ, Squadrito GL, Davies KJA. Free radical biology and medicine, it's a gas, man. Am J Physiol Regulatory Int Com Physiol. 2006;291:491–511.
525. Forman HJ, Fukuto J, Torres M. Redox signaling-chemistry defines which reactive oxygen and nitrogen species can act as second messengers. Am J Physiol Cell Physiol. 2004;287:C246–56.
526. Reiter RJ, Tan DX, Qi W, Manchester LC, Karbownik M, Calvo JR. Pharmacology and physiology of melatonin in the reduction of oxidative stress in vivo. Biol Signals Recept. 2000;9:160–71.
527. Paolocci N, Jackson MI, Lopez BE, Miranda K, Tocchetti CG, Wink DA, Hobbs AJ, Fukuto JM. The pharmacology of nitroxyl (HNO) and its therapeutic potential: not just the janus face of NO. Pharmacol Ther. 2007;113:442–58.
528. Bickar D, Bonaventura C, Bonaventura J. Carbon monoxide-driven reduction of ferric heme and heme proteins. J Biol Chem. 1984;259:10777–83.
529. Valentine WN, Toohey JI, Paglia DE, Nakatani M, Brockway RA. Modification of erythrocyte enzyme activities by persulfides and methanethiol: possible regulatory role. Proc Natl Acad Sci U S A. 1987;84:1394–8.
530. Taoka S, Banerjee R. Characterization of NO binding to human cystathionine β-synthase: possible implications of the effects of CO and NO binding to the human enzyme. J Inorg Biochem. 2001;87:245–51.
531. Lahoute C, Herbin O, Mallat Z, Tedgui A. Adaptive immunity in atherosclerosis: mechanisms and future therapeutic targets. Nat Rev Cardiol. 2011;8:348–58.
532. Berthet J, Damien P, Hamzeh-Cognasse H, Arthaud CA, Eyraud MA, Zeni F, Pozzetto B, McNicol A, Garraud O, Cognasse F. Human platelets can discriminate between various bacterial LPS isoforms via TLR4 signaling and differential cytokine secretion. Clin Immunol. 2012;145:189–200.
533. Hamzeh-Cognasse H, Damien P, Chabert A, Pozzetto B, Cognasse F, Garraud O. Platelets and infections – complex interactions with bacteria. Front Immunol. 2015; doi:10.3389/fimmu.2015.00082.
534. Garraud O, Hamzeh-Cognasse H, Pozzetto B, Cavaillon JM, Cognasse F. Bench-to-bedside review: platelets and active immune functions – new clues for immunopathology? Crit Care. 2013;17:236. doi:10.1186/cc12716.
535. Haaland HD, Holmsen H. Potentiation by adrenaline of agonist-induced responses in normal human platelets in vitro. Platelets. 2011;22:328–37.
536. Boylan B, Gao C, Rathore V, Gill JC, Newman DK, Newman PJ. Identification of FcgammaRIIa as the ITAM-bearing receptor mediating alphaII bbeta3 outside-in integrin signaling in human platelets. Blood. 2008;112:2780–6.
537. Fracchia KM, Walsh CM. Metabolic mysteries of the inflammatory response: T cell polarization and plasticity. Intl Rev of Immunol. 2015;34:3–18.

538. Gagliani N, Hu B, Huber S, Elinav E, Flavell RA. The fire within: microbes inflame tumors. Cell. 2014;157:776–83. doi:10.1016/j.cell.2014.03.006.
539. Burnham V, Thornton J. Luteinizing Hormone as a key player in the cognitive decline of Alzheimer's disease. Horm Behav. 2015; doi:10.1016/j.yhbeh.2015.05.010. pii: S0018-506X(15)00091-4. [Epub ahead of print]
540. Ferreira ST, Clarke JR, Bomfim TR, De Felice FG. Inflammation, defective insulin signaling, and neuronal dysfunction in Alzheimer's disease. Alzheimers Dement. 2014;10(Suppl):S76–83. doi:10.1016/j.jalz.2013.12.010.
541. Searcy DG, Whitehead JP, Maroney MJ. Interaction of Cu, Zn superoxide dismutase with hydrogen sulfide. Arch Biochem Biophys. 1995;318:251–63.
542. Trifunovic A, Wredenberg A, Falkenberg M, Spelbrink JN, Rovio AT, Bruder CE, et al. Premature ageing in mice expressing defective mitochondrial DNA polymerase. Nature. 2004;429:417–23.
543. Smaili SS, Pereira GJ, Costa MM, Rocha KK, Rodrigues L, do Carmo LG, Hirata H, Hsu YT. The role of calcium stores in apoptosis and autophagy. Curr Mol Med. 2013;13:252–65.
544. Hauser CJ, Sursal T, Rodriguez EK, Appleton PT, Zhang Q, Itagaki K. Mitochondrial damage associated molecular patterns from femoral reamings activate neutrophils through formyl peptide receptors and P44/42 MAP kinase. J Orthop Trauma. 2010;24:534–8. doi:10.1097/BOT.0b013e3181ec4991.
545. Shirihai OS, Song M, Dorn GW 2nd. How mitochondrial dynamism orchestrates mitophagy. Circ Res. 2015;116:1835–49.
546. Durcan TM, Fon EA. The three 'P's of mitophagy: PARKIN, PINK1, and post-translational modifications. Genes Dev. 2015;29:989–99.
547. Dela F, Helge JW. Insulin resistance and mitochondrial function in skeletal muscle. Int J Biochem Cell Biol. 2013;45:11–5.
548. Cohen S, Nathan JA, Goldberg AL. Muscle wasting in disease: molecular mechanisms and promising therapies. Nat Rev Drug Discov. 2015;14:58–74. doi:10.1038/nrd4467.
549. Tintignac LA, Brenner HR, Rüegg MA. Mechanisms regulating neuromuscular junction development and function and causes of muscle wasting. Physiol Rev. 2015;95:809–52. doi:10.1152/physrev.00033.2014.
550. Cruz-Jentoft AJ, Landi F, Schneider SM, Zuniga C, Arai H, Boirie Y, Chen LK, et al. Prevalence of and interventions for sarcopenia in ageing adults: a systematic review. Report of the International Sarcopenia Initiative (EWGSOP and IWGS). Age Ageing. 2014;43:748–59.
551. Denison HJ, Cooper C, Sayer AA, Robinson SM. Prevention and optimal management of sarcopenia: a review of combined exercise and nutrition interventions to improve muscle outcomes in older people. Clin Interv Aging. 2015;10:859–69. doi:10.2147/CIA.S55842. eCollection 2015
552. Sayer AA, Dennison EM, Syddall HE, Gilbody HJ, Phillips DI, Cooper C. Type 2 diabetes, muscle strength, and impaired physical function: the tip of the iceberg? Diabetes Care. 2005;28:2541–2.
553. Batsis JA, Mackenzie TA, Barre LK, Lopez-Jimenez F, Bartels SJ. Sarcopenia, sarcopenic obesity and mortality in older adults: results from the National Health and Nutrition Examination Survey III. Eur J Clin Nutr. 2014;68:1001–7.
554. Yang W, Hekimi S. A mitochondrial superoxide signal triggers increased longevity in *Caenorhabditis elegans*. PLoS Biol. 2010;8(12):e1000556.
555. Salminen A, Kaarniranta K, Kauppinen A. Inflammaging disturbed interplay between autophagy and inflammasomes. Aging. 2012;4:166–75.
556. Oláhová M, Taylor SR, Khazaipoul S, et al. A redox-sensitive peroxiredoxin that is important for longevity has tissue- and stress-specific roles in stress resistance. Proc Natl Acad Sci. 2008;105:19839–44.
557. Warburg O. On respiratory impairment in cancer cells. Science. 1956;124:269–70.
558. Warburg O. On the origin of cancer cells. Science. 1956;123:309–14.
559. Warburg O. Ueber den stoffwechsel der tumoren. London: Constable; 1930.

560. Warburg O. Iron, the oxygen-carrier of respiration-ferment. Science. 1925;61:575–82.
561. Palsson-McDermott EM, O'Neill LAJ. The Warburg effect then and now: from cancer to inflammatory diseases. BioEssays. 2013;35:965–73.
562. Racker E. Bioenergetics and the problem of tumor growth. Am Sci. 1972;60:56–63.
563. Lionaki E, Markaki M, Palikaras K, Tavernarakis N. Mitochondria, autophagy and age-associated neurodegenerative diseases: new insights into a complex interplay. Biochim Biophys Acta. 2015; doi:10.1016/j.bbabio.2015.04.010. pii: S0005-2728 (15)00068-7. [Epub ahead of print] Review
564. Shen HM, Mizushima N. At the end of the autophagic road: an emerging understanding of lysosomal functions in autophagy. Trends Biochem Sci. 2014;39:61–71. http://dx.doi.org/10.1016/j.tibs.2013.12.001 24369758
565. Lu H, Li G, Liu L, Feng L, Wang X, Jin H. Regulation and function of mitophagy in development and cancer. Autophagy. 2013;9:1720–36. doi:10.4161/auto.26550. Epub 2013 Sep 26
566. Kongara S, Karantza V. The interplay between autophagy and ROS in tumorigenesis. Front Oncol. 2012;2:171. doi:10.3389/fonc.2012.00171. eCollection 2012
567. Marzetti E, Csiszar A, Dutta D, Balagopal G, Calvani R, Leeuwenburgh C. Role of mitochondrial dysfunction and altered autophagy in cardiovascular aging and disease: from mechanisms to therapeutics. Am J Physiol Heart Circ Physiol. 2013;305:H459–76. doi:10.1152/ajpheart.00936.2012. Epub 2013.
568. Höhn A, Grune T. Lipofuscin: formation, effects and role of macroautophagy. Redox Biol. 2013;11:140–4.
569. Galluzzi L, Pietrocola F, Bravo-San Pedro JM, Amaravadi RK, Baehrecke EH, Cecconi F, Codogno P, Debnath J, Gewirtz DA, Karantza V, Kimmelman A, Kimmelman A, et al. Autophagy in malignant transformation and cancer progression. EMBO J. 2015;34:856–80. doi:10.15252/embj.201490784. Epub 2015 Feb 23
570. Sasaki K, Yoshida H. Organelle autoregulation-stress responses in the ER, Golgi, mitochondria and lysosome. J Biochem. 2015;157:185–95. doi:10.1093/jb/mvv010. Epub 2015 Feb 4
571. Pyo JO, Yoo SM, Ahn HH, Nah J, Hong SH, Kam TI, Jung S, Jung YK. Overexpression of Atg5 in mice activates autophagy and extends lifespan. Nat Commun. 2013;4:2300.
572. Vessoni AT, Filippi-Chiela EC, Menck CF, Lenz G. Autophagy and genomic integrity. Cell Death Differ. 2013;20:1444–54.
573. Sridhar S, Botbol Y, Macian F, Cuervo AM. Autophagy and disease: always two sides to a problem. J Pathol. 2012;226:255–73.
574. Pua HH, Guo J, Komatsu M, He YW. Autophagy is essential for mitochondrial clearance in mature T lymphocytes. J Immunol. 2009;182:4046–55.
575. Roberts EW, Deonarine A, Jones JO, Denton AE, Feig C, Lyons SK, et al. Depletion of stromal cells expressing fibroblast activation protein-alpha from skeletal muscle and bone marrow results in cachexia and anemia. J Exp Med. 2013;210:1137–51.
576. Iverson SL, Orrenius S. The cardiolipin-cytochrome c interaction and the mitochondrial regulation of apoptosis. Arch Biochem Biophys. 2004;423:37–46.
577. Mangalmurti NS, Chatterjee S, Cheng G, Andersen E, Mohammed A, Siegel DL, Schmidt AM, Albelda SM, Lee JS. Advanced glycation end products on stored red blood cells increase endothelial reactive oxygen species generation through interaction with receptor for advanced glycation end products. Transfusion. 2010;50:2353–61.
578. Crabtree HG. Observations on the carbohydrate metabolism of tumours. Biochem J. 1929;23(3):536–45.
579. Krebs H. The Pasteur effect and the relations between respiration and fermentation. Essays Biochem. 1972;8:1–34.
580. Buchanan BB, Arnon DI. A reverse KREBS cycle in photosynthesis: consensus at last. Photosynth Res. 1990;24:47–53.
581. Kim JW, Dang CV. Cancer's molecular sweet tooth and the Warburg effect. Cancer Res. 2006;66:8927–30.

582. Edens WA, Sharling L, Cheng G, et al. Tyrosine cross-linking of extracellular matrix is catalyzed by Duox, a multidomain oxidase/peroxidase with homology to the phagocyte oxidase subunit gp91phox. J Cell Biol. 2001;154:879–91.
583. Wang W, Fang H, Groom L, et al. Superoxide flashes in single mitochondria. Cell. 2008;134:279–90.
584. Kaminskyy V, Zhivotovsky B. Proteases in autophagy. Biochim Biophys Acta. 2012;1824:44–50.
585. Novikoff AB, Essner E. Cytolysomes and mitochondrial degeneration. J Cell Biol. 1962;15:140–6. http://dx.doi.org/10.1083/jcb.15.1.140 13939127
586. Young AR, Narita M, Narita M. Cell senescence as both a dynamic and a static phenotype. Methods Mol Biol. 2013;965:1–13. doi:10.1007/978-1-62703-239-1_1.
587. Ayaz O, Howlett SE. Testosterone modulates cardiac contraction and calcium homeostasis: cellular and molecular mechanisms. Biol Sex Differ. 2015;6:9. doi:10.1186/s13293-015-0027-9. eCollection.
588. Morimoto RI, Driessen AJ, Hegde RS, Langer T. The life of proteins: the good, the mostly good and the ugly. Nat Struct Mol Biol. 2011;18:1–4. doi:10.1038/nsmb0111-1.
589. Ycaza Herrera A, Mather M. Actions and interactions of estradiol and glucocorticoids in cognition and the brain: implications for aging women. Neurosci Biobehav Rev. 2015;55:36–52. doi:10.1016/j.neubiorev.2015.04.005.
590. Halil M, Cemal Kizilarslanoglu M, Emin Kuyumcu M, Yesil Y, Cruz Jentoft AJ. Cognitive aspects of frailty: mechanisms behind the link between frailty and cognitive impairment. J Nutr Health Aging. 2015;19:276–83. doi:10.1007/s12603-014-0535-z.
591. Plas DR, Thompson CB. Cell metabolism in the regulation of programmed cell death. Trends Endocrinol Metab. 2002;13:75–8.
592. Meng R, Tang HY, Westfall J, et al. Crosstalk between integrin αvβ3 and estrogen receptor-α is involved in thyroid hormone-induced proliferation in human lung cancer cells. PLoS One. 2011;6:e27547.
593. De Loof A, Marchal E, Rivera-Perez C, Noriega FG, Schoofs L. Farnesol-like endogenous sesquiterpenoids in vertebrates: the probable but overlooked functional "inbrome" anti-aging counterpart of juvenile hormone of insects? Front Endocrinol. 2015;5(Article 222):1–10.
594. Davis FB, Lin HY, Shih A, et al. Acting via a cell surface receptor, thyroid hormone is a growth factor for glioma cells. Cancer Res. 2006;66:7270–5.
595. Farwell AP, Dubord-Tomasetti SA, Pietrzykowski AZ, Stachelek SJ, Leonard JL. Regulation of cerebellar neuronal migration and neurite outgrowth by thyroxine and 3, 3′, 5′-triiodothyronine. Brain Res Dev Brain Res. 2005;154:121–35.
596. Rutkowski K, Sowa P, Rutkowska-Talipska J, Kuryliszyn-Moskal A, Rutkowski R. Dehydroepiandrosterone (DHEA): hypes and hopes. Drugs. 2014;74:1195–207. doi:10.1007/s40265-014-0259-8.
597. Cohen K, Ellis M, Khoury S, Davis PJ, Hercbergs A, Ashur-Fabian O. Thyroid hormone is a MAPK-dependent growth factors for human myeloma cells acting via αvβ3 integrin. Mol Cancer Res. 2011;9:1385–94.
598. Barbieri M, Bonafè M, Franceschi C, Paolisso G. Insulin/IGFI-signaling pathway: an evolutionarily conserved mechanism of longevity from yeast to humans. Am J Physiol Endocrinol Metab. 2003;285:E1064–71.
599. Gust DA, Wilson ME, Stocker T, Conrad S, Plotsky PM, Gordon TP. Activity of the hypothalamic-pituitary-adrenal axis is altered by aging and exposure to social stress in female rhesus monkeys. J Clin Endocronol Metab. 2000;85:2556–63.
600. Attanasio R, Gust DA, Wilson ME, Meeker T, Gordon TP. Immunomodulatory effects of estrogen and progesterone replacement in a nonhuman primate model. J Clin Immunol. 2002;22:263–9.
601. Kolovou GD, Kolovou V, Mavrogeni S. We are ageing. Biomed Res Int. 2014;808307:2014. doi:10.1155/2014/808307. Epub 2014 Jun 22

602. Van Poznak CH. Bone health in adults treated with endocrine therapy for early breast or prostate cancer. Am Soc Clin Oncol Educ Book. 2015;35:e567–74. doi:10.14694/EdBook_AM.2015.35.e567.
603. Lithgow GJ, Miller RA. Determination of aging rate by coordinated resistance to multiple forms of stress. In: Guarente L, Partridge L, Wallace DC, editors. Molecular biology of aging. New York: Cold Spring Harbor Laboratory Press; 2008. p. 427–81.
604. Kumar V. Innate immune system in sepsis immunopathogenesis and its modulation as a future therapeutic approach. In: Khatami M, editor. Inflammatory diseases; immunopathology, clinical and pharmacological bases. Rijeka: Intech Publishing; 2012. p. 27–56.
605. Koga H, Kaushik S, Cuervo AM. Protein homeostasis and aging: the importance of exquisite quality control. Ageing Res Rev. 2011;10:205–15.
606. Buskirk ER, Hodgson JL. Age and aerobic power: the rate of change in men and women. Fed Proc. 1987;46:1824–9.
607. Evans MC, Buchanan BB, Arnon DI. A new ferredoxin-dependent carbon reduction cycle in a photosynthetic bacterium. Proc Natl Acad Sci U S A. 1966;55:928–934. , 2001. PMC 224252. doi:10.1073/pnas. 55.4.928.
608. Kim JW, Dang CV. Multifaceted roles of glycolytic enzymes. Trends Biochem Sci. 2005;30:142–50.
609. Ralser M, Wamelink MM, Kowald A, et al. Dynamic rerouting of the carbohydrate flux is key to counteracting oxidative stress. J Biol. 2007;6:article (10).
610. Kervinen K, Savolainen MJ, Salokannel J, et al. Apolipoprotein E and B polymorphisms—longevity factors assessed in nonagenarians. Atherosclerosis. 1994;105:89–95.
611. Macauley SH, Stanley M, Caesar EE, Yamada SA, Raichle ME, Perez R, Mahan TM, Sutphen CL, Holtzman DM. Hyperglycemia modulates extracellular amyloid-β concentrations and neuronal activity in vivo. J Clin Investig. 2015; doi:10.1172/JCI79742.
612. Sugden MC, Holness MJ. Recent advances in mechanisms regulating glucose oxidation at the level of the pyruvate dehydrogenase complex by PDKs. Am J Physiol Endocrinol Metab. 2003;284:E855–62.
613. Fitzgerald MD, Tanaka H, Tran ZV, Seals DR. Age-related declines in maximal aerobic capacity in regularly exercising vs. sedentary women: a meta-analysis. J Appl Physiol (1985). 1997;83:160–5.
614. Amir S, Hartvigsen K, Gonen A, Leibundgut G, Que X, Jensen-Jarolim E, Wagner O, Tsimikas S, Witztum JL, Binder CJ. Peptide mimotopes of malondialdehyde epitopes for clinical applications in cardiovascular disease. J Lipid Res. 2012;53:1316–26.
615. Newsholme P, de Bittencourt PI Jr. The fat cell senescence hypothesis: a mechanism responsible for abrogating the resolution of inflammation in chronic disease. Curr Opin Clin Nutr Metab Care. 2014;17:295–305.
616. Edney EB, Gill RW. Evolution of senescence and specific longevity. Nature. 1968;220(5164):281–2.
617. Warner HR. Superoxide dismutase, aging, and degenerative disease. Free Radic Biol Med. 1994;17:249–58.
618. Sun Z. Aging, arterial stiffness, and hypertension. Hypertension. 2015;65:252–6.
619. Paredes SD, Forman KA, García C, Vara E, Escames G, Tresguerres JA. Protective actions of melatonin and growth hormone on the aged cardiovascular system. Horm Mol Biol Clin Investig. 2014;18:79–88.
620. Williams GM, Mattson MP, et al. Biological stress response terminology: Integrating the concepts of adaptive response and preconditioning stress within a hormetic dose-response framework. Toxicol Appl Pharmacol. 2007;222:122–8.
621. Cellini E, Nacmias B, Olivieri F, et al. Cholesteryl ester transfer protein (CETP) I405V polymorphism and longevity in Italian centenarians. Mech Ageing Dev. 2005;126:826–8.
622. Libby P, Ridker PM, Hansson GK. Progress and challenges in translating the biology of atherosclerosis. Nature. 2011;473:317–25.

623. Braig M, Lee S, Loddenkemper C, Rudolph C, Peters AH, Schlegelberger B, Stein H, Dorken B, Jenuwein T, Schmitt CA. Oncogene-induced senescence as an initial barrier in lymphoma development. Nature. 2005;436:660–5.
624. Milinkovic M, Antin JH, Hergrueter CA, Underhill CB, Sackstein R. CD44-hyaluronic acid interactions mediate shear-resistant binding of lymphocytes to dermal endothelium in acute cutaneous GVHD. Blood. 2004;103:740–2. doi:10.1182/blood-2003-05-1500.
625. Bellier A, Chen CS, Kao CY, Cinar HN, Aroian RV. Hypoxia and the hypoxic response pathway protect against pore-forming toxins in C. elegans. PLoS Pathog. 2009;5:e1000689.
626. Akiyama K, Suzuki H, Grant P, Bing RJ. Oxidation products of nitric oxide, NO_2 and NO_3, in plasma after experimental myocardial infarction. J Mol Cell Cardiol. 1997;29:1–9.
627. de la Haba G, Khatami M, Cooper GW, Backlund P, Flaks JG. Alanine or pyruvate is required for the development of myotubes from myoblasts and cortisol satisfies this requirement. Mol Cell Biochem. 1999;198:163–70.
628. DeLorey DS, Kowalchuk JM, Paterson DH. Effect of age on O(2) uptake kinetics and the adaptation of muscle deoxygenation at the onset of moderate-intensity cycling exercise. J Appl Physiol. 2004;97:165–72.
629. Le Blanc K, Ringden O. Immunomodulation by mesenchymal stem cells and clinical experience. J Int Med. 2007;262:509–25.
630. Vogelpoel LTC, Baeten DLP, de Jong EC, den Dunnen J. Control of cytokine production by human Fc gamma receptors: implications for pathogen defense and autoimmunity. Front Immunol. 2015 Feb 24;6:79. doi: 10.3389/fimmu.2015.00079. eCollection 2015.
631. Lenton KJ, Therriault H, Cantin AM, Fulop T, Payette H, Wagner JR. Direct correlation of glutathione and ascorbate and their dependence on age and season in human lymphocytes. Am J Clin Nutr. 2000;71:1194–200.
632. Lee YS, Kang YS, Lee JS, Nicolova S, Kim JA. Involvement of NADPH oxidase-mediated generation of reactive oxygen species in the apoptotic cell death by capsaicin in Hep G2 human hepatoma cells. Free Radic Res. 2004;38:405–12.
633. Bianchi ME, Manfredi AA. High-mobility group box 1 (HMGB1) protein at the crossroads between innate and adaptive immunity. Immunol Rev. 2007;220:35–46. doi:10.1111/j.1600-065X.2007.00574.x.
634. Houthoofd K, Braeckman BP, Lenaerts I, et al. Axenic growth up-regulates mass-specific metabolic rate, stress resistance, and extends life span in *Caenorhabditis elegans*. Exp Gerontol. 2002;37:1371–8.

Chapter 4
THE EYES HAVE IT ALL!

Accidental Systematic Discoveries: Direct Link for Inflammation-Induced Immune Dysfunction toward Multistep Tumorigenesis and Angiogenesis in Models of Allergies

Abstract Lack of systematic studies on the role of inflammation in age-associated chronic diseases, including multistep carcinogenesis has been extremely costly for taxpayers and patients. Recently, unresolved/chronic inflammation was defined as loss of balance between two tightly regulated and biologically opposing arms of acute inflammation (Yin–Yang or immune surveillance). Analyses of a series of data on 'accidental' discoveries that were established in 1980s on models of acute and chronic ocular inflammatory diseases in conjunctival-associated lymphoid tissues (CALTs) revealed at least three stages of clinical and immunological findings including earliest immune disruptor-induced changes in immune response profiles. Inflammation-induced interactions between resident (host) and recruited immune cells included: (a), acute phase, early immune disruptor-induced strong clinical reactions and tearing, activation and effector response from mast cells (MCs) and B/plasma cells, biosynthesis of IgE Abs, release of histamine and biosynthesis of prostaglandin PGF1α; (b), intermediate phase, down-regulation phenomenon, minimal clinical response, exhausted/degranulated MCs, heavy eosinophils (Eos) infiltrations into epithelium and mucus secreting goblet cells (GCs), tissue hypertrophy and neovascularization; and (c), chronic phase; induction of lymphoid hyperplasia, activated macrophages (MΦs), increased (irregular size) B and plasma cells, loss of integrity of lymphoid tissue capsular membrane, presence of histiocytes (activities of dendritic cell phenotype), follicular and germinal center formation, increased ratios of local IgG1/IgG2, epithelial thickening (growth) and/or thinning (necrosis) often noted in the same tissue sections and angiogenesis. Results of these systematic studies are suggestive of first series of evidence for direct association between inflammation and identifiable multistep immune dysfunction in the direction of tumorigenesis. Systematic studies to monitor interactions between resident and recruited cells in site-specific tissues should provide key information not only for identification of immune disruptor-induced early events in the loss of immune surveillance, but they would help making informed decisions for balancing the inherent tumoricidal (Yin) and tumorigenic (Yang) properties of immune system for effective preventive and therapeutic approaches and accurate risk assessment toward improvement of public health.

M. Khatami, *Inflammation, Aging and Cancer*,
https://doi.org/10.1007/978-3-319-66475-0_4

Keywords Adjuvant • Antigen • Angiogenesis • Ascaris Suum • B lymphocytes • CALTs • Conjunctival-associated lymphoid tissues • Direct evidence • Duality • Early responses • Eyes • 'Leaky' MCs • Interactions • Synergies • Developmental Phases • FLOA • Degranulation • Eosinophils • Genetic predisposition • Histamine • IgE • IgE-fεc receptor crosslinking • IgG isotypes • Immune dysfunction • Inflammation • Inflammatory mediators • Macrophages • M-CSF • Mucus secreting goblet cells • Mast cells • Prostacycline • Prostaglandin • Strong and weak ocular responses • Time course kinetics • Tumorigenesis • Tumor promoting agents • Newborn hypersensitivity • Upper and lower bulbar conjunctiva • Yin and Yang

1 Introduction

A hero is an ordinary individual who finds the strength to persevere and endure in spite of overwhelming obstacles. Christopher Reeves

To begin this chapter, it is appropriate to acknowledge the documented historical and fundamental contributions of nineteenth and twentieth century scientists Rudolph Virchow and Paul Ehrlich on the role of inflammation in inflammatory diseases and cancer [1–3]. In his book 'Cellular Pathology' in 1858, Virchow noted that "the signs of inflammation are four; redness and swelling, with heat & pain". He also suggested that arteriosclerosis is an inflammatory and degenerative disease. In 1909, shortly after the microscope was invented, Ehrlich observed that tumor cells are recognized and eliminated by immune/inflammatory cells. Later in 1957, Sir McFarland developed the theory of immune surveillance (cancer surveillance) defining how growth of cancer was controlled, thus the initial concept of immunity [4]. Chapters 1 and 2 of this book provide details of these historical observations, which were practically ignored and minimized by the decision makers in the cancer community. Consequently, while the circumstantial evidence for a role of inflammation in the development of many site-specific cancers have been noted and numerous inflammatory mediators have been identified in pathways of carcinogenesis [4–17], except for our 'accidental' discoveries that were established in 1980s on experimental models of acute and chronic ocular inflammatory diseases, there are little/no reports that systematically demonstrate a direct association between inflammation and multistep tumorigenesis and angiogenesis [18–23].

The ongoing debates, misunderstanding and controversies in the literature, whether inflammation is protective for preventing cancer or it is a cause of carcinogenesis demonstrate lack of comprehending and differentiating the protective ('friend') or destructive ('foe') contributions of immune/inflammatory dynamics in health and diseases of aging, particularly with regard to site-specific cancers and therapeutic approaches [4–39]. Consequently, despite heavy public investment on war against cancer for the last six decades, lack of interest in conducting systematic studies have been very costly for the public, as too many out-of-focus and expensive clinical trials, technologies and drug development repeatedly failed cancer patients.

A simple explanation for the repeatedly failed clinical trials and claims of 'targeted' therapies, 'precision' or 'personalized' medicine is that these approaches are based on identification of too many mutated genes in the molecular chaos of cancer environment. The selected drugs are primarily potent apoptotic factors or inhibitors of specific growth factors that produced life-threatening side-effects for cancer patients [reviewed in 40–46] (details in Chaps. 5 and 6).

In this chapter, details of the systematic analyses of data on the 'accidental' discoveries that were established in 1980s, at the University of Pennsylvania, on experimental models of acute and chronic ocular inflammatory diseases, which resulted in progressive altered immune response dynamics and multistep tumorigenesis will be revisited. The results of these studies show series of first evidence on early changes in immune response profiles when tissue is repeatedly exposed to immune disruptor (antigen). Systematic alterations of immune dynamics at distinct periods of tissue responses that led to tumorigenesis and angiogenesis will be demonstrated. It was suggested that contributions of early changes in host immunity are preventable. Furthermore, we demonstrated that repeated exposures to antigen cause interactions and synergies between host resident and recruiting cells in the direction of tumorigenesis. Future proposed directions toward identification of developmental phases of inflammation-induced altered immune dynamics will be summarized based on recent hypotheses that inflammation is a common denominator in the genesis and progression of nearly all age-associated chronic diseases and site-specific cancers [18–23, 28–30, 40–45]. In 2016, following analyses of data on a wide range of chronic diseases or cancer the author further proposed that nearly all age-associated chronic diseases are manifestation of 'mild', 'moderate' or 'severe' immune disorders. In this context cancer was hypothesized as the severe delayed accumulation of immune responses in susceptible tissues. Histamine was suggested as a blueprint in maintaining oxidative stress and altering the immune dynamics of immune-responsive tissues in the direction of cell growth. Differential roles of Yin and Yang of effective immunity and mitochondrial bioenergetics and function at different stages of life, from fetus orderly growth and development, after birth, adulthood and age-associated chronic diseases were compared (details in Chap. 6) [43, 44].

It should be noted that prior to 1998, few cancer researchers were involved in the role of inflammation in cancer research. These scientists were aware of the circumstantial evidence for an association between chronic irritation or tissue injuries and cancer development and acknowledged lack of a direct evidence for a link between inflammation and tumor development. There were also few reports that desired the need for evidence on systematic developmental phases of tumor growth [21]. In 1998/1999, at the National Cancer Institute (NCI), the author's challenging efforts and struggles to promote the role of inflammation in cancer research met with serious opposition and minimization by decision makers in the upper management at NCI/NIH. In the last decade, appreciation and interest in studying the role of inflammation has significantly increased, as numerous funded projects, clinical and basic science research, therapeutic approaches, technologies and networks are focused on multi-factorial roles of inflammation in cancer research and immunotherapy.

However, many of the current studies are fragmented studies on isolated molecules with reductionist approaches and created further chaos and controversies of what inflammation does in health or diseases of aging, particularly with regard to cancer 'targeted' drugs in clinical trials that produced life-threatening side effects, admitted by governmental and private industry [reviewed in 30, 42–46]. It is disappointing that the professionals in cancer research continue to follow the reductionists and chaotic approaches on identification of too many mutational-derived inflammatory molecules for research and clinical trials 'immunotherapy'. Review of literature shows that the current funded projects and claims of immunotherapy and inflammation and cancer research are practically name-changing, using words of 'inflammation' or 'immunotherapy'. These schemes created additional confusion in all aspects of research and therapy. While clinical conduct for immunotherapy appears logical, there is lack of systematic approach to understand the host tissue complexes of immune and non-immune interactions toward therapy. Immunotherapy studies are based on using specific somatic mutations of defective 'inflammatory' molecules or immune cell checkpoints (e.g., T cells, DCs or NKs) or activation of specific death factors (DFs) in the chaotic molecular landscape of site-specific cancers for treating patients [30, 42–44] (details in Chap. 6).

As emphasized throughout this book, effective cancer preventive strategies, therapeutic approaches and assessment of accurate risk formulation on exposure to a wide range of immune disruptors (antigens, microbiota or pathogen-specific vaccines and adjuvant) are achievable only through systematic and integrative study of the early actions of pathogens, low level carcinogens, allergen or other biological, chemical or environmental hazards that are considered hazardous to effective immunity and disturb the quality of immune and non-immune responses in specific target tissues.

2 Definitions of Acute and Chronic Inflammation in Health and Diseases

Discovery consists of seeing what everyone has seen and thinking what nobody has thought.
Dr. Albert Szent-Gyorgyi

Acute inflammation is a complex self-limiting and natural protective property of immune system (immune surveillance). Immune surveillance is provided through pleiotropic or biphasic properties (polarity or dual function) of acute inflammation that allow organ systems to return to normal physiological function after encountering and neutralizing external or internal unwanted/foreign elements (stimuli or immune disruptors) such as microorganisms (e.g., viruses, bacteria, parasites), allergens, biological, chemical or environmental hazards/toxins, carcinogens, useless and non-functional proteins/enzymes, genetic and epigenetic defects (e.g., mutated DNA/RNA, hypo-, hyper-methylated genes), useless cells (e.g., polyclonal B cell complexes, senescent and cancerous cells), oxidized metabolites (e.g., crystalline uric acid) that are hazardous to body's survival (details in Chaps. 2 and 3)

[28–30, 40–45]. Here, a brief overview of recent definitions on acute and chronic inflammation is provided to discuss the relevance of altered dynamics of host tissues that we found in earlier systematic series of data on time course kinetics of stimuli-induced interactions and synergies between host and recruited cells in multistep tumorigenesis.

Acute inflammation was defined as a highly regulated molecular cross-communications between two biologically opposing arms of immune and non-immune responses termed 'Yin' (apoptosis, initiation, growth-arresting or tumoricidal) and 'Yang' (wound healing, growth-promoting or tumorigenic) [40]. Stimuli-induced cell mediated and humoral immunity (CMI, HI) of activated immune cells are facilitated by appropriate and precise responses from non-immune systems (e.g., vasculature, neuroendocrine, adipose and metabolic response pathways) (Fig. 4.1) [40, 41].

In general, in an acute inflammation, generation of signal transductions and crosstalk between innate and adaptive immune cells and non-immune systems presents a 2-fold principal mission:

(a) Encounter/sense or recognize, process and digest, destroy and eliminate intrinsic or extrinsic foreign elements and the injured host tissue,
(b) Resolve and terminate inflammation and repair, reconstruct or remodel the target (injured) host tissue.

Simply described, in an acute inflammation, apoptosis arm (growth arrest, tumoricidal, initiation, pro-inflammatory) or 'Yin' responses are responsible for high energy-requiring production of ATP hydrolysis from mitochondrial oxidative phosphorylation of activated immune cells, for expression of death signals, oxidants, enzymes and receptor molecules to destroy both the enemy (pathogens, allergen, immune disruptors) and the injured host cells. The wound healing (growth promote, termination, post-inflammatory or tumorigenic) arm of an acute inflammation or 'Yang' responses, the low energy requiring events that utilize glycolysis (Warburg effect) are simultaneously generated from polarized immune and non-immune system, to counteract and neutralize the toxicity that is generated during apoptosis in the 'battle field' and to resolve or terminate inflammation and repair or reconstruct the target host tissue. The major outcomes of an acute inflammation are lymphocyte-derived clonal expansion, increased synthesis of pathogen-, or allergen-specific antibodies and plasma and memory T and B cells that prepare the tissues to appropriately defend the body when exposed to the same hazardous agents [40–44].

A large body of quality data on basic and clinical research on models of chronic inflammatory diseases or human allergies or cancer demonstrate that the immune and non-immune cells, including innate [e.g., natural killer cells (NKs), macrophages (MΦs), dendritic cells (DCs), mast cells (MCs)] or adaptive [e.g., T and B cells, and subpopulations (cytotoxic T cells, Th1, Th2, Treg or plasma cells)], as well as, non-immune response pathways (e.g. vasculature, metabolic, hormonal, neuronal and adipocytes) present shared and specialized biphasic or duality (polarizing or pleiotropy) under acute and chronic inflammation and in cancer environment [47–88]. Analyses of data directly and indirectly support the recent definitions

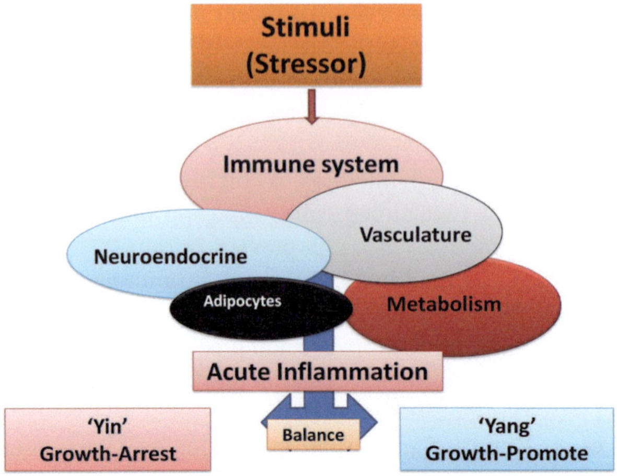

Fig. 4.1 Schematic representation of balance in 'Yin' (growth-arrest) and 'Yang' (growth-promote) properties in acute inflammation. Acute inflammatory processes involve elaborate and precise interdependent crosstalk between immune and non-immune systems (e.g., vasculature, neuroendocrine, metabolic and adipocyte pathways) to combat and destroy foreign elements and injured host tissue and to neutralize, resolve and terminate inflammation and repair and reconstruct the damaged tissues. Modified from Khatami [28]. All rights reserved. See text

on the role of acute and chronic inflammation in health and diseases. Thus, effective immunity is a highly regulated and complex property of defense mechanism (immune surveillance) for maintenance of the balance between two biologically opposing arms of tumoricidal (Yin) and tumorigenic (Yang) pathways provided through self-terminating protective properties of acute inflammation. Polarization of immune cells, during Yang events, is accompanied by expression of mediators whose effects are different from the non-polarized forms (resting status). Therefore, stimuli-induced activation and polarization of immune cells and the expression of mediators are capable of acting as tumor suppressors (growth-arresting) or tumor promoters (growth-promoting) agents (dual properties) [40–44]. Examples of factors and receptor molecules with known dual function include TLRs, MCP-1, CCL2, M-CSF, TGF-β, GM-CSF, histamine, heparin, TNF-α/TNFR, VEGF, CAMs, MMPs, prostaglandins (e.g., prostacyclin to PGE2), surface antigens, adaptor molecules or cell recognition molecules (e.g., CD2, CD11, CD18, CD25, CD 50, CD54, CD63, CD69, CD88), cytokine suppressor molecules (e.g., S100 family of calcium-binding proteins), enzymes (e.g., tryptase/chymase, neutrophil-derived serine proteases, indolamine 2, 3-dioxygenase), peroxynitrite, other cytokines/chemokines, ILs or IFNs (e.g., IFN-γ, Il-2, IL-3, IL-5, IL-10, IL-12, IL-13), ECFA, SCF, c-kit), decoy receptors (e.g., TNFdR, IL1dR, IRAK-M), antibodies (e.g., IgE, IgG isotypes, IgA, IgM), platelet-derived growth factor (PDGF) and related mediators. Numerous reports also demonstrate expression of abnormal proteins/peptides, lipids, metabolites, mutated DNA/RNA, hypo-hyper-methylation of epigenetic modifications (e.g., p53, p27, p16, p70, MAPKs, KRAS, BRAF, ALK, Myc, BCR, ABL, MGMT, TKIs, mTOR/ PI3K/AKT) are identified as potential targets for therapy [4–100].

In the following sections attempts were made to make biological sense of the immunological chaos that disturb effective immunity by demonstrating the results of our systematic studies on experimental models of acute and chronic ocular allergies.

3 Immune Disruptors-Induced Interactions and Synergies between Local and Recruiting Cells Toward Multistep Tumorigenesis

Foreign elements (external or internal components) that disturb effective immunity (immune disruptors) and induce loss of balance in Yin-Yang of acute inflammation (unresolved inflammation, oxidative stress) cause mild, moderate or severe immune responses in tissues. The spectrum of immune responses in susceptible tissues includes responses toward structures and substructures of extrinsic or intrinsic elements that are perceived hazardous to body's survival presents infinite possible response profiles. The general categories of external/extrinsic or internal/intrinsic foreign components that induce certain responses from Yin-Yang of immune system (Fig. 4.1) include the following interdependent list [28–30, 40–44, 91–95] (details in Chaps. 2 and 6):

(a) External Immune Disruptors:

- (i) Specific structures of microorganisms, infective agents or pathogens (e.g., viruses, bacteria, parasites). The specific vaccines against infective agents that impose immune responses and often cause 'antigen overload' for immunity fall into this category;
- (ii) A wide range of allergens and antigens including pollen, mite, dust, certain foods, genetically modified organisms in foods, other biological, chemical or environmental hazards that are considered low level carcinogens or mitogens;

(b) Internal Immune Disruptors:

- (i) Useless and non-functional proteins/enzymes, defective genetic and epigenetic materials (e.g., mutated DNA/RNA, hypo- hypermethylated genetic components), useless cells (e.g., polyclonal B cell complexes, senescent, cancerous cells), oxidized metabolites (e.g., crystalline uric acid),]
- (ii) Aging process and minor or major changes in innate and adaptive immune response profiles, alterations in availability or function of hormones and metabolites (biological rearrangements in organ systems, immunosenescence);

The recognition, uptake and clearance of pathogens by mononuclear phagocytes are crucial events for the protection and defense of host tissue. To achieve infection, pathogens must evade both the natural and specific responses of the host through a variety of mechanisms that would allow them to circumvent (camouflage) the immune responses for their survival. Analyses of relevant data suggest that pathogens (or cancerous cells) take advantage of the natural duality (pleiotropy) of immune and non-immune cell responses, particularly during aging. For example, in immune-responsive tissues, microorganisms or other immune disruptors that cause oxidative stress in host apply multiple mechanisms including induction of decoy receptors to prevent apoptosis and provide signals for wound healing for pathogen survival. Potent pathogens (e.g., pneumococcal bacteria, meningitis) or certain cancer drugs (strong monoclonal antibodies or growth factor inhibitors) can bypass vascular tissue barriers (or gut immune-mucus secreting barriers) and induce expression of overwhelming toxins and apoptotic factors creating 'cytokine storm' or 'immune tsunami', leading to significant destruction of architectural integrity of vasculature and rapid access to multiple organs and induction of severe inflammatory conditions such as sepsis, meningitis or pneumonia and organ failure that are life-threatening to host survival (details in Chap. 6) [reviewed in 40–44].

Analyses of data involving activation of macrophages demonstrate that the receptor molecules provide direct link to NF-kB activation and pro-inflammatory cytokine secretion as preferred mechanisms by M1 phenotype during acute inflammation. Review of reports from human or experimental models of mononuclear cells suggest that IFN-γ stimulates the expression of toll-like receptor 4 (TLR-4) as key factor in the MyD88 signaling pathways, while interleukin-receptor-associated kinase (ILAK-M) in TLR7, or PGE2 and IL-10 expression counteracts these effects and mediate tolerance [5–8, 15–17, 30, 40–43, 56, 57, 101]. These and related findings are perhaps attempts of immunity to terminate apoptosis and inflammation or induce tolerance. Another example of the role of activated/polarized immune cells is the molecular repertoire of M2 versus M1 phenotype and metabolism of arginine. A major discrimination between M1 and M2 phenotypes in mice was demonstrated at the biochemical level, in the metabolism of L-arginine. Furthermore, analyses of data on activation and polarization of macrophages in experimental models of inflammatory diseases or cancer demonstrate that within MΦs, L-Arg is metabolized by three different pathways for production of L-citrulline and NO by inducible iNOS, ureum and L-ornithine by arginase, or agmatin by arginine decarboxylase (ADC). The cross-regulation of the iNOS-arginase balance by Th1 mediators such as IFN-γ and LPS, and by Th2 cytokines such as IL-4 and IL-13, suggest that the measure of NO level and arginase activity in distinct cell populations reflect their activation states [28–30, 40–50, 101–114].

In summary, immune dysfunction is the cumulative impairments of complex immune response networks that result in the loss of balance in critical interactions of CMI and HI and disturb the required bioenergetics of homeostasis between positive and negative control switches of effective immunity or the loss of 2 biologically opposing arms termed tumoricidal (Yin) and tumorigenic (Yang) of protective pathways of acute inflammation. Major known changes in immune response profiles that would lead to multistep tumorigenesis include alterations in the ratios of

Th1:Th2, shifts in 'tumoricidal' (immature) properties of DCs (reduced ratio of DC1: DC2 or TADC), NKs (NK1:NK2), MCs (mature MCs: degranulated or 'leaky' MCs, TAMC), MΦs (M1: M2 or TAM) in tissues that are immune-responsive (details in Chap. 2). In immune-response tissues (e.g., epithelial, endothelial, fibroblast, mucus secreting cells), oxidative stress-induced shifts in tumoricidal properties of innate immune cells very likely alter the bioenergetic quality/power of host defense mechanisms and alter ratios of oxido-reductants (redox potentials) and changes in energy output (ATP/ADP/AMP) that would damage the mitochondrial function and diminish oxidative phosphorylation (high energy production from ATP hydrolysis) [43]. Insufficient ATP production in mitochondria that is generated from oxidative phosphorylation, could lead to progressive alterations in metabolism of host tissues (enhanced glycolysis), induction of hypoxia and expression of VEGF and contribute to retardation of high energy- requiring tumoricidal (Yin) properties toward immune tolerance that facilitate tumor growth (details in Chaps. 2 and 6).

4 'Accidental' Series of Discoveries in Ocular Tissues: Implications for Direct Link Between Inflammation and Multistep Tumorigenesis and Angiogenesis in Conjunctival-Associated Lymphoid Tissues (CALTs)

Circumstantial evidence and meta analyses of the clinical and epidemiological data on an association between prior infections and injuries and the increase risk of site-specific cancers in patients suffering from chronic colitis (or crohn's), pancreatitis, , chronic obstructive pulmonary diseases (COPD), asthma, gastritis (infections with Helicobacter pylori and/or other stomach ulcers), prostatis, thyroiditis, and respective cancers of colon, pancreas, lung, stomach or prostate have been documented for decades [3, 6–8, 10, 11, 14–20, 23, 25–27, 30, 34, 40–44, 104, 110, 112]. However, except for our 'accidental' discoveries that were established in 1980s, little/no data are available to demonstrate a direct association between the role of inflammation in multistep tumorigenesis and angiogenesis. Furthermore, despite the fact that over 20 million articles are available on cancer related topics, there are no reports on how repeated exposure to low level carcinogens (immune disruptors, antigens) can initiate early alterations of immunity, or interactions and synergies between resident and recruiting immune or non-immune cells that cause progressive damages in susceptible site-specific tissues that lead to growth of tissue, tumorigenesis and angiogenesis [40–44, 92].

The following sections describe the extended analyses of data on a series of studies that were established over 35 years ago on ocular inflammatory diseases with emphasis on identification of developmental phases of immune disruption toward tumorigenesis [18–23, 28–30, 40–45, 61, 72, 89–92, 115].

4.1 Background Information on Author's Personal Experience

Courage is the ladder on which all the other virtues mount. (Clare Booth Luce[1])

In 1980s our research team at the University of Pennsylvania, Department of Ophthalmology, was not involved in cancer research and we had no idea of the importance or significance of the original findings for cancer research until I joined the Division of Cancer Prevention (DCP),NCI/NIH, in 1998. At NCI, as a Program Director, Health Science Administrator, I was given the responsibility to review a large amount of data; including questionnaires, clinical forms and a variety of computer-generated information on collected data from patient's biorepositories, statistics and related administrative issues that were gathered by several contracting organizations, under NCI directions. Since 1993, NCI staff and academicians were involved in a peculiar and expensive (over $250 M) clinical project, prostate-lung-colorectal-ovarian (PLCO) Cancer Screening Trials. My formal assignment was to develop concepts for cancer molecular diagnosis and utilization of patient biorepositories (e.g., PLCO), designs of clinical trials for detection and prevention of cancer. After review of enormous amount of published data on cancer-related fields and with much excitements, I learned that the results of our earlier published studies on experimental models of acute and chronic ocular inflammatory diseases, were suggestive of the first and only evidence for a direct link between inflammation and systematic developmental phases of immune dysfunction that led to neoplasia, hyperplasia, tumoigenesis and angiogenesis. Table 4.1 is a growing list of reports on circumstantial evidence that cancer develops at prior site of injuries. The table was a much shorter list in 1998, when I prepared it to promote the important role of inflammation in cancer research. As discussed throughout the book, over the last couple of decades interest in the topic has significantly intensified and extensive epidemiologic, basic and clinical research documented the role of a wide range of inflammatory mediators and immune responses for cancer research and therapy. Details of how the decision makers at NCI downplayed, ignored and minimized the challenging efforts and struggles that I endured to promote the topic are provided in Chaps. 1 and 6 ([40–44], NCI/NIH submitted documents since 1998).

As analyses of our original data continued, it became clear that lack of systematic studies on the roles that inflammation play in multistep tumorigenesis and existence of numerous important knowledge gaps in understanding cancer biology are the principal factors for slow/lack of progress in cancer research, prevention and therapy, despite trillions of dollars that have been invested in cancer research and therapy. In this chapter, analyses of original data and the importance and significance of our 'accidental' discoveries for cancer research and therapy are briefly discussed. In addition, attempts were made to identify a list of important biological gaps for future proposed directions of cancer biology. The goal is to help research-

[1] Clare Booth Luce (1903–1987), American author, politician and a US Ambassador. Source: Internet.

Table 4.1 A growing list of circumstantial evidence on association between cancers and prior tissue sites of injuries or infections

Chronic inflammation and cancer (Retrospective study on prior injuries or infections)	
Site-specific cancers/tumors	Inflammatory disease
Bowel/colon	Ulcerative colitis(Crohn's)
Urinary bladder	Schistomiasis, stones, catheters
Prostate	Prostais—PIA-PIN
Breast	Inflammatory conditions
Cervical	Pericarditis?
Esophagus	Barretts'
Pancreas	Pancreatitis
Stomach	Gastric infection (e.g., Helicobacter Pylori)
	Ulcers/gastritis
Lung	Asthma, emphysema, smoking
Liver	Hepatitis B, C
Thyroid	Thyroiditis
Conjunctiva	Conjunctivitis/CALT(?)
Skin melanomas	Burns/radiations(?)
Uveal melanomas	Uveitis(?)
Others	Cystitis, GALT(?)

In 1998/99 when the author was preparing for oral presentation and submitted written proposals to promote the role of inflammation in cancer research, molecular diagnosis and therapy, the list was not as extensive. Also, as detailed in the text, except for our accidental discoveries, little/no reports were available on inflammation-induced early events in immune dynamic alterations that would lead to tissue damage and functional integrity, toward cell growth promotion, neoplasia/hyperplasia, polyps, or cancer, metastasis and angiogenesis [40–44]. See text ers and clinicians to better understand the importance of immunity and to make informed decisions in promoting immune surveillance and controlling the multistep carcinogenesis. Systematic studies of the role of immunity whose progressive alterations lead to the loss of cancer control mechanisms are essential steps toward design of cost-effective strategies for cancer prevention, assessment of accurate cancer risk calculations, clinical trials and drug development and for better use of public and private funds on selecting science-based technologies.

5 Ocular Tissues: Ideal Targets for Studying Inflammatory Diseases or Tumorigenesis and Angiogenesis. Comparison of Composition and Function of Immune and Non-immune Cells in Conjunctiva and Lung Airways

Among body's organ systems, conjunctiva and lung airways represent ideal systems for demonstration of a wide range of human inflammatory diseases. A major immune function of the conjunctival epithelium and lid architecture is to prevent entry of microorganisms or foreign elements (e.g., infective agents, toxins, allergen, environmental and chemical hazards) into the globe and to clear the eye and prevent damage to the oxidative-sensitive immune-privileged ocular tissues such as the avascular cornea, retina and neuroretina. Major ocular inflammatory conditions include vernal conjunctivitis, keratoconjunctivities, punctuate keratitis, giant papillary conjunctivitis, bechet's disease, Sjogren's syndrome, retinitis or squamous cell carcinoma of conjunctiva [18–23, 40–44, 62–76, 89, 90]. Similarly, an immune function of the epithelial structure of the lung airway is to prevent entry and clearance of inhaled toxins or unwanted particles from the lung tissues [77–81, 83–85].

To perform their functions, both tissues, being accessible to external chemical or environmental hazards (stimuli), have similar diverse cell types, including epithelium, mucus secreting goblet cells (GCs), mast cells (MCs) or dendritic cells (DCs) and depending on the types of immune disruptors (stimuli), they provide somewhat similar cellular and molecular responses. Clinical and histopathological manifestations and immune response mechanisms that are involved in lung allergies or infectious diseases (e.g., asthma, emphysema, COPD, pneumonia) or lung cancers are, to some extent, comparable to those occurring in conjunctival allergic reactions (e.g., vernal and giant papillary conjunctivitis, keratoconjunctivitis, hay fever, atopic eczema, punctuate keratitis) or Behcet's diseases, Sjogren's syndrome and squamous cell carcinomas of the conjunctiva. Stimuli-induced mast cells-IgE activation and degranulation and release of histamine, heparin and other preformed or newly synthesized inflammatory mediators, eosinophil infiltration into epithelium and goblet cells and hyperproduction of thick mucus secretion from GCs have been identified as principal responses during inflammatory conditions in both conjunctiva and lung tissues. Furthermore, abnormalities and diversities in B-cell memory expression of immunoglobulin subclasses have been reported in patients with atopic eczema and Sjogren's syndrome, autoimmune disorders associated with lymphoid follicles and progression to lymphoma are comparable to the mechanisms occurring in asthmatic patients [21, 44, 66, 67, 76–81]. In lung diseases of the respiratory airway, activated epithelial cells, which are coated with a layer of mucus causing a thick barrier has been reported as major contributors in the development of cystic fibrosis, asthma and emphysema that also prevent access to therapeutic drugs [7, 40–44, 62–87, 108–110]. Participation of mast cells (MCs) sensitization and activation (effector function) and release of preformed or newly synthesized mediators, followed by infiltration of eosinophils has been reported in acute and chronic ocular allergies or asthma. Furthermore, activation of mucus secreting goblet cells (GCs) and infiltration of eosinophils into GCs during ocular inflammatory conditions or asthma and the progression of diseases may be considered comparable events. It is also noteworthy that individuals suffering from asthma often manifest ocular allergic reactions and vice versa. While, mast cells are the primary tissue constituent immune cells (effector cells) that respond to many airborne allergens in both conjunctiva and lung airways, exposure of these tissues to specific infective agents may primarily stimulate dendritic cells or macrophages for immunological responses and potentially interact with the release of histamine in host tissue for improving the antigen/pathogen uptake and cross presentation to adaptive immune cells. Therefore, understanding the composition, interactions and synergies of host-antigen (immune disruptor) dynamics at site-specific tissues should be prerequisite when investigating the biology of specific disease processes for effective designs of prevention, drug development and treatment of diseases.

6 Time-Course Kinetics of Inflammation-Induced Immune Dysfunction and Tumorigenesis in Conjunctival Associated Lymphoid Tissues (CALTS)

Experimental models of acute and chronic inflammatory diseases were established in conjunctival-associated lymphoid tissues (CALTs) of guinea pig eyes by topical (unilateral or bilateral) application of fluoresceinyl-ovalbumin (FLOA, antigen, immune disruptor), in the presence or absence of infective agents (A Suum and its extracts), adjuvant or tumor promoting agents (TPAs) for up to 30 months. The major clinical and histopathological findings are summarized in the following sections. Details on experimental procedures, immunization schedules, immunological assays and histological studies for detection of cells, mediators and antibodies are provided in the original publications [18–23]. As detailed in the following sections, further analyses of data on the significance of the original findings relevant to tumorigenesis and angiogenesis, as well as identification of selected biomarkers were reported in recent years [28–30, 40–44, 61, 89–91, 115].

6.1 *Acute Phase (a): Mast Cell (Effector) Response Toward Immune Disruptor*

Clinical findings that initiated after 9 days of repeated topical challenges with antigen (FLOA) produced a range of strong or weak acute (type 1) immediate hypersensitivity reactions including tearing, conjunctival edema, lid scratching or milky (lipid-protein) secretion in tears. Tear production occasionally coagulated and appeared as a thin film covering the sensitized eye (Figs. 4.2, 4.3 and 4.4). The clinical reactions subsided within an hour of the last challenge and eye appeared normal (quiet, resting).

Histopathological and immunological assays of early responses demonstrated IgE-dependent mast cells (MCs) degranulation (effector pharmacological response), release of histamine and prostaglandin (PGs) and vascular hyperpermeability responses. Time course kinetics of histamine and PGs (6-keto-PGF-1α, stable component of PGI2) release in tears demonstrated that the ratios of 6-keto PGF-1α to histamine increased more than 16-folds in the first 2 h of topical antigen challenge, suggesting that histamine was a primary mediator that activated arachidonic acid metabolism and cyclooxygenase pathways for the synthesis and release of prostanoids via constituent and/or infiltrating inflammatory cells [18, 21, 23, 44, 89, 90].

No correlation was found between circulating homocytotropic-IgE and the degree of clinical reactions. This suggested tight binding of IgE-MCs-Fc-ε receptor (IgE-fcεR) molecules by effectively sensitizing MCs in ocular or other distal tissue MCs and removing IgE from circulation. Preliminary observations in animals which produced strong ocular reactions demonstrated wheezing reactions suggesting mast cells sensitization and effector response in lung airways. In addition, preliminary studies with newborn babies of sensitized animals, demonstrated strong ocular responses upon one or 2 challenges with FLOA, suggesting IgE antibody transfer and fetal MCs sensitization and/or fetal genomic predisposition (details in Chap. 6).

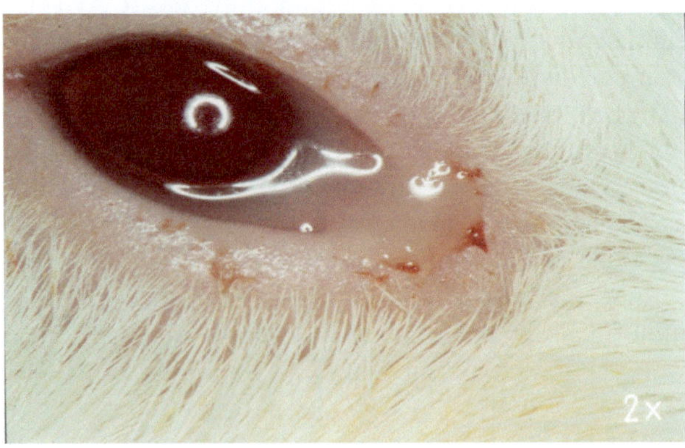

Fig. 4.2 Acute inflammation in an eye repeatedly challenged with FLOA showing milky secretion in tears (Reproduced with permission from Khatami et al. (Ref. [18], 1984) Archives of Ophthalmology, AMA. All rights reserved)

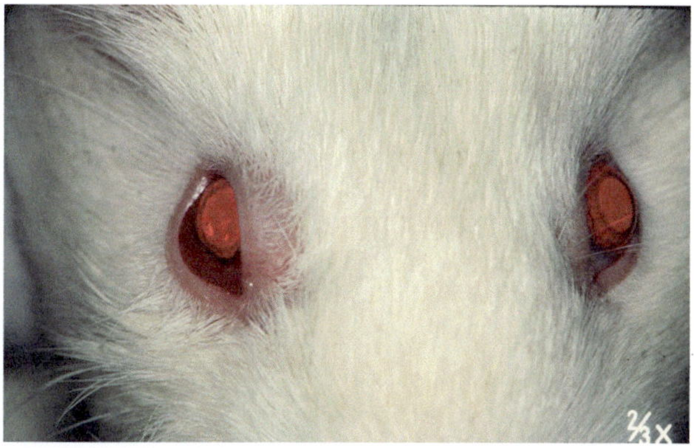

Fig. 4.3 Acute inflammatory response in unilaterally sensitized and challenged eye of guinea pig 30 min after last challenge (Reproduced with permission from Khatami et al (Ref. [18], 1984) Archives of Ophthalmology, AMA. All rights reserved)

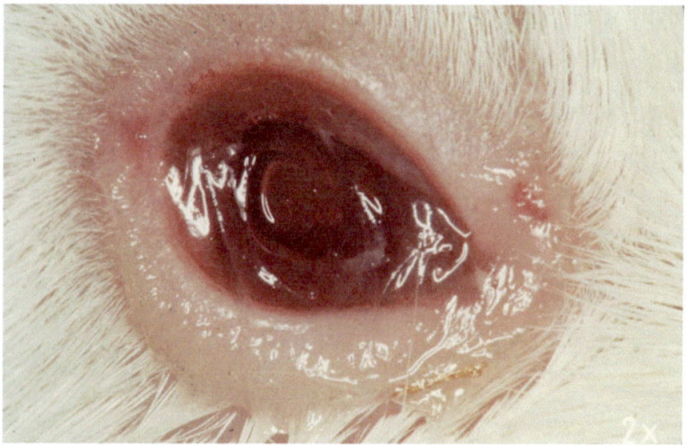

Fig. 4.4 Acute ocular inflammatory responses produced coagulated material in guinea pig eye that was topically sensitized with FLOA and systemically infected with A. Summ parasite (Reproduced with permission from Khatami et al. (Ref. [18], 1984) Archives of Ophthalmology, AMA. All rights reserved)

6.2 Intermediate Phase (Stage b): Down-Regulation Phenomenon

Clinical findings evaluated within 2 months of repeated topical challenges with FLOA included minimal tearing or tissue edema and mild neovascularization and hypertrophy of CALTs. Ocular reactions at this phase seemed reactive at least for a couple of hours after the last antigen challenge. Histological evaluation revealed increased degranulation and loss of mast cell function, increased infiltration of eosinophils into ocular secretion and mucus secreting goblet cells (GCs) and suepithelium accompanied with neovascularization (Fig. 4.5a, b) [18, 19, 21]. A decrease in the number of functional MCs during down-regulation of clinical responses was demonstrated. It was suggested that repeated activation of MCs led to exhaustion of these effector cells. Further examination with topical treatment of the sensitized eyes with histamine produced strong type 1 reactions during down-regulation phenomenon suggesting that histamine receptors were not affected at this stage. In addition, when a mast cell degranulating agent (compound 48/80) was topically applied to the desensitized eye, the minimal clinical reactions were comparable to

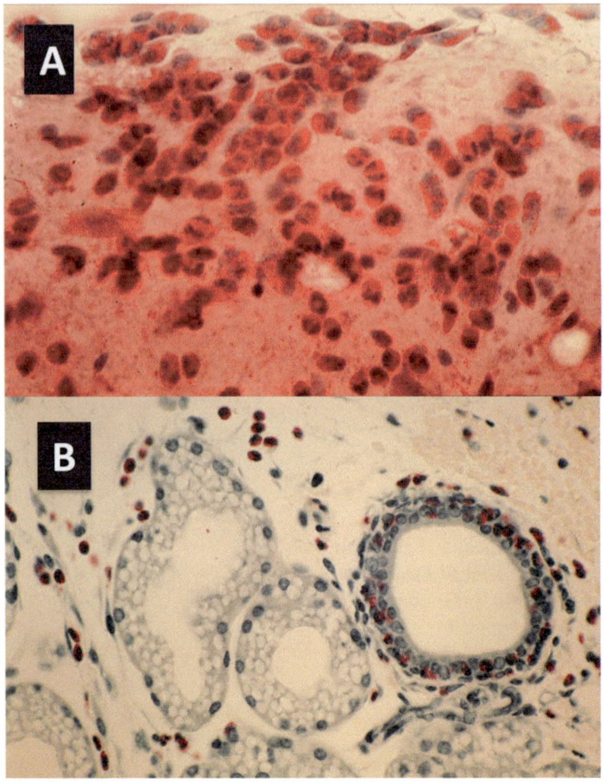

Fig. 4.5 Induction of intermediate inflammatory response in CALTs. A and B panels demonstrate heavy eosinophils infiltration into conjunctival secretions taken from animals that were repeatedly challenged with FLOA, systemically immunized with A. Summ [A]. B panel shows eosinophils infiltration into GCs (Adopted from Ref. [18] American Medical Association @1988, all rights reserved). See text

the eyes that were repeatedly challenged with antigen supporting that repeated stimulation of the tissue reduced the effector function of the MCs [18, 19, 21]. Figure 4.5 demonstrates heavy infiltration of eosinophils in ocular secretion at the intermediate phase of ocular responses toward antigen (A), or in conjunctival mucus secreting GCs (B) in repeatedly sensitized tissue with FLOA.

6.3 Chronic Response (Phase c): Induction of Massive Hyperplasia in CALTs

Massive hyperplasia of CALTs developed in the eyes that were continuously challenged with FLOA for 12–30 months. Little/no clinical hypersensitivity reactions were noted (Figs. 4.6, 4.7 and 4.8). However, tumor-like lesions were prominent features in the conjunctiva (within upper and/or lower lids) along with angiogenesis (Figs. 4.6, 4.7 and 4.8). Cross-sectional areas of massive hyperplastic lymphoid nodules from animals that were continuously challenged with antigen were at least five times greater than lymphoid tissues in normal-untreated animals (Fig. 4.9) [20, 21].

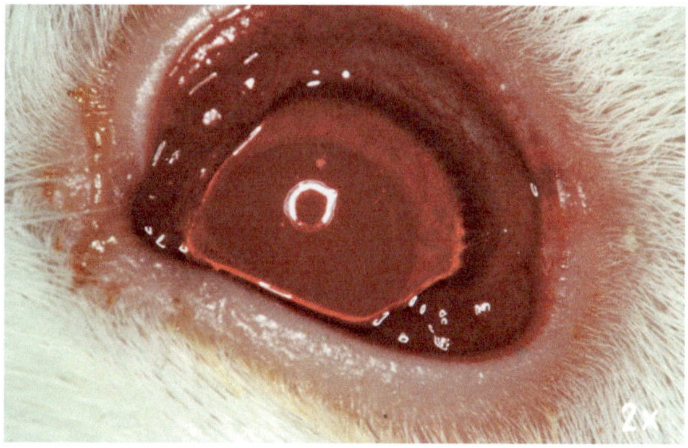

Fig. 4.6 Clinical responses of chronic inflammation-induced massive hyperplasia of conjunctival-associated lymphoid tissue (CALTs) (Reproduced with Permission from Ref. [20] Archives of Ophthalmology, AMA. All rights reserved). See text

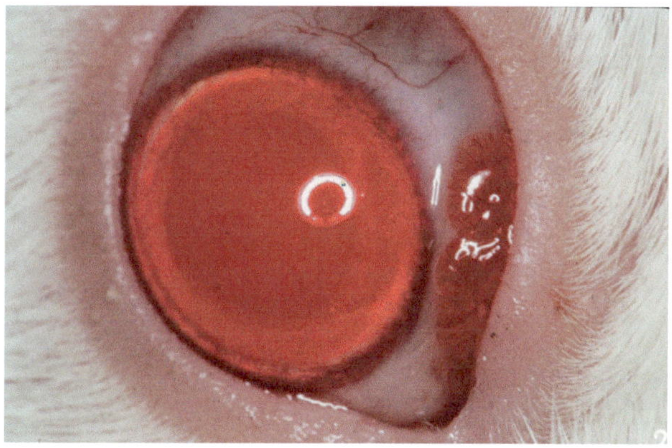

Fig. 4.7 Ocular clinical response to chronic inflammation-induced massive hyperplasia of CALTs after repeated challenges with FLOA (Reproduced with Permission from Ref. [20] Archives of Ophthalmology, AMA. All rights reserved). See text

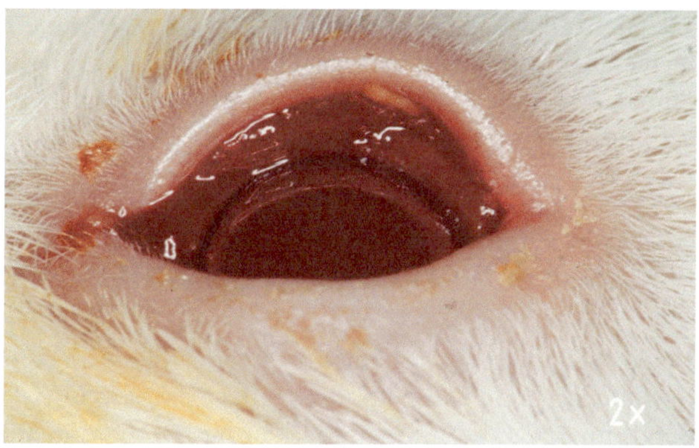

Fig. 4.8 Clinical response to chronic repeated topical challenges of CALTs with FLOA in guinea pigs. It demonstrates extensive angiogenesis, hyperplastic tissue and mucus secretion (Reproduced with Permission from Ref. [20] Archives of Ophthalmol, AMA. All rights reserved. See text

Histopathological examination demonstrated massive lymphoid hyperplasia, follicular formation with germinal centers, activated macrophages, increased swollen GCs, degranulated-partially granulated MCs ('leaky'), involvement of lymphatic channels, extensive epithelial thickening (growth) and/or thinning (necrosis) often

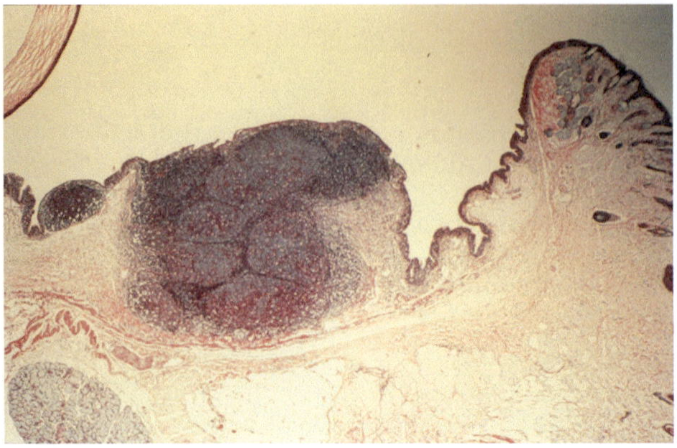

Fig. 4.9 Histopathological findings of hyperplasia of CALTs in the chronic phase of animals repeatedly challenged with FLOA. Reproduced from American Medical Association @1989 [20], all rights reserved. See text

in the same tissue section, suggesting necrosis and/or growth of epithelial tissues [20–22] (Fig. 4.9).

Animals treated with a mixture of FLOA and TPAs showed development of tumor-like lesions within 6 months after commencement of sensitization suggesting shifts in time course kinetics of immune response alterations through activation of protein kinase C (PKC) and perhaps related tumor growth pathways [20, 21, 28, 30].

6.4 Antibody Profiles

Comparison of antibody profiles (i.e., IgE, IgG1/IgG2 isotypes) in ocular and/or splenic tissues in highly sensitized animals during the course of immunization suggested that chronic inflammation-induced site-specific/local alterations in B-plasma or memory cell expression profiles of immunoglobulin subclass (e.g., IgG1/IgG2 ratios). Changes in germinal center reactions could play important role in B cell activities, humoral immunity and tumorigenesis [20–22] (Fig. 4.10).

6.5 Role of Mucus Secreting Goblet Cells in CALTs

Mucus secreting GCs seemed to play a role in developmental phases of immune dysfunction and genesis of tumor-like lesions in CALTs. Heavy eosinophil infiltration into GCs was identified during the intermediate stage of inflammatory responses. The number of swollen GCs also increased in massive hyperplastic CLATs and significant changes in epithelial thickening or thinning. Other studies reported the critical roles of GCs in human or experimental models of inflammatory diseases such as asthma, emphysema, appendicitis, intestinal inflammatory diseases and neoplasia of endocrine system or carcinomas (Fig. 4.5 panel B) [18–22, 28–30, 44, 79, 80].

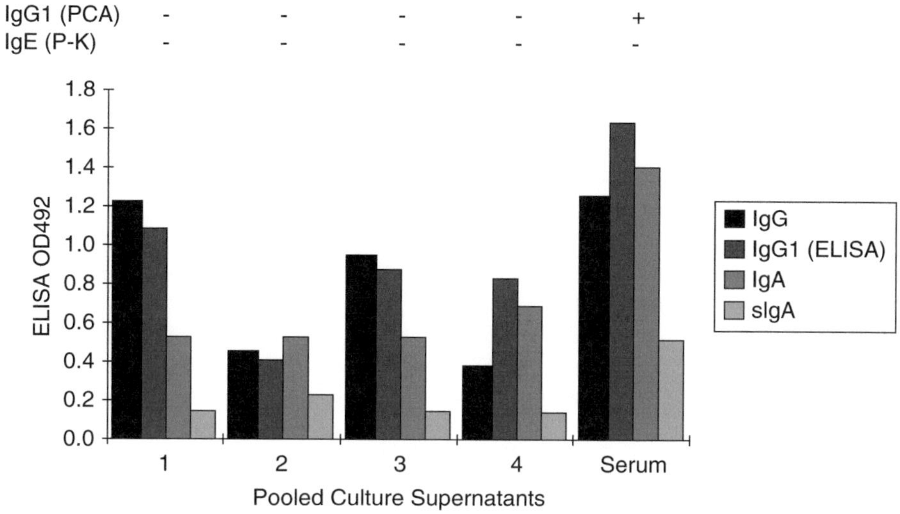

Fig. 4.10 Expression profiles of antibodies detected by ELISA. Data show levels of antibodies in serum and tissue culture supernatants of CALTs from repeatedly challenged guinea pig eyes. Upper panels show detection of IgG isotype (IgG1) by PCA; or IgE by P-K methods in serum. Reproduced from [Ref. 22].

6.6 *Statistical Analyses*

From a total of 400 eyes that were examined, 12/40 (30%) of eyes from animals that were not sacrificed during earlier immunization periods developed tumor-like lesions or hyperplasia of CALTs. It is noteworthy that tumor development in CALTs primarily occurred in animals that produced minimal early type 1 responses toward antigen challenge. Monitoring percentage of tumor-like lesions developed with strong or weak responses during the entire course of immunization is perhaps among the important knowledge gaps that awaits future investigations [20, 21, 28–30, 40–44].

6.7 *Sequential Interactions and Synergies Between Resident MCs and Mucus Secreting GCs and Recruiting Eos and MΦs Toward Multistep Tumorigenesis*

In 2014, further analyses of data resulted in the first report demonstrating systematic time course for progressive interactions and synergies between activated mast cells and recruited Eos (in intermediate phase) and activated/polarized MΦs (TAMs or

M2) in conjunctival-associated lymphoid tissues [30]. It was proposed that such interactions or synergies between resident mast cells and those recruiting eosinophils or macrophages could also occur at various stages of immune responses in lung airways or other tissues (gut-associated lymphoid tissues-GALTs) toward repeated exposures to immune disruptors. The principal resident immune cells in these tissues are also MCs, lymphoid organs and mucus secreting goblet cells. It was suggested that crucial interactions and synergies of the activated cells were responsible for enhancing growth promoting capacities of host toward tumorigenesis [30, 40–44]. It was further proposed that under oxidative stress, M-CSF may produce signals that are cumulative/synergistic with host mediators (e.g., low level release of histamine), facilitating tumor-directed expression of decoy receptors and other immune suppressive factors (e.g., dTNFR, IL-5, IL-10, TGF-β, PGE2). It was also proposed that M-CSF, possessing superior sensitivity and specificity, compared with conventional markers (e.g., CA-125, CA-19-9) was potentially a suitable biomarker for cancer diagnosis and technology development [30, 44, 61, 91].

Systematic monitoring of interactions between resident and recruited cells should provide key information not only about early events in loss of immune surveillance, but it would help making informed decisions for balancing the inherent tumoricidal (Yin) and tumorigenic (Yang) properties of immune system and for effective preventive and therapeutic approaches and accurate risk assessment formulation toward improvement of public health.

The immunopathological data that are reported by a number of investigators on human and experimental models of conjunctivitis as well as squamous cell carcinoma of the conjunctiva produced a range of inflammatory reactions including appearance of yellowish cornea, yellow stringy exudates composed of mucus, activated epithelial cells, activation and infiltration of eosinophils, eosinophil granules, neutrophil and mononuclear cells [21, 28–30, 67–76]. These and related findings on the role of MCs mediators and/or B or plasma cell-derived pro-, and anti-inflammatory mediators in the induction of a wide range of inflammatory conditions, including pathogen-specific vaccines-induced allergies, autoimmune or neurodegenerative diseases or several cancers in human or models of chronic diseases are indirect support of the systematic and progressive presentations of inflammatory conditions that resulted in tumorigenesis and angiogenesis of the 'accidental' discoveries that we established in 1980s [19–27, 40–44, 77–92, 95–144].

Figure 4.11, schematically demonstrates developmental stages of inflammation-induced alterations in immune responses (identified as phases a, b and c) or acute, intermediate and chronic phases, which led to tumor growth and angiogenesis in CALTs. It also represents that while the early stages (a or b) may be reversible (correctable), continuous exposure of host tissue to antigen and aging process increase the risk for induction of advanced stages of carcinogenesis that may not be reversible [40–44].

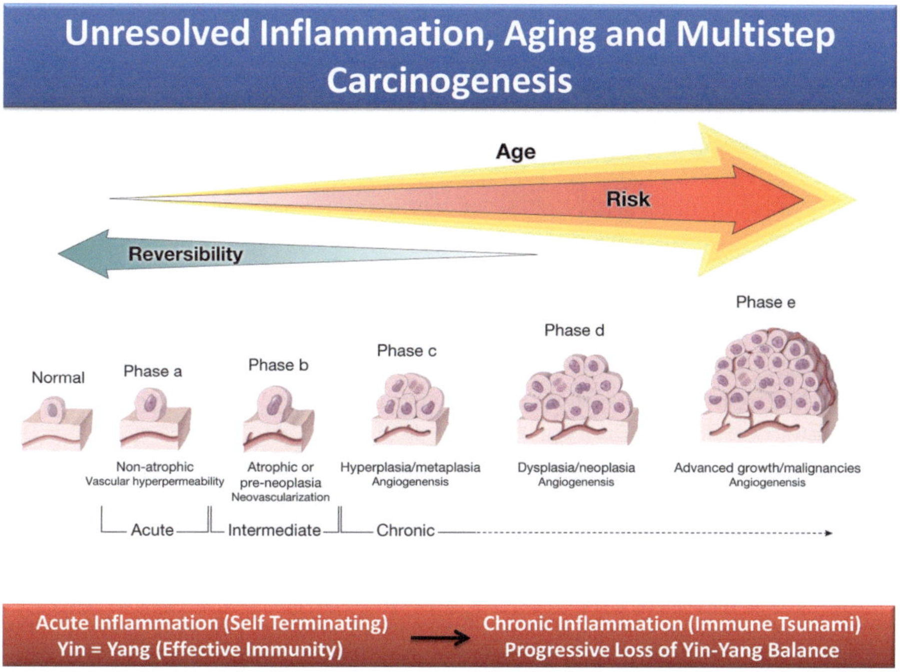

Fig. 4.11 Schematic representation of acute and chronic inflammation and increased risk of carcinogenesis in aging. Left panel depicts acute phase inflammation (**a**) inflammation-induced vascular hyperpermeability and tissue edema followed by tissue repair (reversible, self-terminating phase). Phase (**b**), initiation of tissue atrophy, induction of pre-neoplasia and neovascularization, potentially reversible/correctable phase if inflammatory conditions were removed or if the innate immune cell functions could be stabilized. Phase (**c**) depicts induction of oxidative stress accompanied by altered signals from immune and non-immune cells, expression and co-expression of wound healing and selective apoptotic factors leading to immune dysfunction, loss of tissue integrity and progression towards Phases (**d**) and (**e**) in the direction of tumor growth, metastasis and angiogenesis. See text (Adopted with permission from Khatami [Ref. 41]. All rights reserved)

6.8 *Discussion: Direct Role of Inflammation in Multistep Tumorigenesis*

The results of these studies are the first reported systematic probes into understanding the sequential interactions and synergies between local (host)-resident cells and recruiting immune cells. The results demonstrate a range of immune response dynamics from the earliest (initial) stages of response alterations followed by progressive damages to tissue integrity and function at the intermediate and chronic phases toward development of massive hyperplasia or tumorigenesis and angiogenesis at a site-specific tissue such as the conjunctival-associated lymphoid tissues. Role of MCs and increased levels of histamine in tissue, serum or tears, or expression of IgE antibodies have been demonstrated in isolated reports of human vernal conjunctivitis and other immediate allergic reactions in humans or models of acute or chronic inflammatory (hypersensitivity) conditions or site-specific cancers [18–23, 28–30, 40–44, 71, 86, 98, 99, 110, 119, 129, 135–143].

The dense eosinophil infiltration into epithelial tissues and mucus secreting goblet cells that we observed at the intermediate stages of immune cell responses may directly cause damage at this phase of tissue injury and additionally signal for recruitment of activated macrophages (M2 or TAMs phenotype) into the target tissue. It is also possible that eosinophil-derived expression of apoptotic mediators [e.g., major basic protein (MBP), neurotoxic factors, and/or myeloperoxidase-superoxide anion], directly damage the target tissues and signal for infiltration of macrophages at M2 (TAMs) phenotypes in an attempt to neutralize or induce wound healing and immune suppression. However, recruiting activated MΦs could further damage the host tissue integrity in the direction of cell growth promotion. Synergistic increase in the expression of immune suppressive mediators such as PGE2 from 'leaky' (tumorigenic) MCs and/or TAMs into CALTs could also promote growth properties (Figs. 4.11, 4.12 and 4.13) [20–22, 40–44].

In general, it seems that biological reasons for interdependent interactions between activated or exhausted resident and recruited inflammatory cells that would lead to immune suppression are the attempts of the immune system to resolve inflammatory conditions (oxidative stress) when polarized immune (or non-immune) cells generate mediators from the phenotypes (e.g., M2 or TAMs) that express wound healing factors. The disproportionate expression of wound healing factors create an immunological chaos, by expression and co-expression of apoptotic and wound healing factors that collectively potentiate the immune-suppressive quality of resident immune cells (e.g., exhausted or leaky MCs or TAMs, decreased apoptotic powers) with serious adverse consequences.

There are no other reports to demonstrate systematic analyses of time-course kinetics of stages of developmental phases of inflammation-induced immune dysfunction and sequential interactions and synergies between host resident immune and non-immune cells with those of recruiting cells that would lead to tumor growth and angiogenesis. Majority of cancer-related data report on advanced stages of genetically manipulated experimental models of tumors that are used for identification of a large number of factors for drug development (Fig. 4.11, stage e) (see Chap. 6).

Confirmation and extension of these 'accidental' series of discoveries using systematic studies on the role of infections or carcinogens at site-specific tissues (e.g., CALTs, lung airways or gut-associated lymphoid tissues) are expected to lay solid foundations for better understanding of cellular/molecular and bioenergic mechanisms that are operative during the progressive tissue damage and loss of integrity of epithelial or vascular tissue components in multistep tumorigenesis and angiogenesis. These are logical approaches for targeting and correcting skewed immunity at various stages of tissue response profiles that could lead to effective designs of the balance between Yin-Yang (tumoricidal vs tumorigenesis) of acute inflammation and control of disease processes (see Chaps. 2 and 6).

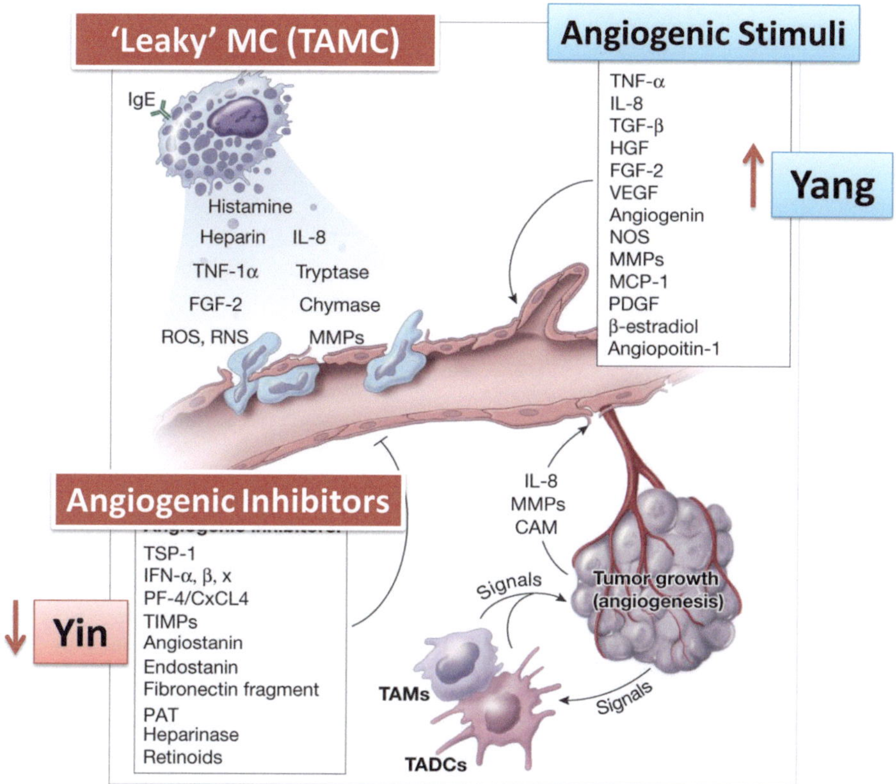

Fig. 4.12 Schematic representation of oxidative stress-induced 'leaky' mast cells (MC, TAMC) and altered expression profiles of angiogenic and anti-angiogenic mediators toward induction of immune suppression and tumorigenesis and angiogenesis. It depicts that repeated tissue stimulation and induction of 'leaky' or tumor associated MCs (TAMC) would lead to expression of low level histamine independent from antigen-IgE-receptor binding and MC degranulation, causing impaired balance in Yin and Yang and signaling for immune suppression and growth promotion by Yang (wound healing, tumorigenesis) that further cause activation, infiltration and polarization of other immune and non-immune cells such as TAMs, TADCs and vasculature toward carcinogenesis. See text (Modified with permission from Khatami [Ref. 40]. All rights reserved)

6.9 *Significance of 'Accidental' Discoveries and Systematic Identification of Stages of Immune Dysfunction in Multistep Tumorigenesis and Angiogenesis*

The author considers the 'accidental' discoveries that were established since 1980s on experimental models of acute and chronic ocular inflammatory diseases that resulted in tumorigenesis and angiogenesis, a real **'Gold Mine'** to further base the future studies. The outcomes of these studies lay a foundation for systematic

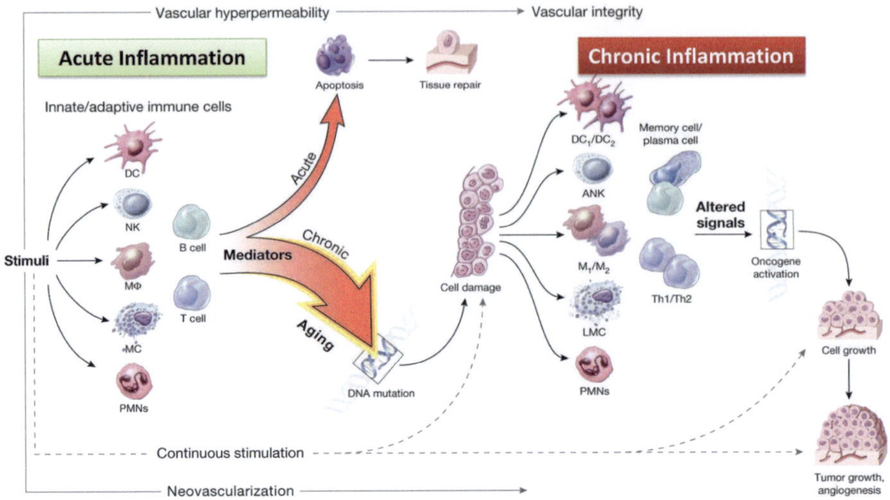

Fig. 4.13 Schematic representation of tissue stimulation during acute and chronic inflammation and aging process toward tumorigenesis. *Left panel* depicts that in acute inflammation, stimuli would activate one or more innate or adaptive immune cells and vasculature for expression of precise quantities of apoptotic and wound healing factors to eliminate hazardous components and injured tissue, resulting in resolution of inflammation, tissue repair and vascular integrity. The *right panel* represents that continuous tissue stimulation (chronic inflammation) and aging process would lead to damage to cell function, such as DNA mutation, polarization of innate and adaptive immune cells followed by abnormal expression and co-expression of apoptotic or wound healing factors from activated cells [e.g., altered/increased ratios of DC2/DC1, M2/M1 (TAMs), 'leaky' MCs (LMC), NKs (ANK), memory and plasma cells, Th2/Th1/Treg] leading to immune suppression and activation of oncogenes and growth of defective cancerous cells. See text. Adopted from Khatami [Ref. 41] with permission. All rights reserved

investigations of the roles of immune disruptors (e.g., wide range of low level carcinogens, infective agents or chemical and biological hazards) in early dynamics of immune dysfunction. These studies deserve confirmation and extension of what other molecular entities are involved in the genesis of tissue damage that would help understanding cancer immunobiology and how to control it.

The summary of the results that were published in 1980s and further analyses of data on the role of inflammation in multistep tumorigenesis (since 1998, during author's initiatives in promoting the role of inflammation in cancer research, and the development of molecular concepts for cancer diagnosis, prevention and designs of clinical trials at NCI/NIH) are listed below ([8–23, 28–30, 40–45, 61, 72, 89–92, 110, 112], NCI submitted proposals since 1998). Highlights of important biological knowledge gaps are also proposed for better understanding of the immunobiology of cancer (details in Chap. 6):

6.9.1 Summary of Data on Models of Acute and Chronic Ocular Inflammatory Diseases in 1980s: Major Knowledge Gaps and Future Research Directions

Experimental models of repeated stimulation of CALTs produced a series of reports on clinical histopathological and immunological changes of immune cell responses. At least three identifiable phases of acute, intermediate and chronic inflammatory responses were demonstrated. The immune responses involved sequential activation and effector function of resident and recruiting immune and non-immune cells that resulted the development of massive lymphoid hyperplasia of CALTs.

The proposed important future studies that deserve confirmation and further studies include:

(i) Initial clinical strong or weak responses toward immune disruptor (FLOA, or other antigens, infective agents) during acute phase of inflammation could potentially influence the onset of stages of inflammatory responses and percentage of tumor growth;

(ii) Altered ratios of IgG antibodies (IgG isotypes) in local vs. distant tissue suggest that extent and potency of factors that are generated during development of hyperplasia of lymphoid tissues determine the fate of tissue damage;

(iii) Preliminary observations that demonstrated strong clinical responses in newly born guinea pigs eyes, upon 1st or 2nd ocular challenges are suggestive of antibody transfer from highly sensitized parents to newly born babies. Confirmation and extension of these observations on details of MCs activation and IgE antibody transfer are important and timely topics for future studies to understand the role of parental genetic predisposition and the basis for the observed increased allergies and anaphylaxis (e.g., asthma, food allergies, vaccines) in younger generation;

(iv) Preliminary observations that mixing antigen with tumor promoting agents shifted the dynamics of immune responses toward earlier timing for tumorigenesis and angiogenesis are important for future understanding of the cumulative roles of immune disruptors or low level carcinogens in immune dynamics;

(v) Cross-sectional areas of massive hyperplastic lymphoid nodules from animals that were continuously challenged with antigen were at least five times greater than lymphoid tissues in normal-untreated animals. To what extend epithelial-mesenchymal transformation alters immune response dynamics toward stages of tissue immune and non-immune damages are important knowledge gaps and deserve further studies;

6.9.2 Summary of Progress and Data Analyses on Inflammation-induced Tumorigenesis and Angiogenesis Since 1998

(i) 1998/1999, at DCP/NCI/NIH, the author initially proposed that inflammatory mediators are ideal targets for molecular diagnosis of cancer (biomarkers) and utilization of biorepositories in clinical trials such as PLCO (Prostate-Lung-Colorectal Ovarian) Cancer Screening Trials[2] [89] (details in Chap. 1);

(ii) 1999, author proposed a number of anti-inflammatory agents such as aspirin, Sulindac and captopril for prevention of cancer to colleagues and decision makers at DCP/NCI/NIH. Aspirin is currently the subject of a number of clinical trials for prevention of several clinical trials such as PLCO Cancer Screening Trials [113][2];

(iii) Statistical analyses of a series of original data using a total of 400 eyes, showed 12/40 (30%) of the animal eyes that were not sacrificed during earlier immunization periods developed tumor-like lesions or hyperplasia of CALTs [20, 21];

(iv) 2005, analyses and integration of a series of published data led to a first publication on time-course kinetics of inflammation-induced at least three identifiable developmental phases of immune dysfunction that led to tumorigenesis and angiogenesis [21];

(v) 2004–2007, standardized criteria of cancer biomarkers ('data elements') for identification of a wide range of published articles on markers reported on clinical and basic research for the purpose of developing a cancer biomarkers database. The work was published as NCI-Invention in Federal Register as research tool for oncology researchers (2005). M-CSF was used as a prototype to test/tailor 'data elements' as a potentially suitable biomarker for technology development when superior sensitivity and specificity of the marker was compared with traditional markers. A detailed article on the topic was published in 2007 [61, 91]. The role of mast cell stabilizers in clinical trials were also proposed in comparison with cyclooxygenase inhibitors (Ketorolac) [90];

(vi) 2008, definitions of acute inflammation as the balance between 2 biologically opposing arms (Yin and Yang) of immunity was introduced [40];

(vii) 2009, oxidative stress or unresolved (chronic) inflammation and altered properties of tumoricidal vs tumorigenic (Yin vs. Yang) of acute inflammation was proposed as a common denominator in the initiation and progression of nearly all age-associated chronic diseases or cancer. An initial roadmap was introduced for identifying and interconnecting the major pathways that are involved in the development of age-associated chronic diseases [29];

---

[2]DCP/NCI, Division of Cancer Prevention, National Cancer Institute; Khatami's challenging efforts to present a number of proposals for molecular diagnosis and prevention of cancer and designs clinical trials including introduction of aspirin, Sulindac and captopril to upper management met with severe opposition and denial and rejections (details in Chap. 1) [21, 44, 45].

(viii) 2011, published differential influence of inflammation in immune-privileged and immune-responsive tissues as the bases for induction of neurodegenerative and autoimmune diseases or cell growth and site-specific cancers [41];
(ix) 2012, assessment of claimed cancer 'targeted' therapy was published, describing why we have not won the war on cancer despite decades of heavy public and private investment for cancer research and therapy [42];
(x) 2012, edited and authored 2 books on cancer and inflammatory diseases and aging, and therapeutic approaches [28, 112, 114];
(xi) 2014/2015, in collaboration/co-authorship with epidemiologists and toxicologists on assessing environmental low level carcinogens and cancer risk, it was found that there are no report on early events of immune response dynamics on a wide range of molecules that are identified as carcinogens and biohazards according to EPA [92–94]. Our earlier data described the role of immune disruptor (FLOA)-induced acute inflammatory responses as the first evidence of the earliest changes in immune dynamics [18–23]. These early stages of immune dysfunction are potentially preventable, reversible or druggable;
(xii) 2014, addressed a major question of how the protective quality of acute inflammation (balance between Yin and Yang) switches to damaging effects of oxidative stress-induced tumorigenesis and angiogenesis. Analyses of earlier data led to a first report that focused on the composition (types) and roles of local or host/resident tissue immune and non-immune cells activities (e.g., mast cells/MCs, B/plasma cells, epithelium, GCs) that sequentially interacted and recruited other inflammatory cells (e.g., Eos, TAMs, histiocytes), in the direction of tumorigenesis and angiogenesis [30];
(xiii) 2016, published an invited perspective hypothesizing that cancer is a severe delayed and cumulative hypersensitivity responses of tissues [43]. A working model on differential bioenergetics of tissues and functionality of mitochondria that parallel the role of Yin-Yang of immunity at different stages of life from orderly fetus growth to adulthood and aging process and disorderly cancer growth was proposed (see Chap. 6). A book was also published on assessment of cancer research and therapy in the last century; provided evidence that the virus-contaminated polio vaccines in 1955s contributed to the sharp increased in cancer incidence and mortality and other chronic diseases in baby boomer generation. Assessment and safety concerns on current emphasis on HPV vaccination of young generation was also reported. A related invited Commentary on the timely topic of safety concerns and hidden agenda behind targeting young generation for HPV vaccination that could potentially increase the population of drug-dependency in America was published [44, 45, 115];

7 Addressing Additional Major Knowledge Gaps in Cancer Biology

Detailed knowledge of how the multistep dysfunction of immunity would allow cancer cells to take over the machinery of the site-specific tissue that result in lawless cell growth and carcinogenesis and metastasize at distant organs causing the death of an individual, is fundamental for optimizing strategies for cancer prevention, designs of logical clinical trials and effective therapeutic approaches. Furthermore, there are numerous important biological knowledge gaps that must be systematically considered in the study of cancer biology. These important biological gaps must be addressed in order to overcome many of the challenges that are currently hinder efforts for accurate risk assessment formulation of cancer and other age-associated chronic diseases and identification of potential reversible/modifiable pathways at early stages of immune dysfunction. Identifying such knowledge gaps is anticipated to enhance our understanding of the biology of cancer as the first logical steps toward design of effective therapeutic approaches and clinical trials.

In addition to what is described above, examples of interdependent major knowledge gaps that hinder our progress in understanding the biology of multistep carcinogenesis are listed in the following. The knowledge gaps identified in this chapter are primarily based on our earlier discoveries that were extended on the roles of acute and chronic inflammation in multistep tumorigenesis. Addressing these intellectually important knowledge gaps are expected to provide a better platform when future studies of cancer research and treatment are strategized (details in Chap. 6):

(a) Sequential identification of immune and non-immune cell composition in site-specific tissues (e.g., lung, prostate, ovarian, breast, thyroid, stomach, colon, esophagus or conjunctiva) that are susceptible to multistep cancer cell growth and metastasis. These tissues are considered immune-responsive and the epithelial-mesenchymal transformation are often reported at the site of initial altered immune response dynamics;

(b) The relationships between stimuli/pathogen and host immunity, nature and potency of immune disruptor and the extent of interactions with host resident and recruiting cells. Quality, potency and nature of pathogenic or mutagenic stimuli, genetic predisposition and vulnerability of site-specific tissues toward exposure to carcinogens could produce heterogeneities in response profiles;

(c) Potential differential influence of strong or weak initial/acute phase responses toward exposure to stimuli during the developmental phases of host immune responses are important in multistage carcinogenesis. In this regard, identification of resident cells (e.g., MCs or other first immune cell responders) profiles of mediator release, biosynthesis and expression of other mediators and bioenergetics in susceptible tissues during induction, down-regulation and chronic phases of responses require detailed studies;

(d) Time-course kinetics of developmental phases of immune disruptor-induced alterations in response dynamics, using site-specific host tissues, specific exposure routs on defined stimuli, identification of expression of mediators at different phases of immune dynamic alterations;
(e) It is important to address how stimuli-induced generations of danger signals (TLRs and decoy receptors) are transmitted in target tissues with specific immune and non-immune composition. For example, epithelial tissues such as conjunctiva, lung airways or gut, whose resident immune defense cells are primarily mast cells, lymphoid tissues and mucus secreting goblet cells, may produce shared or special signals for activation or deactivation (tolerance) in host resident cells and those recruited to the site of tissues;
(f) Little is known about mechanisms of expression of additional shared or specialized mediators from resident or recruited inflammatory cells that result in extensive tissue damage and loss of architectural integrity in immune-privileged or immune-responsive tissues in the induction and manifestation of tissue-specific neurodegenerative or autoimmune diseases and/or cell growth, neoplasia, hyperplasia, polyps, precancer or invasive cancer and angiogenesis.
(g) Role of vasculature mediator response to normal or hypoxic conditions at various stages of inflammatory processes and carcinogenesis;
(h) Antibody profiles expressed during stages of inflammatory responses in target susceptible tissues (e.g., immune-responsive, immune-privileged, insulin-dependent or insulin-independent tissues for glucose transport and metabolism) are perhaps essential steps toward better understanding of the interdependent mechanisms of chronic inflammatory diseases including diabetes and cardiovascular complications, neurodegenerative and cancer biology;
(i) Genetic makeup of immune system and target tissues and the influence of stimuli in induction of genetic mutations at various stages of inflammatory responses;
(j) Susceptibility of target tissues (e.g., immune-responsive, immune-privileged, as well as insulin-dependent and insulin-independent tissues for glucose transport and utilization) toward specific stimuli is anticipated to produce heterogeneities in initial response profiles and outcomes;
(k) Identification of mediators (growth-promoting or growth-arresting) that are abnormally expressed at distinct phases of altered immune dynamics, and which could be potentially reversed or corrected, are expected to provide important clues in better understanding of the complex dynamics of immunity toward maintenance of health and prevention of diseases;
(l) Interrelationships between immune disruptors-(oxidative stress-) induced altered crosstalk in immune and non-immune systems that contribute to alterations of cellular components such as mitochondria and lysosomes, ER or Golgi apparatus and protein-lipid recycling pathways (anabolic/catabolic status of tissues) and altered mitochondria (mitophagy) or bioenergetic status of tissues or autophagy, at early or late phases of immune dynamic alterations;

(m) Monitor percentage of tumor-like lesions as relate to the initial strong or weak responses during the entire course of immunization. Since diversity and heterogeneity of disease processes are considered as major problematic issues for the design of suitable clinical trials, close monitoring of extent of strong or weak acute inflammatory responses is perhaps among the important clues in understanding the influence of immune response dynamics in protecting or damaging the target tissues;

8 Types of Allergies and Immune Disorders: Rational for Promotion of Balance Between Yin (Tumoricidal) and Yang (Tumorigenic) Pathways in Immunity for Prevention of Chronic Diseases

As discussed throughout this book, despite availability of over 20 million publications on a wide range of basic sciences or clinical studies of cancer research and therapies as well as numerous age-associated inflammatory diseases, the peculiar absence of systematic and integrative studies led to existence of numerous key biological gaps and lack of effective progress in understanding the cancer biology or how to prevent or treat it.

In general, allergies such as food allergies, asthma, ocular or skin allergies are clinically considered as symptoms of three types of tissue responses to stimuli, IgE-mediated (acute, immediate or type 1), non-IgE-mediated (cellular or delayed type hypersensitivity) and mixed responses, IgE-mediated and delayed type allergies (details in Chap. 6) [112, 114, 116]. We recently considered that nearly all allergies and age-associated chronic diseases or site-specific cancers may be categorized as 'mild', 'moderate' or 'severe' forms of immune disorders [43–45]. Detailed information on biosynthesis and immune-pharmacological properties of histamine (catecholamine, an alkaline and a vasoactive component) and its direct or indirect influence on organ/tissue metabolism and function in the genesis and progression of nearly all acute hypersensitivity reactions, infections, age-associated chronic immune disorders or site-specific cancers are discussed in Chap. 6 to better appreciate the complexity of histamine role in health and diseases with emphasis on cancer biology [21, 44].

In recent years, a number of drugs such as anti-histamines, mast cell stabilizers or none steroid anti-inflammatory drugs (NSAIDs) and sulfhydryl-containing agents that were originally used for prevention of inflammatory diseases (e.g., asthma or conjunctivitis) or cardiovascular, stroke or kidney complications are being considered as chemopreventive agents for a number of cancers such as gastrointestinal, colorectal and breast cancer [21, 44, 66, 72, 96, 98, 110, 112–114, 121][2].

A fundamental question that should be seriously considered for future research is how the protective and precise crosstalk of immune and non-immune systems (e.g., vasculature, metabolic, hormonal, neuronal) that contribute to tissue physiology and function at different levels (e.g., transport of nutrients and metabolites, proton exchangers, ATPases, bioenergetics from oxidative phosphorylation or glycolysis, protein-lipid degeneration/regeneration pathways) or biological clocks (rhythmic switches of on-off or Yin-Yang) that are involved in guarding the body's health and survival are disturbed by aging process and/or immune disruptors (intrinsic and extrinsic stimuli) to the extent that the inherent duality of immunity favors cell growth promotion, or growth-arrest. Extrinsic or intrinsic stimuli, if not properly removed and neutralized by effective immunity are suggested to take advantage of the inherent duality of immunity, provided through Yin (tumoricidal) and Yang (tumorigenic) properties of self-terminating acute inflammation (body's friend) and would take over the machinery of immunity in the direction of disease process and destruction of organ systems. Conducting systematic and time-course studies of immune response dynamics are essential first steps in understanding details of host tissue interactions with stimuli and extent of damage that specific immune disruptors impose on architectural integrity and function of site-specific tissues in the developmental phases of multistep disease processes [21, 28–30, 40–45].

9 Conclusions and Perspectives

Given the crucial status of immunity that protects the body against a wide range of intrinsic and extrinsic immune disruptors and chronic diseases and cancer, comprehensive understanding of the host composition of resident and recruited immune and non-immune cells and their interactions or synergies during multistage immune dysfunction are essential for effective cancer therapeutics. In this regards, careful identification of multiple interrelated mechanisms of diverse mediators that contribute to the loss of immune surveillance should provide a range of novel targets for promoting the balance between Yin-Yang of acute inflammation and preventing chronic diseases, as well as for effective designs of anti-tumor therapies.

Effective strategies for design of therapies for a wide range of inflammatory diseases or cancer can be achieved only if the biology of immune-surveillance, that was initially theorized several decades ago, are systematically understood and appreciated. Potential reversibility of early stages of inflammation-induced immune dysfunction including alterations in cellular chromosomal/genetic material that would lead to cellular growth promotion and genesis of hyperplasia, neoplasia, polyps, precancer or cancer-malignancy deserve detailed studies. Outcomes of logical and systematic plans for identification of multiple stages of immune regulations are anticipated to lay a foundation for design of accurate risk assessment formulation and effective preventive and/or therapeutics. Proposed interrelated projects for future studies of complex dynamics of immunity that contribute to multistep tumorigenesis and metastasis include understanding the interactions between carcinogens-(antigen-load)-induced altered crosstalk in tissues that alter the functions of lysosomal-derived protein recycling pathways or loss of balance between anabolic/catabolic pathways (autophagy) and energy status of cells (oxidative damage to mitochondria in mitophagy) that lead to skewed/retardation of program cell death (Yin) and wound healing (Yang).

In brief, understanding the detailed heterogeneities of immune response dynamics in site-specific tissues is the essential primary steps toward formulation of more accurate cancer risk assessment and designs of effective diagnostic, preventive and therapeutic strategies.

Acknowledgements The laboratory studies presented in this chapter were established at the University of Pennsylvania, School of Medicine, Department of Ophthalmology, Scheie Eye Institute, with a team of collaborators under the direction of John H. Rockey, MD, PhD. Analyses of data and extension of work were done at the National Cancer Institute (NCI), the National Institutes of Health (NIH) since 1998 and despite tremendous hostility of the NCI upper management who initially opposed, denied and rejected the author's submitted concepts and comprehensive proposals to promote the role of inflammation in cancer research and therapy since 1998. The author is grateful to Mr. Alan Hoofring, at NIH Medical Art Department, for developing the original art work.

References

1. Virchow R. Cellular pathology. London: John Churchill; 1858.
2. Karnovsky ML. Metchnikoff in Messina: a century of studies on phagocytosis. N Engl J Med. 1981;304:1178–80.
3. Ehrlich P. Uber den jetzigen Stand der Karzinomforschung. Ned Tijdschr Geneeskd. 1909;5:273–90. [German]
4. Burnet M. Cancer; a biologic approach. I the processes of control. Br Med Journal. 1957;1(5022):779–86.
5. Werno C, Menrad H, Weigert A, et al. Knockout of HIF-1α in tumor-associated macrophages enhances M2 polarization and attenuates their pro-angiogenic responses. Carcinogenesis. 2010;31:1863–72.
6. Capece D, Fischietti M, Verzella D, Gaggiano A, Cicciarelli G, Tessitore A, Zazzeroni F, Alesse E. The inflammatory microenvironment in hepatocellular carcinoma: a pivotal role for tumor-associated macrophages. Biomed Res Int. 2013;2013:187–204.
7. Tataroğlu C, Kargi A, Ozkal S, Eşrefoğlu N, Akkoçlu A. Association of macrophages, mast cells and eosinophil leukocytes with angiogenesis and tumor stage in non-small cell lung carcinomas (NSCLC). Lung Cancer. 2004;43:47–54.
8. Zhou J, Ding T, Pan W, Zhu LY, Li A, Zheng L. Increased intratumoral regulatory T cells are related to intratumoral macrophages and poor prognosis in hepatocellular carcinoma patients. Int J Cancer. 2009;125:1640–8.
9. Ferrantini M, Capone I, Belardelli F. Dendritic cells and cytokines in immune rejection of cancer. Cytokine and Growth Reviews. 2008;19:93–107.
10. Spear P, Barber A, Rynda-Apple A, Sentman CL. Chimeric antigen receptor T cells shape myeloid cell function within the tumor microenvironment through IFN-γ and GM-CSF. J Immunol. 2012;188:6389–98.
11. Bennewith KL, Huang X, Ham CM, Graves EE, Erler JT, Kambham N, et al. The role of tumor cell-derived connective tissue growth factor (CTGF/CCN2) in pancreatic tumor growth. Cancer Res. 2009;69:775–84.
12. Dvorak HF. Tumors: wounds that do not heal. Similarities between tumor stroma generation and wound healing. N Engl J Medicine. 1986;315:1650–9.

13. Drayton DL, Liao S, Mounzer RH, Ruddle NH. Lymphoid organ development: from ontology to neogenesis. Nat Immunol. 2006;7:344–53.
14. Dempke WC. Targeted therapy for NSCLC--A double-edged sword? Anticancer Res. 2015;35:2503–12.
15. Bonde AK, Tischler V, Kumar S, Soltermann A, Schwendener RA: Intratumoral macrophages contribute to epithelial-mesenchymal transition in solid tumors. BMC Cancer. 12:35. Doi: 10:1186/1471-2407-12-35, 2012.
16. Round JL, Mazmanian SK. The gut microbiota shapes intestinal immune responses during health and disease. Nat Rev Immunol. 2009;9:313–23.
17. Pandol SJ, Edderkaoui M: What are the macrophages and stellate cells doing in pancreatic adenocarcinoma? Front Physiol 6:125, 2015. doi: 10.3389/fphys.2015.00125. eCollection 2015.
18. Khatami M, Donnelly JJ, John T, Rockey JH. Vernal conjunctivitis. Model studies in guinea pigs immunized topically with fluoresceinyl ovalbumin. Arch Ophthalmol. 1984;102:1683–8.
19. Khatami M, Donnell JJ, Rockey JH. Induction and down-regulation of conjunctival type-1 hypersensitivity reactions in guinea pigs sensitized topically with fluoresceinyl ovalbumin. Ophthalmic Res. 1985;17:139–47.
20. Khatami M, Donnelly JJ, Haldar JP, Rockey JH. Massive follicular lymphoid hyperplasia in experimental chronic recurrent allergic conjunctivitis. Arch Ophthalmol. 1989;107:433–8.
21. Khatami M. Developmental phases of inflammation-induced massive lymphoid hyperplasia and extensive changes in epithelium in an experimental model of allergy. Implications for a direct link between inflammation and carcinogenesis. Am J Ther. 2005;12:117–28.
22. Haldar JP, Khatami M, Donnelly JJ, Rockey JH. Experimental allergic conjunctivitis: production of different isotypes of antibody by conjunctival-associated lymphoid tissue in culture. Regional Immunol. 1988;1:92–9.
23. Helleboid L, Khatami M, Wei Z-G, Rockey JH. Histamine and prostacyclin: primary and secondary release in allergic conjunctivitis. Invest Ophthalmol Vis Sci. 1991;32:2281–9.
24. Dranoff G. Immune recognition and tumor protection. Curr Opin Immunol. 2002;14:161–4.
25. Davis BK, Wen H, Ting JP. The inflammasome NLRs in immunity, inflammation and associated disease. Ann Rev Immunol. 2011;29:707–35.
26. Arias JI, Aller MA, Arias J. Cancer cell: using inflammation to invade the host. Mol Cancer. 2007;6:29.
27. Steele CW, Jamieson NB, Evans TR, McKaym CJ, Sansom OJ, Morton JP, Carter CR. Exploiting inflammation for therapeutic gain in pancreatic cancer. Br J Cancer. 2013;108:997–1003.
28. Khatami M. Inflammation, aging and cancer: friend or for? In: Khatami M, editor. Inflammation, chronic diseases and cancer chapter 1, cell and molecular biology, immunology and clinical bases. Rijeka: InTech Publishing; 2012.
29. Khatami M. Inflammation, aging and cancer: Tumoricidal vs tumorigenesis of immunity: a common denominator mapping chronic diseases. Cell Biochem Biophys. 2009;55:55–79.
30. Khatami M. Chronic inflammation: synergistic interactions of recruiting macrophages (TAMs) and eosinophils (Eos) with host mast cells (MCs) and tumorigenesis in CALTs. M-CSF, suitable biomarker for cancer diagnosis! Cancers (Basel). 2014;6:297–322. doi:10.3390/cancers6010297.
31. Goronzy JJ, Wevand CM. T cell development and receptor diversity during aging. Curr Opin Immunology. 2005;17:468–75.
32. Nabel G, Galli SJ, Dvorak AM, Dvorak HF, Cantor H. Inducer T lymphocytes synthesize a factor that stimulates proliferation of cloned mast cells. Nature. 1981;291:332–4.
33. Lu W, Lu L, Feng Y, Chen J, Li Y, Kong X, Chen S, Li X, Chen Q, Zhang P. Inflammation promotes oral squamous carcinoma immune evasion via induced programmed death ligand-1 surface expression. Oncol Lett. 2013;5:1519–26.
34. Metcalfe DD, Baram D, Mekori YA. Mast cells. Physiol Rev. 1997;77:1033–79.
35. Kawakami T, Galli SJ. Regulation of mast-cell and basophil function and survival by IgE. Nat Rev Immunol. 2002;2:773–86.

36. Wouters MM, Vicario M, Santos J: The role of mast cells in functional GI disorders. Gut. 2015 Jul 20. pii: gutjnl-2015-309151. doi: 10.1136/gutjnl-2015-309151.
37. Davalos AR, Coppe JP, Campisi J, Desprez PY: Senescent cells as a source of inflammatory factors for tumor progression. Cancer Metastasis Reviews, 29: 273–283, 2010; 338 (1) 119–125.
38. Ribati D. The crucial role of mast cells in blood-brain barrier alterations. Exp Cell Res. 2015;338(1):119–25.
39. Ribatti D: Mast cells as therapeutic target in cancer. Eur J Pharmacol 2015 pii: S0014–2999(15)00356–8. doi: 10.1016/j.ejphar.201502.056.
40. Khatami M. "Yin and Yang" in inflammation: duality in innate immune cell function and tumorigenesis. Expert Opin Biol Ther. 2008;8:1461–72.
41. Khatami M. Unresolved inflammation: 'immune tsunami' or erosion of integrity in immune-privileged and immune-responsive tissues and acute and chronic inflammatory diseases or cancer. Exp Opin Biol Ther. 2011;11:1419–32.
42. Khatami M. Unresolved inflammation: loss of natural cancer killing ability of immunity as correct 'target' for therapy: seeing the 'elephant' in the light. Cell Biochem Biophys. 2012;62:501–9.
43. Khatami M. Is cancer a severe delayed hypersensitivity reaction and histamine a blueprint? Clin Transl Med 2016 Dec;5(1):35. doi: 10.1186/s40169-016-0108-3. Epub 2016 Aug 23.
44. Khatami M: In: Cancer research and therapy: scam of century–promote immunity [Yin-Yang]. ISBN-10:153043100X; ISBN-13: 978–1530431007; Amazon-Createspace. pp 1–166, 2016.https://www.createspace.com/6123573
45. Khatami M. Book review on cancer research and therapy: safety concerns for HPV vaccination of young generation-paid by Obamacare and V.P. Biden moonshot initiative. Global Vaccines Immunol. 2016;1(3):63–8. doi:10.15761/GVI.1000118.
46. Gøtzsche PC. Deadly medicines and organised crime. In: How big pharma has corrupted health care. London: Radcliffe Publishing; 2013.
47. Keibel A, Singh V, Sharma MC. Inflammation, microenvironment, and the immune system in cancer progression. Curr Pharm Des. 2009;15:1949–55.
48. Medina-Echeverz J, Aranda F, Berraondo P. Myeloid-derived cells are key targets of tumor immunotherapy. Oncoimmunology. 2014;3:e28398. eCollection 2014
49. Gounaris E, Blatner NR, Dennis K, Mahnusson F, Gurish MF, et al. T-regulatory cells shift from a protective anti-inflammatory to a cancer-promoting proinflammatory phenotype in polyposis. Cancer Res. 2009;69:5490–7.
50. Eiró N, Vizoso FJ. Inflammation and cancer. World J Gastrointest Surg. 2012;27(4):62–72.
51. Moore MM, Chua W, Charles KA, Clarke SJ. Inflammation and cancer: causes and consequences. Clin Pharmacol Ther. 2010;87:504–8.
52. Issa LA. Biologic agents for inflammatory bowel disease: the current, the future and the controversy. In: Khatami M, editor. Inflammation, chronic diseases and cancer cell and molecular biology, immunology and clinical bases. Rijeka: InTech Publishing; 2012. p. 417–30.
53. Azim H, Azim HA. Targeting RANKL in breast cancer: bone metastasis and beyond. Expert Rev Anticancer Ther. 2013;13:195–201.
54. Blatner NR, Mulcahy MF, Dennis KL, Scholtens D, Bentrem DJ, Phillips JD, et al. Expression of RORγt marks a pathogenic regulatory T cell subset in human colon cancer. Sci Transl Med. 2012;4:164ra159.
55. Stoecker MM, Wang E. Histiocytic/dendritic cell transformation of B-cell neoplasms: pathologic evidence of lineage conversion in differentiated hematolymphoid malignancies. Arch Pathol Lab Med. 2013;137:865–70.
56. Mantovani A, Sica A. Macrophages, innate immunity and cancer: balance, tolerance, and diversity. Curr Opin Immunol. 2010;22:231–7.
57. Deguine J, Barton GM. MyD88: a central player in innate immune signaling. F1000Prime Rep. 2014 Nov 4;6:97. doi:10.12703/P6-97. eCollection 2014.

58. Arnold-Schrauf C, Berod L, Sparwasser T. Dendritic cell specific targeting of MyD88 signalling pathways in vivo. Eur J Immunol. 2015;45:32–9. doi:10.1002/eji.201444747. Epub 2014 Dec 16
59. Kagan JC, Su T, Horng T, Chow A, Akira S, Medzhitov R. TRAM couples endocytosis of toll-like receptor 4 to the induction of interferon-beta. Nat Immunol. 2008;9:361–8.
60. Yamamoto M, Sato S, Hemmi H, Uematsu S, Hoshino K, Kaisho T, et al. TRAM is specifically involved in the Toll-like receptor 4-mediated MyD88-independent signaling pathway. Nat Immunol. 2003;4:1144–50.
61. Khatami M. Standardizing cancer biomarkers criteria: data elements as foundation of a database. M-CSF (model marker) for early detection of cancer. Cell Biochem Biophys. 2007;47:187–98.
62. Irkeç M, Bozkurt B. Epithelial cells in ocular allergy. Curr Allergy Asthma Rep. 2003;3:352–7.
63. Galicia-Carreon J, Santacruz C, Hong E, Jimenez-Martinez MC. The ocular surface: from physiology to the ocular allergic diseases. Rev Alerg Mex. 2013;60:172–83.
64. Forrester JV, Xu H, Kuffova L, Dick AD, McMenamin PG. Dendritic cell physiology and function in the eye. Immunol Rev. 2010;234:282–304.
65. Hamrah P, Hug SO, Liu Y, Zhang Q, Dana MR. Corneal immunity is mediated by heterogenous population of antigen-presenting cells. J Leukocyte Biology. 2003;74:172–8.
66. Abelson MB, Smith L, Chapin M. Ocular allergic disease: mechanisms, disease sub-types, treatment. Ocul Surf. 2003;1:127–49.
67. Hanson A, Gosemann M, Pruss A, et al. Abnormalities in peripheral B cell memory of patients with primary Sjogren's syndrome. Arthritis Rheum. 2004;50:1897–908.
68. Bonini S, Micera A, Iovieno A, Lambiase A. Expression of toll-like receptors in healthy and allergic conjunctiva. Ophthalmol. 2005;112(1528 discussion):1529–48.
69. Elhers W, Donshik P. Giant papillary conjunctivitis. Curr Opin Allergy Clin Immunol. 2008;8:445–9.
70. Heinz C, Fanihagh F, Steuhl KP. Squamous cell carcinoma of the conjunctiva in patients with atopic eczema. Cornea. 2003;22:135–7.
71. Leonardi A, Di Stefano A, Vicari C, Motterle L, Brun P. Histamine H4 receptors in normal conjunctiva and in vernal keratoconjunctivitis. Allergy. 2011;66:1360–6.
72. Donnelly JJ, Sakla AA, Hill DE, Lok JB, Khatami M, Rockey JH. Effect of diethylcarbamazine citrate and anti-inflammatory drugs on experimental onchocercal punctate keratitis. Ophthalmic Res. 1987;19:129–36.
73. Mimura T, Yamagami S, Kamei Y, Goto M, Matsubara M. Specific IgE in tear fluid and features of allergic conjunctivitis. Curr Eye Res. 2013;38(9):917–25.
74. Donshik P, Ehlers W, Ballow M. Giant papillary conjunctivitis. Immunol Allergy Clin N Am. 2008;28:83–103.
75. Irani AM. Ocular mast cells and mediators. Immunol Allergy Clin N Am. 2008;28:25–42.
76. Akova YA, Gungar SG. Ocular involvement in Behcet's disease. In: Khatami M, editor. Inflammation, chronic diseases and cancer. Cell and molecular biology, immunology and clinical bases. Rijeka: InTech publishing; 2012. p. 391–416.
77. Green RH, Brightling CE, McKenna S, et al. Asthma exacerbations and sputum eosinophil counts: a randomised controlled trial. Lancet. 2002;360:1715–21.
78. Siva R, Green RH, Brightling CE, et al. Eosinophilic airway inflammation and exacerbations of COPD: a randomised controlled trial. Eur Respir J. 2007;29:906–13.
79. Rubin BK, Priftis KN, Schmidt HJ, Henke MO. Secretory hyperresponsiveness and pulmonary mucus hypersecretion. Chest. 2014;146:496–507.
80. Evans CM, Kim K, Tuvim MJ, Dickey BF. Mucus hypersecretion in asthma: causes and effects. Curr Opin Pulm Med. 2009;15:4–11.
81. Evans CM, Williams OW, Tuvim MJ, Nigam R, Mixides GP, Blackburn MR, et al. Mucin is produced by clara cells in the proximal airways of antigen-challenged mice. Am J Respir Cell Mol Biol. 2004;31:382–94.

82. Vardakas KZ, Trigkidis KK, Apiranthiti KN, Falagas ME. The dilemma of monotherapy or combination therapy in community acquired pneumonia. Eur J Clin Investig. 2017 Oct 13. https://doi.org/10.1111/eci.12845. [Epub ahead of print].
83. Liu X, Adams AL. Mucoepidermoid carcinoma of the bronchus: a review. Arch Pathol Lab Med. 2007;131:1400–4.
84. Aoki H, Mogi C, Okajima F. Ionotropic and metabotropic proton-sensing receptors involved in airway inflammation in allergic asthma. Mediat Inflamm. 2014;2014:712962. doi:10.1155/2014/712962. Epub 2014 Aug 13
85. Ordonez CL, Khashayar R, Wong HH, et al. Mild and moderate asthma is associated with airway goblet cell hyperplasia and abnormalities in mucin gene expression. Am J Respir Crit Care Med. 2001;163:517–23.
86. Shim WS, Tak MH, Lee MH, et al. TRPV1 mediates histamine-induced itching via the activation of phospholipase A2 and 12-lipoxygenase. J Neurosci. 2007;27:2331–7.
87. Cruse G, Bradding P: Mast cells in airway diseases and interstitial lung disease. Eur J Pharmacol. 2015 May 8. pii: S0014–2999(15)00408–2. doi: 10.1016/j.ejphar.201504.046.
88. Liu FS. Mechanisms of chemotherapeutic drug resistance in cancer therapy—a quick review. Taiwanese J Obstet Gynecol. 2009;48:239–44.
89. Khatami M: Induction of conjunctival-associated lymphoid hyperplasia by antigen and tumor promoting agents. Targeting mediators of inflammatory responses as biomarkers for early detection of tumor/cancer. Am Assoc Cancer Research; Special Conference Proceedings: The Biology and Genetics of Early Detection and Chemoprevention of Cancer. Bal Harbour, 1999.
90. Khatami M. Cyclooxygenase inhibitor ketorolac or mast cell stabilizers: immunological challenges in cancer therapy. Letters to the. Clin Cancer Res. 2005;11:1350–2.
91. Khatami M: (NCI) standardizing criteria on cancer biomarkers as foundation of a database: creating a common language (data elements) for cancer biomarkers tracking and utilization for professionals in oncology research-- HHS Reference No. E-147-2005/0-Research Tool, 2005.
92. Thompson PA, Khatami M, Baglole CJ, Sun J, Harris S, Moon EY, et al. Environmental immune disruptors, inflammation and cancer risk. Carcinogensis Suppl. 2015;1:S232–53.
93. The Risk Assessment Guidelines of 1986. EPA/600/8–87/045. August. tThe use of these guidelines was phased out in 2002.] and IARC cancer classification groups and descriptions of each category. http://monographs.iarc.fr/ENG/Preamble/currentb6evalrationale0706.php.
94. Guidelines for Carcinogen Risk Assessment. Washington, DC, National Center for Environmental Assessment. EPA/630/P-03/001b. NCEA-F-0644b. http://cfpub.epa.gov/ncea/CFM/nceaQFind.cfm?keyword=Cancer%20Guidelines. U.S. EPA. 2005.
95. Sismanopoulos N, Delivanis DA, Mavrommati D, Hatziagelaki E, Conti P, Theoharides TC. Do mast cells link obesity and asthma? Allergy. 2013;68:8–15.
96. D'Amato G, Salzillo A, Piccolo A, D'Amato M, Liccardi G. A review of anti-IgE monoclonal antibody (omalizumab) as add on therapy for severe allergic (IgE-mediated) asthma. Ther Clin Risk Manage. 2007;3:613–9.
97. Ono SJ, Lane K. Comparison of effects of alcaftadine and olopatadine on conjunctival epithelium and eosinophil recruitment in a murine model of allergic conjunctivitis. Drug Des Devel Ther. 2011;5:77–84.
98. Amaral MM, Davio C, Ceballos A, et al. Histamine improves antigen uptake and cross-presentation by dendritic cells. J Immunol. 2007;179:3425–33.
99. Brown J, Wilson T, Metcalfe D. The mast cell and allergic diseases: role in pathogenesis and implications for therapy. Clin Exp Allergy. 2008;38:4–18.
100. Matsuda H, Kawakita K, Kiso Y, Nakano T, Kitamura Y. Substance P induces granulocyte infiltration through degranulation of mast cells. J Immunol. 1989;142:927–31.
101. Harvey BP, Quan TF, Rudenga BJ, Roman RM, et al. Editing antigen presentation: antigen transfer between B lymphocyte and macrophages mediated by class a scavenger receptors. J Immunol. 2008;181:4043–51.

102. Mages J, Dietrich H, Lang RA. Genomewide analysis of LPS tolerance in macrophages. Immunobiology. 2007;212:723–37.
103. Hassan F, Islam S, Tumurkhuu G, et al. Involvement of interleukin-1 receptor-associated kinase (IRAK)-M in toll-like receptor (TLR) 7-mediated tolerance in RAW 264.7 macrophage-like cells. Cell Immunol. 2009;256:99–103.
104. Zhao HF, Wang J, Tony SS. The phosphatidylinositol 3-kinase/Akt and c-Jun N-terminal kinase signaling in cancer: alliance or contradiction? (review). Int J Oncol. 2015;48(2):765–73. doi:10.3892/ijo.2015.3052. Epub 2015 Jun 16
105. Ganz M, Csak T, Nath B, Szabo GLPS. Stimulation induces and activates the Nalp3 inflammasome in the liver. World J Gastroenterol. 2011;17:4772–8.
106. Gallegos AM, Bevan MJ. Central tolerance: good but imperfect. Immunol Rev. 2006;209:290–6.
107. Harrois A, Huet O, Duranteau J. Alterations of mitochondrial function in sepsis and critical illness. Curr Opin Anesthesiol. 2009;22:143–9.
108. Wright RJ, Cohen RT, Cohen S. The impact of stress on the development and expression of atopy. Curr Opin Allergy Clin Immunol. 2005;5:23–9.
109. Alkhouri H, Hollins F, Moir LM, Brightling CE, Armour CL, Hughes JM. Human lung mast cells modulate the functions of airway smooth muscle cells in asthma. Allergy. 2011;66:1231–41.
110. Cundell DR, Mickle KE: Developing the perfect antihistamine for use in allergic conditions: a voyage in H1 selectivity. eBook, Front Clin Drug Res-Anti Allergy Agents; 2016.
111. Sriskandan S, Cohen J. Gram-positive sepsis. Mechanisms and differences from gram-negative sepsis. Infect Dis Clin N Am. 1999;13:397–412.
112. Book: Inflammation, Chronic Diseases and Cancer-Cell and Molecular Biology, Immunology and Clinical Bases (edited by Mahin Khatami), pp-1-430, InTech, ISBN978-953-51-0102-4, 2012, Rijeka, Croatia, http://www.intechopen.com/books/editor/inflammation-chronic-diseases-and-cancer-cell-and-molecular-biology-immunology-and-clinical-bases
113. Bradley MC, Black A, Freedman AN, Barron TI: Prediagnostic aspirin use and mortality in women with stage I to III breast cancer: a cohort study in the prostate, lung, colorectal, and ovarian cancer screening trial. Cancer. 2016 Jul 1;122(13):2067–75. doi: 10.1002/cncr.30004. Epub 2016 May 3
114. Book: Inflammatory Diseases-Immunopathology, Clinical and Pharmacological Basis (edited by Mahin Khatami); InTech; pp1–396; ISBN 978-953-307-911-0, 2012, Rijeka, Croatia, http://www.intechopen.com/books/editor/inflammation-chronic-diseases-and-cancer-cell-and-molecular-biology-immunology-and-clinical-bases
115. Khatami M. Safety concerns and hidden agenda behind HPV vaccines: another generation of drug-dependent society? Clin Transl Med. 2016;5(1):46. Epub 2016 Dec 5. doi: 10.1111/j.1365-2249.2008.03713.x PMCID: PMC2515351
116. Vighi G, Marcucci F, Sensi L, DiCara G, Frati F. Allergy and the gastrointestinal system. Clin Exp Immunol. 2008;153(Suppl 1):3–6.
117. Patrono C. The multifaceted clinical readouts of platelet inhibition by low-dose aspirin. J Am Coll Cardiol. 2015 Jul 7;66(1):74–85. doi:10.1016/j.jacc.2015.05.012.
118. Usman MW, Luo F, Cheng H, Zhao JJ, Liu P. Chemopreventive effects of aspirin at a glance. Biochim Biophys Acta. 2015;1855:254–63. doi:10.1016/j.bbcan.2015.03.007.
119. García-Martín E, Ayuso P, Martínez C, et al. Histamine pharmacogenomics. Pharmacogenomics. 2009;10:867–83.
120. Crusz SM, Balkwill FR. Inflammation and cancer: advances and new agents. Nat Rev Clin Oncol. 2015;12(10):584–96. doi:10.1038/nrclinonc.2015.105. Epub 2015 Jun 30
121. Yalcin AD. Advances inAnti-IgE therapy. Biomed Res Int. 2015;2015:317–465.
122. Blank U, Rivera J. The ins and outs of IgE-dependent mast-cell exocytosis. Trends Immunol. 2004;25:266–73.
123. Angelis N, Porpodis K, Zarogoulidis P, Spyratos D, Kioumis I, Papaiwannou A, Pitsiou G, Tsakiridis K, Mpakas A, Arikas S, Tsiouda T, Katsikogiannis N, Kougioumtzi I, Machairiotis

N, Argyriou M, Kessisis G, Zarogoulidis K. Airway inflammation in chronic obstructive pulmonary disease. J Thorac Dis. 2014;6(Suppl 1):S167–72.
124. Bienenstock J, Tomioka M, Matsuda H, Stead RH, Quinonez G, Simon GT, Coughlin MD, Denburg JA. The role of mast cells in inflammatory processes: evidence for nerve mast cell interactions. Intl Arch Allergy Appl Immunol. 1987;82:238–43.
125. Hammad H, Lambrecht BN. Barrier epithelial cells and the control of type 2 immunity. Immunity. 2015;43:29–40.
126. Gurish F, Boyce JA. Mast cells: ontogeny, homing, and recruitment of a unique innate effector cell. J Allerg Clin Immunol. 2006;117:1285–91.
127. Bischoff SC. Role of mast cells in allergic and non-allergic immune responses: comparison of human and murine data. Nat Rev Immunol. 2007;7:93–104.
128. Redegeld FA, Nijkamp FP. Immunoglobulin free light chains and mast cells: pivotal role in T-cell-mediated immune reactions? Trends Immunol. 2005;24:181–5.
129. Damaj BB, Becerra CB, Esber HJ, Wen Y, Maghazachi AA. Functional expression of H4 histamine receptor in human natural killer cells, monocytes, and dendritic cells. J Immunol. 2007;179:7907–15.
130. Leiper K, Cambell BJ, Jenkinson MD, Milton, et al. Interaction between bacterial peptides, neutrophils and goblet cells. A possible mechanism for neutrophil recruitment and goblet cell depletion in colitis. Clin Sci (Lond). 2001;101:395–402.
131. Barcante JMP, Barcante TA, Peconick AP, Pereira LJ, Lima WS. Parasitic infections and inflammatory diseases. In: Khatami M, editor. Inflammation, chronic diseases and cancer cell and molecular biology, immunology and clinical bases. Rijeka: InTech Publishing; 2012. p. 205–18.
132. Afrin LB, Pöhlau D, Raithel M, Haenisch B, Dumoulin FL, Homann J, Mauer UM, Harzer S, Molderings GJ: Mast cell activation disease: an underappreciated cause of neurologic and psychiatric symptoms and diseases. Brain Behav Immun. 2015 Jul 8. pii: S0889–1591 (15)00236–6. doi: 10.1016/j.bbi.2015.07.002.
133. Shore SA, Schwartzman IN, Mellema MS, Flynt L, Imrich A, Johnston RA. Effect of leptin on allergic airway responses in mice. J Allergy Clin Immunol. 2005;115:103–9.
134. McLeod JJ, Baker B, Ryan JJ: Mast cell production and response to IL-4 and IL-13. Cytokine. 2015 Jun 15. pii: S1043–4666 (15)00205–7. doi: 10.1016/j.cyto.2015.05.019.
135. Saravanan C, Bharti SK, Jaggi S, Singh SK. Histamine H(4) receptor: a novel target for inflammation therapy. Mini Rev Med Chem. 2011;11:143–58.
136. Fajardo AM, Piazza GA. Chemoprevention in gastrointestinal physiology and disease. Anti-inflammatory approaches for colorectal cancer chemoprevention. Am J Physiol Gastrointest Liver Physiol. 2015;309:G59–70.
137. Enoksson M, Lyberg K, Moller-Westerberg C, Fallon PG, Nilsson G, Lunderius-Andersson C. Mast cells as sensors of cell injury through IL-33 recognition. J Immunol. 2011;186:2523–8.
138. Theoharides TC. Mast cell: a neuroimmunoendocrine master player. Int J Tissue React. 1996;18:1–21.
139. Hundley TR, Gilfillan AM, Tkaczyk C, Andrade MV, Metcalfe DD, Beaven MA. Kit and Fc epsilonRI mediate unique and convergent signals for release of inflammatory mediators from human mast cells. Blood. 2004;104:2410–7.
140. Sansonetti PJ. War and peace at mucosal surfaces. Nat Rev Immunol. 2004;4:953–64.
141. Aprahamian T. Autoimmunity, atherosclerosis and apoptic cell clearance. In: Khatami M, editor. Inflammation, chronic diseases and cancer. Cell and molecular biology, immunology and clinical bases. Rijeka: InTech Publishing; 2012. p. 75–96.
142. McCurdy JD, Olynych TJ, Maher LH, Marshall JS. Cutting edge: distinct toll-like receptor 2 activators selectively induce different classes of mediator production from human mast cells. J Immunol. 2003;170:1625–9.
143. Kmiecik T, Otocka-Kmiecik A, Gorska-Ciebiada M, Ciebiada M. T lymphocytes as a target of histamine action. Arch Med Sci. 2012;8:154–61.
144. Hsieh SL, Lin WW. Decoy receptor 3: an endogenous immunomodulator in cancer growth and inflammatory reactions. J Biomed Sci. 2017;24(1):39. https://doi.org/10.1186/s12929-017-0347-7.

Chapter 5
Cancer Statistics and Concerns for Safety of Drugs or Vaccines: Increased Population of Drug-Dependent Sick Society!

It is better to deserve honors and not have them than to have them and not deserve them.

Mark Twain

Abstract Statistical analyses of a number of data from 1946 to 2010 on baby boomers show that despite the improved hygiene and eradication of many infectious diseases, or reduction of cigarette smoking and longer life expectancy over previous generations, the baby boomers in USA have higher rates of chronic disease. In particular there is a disproportionate increased in rates of many types of cancers and neurodegenerative diseases and related disabilities when baby boomer generation health is compared with the previous two generations at the same age. In 2010 the baby boomers made up 26.1% of the total population of USA. In 2013, American Association for Cancer Research (AACR) announced that 33% of women and 50% of men will develop cancer in their life time.

The focus of this chapter is to discuss analyses of data on health status, with emphasis on the models used for estimation of cancer incidence, mortality and survival rates in different parts of the world by governmental and private organizations on epidemiological reports. The estimated distribution of deaths by site-specific cancers along with what is officially known as risk factors for induction of chronic diseases will be presented. The outlines of epidemiological logics and missing information on bases for reported increased in chronic illnesses are presented for future considerations of research and formulation of accurate risk assessment and effective strategies for prevention and treatment of chronic diseases and cancer. In this context, the role of aging process and impact of immune-disruptors or low level carcinogens, including the potential impact of viral or bacterial components in pathogen-specific vaccines in induction of antigen-load and chronic inflammation that increase the risk of age-associated chronic diseases and site-specific cancers will be discussed.

Developing a universal vaccine, a prophylactic agent that generally boosts immunity and prevent chronic diseases, rather than preventing specific disease is proposed for future studies. Due to the current philosophy of reductionist approaches to all aspects of medical sciences developing universal vaccines has yet to be thought of.

M. Khatami, *Inflammation, Aging and Cancer*,
https://doi.org/10.1007/978-3-319-66475-0_5

Keywords American health status • Big pharma • Cancer establishment • Cancer myth • Cancer risk factors • Cancer statistics • Chaos in cancer research • Contaminated polio vaccines • Failed therapies • Health hazard of specific vaccines • Health Risk hazards • HPV vaccines • National Cancer Institute • Personalized or precision medicine • SEER • Statistics • Targeted therapy • Viruses • World Health Organization

1 Introduction

A chief event of life is the day in which we have encountered a mind that startled us. Ralph Valdo Emerson

Statistical analyses of data sponsored and reported by various governmental agencies (e.g., NCI-SEERS*Stat, CDC, ACS, National Health and Nutrition Surveys-NHANES) and private epidemiological and clinical studies from 1946 to 2010 show that despite the improved hygiene and eradication of many infectious diseases, less cigarette smoking and longer life expectancy over previous generation, the baby boomers in USA have higher rates of chronic diseases, particularly disproportionate increased in incidence and mortality of many cancers and related disabilities, compared with the previous generation at the same age [1–22]. Despite the fact that medicine and detection technologies have improved significantly during the baby boomers' lifetimes that increased life expectancy, the health status of aging baby boomers seem poorer with regard to several diseases such as obesity, autoimmune and neurodegenerative illnesses, hypertension, diabetes and cardiovascular complications, osteoporosis and malnutrition, compared with prior generations [4–14, 23–38]. A major factor that has not been included or analyzed in the majority of reports on statistical analyses is the sharp increase in site-specific cancer incidence and mortality (particularly in America) between 1955s and 1960s, the period that public was vaccinated with virus-contaminated polio vaccines [31–33, 39–49]. American health ranks last among many other developed nations, despite the fact that America spends the highest amount of public and private funds for healthcare. In addition, racial and ethnic disparities including economic inequality impact the outcomes of diseases such as obesity, malnutrition, infectious diseases and cancer [31–33, 43–71][1,2,3]

[1] a.Sharon Begley (2008-09-05). "Rethinking the War on Cancer". *Newsweek*. http://www.newsweek.com/rethinking-war-cancer-88941;

b.Bernadine Healy (2008-06-12). "We Need a New War on Cancer". U.S. News and World Report;

c."LIVESTRONG Global Cancer campaign announces Hashemite Kingdom Of Jordan's commitment of $300 million to fund three cancer control initiatives."

[2] Kolata, Gina (April 24, 2009). "As Other Death Rates Fall, Cancer's Scarcely Moves". *The New York Times*.

[3] Apostolides AD, Apostolides,IK: The United States Program on Cancer, 1975–2006: A Failure

In this chapter, reported statistical data, definitions and the models that are used for estimation of cancer incidence, mortality and survival rates in different parts of the world will be overviewed with emphasis on data for the distribution of site-specific cancer mortality. The existence of important knowledge gaps and missing information or misinformation that obscure accurate statistics and risk assessment formulation will be discussed for future considerations. Among important knowledge gaps are the strange absence of systematic studies on the relationships between host-pathogens or the cumulative role of environmental hazards that would increase the risk of cancer and other age-associated chronic diseases (details in Chaps. 1 and 6).

2 Statistical and Epidemiologic Data on Disease Mortality and Morbidity Around the World: Why Americans Health Rank Last?

Noise proves nothing. Often a hen who has merely laid an egg cackles as if she laid an asteroid. Mark Twain

Reports from governmental and private sources similarly demonstrate that the Americans (baby boomers) health has fallen behind many other developed countries [4–8, 31–33, 52–66][4,5]. From 1946 through 1964, 78 million children were born in the United States that are considered the "baby boomers". In 2010, baby boomers made up 26.1% of the US population [4–9, 31]. Figure 5.1, is a comparison of the health status of American baby boomers with previous generation, with regard to hypertension, increased cholesterol, diabetes and obesity [6].

In another study, analyses of poor health in America were reported by a panel of experts who found that American ranked last among 16 other developed countries. The group's remarks included "… *Is it Americans' rugged individualism and the sense that most important thing is the individual's freedom, and that's so much more important than doing what is right for society… American are less likely to smoke or may drink less heavily than their counterparts in peer countries, but they consume the most calories per capita, abuse more prescription and illicit drugs…. Yet even fit, nonsmoking Americans have higher disease rates than those elsewhere…*".[6]

The above report was prepared by a group of physicians, epidemiologists, demographers and other researchers charged by the National Research Council and the Institute of Medicine to better understand American's comparative health status. Figure 5.2, demonstrates data on the rate of deaths from all causes by 17 developing

(Part 2), Townsend Letter. The Examiner of Alternative Medicine. August/September 2010.

[4] Mirror, Mirror on the Wall, 2014 Update: How the U.S. Health Care System Compares Internationally. Executive Summary.

[5] USA Today (1994) reflected an article that was published in JAMA: 'Baby boomers are much more likely to get cancer than their grandparents were at the same age.'

[6] Grace Rubenstein: New Health Rankings: Of 17 Nations, U.S. is Dead Last….Jan 10, 2013.

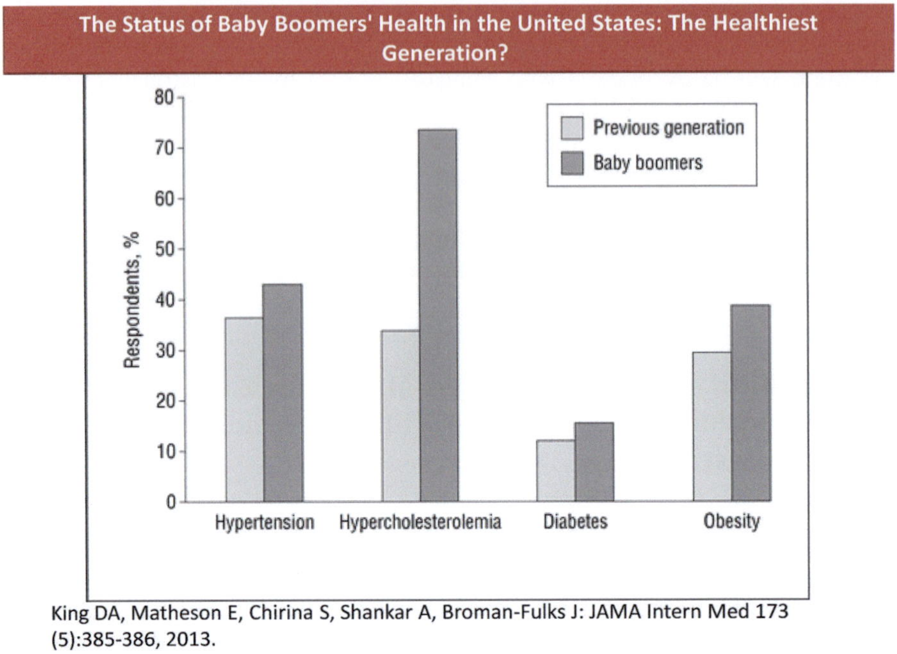

Fig. 5.1 Comparison of health status for hypertension, hypercholesterolemia, diabetes and obesity in baby boomers and previous generation (Adopted from JAMA Intern Med. (Ref. [6]) with permission)

countries, using data on 2008 report from World Health Organization (WHO) in 2012/2013 publications [31–33, 55–58].[6] It shows death from all causes; and that Americans' health ranked last, despite the fact that America invest highest amount of money under the claim of healthcare!

The panel examined when and why people die in the United States and 16 other nations (e.g., Australia, Japan, Canada and Western European countries) using the data that reported by the WHO for Economic Cooperation and Development. Outlines of data that were reported for death in the USA showed the following surprising factors:

(a) Highest rate of death occurred by violence;
(b) Highest rate of death was due to car accident;
(c) Highest chance that a child dies before the age of 5;
(d) Second (2nd) highest rate of death by coronary heart disease;
(e) The 2nd highest rate of death by lung diseases;
(f) Highest teen pregnancy and death due to childbirth
(g) Even white and the "*well-off Americans live sicker and die sooner than similarly situated people elsewhere…*"[6]

According to another report "*The United States healthcare system is the most expensive in the world, but this report and prior editions consistently show the U.S.*

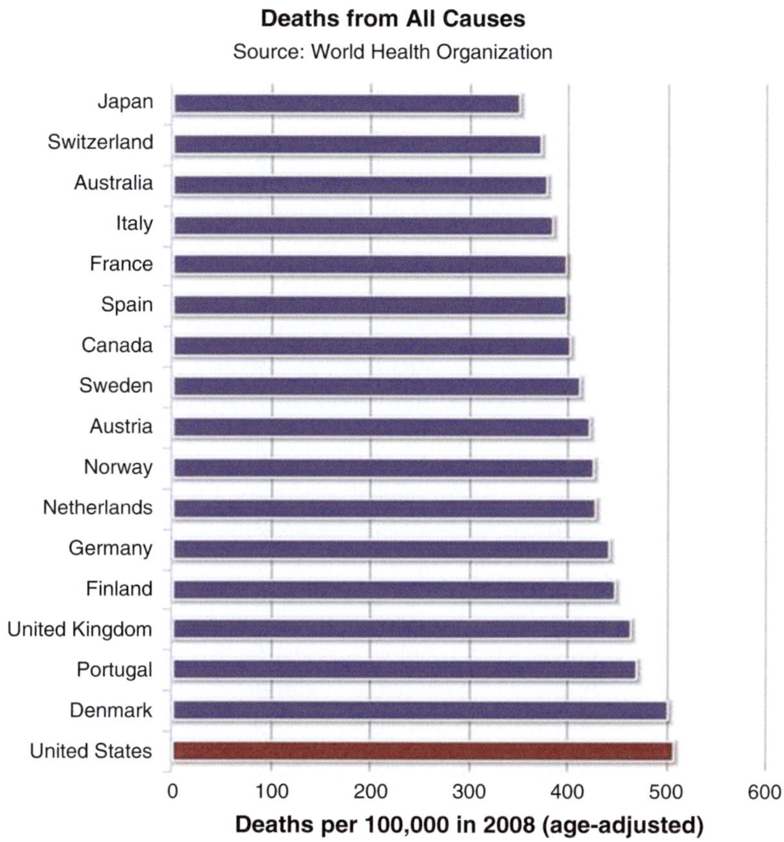

Fig. 5.2 Age-adjusted death among 17 developed nations.[1] It shows lifespan among various developed nations regardless of income or level of education

underperforms relative to other countries on most dimensions of performance. Among the 11 nations studied …Australia, Canada, France, Germany, the Netherlands, New Zealand, Norway, Sweden, Switzerland, and the United States—the U.S. ranks last, as it did in the 2010, 2007, 2006, and 2004 edition of Mirror, Mirror….".[4] [See Chap. 1]

2.1 Anatomy of a Sick Care Nation (America): Power of Advertisement-Creation of 'Magical Reality' Culture for Selling Drugs and Unhealthy Food Products

The above reports neglected to identify the important factors that contribute to the increased disease status of Americans. In addition to the roles that virus-contaminated polio vaccines or other pathogen-specific vaccines and environmental hazards played in sharp increase in cancer incidence and neurodegenerative and autoimmune diseases around the globe (see below) [31–33, 39–41, 47–49, 62, 67–88], the available publications underestimate the power of advertisement and propaganda in all aspects of American lives as major contributors to the higher disease status [31–33]. The militarized power of medical establishment that includes the Government (NIH, FDA, CDC-DHHS), major health/medical/cancer organizations, food industries, Big Pharma and their powerful lobbying groups, collectively control major media. The establishment has been able to heavily advertise and publicize all types of packaged foods that are fortified with hormones, antibiotics, preservatives, salt, sugars or imitation fats or sweeteners; or a wide range of genetically modified microorganisms (GMOs) foods, herbicides-, pesticide-(carcinogen)-laced fruits and vegetables, drinks (e.g., energy, diet, sugarless), as well as a variety of prescription or over-the-counter drugs as 'choices' for individuals who may experience minor or major health discomfort or mental problems [31–33]. The system has cleverly and gradually created a different, magical or virtual culture in America by pushing Americans to be consumers of a wide range of what is marketed and call it 'freedom of choice'! The foods and drugs are heavily publicized in such a way that maximize and exaggerate their pleasures and positive effects while minimize the short-, or long-term health hazards. The wide range of chemical, biological and environmental hazards that are in the food and household products and are routinely advertised and consumed by the public has created a 'magical reality' for Americans, while these products gradually caused a wide range of chronic diseases that require more medications [31–33, 89–148]. The power of medical establishment, which was formed over a century ago, increased since the 1955s, by deceiving the public and injecting Americans with virus-contaminated polio vaccines, claiming to eradicate polio. It is estimated that for every case of polio that the vaccine prevented, 15 cases of cancer and untold number of other diseases were induced since 1955 [31–33, 39–61, 67].[1–6] This created a huge business advantage for the establishment that continues to its current scary state. The establishment has absolute power to control, design and direct not only the research and clinical projects, and drug development, but it controls and publicizes the majority of food and household products that are routinely consumed by Americans.

3 Cancer Global Burden: Statistics on Incidence and Mortality

There are lies and damned lies and statistics. Mark Twain

The following sections reflect review of data on examples of procedures and epidemiological methods that were used for estimation of cancer burden on a global scale. The calculations of cancer incidence and mortality rates were based on the reports from the World Health Organization (WHO) and International Agency on Research in Cancer (IARC, 2000, 2012, 2014), Global Burden of Disease (GBD, 2000) [31, 38, 39, 58–88]. The data sources for cancer death and survival also derived from the cancer survival models developed by the National Cancer Institute Surveillance, Epidemiology, and End Results (SEER)[7] and SEER statistical program (SEER *Stat), the Connecticut survival data from Cancer in Connecticut – Survival Experience, 1935–1962 and the US vital statistics. The data for SEER statistical program is considered as the standard for quality among cancer registries around the world, being the most authoritative source of information on cancer incidence and survival in the United States. The SEER-related information includes data from population-based cancer registries, which collect cancer data on a routine basis and covers approximately 14% or 30% of US population (2015 report, see below) [58, 63, 64].[7] It should be noted that the SEER program is funded by NCI and initiated in 1973, apparently as the results of the significant rise of cancer incidence in America following public vaccination with virus-contaminated polio vaccines in the 1955s/1960s [31–33, 36, 44, 45]. However, except for numerous incomplete and isolated reports on circumstantial evidence for relationship between contaminated vaccines or low level carcinogens and environmental biohazards with chronic diseases or site-specific cancers [31–37, 49–53, 62, 64–88],[7] there is a disconnect on statistics between the decades of 1930s to 1960s to make a better comparison on the influence of virus-contaminated polio vaccines in the increased cancer incidence and mortality and other autoimmune and neurodegenerative diseases of 'Baby Boomers' and the subsequent 2 generations that are likely more vulnerable toward chronic illnesses (e.g., asthma, diabetes, obesity, neurodegenerative and autoimmune diseases) [31–33]. The review of data on statistics and epidemiologic reports are presented to collectively demonstrate potential relationships between viral/bacterial infections, specific vaccines, chemical, biological and environmental hazards with site-specific cancers in specified regions around the world, including increased diseases in younger population in America that is becoming drug-dependent.

To build survival models and prediction of cancer incidence researchers used primarily information from SEER*Stat and related cancer databases. The results provided information on frequencies, death and survival rates, as well as data on state/local information (e.g., Connecticut State Department of Health on Tumor Registry on survival and causes of death followed up by decades, since 1935).

The summary of key points from latest SEER report that was published in the JNCI, includes the following [58, 63] [7,8]:

---

[7] SEER updated information presented at a joint meeting of NCI Board of Scientific Advisor (BSA) and National Cancer Advisory Board (NCAB), December 1, 2015, 'Challenges to cancer surveillance' and 'New initiatives to address the challenges'. etc..

[8] JNCI: Journal of National Cancer Institute, March 30, 2015.

- ***The report highlights the period from 1975–2011 to provide the best perspective on long-term trends in cancer incidence (new cases) and mortality (death) rates for all races combined.***
- ***Researchers found continued declining mortality rates for men, women, and children.***
- ***The incidence rate of thyroid cancer is increasing among both men and women, as well as the mortality rate for liver cancer.***
- ***The incidence rate of oral/oropharyngeal cancers is increasing among white men despite a decline in oral cancers that are more closely associated with tobacco use.***
- ***With a focus on breast cancer, the researchers used comprehensive national data on hormone receptor (HR) and HER2 status to determine the incidence of the four major molecular subtypes of breast cancer by age, race/ethnicity, poverty level, and several other factors.***
- ***Moreover, researchers found unique racial/ethnic group-specific patterns by age, poverty level, geography, and by specific breast tumor characteristics.***

4 Statistical Definitions for Cancer Mortality and Morbidity

Highlights of selected basic guidelines of WHO Cancer Mortality Database or SEER on definitions, surveys, classifications and terms that are commonly reported, applied and extended for disease risk assessment formulation, estimated cancer incidence and mortality or survival outcomes in studies by clinicians, researchers, statisticians, epidemiologists or demographers are shown below [1, 4, 10, 16–21, 35, 36, 42, 43, 54–65, 70, 79–81, 149–152].

(a) ***Mortality***: Mortality is the number of deaths occurring in a given period in a specified population. It can be expressed as an absolute number of deaths per year or as a rate per 100,000 persons per year.
(b) ***Population at risk***: The population at risk includes all individuals susceptible to a specific cancer. It is defined on the basis of demographic variables, such as place of residence, sex, age group. Years of risk duration are counted in person-years.
(c) ***Age-specific rate***: The age-specific rate is calculated simply by dividing the number of cancer deaths observed in a given age category during a given time period by the corresponding number of person years in the population at risk in the same age category and time period. For cancer, the result is usually expressed as an annual rate per 100,000 person-years.
(d) ***Crude rate***: Data on mortality are often presented as rates. For a specific tumor and population, a crude rate is calculated simply by dividing the number of cancer deaths observed during a given time period by the corresponding number of person years in the population at risk. For cancer, the result is usually expressed as an annual rate per 100,000 persons at risk.

(e) ***Age-standardized rate (ASR)***: An age-standardized rate (ASR) is a summary measure of the rate that a population would have if it had a standard age structure. Standardization is necessary when comparing several populations that differ with respect to age because age has a powerful influence on the risk of dying from cancer. The ASR is a weighted mean of the age-specific rates; the weights are taken from population distribution of the standard population. The most frequently used standard population is the World Standard Population. The calculated mortality rate is then called age-standardized mortality rate (world).[9] The ASR is also expressed per 100,000.' Other definition for Age-standardized rate is the number of new cases or deaths per 100, 000 persons per year, which a population would have if it had a standard age structure. Standardization is necessary when comparing several populations that differ with respect to age because age has a powerful influence on the risk of cancer.

(f) ***Risk of getting or dying from the disease before age 75 (%)***: The probability or risk of individuals getting/dying from cancer. It is expressed as the number of new born children (out of 100) who would be expected to develop/die from cancer before the age of 75 if they had cancer (in the absence of other causes of death).

(g) ***Method***: Population weighted average of the area-specific rates applied to the 2012 area population.

(h) ***Prevalence***: Sum of area-specific prevalent cases. Causes of death for the WHO subregions and the world have been estimated based on data from national vital registration systems that capture about 17 million deaths annually. In addition, information from sample registration systems, population laboratories and epidemiological analyses of specific conditions have been used to improve estimates of the cause of death patterns. Cause of death data have been carefully analyzed to take into account incomplete coverage of vital registration in countries and the likely differences in cause of death patterns that would be expected in the uncovered and often poorer sub- populations.

For majority of such reports algorithms were developed to estimate region-specific cancer incidence, survival and death distributions, rates and absolute numbers of cases for the year 2000 using the available published information on age-, sex-, and site-specific cancer incidence and survival. These data have been used to estimate the global burden of cancer (GBC) as part of the Global Burden of Disease (GBD or GD) for 2000 [36–38, 54–60, 63–65, 150–152, 160]. Cancer sites primarily identified with codes; i.e., mouth and pharynx [ICD-9 140–149], oesophagus [ICD-9 150], stomach [ICD-9 151], colon and rectum [ICD-9 153, 154], liver (ICD-9 155), pancreas [ICD-9 157], lung [ICD-9 162], melanoma of skin [ICD-9 172], female breast [ICD-9 174], cervix uterine [ICD-9 180], corpus uteri [ICD-9 182], ovary [ICD-9 183], prostate [ICD-9 185], bladder [ICD-9 188], lymphomas [ICD-9 200–203], leukemia [ICD-9 204–208], and other cancers with related con-

[9] The world standard population used within the application as proposed by Segi (1960) and modified by others [150–152].

troversies or disagreements on such topics as mortality patterns with various registries or diseases surveillance systems [balance of ICD-9 140–208] [54–60, 63–65, 150–152, 160].

According to these reports, the techniques to undertake the analyses were developed based on the global burden of disease study and further refined using a more extensive database and more robust modeling techniques. The resulting estimates of death were systematically corrected on the basis of other epidemiological evidence from registries, community studies, and disease surveillance systems. For China and India, cause patterns of mortality were based on existing mortality registration systems, namely the Disease Surveillance Points system (DSP) and the Vital Registration System of the Ministry of Health in China, and the Medical Certificate of Cause of Death (MCCD) for urban India and the Annual Survey of Causes of Death (SCD) for rural areas of India. For all other countries lacking vital registration data, cause of death models were used to estimate the maximum likelihood distribution of deaths across the broad categories of communicable, non-communicable and injuries, based on estimated total mortality rates and income. A regional model pattern of specific causes of death was then constructed based on local vital registration and verbal autopsy data and this proportionate distribution was then applied within each broad cause group. Finally, the resulting estimates were then adjusted based on other epidemiological evidence from specific disease studies [4, 55–60, 64, 65, 73, 74, 78–81, 88].

It should be noted that according to the 2015 SEER update, national population-based registries covering 30% of the US population; reported 400,000+ cases of cancer incidence annually.[7] SEER identified that from the $87 M funded in 2011–2012 for research projects, 112 used SEER data as 'critical to the grant', and that '40,000 manuscripts referencing to SEER data'.[7]

As a general rule, the information provided by various sources on vital registration data are accepted to suitably correct for ill-defined coding and probable systematic biases in certifying deaths to non-specific vascular, cancer and injury codes when estimated number of the cause of death pattern were considered (Figs. 5.3, 5.4, 5.5, 5.6, 5.7, 5.8, 5.9, 5.10, 5.11 and 5.12).

It should also be noted that, although the statistical analyses between 1940s and 1960s on the cancer incidence and mortality rates are not detailed, there is sufficient evidence to show that the cancer became a deadly disease since 1960s/1970s, after the consumption of virus-contaminated polio vaccines in 1955–1960s [31–33, 40, 41, 42, 67]. In 1955 and before the public consumed virus-contaminated polio vaccines Bernice Eddy who discovered that the polio vaccines were contaminated with live viruses warned the authorities and predicted that consumption of vaccines could cause a cancer epidemic. However, because million doses of vaccines were already prepared, decision makers decided to sell the contaminated vaccines to the public with little regard to the health hazards that led to the sharp increase in cancer incidence and death that followed by heavy cost of cancer drug development with outcome failure rates of 90% (+/−5) (details in Chaps. 1 and 6) [31–33, 44–54].

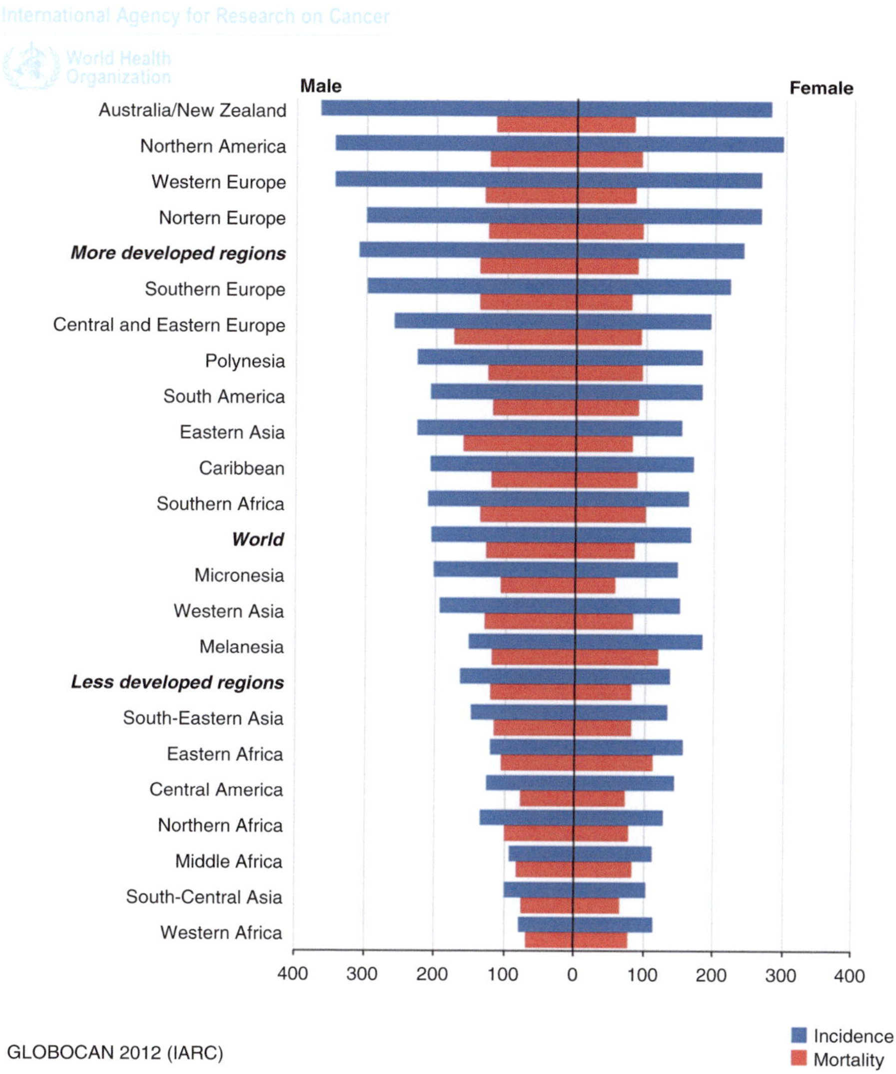

Fig. 5.3 Estimated incidence and mortality of all cancers (excluding non-melanoma skin cancer) worldwide in 2012. Globocan-IARC-WHO report 2012

5 Results and Analyses of Cancer-Related Statistics on Incidence, Mortality and Morbidity

Facts are stubborn, but statistics are more pliable. Mark Twain

Estimated data on cancer incidence, mortality and morbidity reported by WHO (IARC, Globocan) or GBD are demonstrated in Figs. 5.3, 5.4, 5.5, 5.6, 5.7, 5.8, 5.9, 5.10 and Tables 5.1, 5.2 5.3, 5.4. Vital registration data from 65 countries was

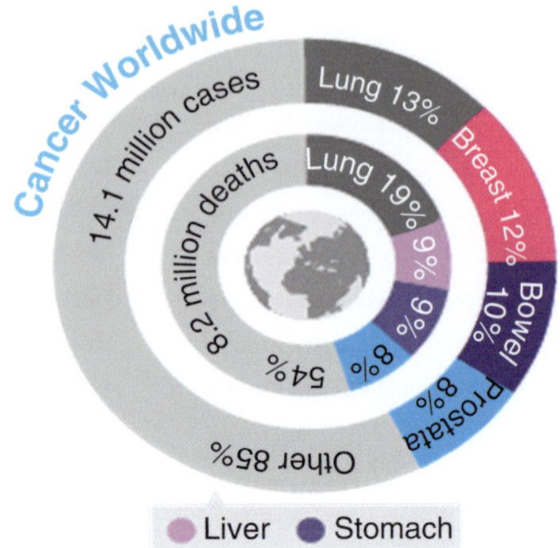

Fig. 5.4 Estimated rate of cancer incident and mortality globally (Source: WHO-IARC, 2012. The figure projected that from 14.1 million cases of cancers, 8.2 million people die of different site-specific cancers in one year)

available for majority of the analyses. In 28 countries, cause of death models were used to correct vital registration data by age and sex to yield more plausible patterns across different population (e.g., Groups I, II and III) and to calculate estimated distribution or profiles of specific causes of death obtained from recorded vital registration data [28, 55–60].

According to the 2012 report by IARC-Globocan (WHO), the estimated cancer incidence, mortality and morbidity for all cancers and some site-specific (e.g., lung colorectal and breast) cancers are summarized below [55–59]:

(a) **All Cancers:** The summary of reports indicated that in 2008, there were 14. 1 million new cancer cases, of which 8.2 million died. The cumulative number of people living with cancer (within 5 years of diagnosis worldwide) was 32.6 million. Fifty seven percent (57%) of new cases of cancer, and 65% (5.3 million) of the cancer deaths and 48% (15.6 million) of the 5-year prevalent cancer cases occurred in less developed countries. The report demonstrates that the overall age-standardized (adjusted) cancer incidence rate is about 25% higher in men than in women, with rates of 205 and 165/100,000, respectively. The cancer rate in men was shown to be highest in Central and Eastern Europe (173/100,000) and lowest in Western Africa (69/100,000). In contrast, the highest rates in women are in Melanesia (119/100,000) and Eastern Africa (111/100,000), and the lowest in Central America (72/100,000) and South-Central Asia (65/100,000) (Table 5.1 and Fig. 5.5).

(b) **Lung Cancer:** Lung cancer has been the most common cancer in the world for the last few decades. Lung cancer is also the most common cause of death from

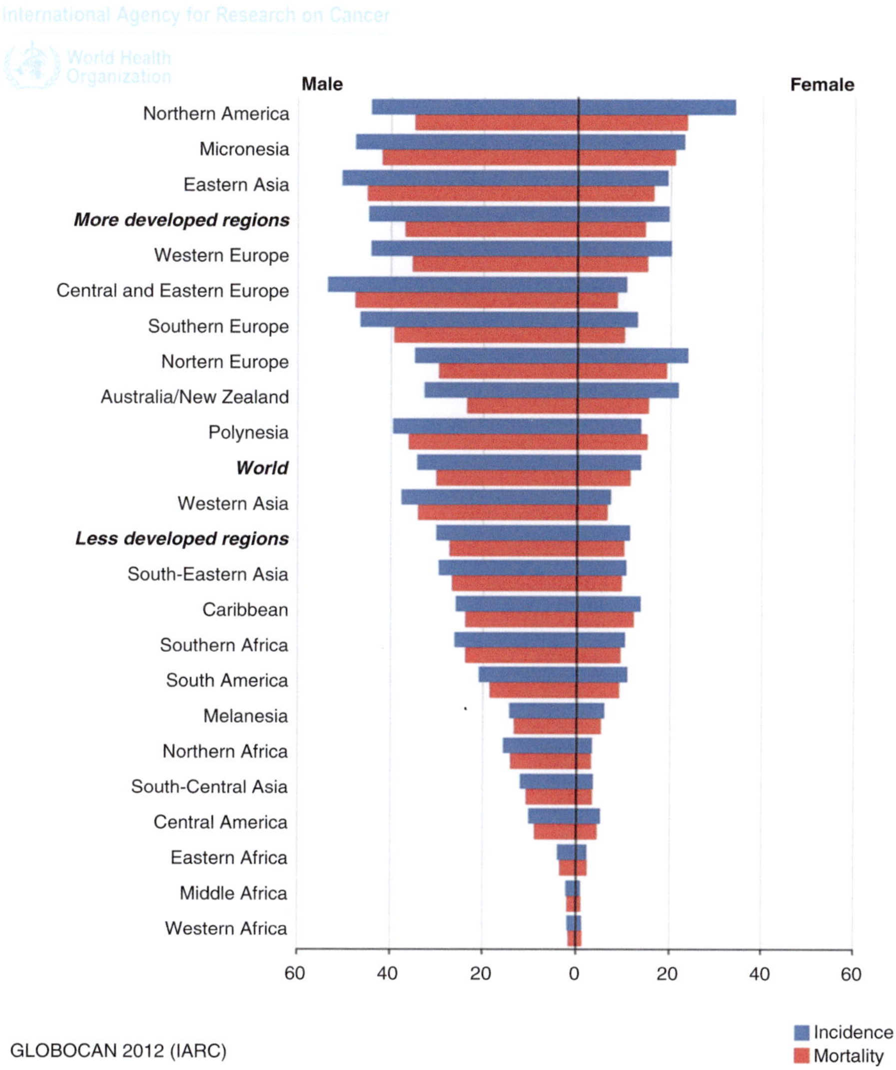

Fig. 5.5 Lung cancer data. Estimated incidence, mortality and prevalence by regions, reproduced from Globocan 2012 [54]

cancer worldwide. The 2012 estimated number of new cases is 1.8 million (12.9%) of total new cases of cancers. Fifty eight percent (58%) of cases occurred in less developed regions. Lung cancer remains the most common in men worldwide (1.2 million or the 16.7% of total cases) with the highest estimated age-standardized incidence rates in Central and Eastern Europe (53.5/100,000) and Eastern Asia (50.4/100,000). The incidence rates were

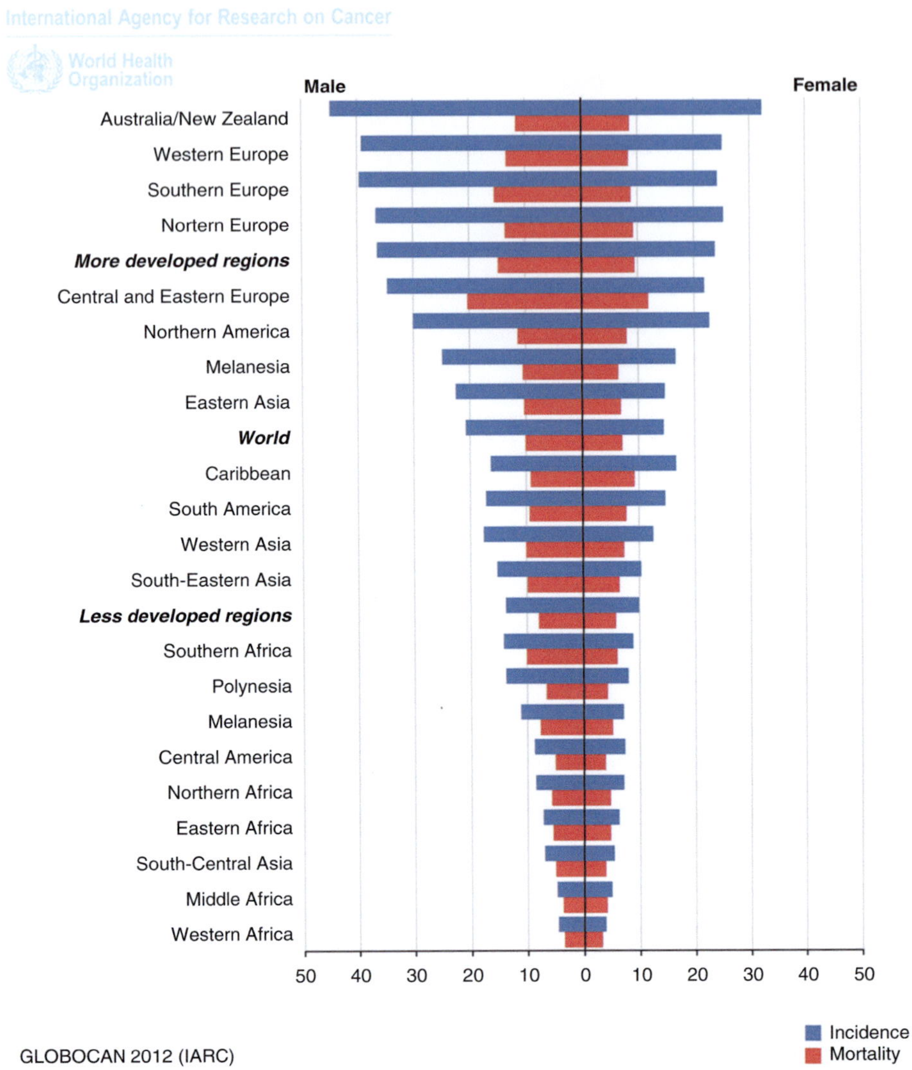

Fig. 5.6 Colorectal cancer. Estimated incidence, mortality and prevalence worldwide in men and women (Source: Globocan-IARC–WHO, 2012)

observed to be lower in Middle and Western Africa (2.0 and 1.7/100,000) respectively. Also the incidence rates as reported are generally lower and the geographical pattern is a little different, which suggested to reflect different historical exposure to tobacco smoking. Thus the highest estimated rates are in North America (33.8) and Northern Europe (23.7) with a relatively high rate in Eastern Asia (19.2) and the lowest rates again in Western and Middle Africa (1.1 and 0.8) respectively. Due to its high fatality (ratio of mortality to incidence is about 0.87) and the relative lack of variability in survival in different regions

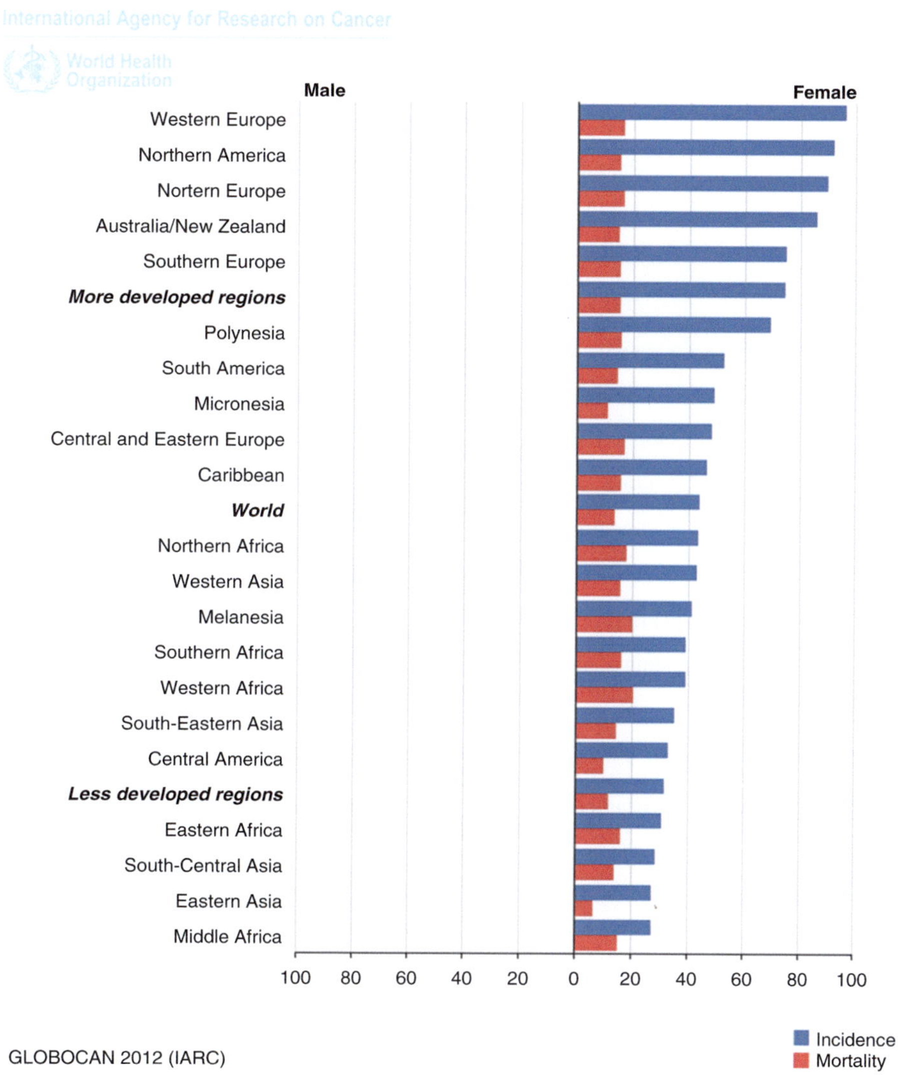

Fig. 5.7 Breast Cancer: Estimated incidence, mortality and prevalence worldwide in 2012

of the world, the geographical patterns in mortality closely follow those in incidence. (Table 5.2 and Fig. 5.5).

(c) **Colorectal Cancer:** Colorectal has been reported as the third most common cancer in men (746,000 cases or 10.0% of the total) and the 2nd in women (614,000 cases or 9.2% of total) worldwide. Nearly 55% of the colorectal cancers occur in more developed countries and incidence rate vary 10-fold in both sexes worldwide, the highest estimated rates shows in Australia-NewZealand

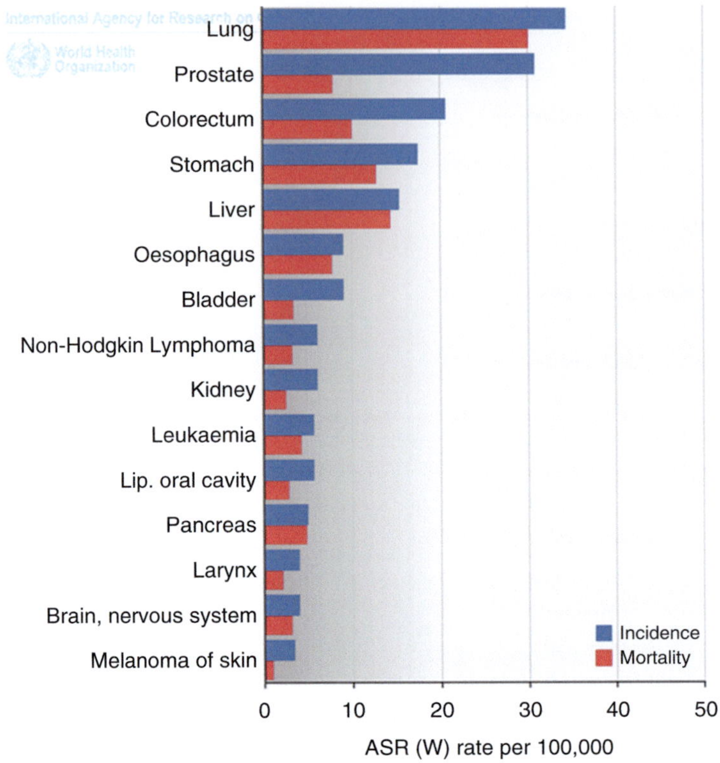

Fig. 5.8 Estimated age-standardized incidence and mortality rates in men. Data reproduced from WHO/IARC-Globacan 2012 (IARC) Section of Cancer Surveillance accessed October 19, 2015

(ASR 44.8 and 32.2/100,000 in men and women, respectively) and the lowest in Western Africa (4.5 and 3.8/100,000). Table 5.3 and Fig. 5.8 show that mortality is lower (694,000 deaths, 8.5% of the total) with more deaths (52%) in the less developed regions of the world, reflecting a poorer survival in these regions. There is less variability in mortality rates worldwide (six-fold in men, four-fold in women), (Table 5.3 and Figs. 5.6 and 5.8).

(d) **Breast Cancer.** Breast cancer ranks as the 5th cause of death from cancer (522,000 deaths) and while it is the most frequent cause of cancer, death in women seems lower in less developed regions (324,000 deaths or 14.3% of total death from cancer). In recent years breast cancer is the 2nd cause of cancer death in more developed region of world (198,000 deaths or 15.4%) after lung cancer. As shown in Table 5.4 and Fig. 5.7 and 5.9, breast cancer is the 2nd most common cancer in the world and, by far, the most frequent cancer in women with an estimated 1.67 million new cancer cases diagnosed in 2012 (25% of all cancers). According to IARC-WHO breast cancer cases reported to slightly increase in less developed regions compared with more developed countries (883,000 v 794,000) respectively. The incidence rates vary four-fold across the

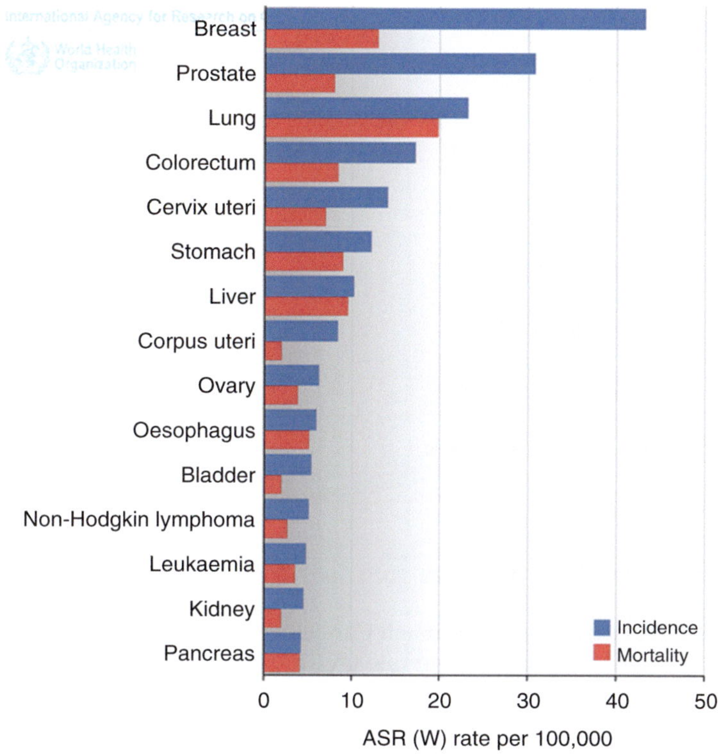

Fig. 5.9 Estimated age-standardized incidence and mortality rates: both sexes. Data reproduced from WHO/IARC–Globacan 2012 (IARC) Section of Cancer Surveillance accessed October 19, 2015

world regions, ranging from 27/100,000 in Middle Africa and Eastern Asia to 96 in Western Europe (Table 5.4 and Figs. 5.9 and 5.11).

Figures 5.7, 5.8, 5.9, 5.10 and 5.11 show estimated age-standardized incidence and mortality of site-specific cancers. Details of data on cancer incidence, mortality and prevalence and the age-adjusted site-specific cancers are reported by governmental agencies and other publications [55–58].[7,8]

Figure 5.10a, b, c represents age-adjusted trends in stomach cancer in men at different regions of the world as reported by Globocan-IARC-WHO.[9] Details of methods and procedures and age-adjusted calculation are provided in a number of publications [1, 4, 55–60]

Figures 5.7 and 5.9 and Tables 5.4 and 5.5 show data on incidence, mortality and 5-year survival (prevalence) of cancers in women around the world, according to Globocan-IARC-WHO [53–57].[7,8]

According to the 2000 calculated estimation of Global Burden of Disease (GBD), the sum of deaths from all specific causes for any sex-age group must sum to the total number of deaths for that age-sex group via the data sources and methods used

Trends in Incidence of Stomach Cancer in Selected Countries-Age-standardized rate (W)/100,000, Men.

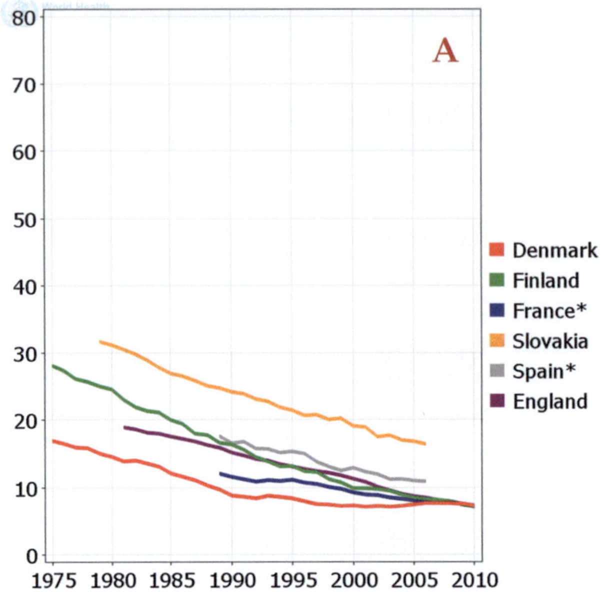

Trends in Incidence of Stomach Cancer in Selected Countries-Age-standardized rate (W)/100,000, Men.

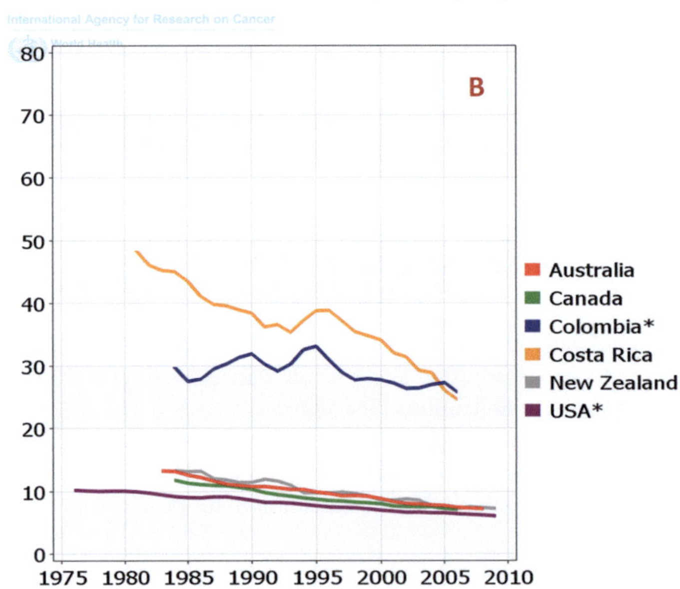

Fig. 5.10 (**a**, **b**, **c**) Trends in incidence of stomach cancer in selected countries (A, B and C regional countries): age-standardized rate (W) per 100,000 for men. Data show in a, b and c countries. Estimated age-standardized rates (World) per 100,000 — Data reproduced from WHO/IARC- Globacan 2012 (IARC) Section of Cancer Surveillance accessed October 19, 2015 (Regional data derived from-NORDCAN-C15.iarc.fr; Australia: www.aihw.gov.au; New Zealand: www.health.govt.nz; England: www.ons.gov.uk USA: seer.cancer.gov NORDCAN: www.ancr.nu--2012 and 2015-IARC)

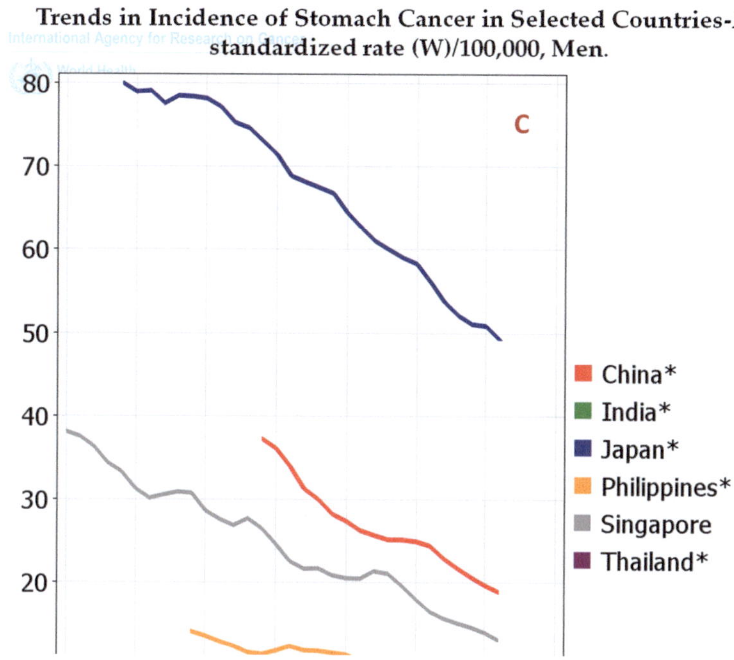

Fig. 5.10 (continued)

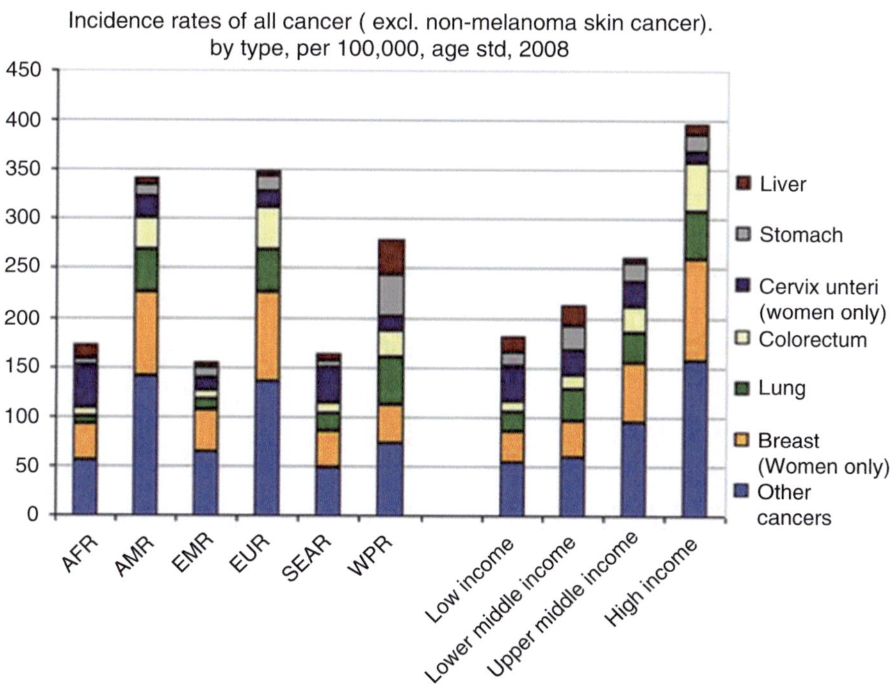

Fig. 5.11 Incidence rates of all cancers around the globe for 2008 (Source: IARC-WHO)

Table 5.1 Estimated incidence, mortality and prevalence for all cancers (excluding non-melanoma skin cancer), worldwide in 2012

	Men			Women			Both sexes		
Estimated numbers (thousands)	Cases	Deaths	5-year prev.	Cases	Deaths	5-year prev.	Cases	Deaths	5-year prev.
World	7410	4653	15,296	6658	3548	17,159	14,068	8202	32,455
More developed regions	3227	1592	8550	2827	1287	8274	6054	2878	16,823
Less developed regions	4184	3062	6747	3831	2261	8885	8014	5323	15,632
WHO Africa region (AFRO)	265	205	468	381	250	895	645	456	1363
WHO Americas region (PAHO)	1454	677	3843	1429	618	4115	2882	1295	7958
WHO East Mediterranean region (EMRO)	263	191	461	293	176	733	555	367	1194
WHO Europe region (EURO)	1970	1081	4791	1744	852	4910	3715	1933	9701
WHO South-East Asia region (SEARO)	816	616	1237	908	555	2041	1724	1171	3278
WHO Western Pacific region (WPRO)	2642	1882	4493	1902	1096	4464	4543	2978	8956
IARC membership (24 countries)	3689	1900	9193	3349	1570	9402	7038	3470	18,595
United States of America	825	324	2402	779	293	2373	1604	617	4775
China	1823	1429	2496	1243	776	2549	3065	2206	5045
India	477	357	665	537	326	1126	1015	683	1790
European Union (EU-28)	1430	716	3693	1206	561	3464	2635	1276	7157

Data from Globocan/IARC-WHO 2012

Table 5.2 Lung cancer: Estimated incidence, mortality and prevalence of lung cancer worldwide in 2012-Globocan-IARC-WHO 2012

	Men			Women			Both sexes		
Estimated numbers (thousands)	Cases	Deaths	5-year prev.	Cases	Deaths	5-year prev.	Cases	Deaths	5-year prev.
World	1242	1099	1267	583	491	626	1825	1590	1893
More developed regions	490	417	593	268	210	341	758	627	933
Less developed regions	751	682	674	315	281	286	1066	963	960
WHO Africa region (AFRO)	12	11	10	6	6	5	18	16	15
WHO Americas region (PAHO)	178	149	208	146	113	175	324	262	383
WHO East Mediterranean region (EMRO)	26	23	22	7	6	6	33	29	28
WHO Europe region (EURO)	323	283	343	126	105	133	449	388	476
WHO South-East Asia region (SEARO)	116	104	79	46	42	34	162	146	113
WHO Western Pacific region (WPRO)	588	528	605	251	220	273	839	748	878
IARC membership (24 countries)	514	438	582	279	219	343	794	657	925
United States of America	112	92	140	102	76	128	214	168	269
China	459	422	431	193	175	179	653	597	610
India	54	49	24	17	15	8	70	64	32
European Union (EU-28)	214	186	234	99	82	106	313	268	340

Table 5.3 Colorectal cancer: Estimated incidence, mortality and prevalence worldwide in 2012

	Men			Women			Both sexes		
Estimated numbers (thousands)	Cases	Deaths	5-year prev.	Cases	Deaths	5-year prev.	Cases	Deaths	5-year prev.
World	746	374	1953	614	320	1590	1361	694	3544
More developed regions	399	175	1164	338	158	966	737	333	2130
Less developed regions	347	198	789	276	163	624	624	361	1414
WHO Africa region (AFRO)	16	11	32	15	11	31	31	22	63
WHO Americas region (PAHO)	125	57	362	121	55	342	246	112	705
WHO East Mediterranean region (EMRO)	18	12	40	15	10	33	33	21	73
WHO Europe region (EURO)	255	120	686	216	108	573	471	228	1258
WHO South-East Asia region (SEARO)	68	48	122	52	37	93	120	85	216
WHO Western Pacific region (WPRO)	264	125	711	195	100	518	460	225	1229
IARC membership (24 countries)	418	187	1181	351	167	976	769	353	2157
United States of America	69	29	214	65	27	199	134	55	413
China	147	79	338	107	60	245	253	139	583
India	37	28	50	27	21	37	64	49	87
European Union (EU-28)	193	83	536	152	69	417	345	152	953

Table 5.4 Breast cancer: Estimated incidence, mortality and prevalence worldwide in 2012

Estimated numbers (thousands)	Cases	Deaths	5-year prev.
World	1671	522	6232
More developed regions	788	198	3201
Less developed regions	883	324	3032
WHO Africa region (AFRO)	100	49	318
WHO Americas region (PAHO)	408	92	1618
WHO East Mediterranean region (EMRO)	99	42	348
WHO Europe region (EURO)	494	143	1936
WHO South-East Asia region (SEARO)	240	110	735
WHO Western Pacific region (WPRO)	330	86	1276
IARC membership (24 countries)	935	257	3591
United States of America	233	44	971
China	187	48	697
India	145	70	397
European Union (EU-28)	362	92	1444

for such estimation. GBD-2000 described that complete or incomplete vital registration data together with sample registration systems covered 74% of global mortality in 128 countries. Survey data and indirect demographic techniques provide information on levels of child and adult mortality for the remaining 26% of estimated global mortality. Causes of death for the WHO sub-regions and the world have been estimated based on data from national vital registration systems that capture about 17 million deaths annually. In addition, information from sample registration systems, population laboratories and epidemiological analyses of specific conditions have been used to improve estimates of the cause of death patterns [12–15, 35, 37, 38, 63–65].

The 2000 GBD estimate for global cancer deaths is 11% higher than the GLOBOCAN 2000 estimate. This difference has been explained to be predominantly due to the very large difference in the regional/local data estimation (e.g., AFRO and SEARO regions), suggesting GBD estimates are almost double that of GLOBOCAN and adjustment to cancer deaths attributable to HIV/AIDS. For these and related reasons on estimation of deaths by other diseases, the expected GBD estimates of cancer deaths were higher than those of GLOBOCAN estimates. For other regions, the GLOBOCAN estimates are based on either cancer incidence data from cancer registries in the region (with a survival model used to estimate deaths) or on mortality data collected by regional cancer registries or other sources. As suggested by the sources of information the current data are likely incomplete and the result may be underestimation of cancer deaths [30, 31, 34, 35, 55–59].[7]

In general, the proportional representation in the cancer literature of individual cancers has been difficult, if not confusing, to establish. The principal repositories for medical research publications are the Web of Science (WoS) (Thompson Reuters), and PubMed [the National Library of Medicine (NLM)], the latter recognised as the most frequently used source for information in the medical field. Recently developed internet-based analytical tools now allow for interrogation of these online databases

Table 5.5 Estimated incidence, mortality and 5-year prevalence for women for all site-specific cancers except non-melanoma skin cancers

	Incidence			Morality			5-year prevalence	
Cancer	Number	(%)	ASR (W)	Number	(%)	ASR (W)	Number	(%)
Lip, oral cavity	101,398	1.5	2.5	47,413	1.3	1.2	234,992	1.4
Nasopharynx	25,795	0.4	0.7	15,075	0.4	0.4	66,799	0.4
Other pharynx	27,256	0.4	0.7	18,507	0.5	0.5	58,873	0.3
Oesophagus	132,776	2.0	3.1	118,952	3.4	2.7	127,528	0.7
Stomach	320,301	4.8	7.5	254,103	7.2	5.7	507,340	3.0
Colorectum	614,304	9.2	14.3	320,294	9.0	6.9	1,590,151	9.3
Liver	228,082	3.4	5.3	224,492	6.3	5.1	179,825	1.0
Gallbladder	101,257	1.5	2.3	82,484	2.3	1.8	115,278	0.7
Pancreas	159,711	2.4	3.6	156,564	4.4	3.4	97,110	0.6
Larynx	18,775	0.3	0.5	10,115	0.3	0.2	53,082	0.3
Lung	583,100	8.8	13.6	491,223	13.8	11.1	626,382	3.7
Melanoma of skin	111,481	1.7	2.8	24,098	0.7	0.6	417,080	2.4
Kaposi sarcoma	15,225	0.2	0.4	9616	0.3	0.3	25,058	0.1
Breast	1,671,149	25.1	43.1	521,907	14.7	12.9	6,232,108	36.3
Cervix uteri	527,624	7.9	14.0	265,672	7.5	6.8	1,547,161	9.0
Corpus uteri	319,605	4.8	8.3	76,160	2.1	1.8	1,216,504	7.1
Ovary	238,719	3.6	6.1	151,917	4.3	3.8	586,624	3.4
Kidney	123,936	1.9	3.0	52,604	1.5	1.2	326,046	1.9
Bladder	99,413	1.5	2.2	42,033	1.2	0.9	301,334	1.8
Brain, nervous system	116,605	1.8	3.0	83,006	2.3	2.1	152,903	0.9
Thyroid	229,923	3.5	6.1	27,145	0.8	0.6	934,805	5.4
Hodgkin lymphoma	27,430	0.4	0.7	10,006	0.3	0.3	80,237	0.5
Non-Hodgkin lymphoma	168,098	2.5	4.1	84,266	2.4	2.0	369,475	2.2
Multiple myeloma	51,782	0.8	1.2	36,928	1.0	0.8	104,483	0.6
Leukaemia	151,289	2.3	3.9	114,150	3.2	2.8	216,137	1.3
All cancers excl. non-melanoma skin cancer	6,657,518	100.0	165.2	3,548,190	100.0	82.9	17,159,060	100.0

Incidence and mortality data for all ages. 5-year prevalence for adult population only. ASR (W) and proportions per 100,000. Source: IARC-WHO. See text[4]

and for the provision of reports that are comparable within and between datasets. However, interpretation and integration of generated data are chaotic and somewhat confusing (if not misinforming), due to disproportionate rapid increase in research publications, facilitated by the development of the internet, search engines, computational biology reports and on-line publishing compared with accurate assessment of data for cancer risk formulation to design follow up studies.

Limitations in Analyses of Data Sifting through the various incomplete reported data for 2008, 2010 and 2012 from governmental (e.g., WHO/IARC and SEER) and private organizations, on the number of chronic diseases or site-specific cancers since the 1940's (with limited cancer statistics until 1970's, post polio vaccines [31]) the following conclusions and perspectives are outlined:

(a) Lung, breast, colorectal, stomach, liver and prostate cancers seem to be causes of the majority of cancer deaths around the world;
(b) There are several intrinsic problems and potential misinformation with such reports. As an example, the reported data on breast cancer are examined here. It has been reported that over 2.2 million women are living with breast cancer (beyond 5-year survival), suggesting a decrease in the breast cancer death. However, the data is misleading because while the 2.2 million survival number is the cumulative number of breast cancer, the data do not reflect that well over 30 millions died from breast cancer when reported data are analyzed in more details. According to Globacan (2000), the estimated incidence and mortality for breast cancer (in thousands) per 1 year, were 1,671 and 522, respectively (Tables 5.4 and 5.5), showing, that over 35% of newly diagnosed breast cancers patients died of the disease [55–58].[9] In addition, the data do not account for the number of over-, or mis-diagnosed patients who could better, tolerated or discontinued the treatment. Furthermore, the SEERS updated report admits that the cancer '*Population-based registries covering 30% of the US population*'.[7] The estimated number that over 30 million women died from breast cancer since the 1940s comes from extrapolation of data on the numbers reported by WHO (Tables 5.4 and 5.5 and Fig. 5.11) and the cumulative number of breast cancer incidence around the world reported separately by WHO in 2008, showing approximately over a total of 1.4 millions cases of breast cancer incidence occurred (sum number by various regions of the world, or by economic status), and the number of death provided by WHO in 2012 alone (age-adjusted) (Fig. 5.11, and Tables 5.4 and 5.5). The 30 million deaths from breast cancer is an estimated figure and could be off by10-20%, because little data on yearly incidence of breast cancer are documented prior to 1940's and since 1950s and 1960s. The author's estimated number of death from breast cancer has other limitations because extrapolation of data is from analyses of only 2 years (2008 and 2012, Fig. 5.11 and Tables 5.4 and 5.5), breast cancer cases rising from approximately 1.4 million (2008) to 1.67 million (2012). The total numbers in each column in Fig. 5.11 are gross estimation (yellow bars)/100,000 and the parameters used may not be comparable. The next challenge for statisticians, epidemiologists and demographers is to investigate detailed analyses and comparison of the number of incidence and cancer deaths in 1930s to 1940s and

compare the data with those incidences after 1950s/1960s, which are pre- and post- vaccination of the public with virus-contaminated polio vaccines or perhaps other vaccinations, (e.g., swine flu, HPV), which become compulsory for the public under the propaganda to prevent diseases and improve public health (see the following) [31–33][10]

(c) Since 1940's (Baby Boomer generation), over 20 million women developed hypertension and coronary disease complications. These data do not provide the potential increase in the rate of coronary diseases after 1960s (post polio vaccines era), although analyses of data from few reports suggest such association for baby boomers (Fig. 5.1, see Chap. 6) [1–8].

(d) Since the 1940s, aside from increased in cancer incidence and mortality, over 20 million women are afflicted with several common autoimmune and neurodegenerative diseases (e.g., rheumatoid arthritis, multiple sclerosis, lupus, scleroderma, inflammatory bowl diseases, Sjogren's, type 2 diabetes, obesity, stroke and Alzheimer's) [4–14, 23–25, 30–34]. The estimated number of such health conditions for men in the same time-frames are also provided in a number of publications [1–8] (data not analyzed).

(e) Proportion of various cohort on comparison of baby boomers and the previous generation at age 46–64, with regard to increased diseases such as hypertension, hypercholesterolelimia, diabetes, obesity and other chronic illnesses reported in various studies suggest significantly poorer health status (2–8 times) between the current and previous two generations, despite much higher expenditure in medicine, diagnostic technologies and improved hygiene since a century ago [6–10, 31, 32].

6 Cancer Risk Factors: Impact of Aging Process, Chronic Infections, Pathogen-Specific Vaccines, Carcinogens and Chemicals

In the last few decades, cancer prevention community has focused on the contribution of "lifestyle" factors (primarily smoking habits) as the principal modifiable causes of cancer. However, increasing number of pollutants, biological and chemicals that are identified in the environment we live and breathe, such as commonly used products, pesticides, herbicides, hormones, steroids, food additives and preservatives, gasoline exhausts, genetically modified foods, plastic containers, cosmetics care products, over-the-counter remedies, asbestos, house paints, chemicals in artificial rains and drinking water or pathogen-specific vaccines and adjuvant, as well as direct and indirect exposures to high radiofrequency electronics, are considered health-hazard concerns that could increase the risk of carcinogenesis. Extensive access/exposure to advanced technologies and electronic devices and games (e.g., cell/smart/iphones, household gadgets, medical diagnostics tools, microwaves etc)

[10] Tom Valentine: Polio vaccine spreads cancer. Dark Politricks. Part II, SHOAH, June 21, 2011.

may be considered potential hazards whose additive impacts in biology and function of tissues are not well understood [110–147].

According to governmental and academic reports, the important risk factors for cancer incidence, in both developed and developing countries include the tobacco use, unhealthy diet, several known carcinogens, physical inactivity and excessive use of alcohol. As noted above, the reports indicate that the developed countries such as the Europe and the Americas had the highest incidence of all types of cancer combined for both sexes, while countries in Eastern Mediterranean Region had the lowest cancer incidence (see above). The reported exposures to known agents such as cadmium, o-toluidine, trichloropropane, thiourea, 4-chloro-1,2-benzenediamine 1,3-dihydroxybenzene (resorcinol), diethylene glycol dimethyl ether, p-chloroaniline (parachloroaniline), expoxybutane, dichlorobenzidine, chloroprene, chloromethyl methyl ether, L-lewisite, methylenedianiline, coal tar, nickel chloride, nickel sulfate, copper components, diacetone alcohol (DAA), 2-ethylhexanoic acid, n-nitroso-n-methylethylamine, soluble nickel, n-nitrosodi-n-propylamine, are among risk factors in carcinogenesis, particularly for the older population around the globe (NIEHS or EPA websites and databases). Table 5.6, is a list of examples of biological and environmental components that are known as potential risk factors (immune disruptors) that at low levels act as carcinogens. The information is provided from overall analyses of reported data on a wide range of isolated experiments in animal models of inflammatory diseases, genotoxicity, carcinogenesis or in clinical trial. The results also reflect continued confusion, inconsistency and misunderstanding on the actions of various agents that are reported in different labs or clinical trials including efficacy of drugs, safety of pathogen-specific vaccines, hormonal replacement therapy, use of steroids and antibiotics in the induction of chronic diseases (Table 5.6) [31–33, 56, 71, 84–212].

Analyses of reported data demonstrate that majority of these agents are stimuli that affect combination of the complex molecular components of immune/inflammatory response processes. It should be emphasized that despite the facts that the chemical, structural and biological properties of numerous carcinogens are well known in the literature, there is a peculiar absence of systematic studies to demonstrate how these chemical structure can cause early disturbance of immune response profiles in the direction of tumorigenesis or angiogenesis. Identification of early events of immune responses is important as these responses are potentially reversible or correctable. However, the cumulative roles of these potential carcinogens or the mixtures of carcinogens that could contribute to mutagenesis in susceptible or site-specific tissues toward multistep carcinogenesis are yet to be determined.

In general, the reported actions of all known carcinogens fall into the two categories of disturbing the effective immunity or the loss of Yin and Yang balance of acute inflammation and causing over-, or under-expression of hundreds or thousands of proteins, enzymes or receptor molecules that contribute to the control of cancer or any other diseases processes. In general, the identified carcinogens belong to the following interdependent biological categories that would likely alter effective immunity (details in Chap. 6) (Fig. 5.12) [31–33, 82–84, 95, 99, 107, 82–84, 111, 112, 119–125, 180–183]:

Table 5.6 Examples of immune disruptors or carcinogens and inconsistency in reported inflammatory responses [31–33, 96–212]

Agent/Carcinogen Immune disruptor	Nature/ Property/Tissue	Reported paradoxical actions-controversy of risk factors in carcinogenesis
Bisphenol A (BPA); Brominated BPA;	Intracellular signaling; Mitochondrial oxidative metabolism; Endocrine-Estrogen disruptor	ER-- Activate mTOR (mammalian target of rapamycin); Block P53, Promote growth signal and angiogenesis; Genetic instability; Estrogen Activity (ER); Upregulation of hTERT transcription factor complex to Fos/Jun; Replicative immortality; DNA and chromosomal instability-reprogramming; Induce neoplasia (prostate); Genotoxic; Cell proliferation; Polarization; Endocrine disruption; PPARs antagonist
Polybrominated diphenyl ethers (PBDEs) +17v-estradiol	Disrupt glucose and lipid metabolism (MCSF); Present in breast milk; Placenta; Amniotic fluid, Umbelical cord blood; Mutagen	iNOS--Genetic instability, Pro- and anti-apoptotic (IL-1β, TNFα, PGE2), Risk for breast cancer;
NO and iNO Permissive factor	Genotoxic	Angiogenesis; Tumor metastasis
Vinclozolin & Dicarboximide (fungicide)	Endocrine disruptor, Amide-	NFkB--Promote evasion of anti-growth signals; Oxidative damage; AR and ER expression (prostate gland)/prostatitis; Phosphorylation and Nuclear Translocation of NFkB (expression of IL8 andTGFβ1);
Nonylphenol (NP), 4-NP	Estrogenic action Genotoxic Saccharomyces cervisiae	IL-6–Proliferation in estrogen responsive ovarian cancer PEO4 and Anti-cancer or enhancing apoptosis, TNF-α and suppress regulatory cytokines e.g., IL-10, IFB-g, IFB-β; Enhance replicative immortality- altered telomerase activity; Pro-epigenetic; decrease in ERα; Expression of COX-2-PGE2; lung allergies;

(continued)

Table 5.6 (continued)

Agent/Carcinogen Immune disruptor	Nature/ Property/Tissue	Reported paradoxical actions-controversy of risk factors in carcinogenesis
Phthalates; Di-isonoyl phthalate, Benzyl butyl, or di-n-buthyl phathalate; Diethylhexyl Phthalate (DEHP)	Vinyl products; plastic wrapping	TNF-α–Increase proliferation; Reproductive system (spermatogenesis); Evasion of Anti-growth signals; Decrease Smad regulation of Cyclin D; Increase palmitoyl-CoA oxidase activity; Increase β-and ω-oxidation of fatty acids; Nuclear receptor-PPARa in hepatocytes; Asthma; Prostate; Uterus; Ovary; Breast
Atrazine; Herbicide; Pesticide (copper 8-hydroxyquinoline)	Contaminate water; Endocrine disruptor; (diaminochlorotriazine, major metabolite); weak mutagen;	Induction of mammary gland tumors; Reproductive/endocrine disruptors; Suppression of anti-oxidant in liver; decrease testosterone gene transcription; NO regulation; Angiogenesis; Immunotoxicity; Decrease TNFα, IFNγ
Copper (C), C. sulfate, C. gluconate, C. ore (silica, iron, manganese, arsenic, titanium, sulfur) C. hydroxide, C. ammonium carbonate, C.oxychloride +sulfate	Copper miner, Cumulative contaminated food or water/ beverage, Radon emission (??), Fungicide, Crop [citrus fruits, peanuts, deciduous fruits (other than apples), potatoes, vegetables]	Increased Metallothionein, 5-HT3,4Rs (?), Atherosclerosis, Cardiovascular, Hypertension, CNS, Hepatic (Wilson's diseases), Renal, Gastrointestinal, Children's cirrhosis, Hyperplasia, Hyperkeratosis of squamous mucosa in stomach, Lung cancer
Aluminum, Mercury, L-histidine	Pathogen-specific vaccines (HPV) and Adjuvant	Histidine-protein metabolism, histamine synthesis, Autoimmune and neurodegenerative diseases or cancers (?)

(a) Carcinogens that are known to interrupt the endocrine and hormonal activities (e.g., insulin, estrogen or DHT receptors, enzymes) are often facilitators of wound healing and growth (anabolic) pathways. In such pathways all metabolic and growth factors contribute to the loss of balance in tumoricidal vs tumorigenic properties of immunity in favor of growth promotion. Among altered activities of such pathways are expression of kinases, NADP/NADPH regeneration, COX/LOX pathways and induction of PGE2, mTOR/PI3K, induction of IRA-M for tolerance, altered mitochondrial oxidative phosphorylation (mitophagy); hypoxic conditions and induction of vascular growth pathways; nuclear and genomic toxicity and instability affecting pathways such as DNA/RNA repair mechanisms, genomic mutations, chromatin, transcription, epigenetic (hypo-, and hyper methylation), impaired p53 and other growth suppressor genes activities that lead to immune suppression and initiation of growth in susceptible tissues;

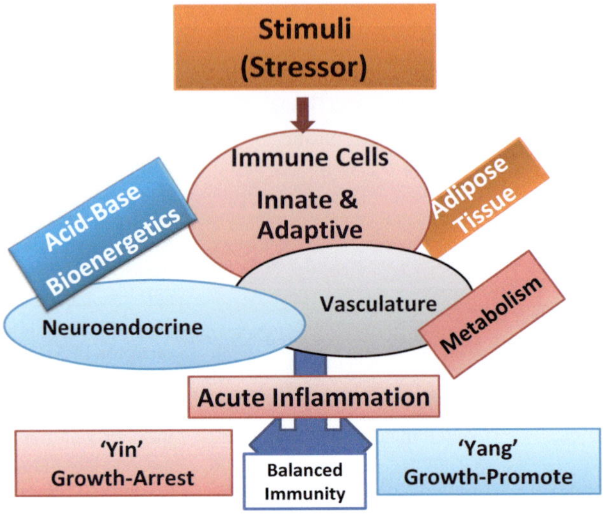

Fig. 5.12 Schematic representation of effective immunity (immune surveillance) provided by acute inflammation. Immune disruptor (stimuli) causes activation of self-terminating and protective mechanisms of acute inflammation for maintenance of health. Acute inflammation is depicted as the precise balance between 2 biologically opposing arms, Yin (growth-arresting or tumoricidal) and Yang (growth promoting or tumorigenic) properties of immunity. Acute inflammation involves crosstalks between immune and non-immune systems such as vasculature, adipose tissue, metabolism of mitochondrial and ribosomal bioenergetics and acid-base balance See text (details in Chaps. 2 and 6)

(b) Carcinogens or immune disruptors that are reported to alter the activities or expression of apoptotic factors such as TNFs/TNFR, ILs, toxins, decoy receptors, accumulation of ROS/RNS, oxidants, vasoactive components (e.g., histamine and receptor molecules) similarly contribute to the dysfunction of acute inflammation and their actions disturb the function of effective immunity that also lead to immune suppression;

Our 'accidental' discoveries on experimental models of acute and chronic inflammatory diseases seem to be the only evidence on the systematic series of data showing identifiable sequential changes of immune responses, that also revealed the time course interactions and synergies between host immune and non-immune cells (e.g., mast cells, B and goblet cells, and epithelial) with recruiting cells (e.g., eosinophils and tumor-associated macrophages/TAMs) in the direction of tissue growth promotion, tumorigenesis and angiogenesis [31–33, 175–183]. Therefore, understanding the biology of host toward exposure to various carcinogens that alter the activities of endocrine, neuronal, metabolic or immune systems and signal transductions require systematic, detailed study of initial events toward multistep immune dysfunction. The outcomes of such studies are expected to be highly effective for detection, prevention and therapy of cancer and for accurate risk assessment formulation (details in Chap. 6).

7 Misrepresented Information and Knowledge Gaps on Cancer Triggers: Viral Oncogene Sub-structures in Vaccines and Sharp Increase in Cancer Incidence or Chronic Neurodegenerative and Autoimmune Diseases

Wisdom has never made a bigot, but learning has. Josh Billings[11]

The available statistical and epidemiological reports and the models that are established for estimation of disease-related deaths, particularly SEER data on cancer incidence and mortality or morbidity in America lack fundamental information on the causes of cancer, particularly with regard to comparison of detailed statistics in cancer incidence and mortality, prior to 1940s and after 1970s. These statistics ignore the contribution of virus-causing cancers on sharp increased in cancer incidence and death and other chronic diseases that are due to the vaccination of public with virus-contaminated polio vaccines in 1955s and early 1960s that affected millions of baby boomers, particularly in America [4–8, 25, 28, 31–33, 39–41, 47–49, 67, 68].

The current epidemiological data on major risk factors in the induction of mortality and morbidity of cancer and other chronic diseases, as well as, strategies in vaccine production that aim to prevent specific infectious diseases or site-specific cancers lack the following fundamental information:

1. As early as a century ago, Rous presented evidence that viruses are triggers of cancer [31–33, 184, 185].
2. Analyses of data on viral/bacterial infections and many vaccines suggest that the viral or bacterial oncogenes and their substructures have stronger additive influence for triggering cancer, compared with low level carcinogens or environmental hazards such as smoking or drinking alone for facilitating changes in biological dynamics of cellular and sub-cellular functions of susceptible tissues (e.g., lung airways). The association between smoking and environmental hazards in the increased risk of site-specific cancers (e.g., lung) is still controversial. Results of several studies suggest that not all smokers, even heavy smokers, may be prone to lung cancer. Reports on none-smokers or never smokers who develop lung cancer further suggest that such data overlook other participating factors, such as infective agents or virus- or bacteria-specific vaccines in the development of asthma, tuberculosis, lung or other site-specific cancers [31–33, 184–207]. Even the BCG (Mycobacterium bovis bacillius calmette-Guerin) vaccines that are considered the most successful bacterial pathogen that is safe for prevention of tuberculosis have adverse and diverse effects in the induction of diseases such as vasculitis, secondary infections, diabetes complications, immunological problems with T or B cell function and production of anti-

[11] Josh Billings (pen name), born Henry Wheeler Shaw, American author, humorist, Poet, Nonfiction (1818–1885). Known as the second most humor writer and lecturer in USA, after Mark Twain, although his reputation has not fared so well with later generations.

bodies, and the increased risk of cancers and diseases in children and adults. There are estimated two billion people that are exposed to Mycobacterium tuberculosis around the globe, where approximately eight million patients present active disease and die from it each year. With the emergence of HIV, people exposed to Mycobacterium tuberculosis are shown to be more vulnerable to die of TB or become more resistant to drug [186–205]. While the need for developing new TB vaccines to boost or replace BCG has been expressed in recent publications, progress has been slow and the result of one candidate vaccine in phase IIb efficacy trials have been inconclusive and disappointing [195–198, 203–205].

3. With regard to the politics of smoking and lung cancer, in an interesting letter to then VP and Counsel for Philip Morris Inc. (1965),[12] Holtzman writes '*He* [Dr. Dmochowski] *is not impressed with the fact that tobacco con* [not legible] *will produce tumors in animals…that isoniazid, a drug used in the standard treatment for tuberculosis, has been to be proved to be carcinogenic for animals. He also mentioned that an organisim commonly found in milk (PPLO) has been found in the blood of leukemia patients and that if attention were directed to that fact the drinking of milk might well be curtailed…Dr. Dmochowski worked under Dr. Passey at the University of Leeds for many years and he mentioned that Dr. Passey was for many years contemptuous of the cigarette theory. At the University of Leeds two out of 57 doctors in a professional society had died of lung cancer and neither had ever smoked…*'.[12] However, Holtzman described how Dr. Lee Clark intimidated Dr. Dmochowski out of testifying before the Congress on the evidence that human cancers are potentially caused by viruses, an issue that was noted in virus-contaminated polio vaccines since 1955s. The contaminated vaccines caused numerous death and diseases followed by several law suits against NIH and DHHS directors that led to their resignation [31–33] [12,13,14]
4. The current data still lack details on the link between virus-contaminated vaccines or frequent infections as cancer triggers that would enhance the risk of induction of chronic diseases or site-specific cancers such as the lung or liver.
5. For the same rational, other viral-substructures or oncogene-induced vulnerability of tissue could lead to site-specific cancers or the induction of hepatitis B or C infections and integration of viral components in host tissues. These viruses could be strong triggers in facilitating the induction of liver cancers in alcoholics.

---

[12] Holtzman A: Dr. Leon Dmochowski and Dr. R. Lee Clark-- Truth Tobacco Industry Documents. 5-page Letter, to Paul D. Smith, VP and General Counsel, Philip Morris Inc., January 06, 1965. https://industrydocuments.library.ucsf.edu/tobacco/docs/[ID], Ness Motley Law Firm. https://industrydocuments.library.ucsf.edu/tobacco/docs/qymd0040---Bates Number: 1005100176100510018O.

[13] The Charles A LeMaistre Page—The Conspiracy Against Tobacco-- www.smokershistory.com/LeMaistr.htm - **Since** its establishment, the NUATRC has been led by an interim Board of Directors, ... Emerson Foote; Mrs. Anna Rosenberg Hoffman; Alton Ochsner; Ann Landers. ..... John Mendelsohn, Alan S. Rabson of the NCI (former acting NIH Director Ruth ... a Public Health Service pathologist) before they came to NIH in 1955.

[14] Tom-Valentine.doc - … real story behind the Polio vaccine. - Vaccine ... vaccineliberationarmy.com/wp-content/.../By-... scourge prior to the 1950's (polio vaccine first arrived in 1955)... (Mary Sherman is the Mary in the book title [Dr. Mary's Monkeys] …and Alton Ochsner was ... Due to this, she was not well accepted by the NIH or NCI staffs who ...).

Other infections with viruses (e.g., Epstein Barr Virus/EBV or HPV), or bacteria (e.g., Helicobacter pylori) are likely the initiators of site-specific cancers [31–33, 75–78. 186, 206–211].

6. In all likelihood, the viral/bacterial structures (oncogenes or proteins) are additional antigen-load for the immune surveillance to handle and neutralize. The virus-substructures could alter the balance in Yin and Yang of acute inflammation to the extent of disrupting the activities of immune and non-immune (vasculature, metabolism, neuronal) response profiles and inducing a wide range of chronic diseases or site-specific cancers. In other words, the viral particles (oncogenes) that are in the vaccines and their adjuvant or stabilizers (e.g., L-histidine, mercury, aluminum) could disrupt the highly ordered structure and function of host tissues and facilitate the induction of disease processes, rather than being prophylactic, particularly in the older population who normally develop minor or major altered immune responses (immunosenescence) [31–33, 175–183]. Therefore, in the production of prophylactic (vaccines) candidates, the key question is whether, and to what extent the integration of various viral or bacterial oncogenes into the host modifies the integrity of host sub-anatomical or subcellular organelles that could cause additional disruption in effective immunity. Analyses of the reported data on the role of viruses (e.g., Rous sarcoma, polio, HIV, meningitis, human papilloma, Epstein-Barr, hepatitis B, C), bacteria (e.g., Mycobacterium tuberculosis, helicobacter pylori) and/or viral and bacterial oncogene sub-structures in the induction of site-specific cancers and neurodegenerative or autoimmune diseases and many other inflammatory diseases have not be emphasized or considered in the statistical calculations as important cancer risk factors [31–33].
7. The vaccines that carry segmented bacterial or viral oncogenes, in addition to induction of neutralizing antibodies, are likely to damage and/or be incorporated into the chromosomal and DNAs/RNAs substructures causing genomic instabilities that would lead to abnormal expression profiles of important functional proteins/enzymes or membrane structures and alter the repair mechanism pathways or cellular function in susceptible tissues.
8. It was suggested that the long-term consequences of integration of viral oncogenes in host sub-anatomical structures influence not only the individual vulnerability toward diseases but also influence the next generation (off springs) having genetic disorders! [31–33].

In brief, the viral/bacterial oncogenes-induced altered sub-anatomical behaviors of host tissue could cumulatively facilitate minor or major altered architectural and functional integrity of tissues/organs and enhance the risks of induction of chronic diseases (autoimmune and neurodegenerative diseases) in immune-privileged tissues, or site-specific cancers in immune-responsive tissues [31–33]. In order to better assess the risk for cancer and a wide range of autoimmune and neurodegenerative diseases, the statisticians and oncology professionals should focus on gathering and including relevant information on the frequency and quality of individual exposures to viruses/bacteria and the many vaccines with adverse effects on biology of host tissues that potentiate the initiation and progression of chronic illnesses.

8 Challenges in Formulation of Accurate Risk Assessment: Immune Disruptor-(Antigen)-Induced Chronic Inflammation as Precancerous State of Tissues

A person with a new idea is a crank until the idea succeeds. Mark Twain

Ongoing debates, misunderstanding and downplaying the important role that inflammation play in carcinogenesis are perhaps the most damaging factors in the extreme slow progress in the cancer prevention, therapeutic approaches and formulation of accurate risk assessment. A role for acute or chronic inflammation in controlling or inducing cancer, has been noted in isolated reports for over a century [31–33]. However, the formal acceptance and appreciation of the author's submitted concepts that chronic inflammation is a prerequisite in carcinogenesis; that inflammatory mediators are ideal targets (biomarkers) for diagnosis, prevention and therapy of cancer, which awakened the cancer community has been recognized in the last couple of decades (Khatami, submitted scientific and legal documents, NCI/NIH, since 1998) [31–33, 175–183].

Aging and long-term exposures to inflammatory conditions are considered 'co-conspirators' in increasing the risk of tumorigenesis and angiogenesis or other chronic diseases such as neurodegenerative and autoimmune diseases. However, the rates and susceptibilities toward diseases vary in aging individuals. In general, the principal challenges and complexities in the formulation of accurate disease risk assessment fall into the following confounding and interdependent categories and deserve systematic studies:

1. Heterogeneities in immune-biological-genomic response dynamics of individuals toward potential carcinogens or immune disruptors;
2. Heterogeneities in reported outcomes of case-control, prospective or meta-analysis when risk values toward a wide range of hazards are estimated and formulated;
3. Lack of suitable models to systematically monitor the initial signals/events that disturb the immunity in multistep pathways toward loss of balance in Yin-Yang of acute inflammation, the inherent property of effective immunity;
4. Comprehending that cancer cells become a threat when the dynamics of immune system (immune surveillance) responses significantly shift in favor of growth promotion pathways, particularly during the aging process.

The inherent heterogeneities/diversities, duplicities and/or compensating biological responses toward exposures to combination of hazardous components can further complicate risk assessment calculations that are the results of reported bias and heterogeneities in study designs and outcomes. The case control vs. prospective studies or meta-analysis where diverse clinical and neurological methodologies consider using heterogeneous parameters such as sample size analyses, emphasis on types of exposures (occupational vs non-occupational hazards) or specific components (e.g., pesticides, food additives/preservatives, radiation exposures, or other commonly used products) are challenges and hurdles that complicate accurate risk assessment values. One should also keep in mind that the risk values that are reported on many chemicals or environmental hazards generally reflect the properties of molecular entities in isolation and have little values on their own for risk assessment purposes to benefit the public, as several compensating biological factors in immune and non-immune systems can easily skew such risk assessment formulations.

In summary, effective immunity is an elaborate and precise involvement of coordination of biological signals, with opposing properties, from immune and non-immune systems (e.g., vasculature, hormonal, neuronal and metabolic pathways) that are required for maintenance of health throughout life (Fig. 5.12). The genetic makeup of immune and non-immune systems generally plays the most important roles in maintaining health or disturbing well being of individuals. The heterogeneities of response profiles in site-specific tissues toward internal/intrinsic or external/extrinsic stimuli (immune disruptors or risk factors), present challenges for better understanding of the initiation and progression of disease processes, design of accurate risk assessment formulations, prevention and therapeutic strategies.

As emphasized throughout this book the bases for the reported controversies, debates and misunderstandings on the role of immune disruptors in the induction of cancer are primarily the results of the following important factors:

(a) Lack of systematic study on the role of acute and chronic inflammation that would include understanding of immune disruptor-(antigen)induced early changes in biphasic properties of effective immunity that we proposed as the loss of Yin and Yang of acute inflammation.
(b) Tremendous knowledge gaps to logically understand the extent of host-immune disruptor interactions or potential synergies in enhancing tissue growth or necrosis at site-specific tissues that would lead to carcinogenesis or induction of autoimmune and neurodegenerative diseases.
(c) Lack of understanding of the heterogeneity between vulnerable host/target tissues and cumulative role of exposures to a wide range of immune disruptors.

9 Proposed Future Directions: Risk Reduction and Control of Cancer

There are basically two types of people; those who accomplish the things, and those who claim to have accomplished things. The first group is less crowded. Mark Twain

Detailed understanding of how carcinogenesis can destroy the multilayer organization of tissues is fundamentals in optimizing cancer molecular/cellular diagnosis, prevention or therapeutic approaches. The multistep carcinogenesis occur several steps distance from the time cancer cells are able to destroy and take over the machinery of well-organized multilayer structures of tissue and alter physical and mechanical forces of tissues. As emphasized throughout this book, future proposed studies toward effective diagnostic, preventive or therapeutic measures are outlined below on the notion that unresolved inflammation is a common denominator in the genesis and progression of nearly all age-associated diseases or cancer:

(a) Systematic studies on the role of unresolved inflammation in loss of balance between inherent 'tumoricidal' vs 'tumorigenic'(Yin vs Yang) protective properties of immune cells is suggested as the primary focus in comprehending the cancer biology or other chronic diseases,
(b) Time-course kinetics of developmental phases of inflammation-induced alterations in immune dynamics in site-specific host tissues with specific exposure routs and defined stimuli;
(c) Determination of composition and heterogeneity of immune and non-immune cells in site-specific tissues and influence of immune disruptors in altering immune dynamics;
(d) Dose-response relationships between stimuli and altered inflammatory dynamics (e.g., cell and mediator response profiles);
(e) Pathogen-host interaction profiles that include identification of principal response features on pathogen-, allergen-induced activation of resident or recruited immune cells in target tissues;
(f) Identification of molecular components that are over-, or under-expressed during developmental phases of tumorigenesis. Potential reversibility at early stages of immune dysfunction designed to monitor by such parameters as altered cellular oxidative stress, chromosomal and genetic/epigenetic components, mediator profiles in immune and non-immune cells in models of site-specific tumors;
(g) Sequential monitoring of clinical, histopathological and expression profiles of the initial strong or weak responses toward stimuli. Preliminary analyses of data on experimental models of acute and chronic ocular inflammatory diseases suggested that initial strong reactions (type I hypersensitivity) such as tissue edema, tearing, scratching/itching, vascular hyperpermeability, mast cells degranulation, production of histamine and prostaglandins, could potentially be protective in preventing tumorigenesis. However, tissues with low (weak) initial responses could show progressive cellular changes, such as interactions and synergies with other infiltrated and activated cells (e.g., eosinophils, mucus secreting goblet cells and macrophages), toward induction of hyperplasia of lymphoid tissues, thickening and/or thinning of epithelial surfaces (necrosis and/or cell growth) and angiogenesis as we observed in a series of studies on experimental models of tumorigenesis and angiogenesis in conjunctival-associated lymphoid tissues (details in Chaps. 4 and 6),
(h) Role of unresolved inflammation or oxidative stress in the induction of immune dysfunction in tissues that are naturally immune-privileged or immune-responsive as well as insulin-dependent or insulin-independent tissues for glucose transport and metabolism;
(i) Tissues susceptibility toward oxidative stress-induced damage to genetic and epigenetic modifications of immune and non-immune systems;

(j) Potential reversibility of early stages of inflammation-induced immune dysfunction (e.g., in the developmental phases of immune disruptors during acute and/or intermediate phases) that include altered initial immune responses and cellular chromosomal/genetic material that lead to cellular growth and induction of hyperplasia, neoplasia/precancer or cancer-malignancy.

It is anticipated that the outcomes of systematic investigations of immune disruptors-induced altered response dynamics of immunity toward multistep tissue damage and initiation of disease processes and site-specific cancers would help advance comprehensive understanding of tumor biology. The overall outcomes are expected to improve the following integrated medical sciences:

(a) Improved accuracy of risk assessment formulation for chronic diseases or cancer;
(b) Accuracy on cancer diagnosis and minimizing the costly over-, or under diagnosis of site-specific cancers;
(c) Effective decision making for prevention strategies of age-associated chronic illnesses and cancer;
(d) Effective designs of drug development for suitable clinical trials and therapy with the goal to minimize life-threatening side effects of drugs.

10 Author's Final Comments on Future Perspectives

The real voyage of discovery consists not in seeking new landscapes, but in having new eyes. Marcel Proust.[15]

Body's tolerance and defense mechanism toward adverse reactions of extrinsic and intrinsic factors is limited. This chapter primarily raised questions on fundamental knowledge gaps that are reported for the methods used for statistical assessment of risk factors and epidemiological data that influenced the scientific outputs in the field of oncology. There are fundamentally different philosophies that author proposes for supporting research on systematical and logical search for causes of disease initiation. The mindset is a new way of searching the truth in medical sciences and different from reductionist approaches that created a costly sick and drug dependent society, particularly in America. The outcomes of proposed systematic and logical approaches to study early events in alterations of immune response profiles are very likely reversible, correctible or drugable.

The primary topic in promoting health is to first understand how the amazing defense mechanisms that routinely monitor, neutralize and control adverse effects of pathogens and kill defective cells such as cancerous cells are weakened or lost

[15] Marcel Proust:Valentin Louis Georges Eugène (1871–1922), known as Marcel Proust, French novelist, critic, and essayist best known for his monumental novel À la recherche du... Book: 'In Search of Lost Time' "http://en.wikipedia.org/wiki/Marcel_Proust" Wikipedia

during aging or disease processes. The cancer literature is overcrowded with continuously 'new' information on molecular entities that are identified in the environment of site-specific cancers, and related chaotic data on statistics or methods of risk assessment formulation and epidemiological reports. Careful analyses of cancer research and therapy show that the organized system in power structure of medical establishment vs. anti-system and chaos in conducting science is a potent recipe for failed therapeutics that kills patients but generates huge corporate profit. Health status of Americans ranks last compared with other developed nations, while America invests the highest resources for healthcare [31, 32, 82, 83].

Future studies require logical systematic understanding of risk factors that alter the dynamics of Yin and Yang (tumoricidal vs tumorigenic) properties of effective immunity. There are wide ranges of molecular hazards that often possess shared features in changing the proper response profiles of site-specific host tissues at the early phases of altered immune dynamics. Among such risk factors, researchers should seriously consider the adverse influence of pathogens- (virus, or bacteria) specific vaccines that are claimed to prevent certain diseases or cancers. Introduction of viral or bacterial genomic materials and vaccine stabilizer that are used as adjuvant (e.g., aluminum, mercury or L-histidine) are perhaps the most hazardous risk factors in altering the defense of body. These factors are rarely reported in statistical or epidemiological data or clinical studies.

It is reasonable to anticipate that the designs of logical and systematic investigations provide important biological clues that would lead to minimizing or correcting the defects in the interdependent molecular village that constitute immune surveillance for guarding body's health throughout life. The outcomes of such studies are also expected to provide statisticians and epidemiologists to make informed decisions on formulating accurate risk assessments and better interpretations and analyses of data for a wide range of chronic diseases or cancer.

References

1. Torre LA, Bray F, Siegel RL, Ferlay J, Lortet-Tieulent J, Jemal A. Global cancer statistics. CA Cancer J Clin. 2012;65(2):87–108. doi:10.3322/caac.21262. Epub 2015 Feb 4.
2. Hewitt M, Simone JV. Ensuring quality cancer care. Institute of Medicine (US) and National Research Council (US) National Cancer Policy Board; Hewitt M, Simone JV, Washington (DC): National Academies Press (US); 1999.
3. Atun R. Health systems, systems thinking and innovation. Health Policy Plan. 2012;27(Suppl 4):iv4–8.
4. WHO. Everybody's Business: Strengthening Health Systems to Improve Health Outcomes. WHO's framework for action. Geneva: World Health Organization; 2007.
5. US Census Bureau. Selected characteristics of baby boomers 42 to 60 years old in 2006. http://www.census.gov/population/age/publications/files/2006babyboomers.pdf. [Accessed 1 Aug 2012].
6. King DE, Matheson E, Chirina S, Shankar A, Broman-Fulks J. The status of baby boomers' health in the United States: the healthiest generation? JAMA Intern Med. 2013;173(5):385–6. doi:10.1001/jamainternmed.2013.

7. King DE, Xiang J, Brown A. Intake of key chronic disease-related nutrients among baby boomers. South Med J. 2014;107(6):342–7. doi: 10.14423/01.SMJ.0000450706.44388.45
8. King DE, Mainous AG, Geesey ME. Turning back the clock: adopting a healthy lifestyle in middle age. Am J Med. 2007;120:598–603.
9. Robinson WR, Utz RL, Keyes KM, Martin CL, Yang Y. Birth cohort effects on abdominal obesity in the United States: the Silent Generation, Baby Boomers and Generation X. Int J Obes (Lond). 2013;37(8):1129–34. doi:10.1038/ijo.2012.198. Epub 2012 Dec 11
10. National Center for Health Statistics. Plan and operation of the health and nutrition examination survey. United states–1971–1973. Vital and Health Statistics. 1–407, 1978.
11. US Department of Agriculture, Center for Nutrition Policy and Promotion. Dietary guidelines for Americans. [Accessed April 15, 2014]; http://www.cnpp.usda.gov/dietaryguidelines.htm
12. National Center for Health Statistics. Plan and operation of the Third National health and nutrition examination survey, 1988–94. Series 1: programs and collection procedures. Vital and Health Statistics. 1–46, 1994.
13. National Institutes of Health, National Heart, Lung and Blood Institute. Clinical guidelines on the identification, evaluation, and treatment of overweight and obesity in adults–the evidence report. Obes Res. 1998;6(Suppl 2):S51–209.
14. Flegal KM, Carroll MD, Ogden CL, Curtin LR. Prevalence and Trends in Obesity Among US Adults, 1999–2008. JAMA 2010 2009. 2014.
15. Bieri U, Moch H, Dehler S, Korol D, Rohrmann S. Changes in autopsy rates among cancer patients and their impact on cancer statistics from a public health point of view: a longitudinal study from 1980 to 2010 with data from cancer registry Zurich. Virchows Arch 2015 Jun;466(6):637–43. doi: 10.1007/s00428-015-1734-7. Epub 2015 Mar 7.
16. Ryder NB. The cohort as a concept in the study of social change. Am Sociol Rev. 1965;30(6):843–61.
17. Keyes KM, Li G. A multiphase method for estimating cohort effects in age-period contingency table data. Ann Epidemiol. 2010;20(10):779–85.
18. Keyes KM, Li G. Age-period-cohort analysis in injury epidemiology. In: Li G, Baker SP, editors. Injury research: theories, methods, approaches. New York: Springer; 2011.
19. Yang Y, Land KC. A mixed models approach to age-period-cohort analysis of repeated cross-section surveys: trends in verbal test scores. Sociol Methodol. 2006;36:75–97.
20. Eggebeen DJ, Lichter DT. Race, family structure, and changing poverty among American children. Am Sociol Rev. 1991;56(6):801–17.
21. Ghaffar A, Tran NT, Reddy KS, Kasonde J, Bajwa T, Ammar W, Ren M, Rottingen JA, Mills A. Changing mindsets in health policy and systems research. Lancet. 2013;381:436–7. doi:10.1016/S0140-6736(12)61858-3.
22. Adam T, Hsu J, de Savigny D, Lavis JN, Rottingen JA, Bennett S. Evaluating health systems strengthening interventions in low-income and middle-income countries: are we asking the right questions? Health Policy Plan. 27(Suppl 4):iv 9–19, 2012.
23. Brenner DR, Tepylo K, Eny KM, Cahill LE, El-Sohemy A. Comparison of body mass index and waist circumference as predictors of cardiometabolic health in a population of young Canadian adults. Diabetol Metab Syndr. 2010;2(1):28.
24. Dallman MF, Pecoraro NC, la Fleur SE. Chronic stress and comfort foods: self-medication and abdominal obesity. Brain Behav Immun. 2005;19(4):275–80.
25. Worsley A, Wang WC, Hunter W. The relationships between eating habits, smoking and alcohol consumption, and body mass index among baby boomers. Appetite. 2012;58(1):74–80. doi:10.1016/j.appet.2011.09.003. Epub 2011 Sep 29
26. Frey WH, Abresch B, Yeasting J. America by the numbers: a field guide to the US population. 1st ed. New York: New Press; 2001.
27. Li C, Ford ES, McGuire LC, Mokdad AH. Increasing trends in waist circumference and abdominal obesity among US adults. Obesity (Silver Spring). 2007;15(1):216–24.
28. U.S. EPA. Guidelines for Carcinogen Risk Assessment. Washington, DC, National Center for Environmental Assessment. EPA/630/P-03/001b. NCEA-F-0644b. 2005. http://cfpub.epa.gov/ncea/CFM/nceaQFind.cfm? keyword=Cancer%20 Guidelines

29. Leung CW, Ding EL, Catalano PJ, et al. Dietary intake and dietary quality of low-income adults in the supplemental nutrition assistance program. Am J Clin Nutr. 2012;96:977–88.
30. Olshansky SJ, Goldman DP, Zheng Y, et al. Aging in America in the twenty-first century: demographic forecasts from the MacArthur Foundation research network on an aging society. Milbank Q. 2009;87:842–62.
31. Khatami, M: In Cancer Research and Therapy: Scam of Century–Promote Immunity [Yin-Yang], 2016; ISBN-10:153043100X;ISBN-13:978-1530431007; Amazon-Createspace p1–166, http://www.createspace.com/6123573, 2016.
32. Khatami M. Safety concerns and hidden agenda behind HPV vaccines: another generation of drug-dependent society? Clin Transl Med. 2016;5(1):46. Epub 2016 Dec 5
33. Khatami M. Book review on cancer research and therapy: safety concerns for HPV vaccination of young generation, paid by Obamacare and V.P. Biden moonshot initiative. Global Vaccines and Immunol; 2016, 1(3.) ISSN: 2397-575X https://oatext.com/pdf/GVI-1-118.pdf
34. Park J, Myers D, Kao D, Min S. Immigrant obesity and unhealthy assimilation: alternative estimates of convergence or divergence, 1995–2005. Soc Sci Med. 2009;69(11):1625–33.
35. Selvin S. Statistical analysis of epidemiologic data. 2. New York: Oxford University Press; 1996.
36. Keyes KM, Utz RL, Robinson W, Li G. What is a cohort effect? Comparison of three statistical methods for modeling cohort effects in obesity prevalence in the United States, 1971–2006. Soc Sci Med. 2010;70(7):1100–8.
37. Robinson WR, Keyes KM, Utz RL, Martin CL, Yang Y. Birth cohort effects among US-born adults born in the 1980s: foreshadowing future trends in US obesity prevalence. Int J Obes. 2012;
38. Reither EN, Hauser RM, Yang Y. Do birth cohorts matter? Age-period-cohort analyses of the obesity epidemic in the United States. Soc Sci Med. 2009;69(10):1439–48.
39. Barbanti-Brodano G, Sabbioni S, Martini F, Negrini M, Corallini A, Tognon M. Simian virus 40 infection in humans and association with human diseases: results and hypotheses. Virology. 2004;318(1):1–9.
40. Day A. 'An American tragedy', the cutter incident and its implications for the Salk polio vaccine in New Zealand 1955–1960. Health Hist. 2009;11:42–61.
41. Pietruska JR, Kane AB. SV40 oncoproteins enhance asbestos-induced DNA double-strand breaks and abrogate senescence in murine mesothelial cells. Cancer Res. 2007;67(8):3637–45.
42. Bosetti C, Malvezzi M, Chatenoud L, Negri E, Levi F, La Vecchia C. Trends in cancer mortality in the Americas, 1970–2000. Ann Oncol. 2005;16:489–511.
43. Doll R. Progress against cancer: an epidemiologic assessment. The 1991 John C. Cassel memorial lecture. Am J Epidemiol. 134(675–88):1991.
44. Faguet G. *In* The war on cancer: an anatomy of failure, a blueprint for the future. Dordrecht: Springer; 2005.
45. Bailar JC III, Gornick HL. Cancer undefeated. N Engl J Med. 1997;336(22):1569–74.
46. LaDou J, Bailar JC 3rd. Cancer and reproductive risks in the semiconductor industry. Int J Occup Environ Health. 2007;13(4):376–85.
47. Bonetto C, Trotta F, Felicetti P, Alarcón GS, Santuccio C, et al. Vasculitis as an adverse event following immunization: systematic literature review. [Brighton Collaboration Vasculitis Working Group]. Vaccine. 2015;34(51):6641–51. http://dx.doi.org/10.1016/j.vaccine.2015.09.026
48. Virendra B. Problems with the oral polio vaccine. Nat Med. 2008;14:9.
49. Eddy BE, Stewart SE, Stanton MF, Marcotte JM. Induction of tumors in rats by tissue-culture preparations of SE polyoma virus. J Natl Cancer Inst. 1959;22:161–71.
50. Schnipper LE, Davidson NE, Wollins DS, Tyne C, Blayney DW, Blum D, Dicker AP, Ganz PA, Hoverman JR, et al. American Society of Clinical Oncology statement: a conceptual framework to assess the value of cancer treatment options. J Clin Oncol. 2015;33(23):2563–77. doi:10.1200/JCO.2015.61.6706. Epub 2015 Jun 22
51. Schnipper LE, Meropol NJ, Brock DW. Value and cancer care: toward an equitable future. Clin Cancer Res. 2010;16(24):6004–8. doi:10.1158/1078-0432.CCR-10-1643.

52. Wagstaff A, Culyer AJ. Four decades of health economics through a bibliometric lens. J Health Econ. 2012;31:406–39. doi:10.1016/j.jhealeco.2012.03.002.
53. Greenberg D, Rosen AB, Wacht O, Palmer J, Neumann PJ. A bibliometric review of cost-effectiveness analyses in the economic and medical literature: 1976–2006. Med Decis Mak. 2010;30(3):320–7. doi:10.1177/0272989X09360066. Epub 2010 Mar 12
54. Bandera EV, Maskarinec G, Romieu I, John EM. Racial and ethnic disparities in the impact of obesity on breast cancer risk and survival: a global perspective. Adv Nutr. 2015;6(6):803–19. doi:10.3945/an.115.009647. Print 2015 Nov
55. WHO-Research Groups – Section of Cancer Surveillance – IARC www.iarc.fr Research Cancer Surveillance Publications- Research Groups – Section of Cancer Surveillance ... – IARC... patterns in GLOBOCAN 2012.
56. IARC. Monographs on the evaluation of carcinogenic risks to humans Vol. 100E Personal Habits and Indoor Combustions. 2012.
57. International Agency for Research on Cancer (IRAC-WHO). IARC Monographs of carcinogenic risk to human and cancer classification groups and descriptions of each category. 2008. http://monographs.iarc.fr/ENG/Preamble/currentb6evalrationale0706.php
58. Ferlay J, Bray F, Pisani P, Parkin DM. Globocan 2000: Cancer Incidence, Mortality and Prevalence Worldwide, Version 1.0. IARC Cancer Base No. 5. 2001. Lyon, IARCPress. [Regional data derived from-NORDCAN-C15.iarc.fr; Australia: www.aihw.gov.au; New Zealand: www.health.govt.nz; England: www.ons.gov.uk USA: seer.cancer.gov, NORDCAN: www.ancr.nu--2012 and 2015-IARC.].
59. Ferlay J, Steliarova-Foucher E, Lortet-Tieulent J, Rosso S, Coebergh JW, Comber H, Forman D, Bray F. Cancer incidence and mortality patterns in Europe: estimates for 40 countries in 2012. Eur J Cancer. 2013;49(6):1374–403.
60. World Health Organization- IARC. Cancer mortality database; 2013 June 2013; http://www-dep.iarc.fr/WHOdb/WHOdb.htm
61. Wu X, Elkin EE, Marghoob AA. Burden of basal cell carcinoma in USA. Future Oncol. 2015;11(22):2967–74. doi:10.2217/fon.15.180. Epub 2015 Oct 15
62. Rose RF, Boon A, Forman D, Merchant W, Bishop R, Newton-Bishop JA. An exploration of reported mortality from cutaneous squamous cell carcinoma using death certification and cancer registry data. Br J Dermatol. 2013;169(3):682–6. PMID: 24381068
63. SEER: Database. http://seer.cancer.gov/csr/1975_2006/. Last Accessed 28 Sept 2010
64. Ferlay J, et al. Cancer Incidence and Mortality Worldwide: Sources, Methods and Major Patterns in GLOBOCAN 2012. Int J Cancer. 136(5):E359–86. and SEERS Results: http://seer.cancer.gov/csr/1975_2003/results--topics_annualrates.pdf.. View info at http://seer.cancer.gov/csr/1975_2007/sections.html
65. Australian Institute of Health and Welfare (AIHW). Australian cancer incidence and mortality books; 2011 [cited 2012 September 13]; http://www.aihw.gov.au/acim-books/
66. Bailar JC 3rd, Ballal SG, Boback M, Castleman B, Chee HL, Cherniack M, Christiani D, Cicolella A, Fernández de D'Pool J, Egilman D, et al. FIOH-sponsored newsletter misrepresents asbestos hazards in Zimbabwe. Int J Occup Environ Health. 2006;12(3):254–8.
67. Cutrone R, Lednicky J, Dunn G, et al. Some oral poliovirus vaccines were contaminated with infectious SV40 after 1961. Cancer Res. 2005;65(22):10273–9.
68. McShane H, Jacobs WR, Fine PE, Reed SG, McMurray DN, Behr M, Williams A, Orme IM. BCG: myths, realities, and the need for alternative vaccine strategies. Tuberculosis (Edinb). 2012;92:283–8. doi:10.1016/j.tube.2011.12.003.
69. Coleman MP, Forman D, Bryant H, Butler J, Rachet B, Maringe C, Nur U, Tracey E, Coory M, Hatcher J, McGahan CE, Turner D, Marrett L, et al. Cancer survival in Australia, Canada, Denmark, Norway, Sweden, and the UK, 1995–2007 (International Cancer Benchmarking Partnership): an analysis of population-based cancer registry data. Lancet. 2011;377(9760):127–38. PMID: 21183212
70. Arnold M, Moore SP, Hassler S, Ellison-Loschmann L, Forman D, Bray F. The burden of stomach cancer in indigenous populations: a systematic review and global assessment. Gut. 2014;63(1):64–71. PMID: 24153248

71. Centers for Disease Control and Prevention. Women and smoking: a report of the surgeon general. Rockville: U.S. Department of Health and Human Services, Centers for Disease Control and Prevention, National Center for Chronic Disease Prevention and Health Promotion, Office on Smoking and Health; 2001.
72. Chaabna K, Bray F, Wabinga HR, Chokunonga E, Borok M, Vanhems P, Forman D, Soerjomataram I. Kaposi sarcoma trends in Uganda and Zimbabwe: a sustained decline in incidence? Int J Cancer. 2013;133(5):1197–203. PMID: 23436712
73. Crawford SM, Sauerzapf V, Haynes R, Forman D, Jones AP. Social and geographical factors affecting access to treatment of colorectal cancer: a cancer registry study. BMJ Open. 2012;2(2):e000410. PMID: 22535788
74. Cvancarova M, Aagnes B, Fossa SD, Lambert PC, Moller B, Bray F. Proportion cured models applied to 23 cancer sites in Norway. Int J cancer. 2013;132(7):1700–10. PMID: 22927104
75. Chaabna K, Soerjomataram I, Rouabhia S, Chichoune S, Scholtes C, Vanhems P, Saidi M, Forman D. Co-occurrence of diffuse large B cell non-hodgkin lymphoma and chronic hepatitis C in Algerian patients: two case reports. J Cancer ResTher. 2013;9(3):532–3.
76. Kang J, Cho JH, Suh CW, Lee DH, Oh HB, Sohn YH, Chi HS, Park CJ, Jang SS, Lee KH, Lee JH, Lee JH, Lee SW, Chung YH, Kim TH, Shin H.R, Huh J: High prevalence of hepatitis B and hepatitis C virus infections in Korean patients with hematopoietic malignancies Ann Hematol; 90(2):159–164, 2011. PMID: 20821327
77. Bray F, Lortet-Tieulent J, Znaor A, Brotons M, Poljak M, Arbyn M. Patterns and trends in human papillomavirus-related diseases in central and eastern Europe and central Asia. Vaccine. 2013;31(suppl 7):H32–45. PMID: 24332296
78. Ribeiro KB, Levi JE, Pawlita M, Koifman S, Matos E, Eluf-Neto J, Wunsch-Filho V, Curado MP, Shangina O, Zaridze D, Szeszenia-Dabrowska N, Lissowska J, et al. Low human papillomavirus prevalence in head and neck cancer: results from two large case-control studies in high-incidence regions. Int J Epidem. 2011;40(2):489–502. PMID: 21224273
79. Pineros M, Gamboa O, Hernandez-Suarez G, Pardo C, Bray F. Patterns and trends in cancer mortality in Colombia 1984–2008. Cancer Epidemiol. 2013;37(3):233–9. PMID: 23499325
80. van den Broek EC, Liu L, Posthuma EF, Janssen-Heijnen ML, Coebergh JW, Soerjomataram I. Increased risk of chronic lymphocytic leukaemia among cancer survivors in the Netherlands: increased detection, causal factors or both? Ann Hematol. 2014;93(1):157–62. PMID: 24381068
81. Lambert PC, Holmberg L, Sandin F, Bray F, Linklater KM, Purushotham A, Robinson D, Moller H. Quantifying differences in breast cancer survival between England and Norway. Cancer Epidemiol. 2011;35(6):526–33.
82. Khatami M. Unresolved inflammation and cancer: loss of natural immune surveillance as the correct “target” for therapy! Seeing the “elephant” in the light of logic. Cell Biochem Biophys. 2012;62:501–9.
83. Khatami M. Chronic inflammation: synergistic interactions of recruiting macrophages (MFs) and eosinophils (Eos) with host mast cells (MCs) and tumorigenesis in CALTs. M-CSF, suitable biomarker for cancer diagnosis! Cancers. 2014;6:297–322.
84. Thompson PA, Khatami M, Baglole CJ, Sun J, Harris S, Moon EY, Al-Mulla F, Al-Temaimi R, Brown D, Colacci A, Mondello C, Raju J, Ryan E, Woodrick J, Scovassi I, Singh N, Vaccari M, Roy R, Forte S, Memeo L, Salem HK, Amedei A, Hamid RA, Lowe L, Guarnieri T, Bisson WH. Environmental immune disruptors, inflammation and cancer risk. Carcinogenesis. 2015;1(Suppl):S232–53.
85. IARC. Monograph on the evaluation of carcinogenic risk to humans. Some industrial chemicals. Di(2-ethylhexyl) phthalate. Lyon: International Agency for Research and Cancer; 2000. p. 41–148.
86. Eriksen M, Mackay J, Ross H. The tobacco atlas. 4th ed. American Cancer Society: Atlanta; 2012.
87. National Cancer Institute. NCI Tobacco Control Monograph Series 20-Phenotypes and Endotypes. Foundations for Genetic Studies of Nicotine Use and Dependence. US Department of Health and Human Service, National Institutes of. Health, 625 p 2009.

88. Spitz MR, Wu X, Wilkinson A, Wei Q. Cancer of the lung. In: Schottenfeld D, Fraumeni Jr J, editors. Cancer epidemiology and prevention. 3rd ed. New York: Oxford University Press; 2006. p. 638–58.
89. U.S. EPA, 1986. Classifications: A-human carcinogen; B-probable human carcinogen; B1-limited evidence of carcinogenicity in humans; B2-sufficient evidence of carcinogenicity in animals with inadequate or lack of evidence in humans; C-possible human carcinogen; D-not classifiable as to human carcinogenicity; E-evidence of noncarcinogenicity for humans. The risk assessment guidelines of 1986. EPA/600/8-87/045. August. [the use of these guidelines was phased out in 2002.]
90. Ren JS, Kamangar F, Forman D, Islami F. Pickled food and risk of gastric cancer–a systematic review and meta-analysis of English and Chinese literature. Cancer Epidemiol Biomarkers Prev. 2012;21(6):905–15. PMID: 22499775
91. Cross AJ, Freedman ND, Ren J, Ward MH, Hollenbeck AR, Schatzkin A, Sinha R, Abnet CC. Meat consumption and risk of esophageal and gastric cancer in a large prospective study. Am J Gastroenterol. 2011;106(3):432–42.
92. Gómez-Martín A, Amores J, Paterna A, De la Fe C. Contagious agalactia due to Mycoplasma spp. in small dairy ruminants: epidemiology and prospects for diagnosis and control. Vet J. 2013;198(1):48–56.
93. Suen JL, Hsu SH, Hung CH, Chao YS, Lee CL, et al. A common environmental pollutant, 4-nonylphenol, promotes allergic lung inflammation in a murine model of asthma. Allergy. 2013;68:780–7.
94. Uzumcu M, Suzuki H, Skinner MK. Effect of the anti-androgenic endocrine disruptor vinclozolin on embryonic testis cord formation and postnatal testis development and function. Reprod Toxicol. 2004;18:765–74.
95. Cupp AS, Skinner MK. Actions of the endocrine disruptor methoxychlor and its estrogenic metabolite on in vitro embryonic rat seminiferous cord formation and perinatal testis growth. Reprod Toxicol. 2001;15(3):317–26.
96. Frassinetti S, Barberino C, Caltavuturo L, Fava F, Di Gioia D. Genotoxicity of 4-nonylphenol and nonylphenol ethoxylate mixtures by the use of Saccharomyces Cerevisiae D7 mutation assay and use of this text to evaluate the efficiency of biodegradation treatments. Ecotoxicol Environ Saf. 2011;74:253–8.
97. Dea S, Zhoub H, DeSantisc D, Cronigerc CM, Lib X, George R, Starka GR. Erlotinib protects against LPS-induced endotoxicity because TLR4 needs EGFR to signal. Proc Natl Acad Sci. 2015;112:9680–5.
98. Nakahara T, Moroi Y, Uchi H, Furue M. Differential role of MAPK signaling in human dendritic cell maturation and Th1/Th2 engagement. J Dermatol Sci. 2006;42:1–11.
99. Stossi F, et al. Defining estrogenic mechanisms of bisphenol a analogs through high throughput microscopy-based contextual assays. Chem Biol. 2014;21:743–53.
100. Lopez-Espinosa MJ, Freire C, Arrebola JP, Navea N, Taoufiki J, et al. Nonylphenol and octylphenol in adipose tissue of women in southern Spain. Chemosphere. 2009;76:847–52.
101. Goodson WH 3rd, Luciani MG, Sayeed SA, Jaffee IM, Moore DH 2nd, Dairkee SH. Activation of the mTOR pathway by low levels of xenoestrogens in breast epithelial cells from high-risk women. Carcinogenesis. 2011;32:1724–33.
102. Hung CH, Yang SN, Wang YF, Liao WT, Kuo PL, Tsai EM, Lee CL, Chao YS, Yu HS, Huang SK, Suen JL. Environmental alkylphenols modulate cytokine expression in plasmacytoid dendritic cells. PLoS One. 2013;8:e73534.
103. Kolarik B, Naydenov K, Larsson M, Bornehag CG, Sundell J. The association between phthalates in dust and allergic diseases among Bulgarian children. Environ Health Perspect. 2008;116:98–103.
104. Sabbieti MG, Agas D, Santoni G, Materazzi S, Menghi G, Marchetti L. Involvement of p53 in phthalate effects on mouse and rat osteoblasts. J Cell Biochem. 2009;107:316–27.
105. Erkekoğlu P, et al. Induction of ROS, p53, p21 in DEHP- and MEHP-exposed LNCaP cells-protection by selenium compounds. Food Chem Toxicol. 2011;49:1565–71.

106. Kleinsasser NH, Kastenbauer ER, Weissacher H, Muenzenrieder RK, Harreus UA. Phthalates demonstrate genotoxicity on human mucosa of the upper aerodigestive tract. Environ Mol Mutagen. 2000;35:9–12.
107. Singh B, et al. Cyclooxygenase-2 expression induces genomic instability in MCF10A breast epithelial cells. J Surg Res. 2007;140:220–6.
108. Persson C, Canedo P, Machado JC, El-Omar EM, Forman D. Polymorphisms in inflammatory response genes and their association with gastric cancer: A HuGE systematic review and meta-analyses. Am J Epidemiol. 2011;173(3):259–70.
109. Veldhoen M, Hirota K, Westendorf AM, Buer J, Dumoutier L, et al. The aryl hydrocarbon receptor links TH17-cell-mediated autoimmunity to environmental toxins. Nature. 2008;453:106–9.
110. Lalah JO, Behechti A, Severin GF, Lenoir D, Gunther K, et al. The bioaccumulation and fate of a branched 14C-p-nonylphenol isomer in Lymnaea stagnalis L. Environ Toxicol Chem. 2003;22:1428–36.
111. Chalubinski M, Kowalski ML. Endocrine disrupters–potential modulators of the immune system and allergic response. Allergy. 2006;61:1326–35.
112. Kato T, Tada-Oikawa S, Takahashi K, Saito K, Wang L, et al. Endocrine disruptors that deplete glutathione levels in APC promote Th2 polarization in mice leading to the exacerbation of airway inflammation. Eur J Immunol. 2006;36:1199–209.
113. Laws SC, et al. Chlorotriazine herbicides and metabolites activate an ACTH-dependent release of corticosterone in male Wistar rats. Toxicol Sci. 2009;112:78–87.
114. Rusyn I, et al. Modes of action and species-specific effects of di-(2-ethylhexyl)phthalate in the liver. Crit Rev Toxicol. 2006;36:459–79.
115. Cavas T. In vivo genotoxicity evaluation of atrazine and atrazine-based herbicide on fish Carassius Auratus using the micronucleus test and the comet assay. Food Chem Toxicol. 2011;49:1431–5.
116. Chua AC, Klopcic BR, Ho DS, Fu SK, Forrest CH, et al. Dietary iron enhances colonic inflammation and IL-6/IL-11-Stat3 signaling promoting colonic tumor development in mice. PLoS One. 2013;8(11):e78850. doi:10.1371/journal.pone.0078850. eCollection 2013
117. Benninghoff AD, Bisson WH, Koch DC, Ehresman DJ, Kolluri SK, Williams DE. Estrogen-like activity of perfluoroalkyl acids in vivo and interaction with human and rainbow trout estrogen receptors in vitro. Toxicol Sci. 2011;120:42–58.
118. Rossouw JE, Prentice RL, Manson JE, et al. Postmenopausal hormone therapy and risk of cardiovascular disease by age and years since menopause. JAMA. 2007;297(13):1465–77.
119. Schwartz AG, Wenzlaff AS, Prysak GM, et al. Reproductive factors, hormone use, estrogen receptor expression and risk of non small-cell lung cancer in women. J Clin Oncol. 2007;25(36):5785–92.
120. Pike MC, Peters RK, Cozen W, et al. Estrogen-progestin replacement therapy and endometrial cancer. J Natl Cancer Inst. 1997;89:1110–6.
121. Chlebowski RT, Wactawski-Wende J, Ritenbaugh C, et al. Estrogen plus progestin and colorectal cancer in postmenopausal women. N Engl J Med. 2004;350:991–1004.
122. Calandra T, et al. MIF as a glucocorticoid-induced modulator of cytokine production. Nature. 1995;377:68–71.
123. Bucala R. MIF rediscovered: cytokine, pituitary hormone, and glucocorticoid-induced regulator of the immune response. FASEB J. 1996;10:1607–13.
124. Lee E, Kim TH, Choi JS, Nabanata P, Kim NY, Ahn MY, Jung KK, et al. Evaluation of liver and thyroid toxicity in Sprague Dawley rats after exposure to polybrominated diphenyl ether BDE-209. J Toxicol Sci. 2010;35:535–45.
125. Martin PA, Mayne GJ, Bursian FS, Tomy G, Palace V, Pekarik C, Smits J. Immunotoxicity of the commercial polybrominated diphenyl ether mixture DE-71 in ranch mink (Mustela Vison). Environ Toxicol Chem. 2007;26:988–97.
126. Chen F, Zhou L, Bai Y, Zhou R, Chen L. Sex differences in the adult HPA axis and affective behaviors are altered by perinatal exposure to a low dose of bisphenol a. Brain Res. 2014;1571:12–24.

127. Panagiotidou E, Zerva S, Mitsiou DJ, Alexis MN, Kitraki E. Perinatal exposure to low-dose bisphenol a affects the neuroendocrine stress response in rats. J Endocrinol. 2014;220:207–18.
128. Ames BN. Identifying environmental chemicals causing mutations and cancer. Science. 1979;204:587–93.
129. McLachlan JA. Environmental signaling: what embryos and evolution teach us about endocrine disrupting chemicals. Endocr Rev. 2001;22:319–41.
130. Eklind Y, Beck-Friis B, Bengtsson S, et al. Chemical characterization of source-separated organic household wastes. Swed J Agric Res. 1997;27:167–78.
131. Epstein O, Spisni R, Parbhoo S, et al. The effect of oral copper loading and portasystemic shunting on the distribution of copper in the liver, brain, kidney, and cornea of the rat. Am J Clin Nutr. 1982;35:551–5.
132. Ettinger MJ, Darwish HM, Schmitt RC. Mechanism of copper transport from plasma to hepatocytes. Fed Proc. 1986;45:2800–4.
133. Fernandes AC, Filipe PM, Manso CF. Protective effects of a 21-aminosteroid against copper induced erythrocyte and plasma lipid peroxidation. Eur J Pharmacol. 1992;220(2-3):211–6.
134. Fernandes A, Mira ML, Azevedo MS, Manso C. Mechanisms of hemolysis induced by copper. Free Radic Res Commun. 1988;4(5):291–8.
135. Fewtrell L, Kay D, MacGill S. A review of the science behind drinking water standards for copper. Int J Environ Health Res. 2001;11(2):161–7.
136. Evering WE, Haywood S, Bremner I, et al. The protective role of metallothionein in copperoverload. II. Transport and excretion of immunoreactive MT-1 in blood, bile and urine of copper-loaded rats. Chem Biol Interact. 1991;78(3):297–305.
137. US Environmental Protection Agency. EPA600282001a, I4.7-1 to I.4.—5. Methods for chemical analysis of water and wastes. Washington DC, 1983.
138. U.S. Environmental Protect Agency. Copper. Water-related environmental fate of 129 priority pollutants. Fed Regist. 1979;40(143):373–4.
139. U.S. Environmental Protection Agency. EPA600479020. Air quality data for metals 1977 through 1979 from The National Air Surveillance Networks. 1984.
140. U.S. Environmental Protection Agency. Assessment of copper as a potentially toxic air pollutant. U.S. Environmental Protection Agency. Fed Regist. 1987;(35):52, 5496–5499.
141. U.S Food and Drug Administration. Code of Federal Regulations. 21 CFR 184.1261. http://www.frwebgate.accessgpo.gov/cgi. 10 Apr 2002. FDA. 2001. Food labeling. Nutritional labeling of food.
142. U.S. Food and Drug Administration. Code of Federal Regulations. 21 CFR 101.9(c)(8). http://www.frwebgate.accessgpo.gov/cgi. 09 Apr 2002. FDA. 2001. Listing of color additives exempt from certification. Copper powder. U.S. Food and Drug Administration. Code of Federal Regulations 21 CFR 73.1647. http://www.frwebgate.accessgpo.gov/cgi. 09 Apr 2002.
143. Goldfrank LR, Flomenbaum FE, Lewin NA, et al. Goldfrank's toxicologic emergencies. 6th ed. Stamford: Appleton & Lange; 1998. p. 1339–40.
144. Haddad LM, Shannon MW, Winchester JF, editors. Clinical management of poisoning and drug overdose. 3rd ed. Philadelphia: WB Saunders; 1998. p. 165.
145. Farrah H, Pickering WF. Factors influencing the potential mobility and bioavailability of metals in dried lake sediments. Chem Speciat Bioavailab. 1993;5(3):81–96.
146. Farrer P, Mistilis SP. Absorption of exogenous and endogenous biliary copper in the rat. Nature. 1967;213:291–2.
147. Huovinen E, Kapiro J, Vesterinen E, Koshenvuo M. Mortality of adults with asthma: a prospective cohort study. Thorax. 1997;52:49–54.
148. Vesterinen E, Oukkala E, Timonen T, Aromaa A. Cancer incident among 78000 asmatic patients. Int J Epidemiol. 1993;22:976–82.
149. Barnard J, Frangakis CE, Hill JL, Rubin DB. Principal stratification approach to broken randomized experiments. J Am Stat Assoc. 2003;98:299–323.

150. Baker SG, Kramer BS, Lindeman KS. Latent class instrumental variables: a clinical and biostatistical perspective. Stat Med 2016 Jan 15;35(1):147–60. doi: 10.1002/sim.6612. Epub 2015 Aug 4.
151. Bray F, Guilloux A, Sankila R, Parkin DM. Practical implications of imposing a new world standard population. Cancer Causes Control. 2002;13(2):175–82.
152. World Health Organization. Global tuberculosis report. Geneva: World Health Organization; 2013. http://apps.who.int/iris/bitstream/10665/91355/1/9789241564656_eng.pdf.
153. Hung CH, Chu YT, Suen JL, Lee MS, Chang HW, et al. Regulation of cytokine expression in human plasmacytoid dendritic cells by prostaglandin I2 analogues. Eur Respir J. 2009;33:405–10.
154. Gomez D, Lemarteleur T, Lacroix L, Maillient P, et al. Telomerase downregulation induced by the G-quadruplex ligand 12459 in A549 cells is mediated by hTERT RNA alternative splicing. Nucleic Acids Res. 2004;32:371–9.
155. Straus DS. TNFα and IL-17 cooperatively stimulate glucose metabolism and growth factor production in human colorectal cancer cells. Mol Cancer. 2013;12:78.
156. Chau BN, Chen TT, Wan YY, DeGregori J, Wang JY. Tumor necrosis factor alpha-induced apoptosis requires p73 and c-ABL activation downstream of RB degradation. Mol Cell Biol. 2004;24:4438–47.
157. Pastor DM, Irby RB, Poritz LS. Tumor necrosis factor alpha induces p53 up-regulated modulator of apoptosis expression in colorectal cancer cell lines. Dis Colon Rectum. 2010;53:257–63.
158. Zhang Z, et al. Interleukin-17A- or tumor necrosis factor α-mediated increase in proliferation of T cells cocultured with synovium-derived mesenchymal stem cells in rheumatoid arthritis. Arthritis Res Ther. 2013;15:R169.
159. Li W, Mao Z, Fan X, Cui L, Wang X. Cyclooxygenase 2 promoted the tumorigenecity of pancreatic cancer cells. Tumour Biol. 2014;35(3):2271–8.
160. Sriplung H, Kantipundee T, Tassanapitak C. Disagreement of ICD-10 codes between a local hospital information system and a cancer registry. Asian Pac J Cancer Prev. 2015;16(1):259–63.
161. Touboul C, Lis R, Al Farsi H, Raynaud CM, Warfa M, Althawadi H, Mery E, Mirshahi M, Rafii A. Mesenchymal stem cells enhance ovarian cancer cell infiltration through IL6 secretion in an amniochorionic membrane based 3D model. J Transl Med. 2013;11:28.
162. Yadav A, Kumar B, Datta J, Teknos TN, Kumar P. IL-6 promotes head and neck tumor metastasis by inducing epithelia–mesenchymal transition via the JAK-STAT3- SNAIL signaling pathway. Mol Cancer Res. 2011;9:1658–67.
163. Na YR, Lee JS, Lee SJ, Seok SH. Interleukin-6-induced twist and N-cadherin enhance melanoma cell metastasis. Melanoma Res. 2013;23:434–43.
164. Fosslien E. Cancer morphogenesis: role of mitochondrial failure. Ann Clin Lab Sci. 2008;38:307–29.
165. Tang HY, Shih A, Cao HJ, Davis FB, Davis PJ, Lin HY. Resveratrol-induced cyclooxygenase-2 facilitates p53-dependent apoptosis in human breast cancer cells. Mol Cancer Ther. 2006;5:2034–42.
166. Subbaramaiah K, Altorki N, Chung WJ, Mestre JR, Sampat A, Dannenberg AJ. Inhibition of cyclooxygenase-2 gene expression by p53. J Biol Chem. 1999;274:10911–5.
167. Corcoran CA, et al. Cyclooxygenase-2 interacts with p53 and interferes with p53-dependent transcription and apoptosis. Oncogene. 2005;24:1634–40.
168. Berry M, Brightling C, Pavord I, Wardlaw A. TNF-alpha in asthma. Curr Opin Pharmacol. 2007;7:279–82.
169. Lee JY, Kim NA, Sanford A, Sullivan KE. Histone acetylation and chromatin conformation are regulated separately at the TNF-alpha promoter in monocytes and macrophages. J Leukoc Biol. 2003;73:862–71.
170. Kuo CH, Lin CH, Yang SN, Huang MY, Chen HL, et al. Effect of prostaglandin I2 analogs on cytokine expression in human myeloid dendritic cells via epigenetic regulation. Mol Med. 2012;18:433–44.
171. Wang SW, Sun YM. The IL-6/JAK/STAT3 pathway: potential therapeutic strategies in treating colorectal cancer (review). Int J Oncol. 2014;44:1032–40.

172. Ellenhorn MJ, Schonwald S, Ordog G, et al., editors. Medical toxicology: diagnosis and treatment of human poisoning. 2nd ed. Baltimore: Williams & Wilkins; 1997. p. 1554–6.
173. Fitzgerald DJ. Safety guidelines for copper in water. Am J Clin Nutr. 1998;67 (Suppl):1098S–102S.
174. Evans DW, Dodoo DK, Hanson PJ. Trace elements concentrations in fish livers: implications of variations with fish size in pollution monitoring. Mar Pollut Bull. 1993;26(6):329–34.
175. Khatami M, Donnelly JJ, John T, et al. Vernal conjunctivitis. Model studies in guinea pigs immunized topically with fluoresceinyl ovalbumin. Arch Ophthalmol. 1984;102:1683–8.
176. Khatami M, Donnelly JJ, Rockey JH. Induction and down-regulation of conjunctival type-1 hypersensitivity reactions in guinea pigs sensitized topically with fluoresceinyl ovalbumin. Ophthalmic Res. 1985;17:139–47.
177. Khatami M, Donnelly JJ, Haldar JP, Rockey JH. Massive follicular lymphoid hyperplasia in experimental chronic recurrent allergic conjunctivitis. Arch Ophthalmol. 1989;107:433–8.
178. Haldar JP, Khatami M, Donnelly JJ, Rockey JH. Experimental allergic conjunctivitis: production of different isotypes of antibody by conjunctival-associated lymphoid tissue in culture. Regional Immunol. 1988;1:92–9.
179. Khatami M. Cyclooxygenase inhibitor ketorolac or mast cell stabilizers: immunological challenges in cancer therapy. Letters to the editor. Clin. Cancer Res. 2005;11:1350–2.
180. Khatami M. Developmental phases of inflammation-induced massive lymphoid hyperplasia and extensive changes in epithelium in an experimental model of allergy. Implications for a direct link between inflammation and carcinogenesis. Am J Ther. 2005;12:117–28.
181. Khatami M. "Yin and Yang" in inflammation: duality in innate immune cell function and tumorigenesis. Exp Opin Biol Ther. 2008;8:1461–72.
182. Khatami M. Inflammation, aging and cancer: Tumoricidal vs tumorigenesis of immunity: a common denominator mapping chronic diseases. Cell Biochem Biophys. 2009;55:55–79.
183. Khatami M. Unresolved inflammation: "Immune tsunami" or erosion of integrity in immune-privileged and immune-responsive tissues and acute and chronic inflammatory diseases or cancer. Exp Opin Biol Ther. 2011;11:1419–32.
184. Rous P. A sarcoma of the fowl transmissible by an agent separable from the tumor cells. J Exp Med. 1911;13:397–411. doi:10.1084/jem.13.4.397.
185. Rous P. A transmissible avian Neoplasm. (SARCOMA OF THE COMMON FOWL) J Exp Med. 1910 Sep 1; 12(5):696–705. PMCID: PMC2124810.
186. Orme IM. The search for new vaccines against tuberculosis. J Leukoc Biol. 2001;70:1–10.
187. Orme IM. Vaccines to prevent tuberculosis infection rather than disease: physiological and immunological aspects. Tuberculosis (Edinb); 27 November 2014. doi:10.1016/j.tube.2014.10.008
188. Williams A, Reljic R, Naylor I, Clark SO, Falero-Diaz G, Singh M, Challacombe S, Marsh PD, Ivanyi J. Passive protection with immunoglobulin a antibodies against tuberculous early infection of the lungs. Immunology. 2004;111:328–33.
189. Tameris MD, Hatherill M, Landry BS, Scriba TJ, Snowden MA, Lockhart S, Shea JE, McClain JB, Hussey GD, Hanekom WA, Mahomed H. McShane H: [Team MATS] Safety and efficacy of MVA85A, a new tuberculosis vaccine, in infants previously vaccinated with BCG: a randomised, placebo-controlled phase 2b trial. Lancet. 2013;381:1021–8. doi:10.1016/S0140-6736(13)60177-4.
190. McShane H, Williams A. A review of preclinical animal models utilised for TB vaccine evaluation in the context of recent human efficacy data. Tuberculosis (Edinb). 2014;94:105–10. doi:10.1016/j.tube.2013.11.003.
191. Moliva JI, Turner J, Torrelles JB. Prospects in Mycobacterium Bovis Bacille Calmette et Guérin (BCG) vaccine diversity and delivery: why does BCG fail to protect against tuberculosis? Vaccine. 2015;33(39):5035–41. doi:10.1016/j.vaccine.2015.08.033. Epub 2015 Aug 28
192. Ernst JD. The immunological life cycle of tuberculosis. Nat Rev Immunol. 2012;12:581–91. doi:10.1038/nri3259.

193. Mahmoudi S, Khaheshi S, Pourakbari B, Aghamohammadi A, Keshavarz Valian S, Bahador A, Sabouni F, Ramezani A, Mamishi S. Adverse reactions to Mycobacterium bovis bacille Calmette-Guérin vaccination against tuberculosis in Iranian children. Clin Exp Vaccin Res. 2015;4(2):195–9.
194. Nell AS, D'Lom E, Bouic P, Sabate M, Bosser R, Picas J, Amat M, Churchyard G, Cardona PJ. Safety, tolerability, and immunogenicity of the novel antituberculous vaccine RUTI: randomized, placebo-controlled phase II clinical trial in patients with latent tuberculosis infection. PLoS One. 2014;9:e89612. doi:10.1371/journal.pone.0089612.
195. Dockrell HM, Smith SG. What have we learnt about BCG vaccination in the last 20 years? Front Immunol. 2017;8:1134. https://doi.org/10.3389/fimmu.2017.01134. eCollection 2017
196. Orme IM. Tuberculosis vaccine types and timings. Clin Vaccine Immunol. 2015;22(3):249–57. doi:10.1128/CVI.00718-14. Epub 2014 Dec 24
197. Orme IM. Safety issues regarding new vaccines for tuberculosis, with an emphasis on post-exposure vaccination. Tuberculosis (Edinb). 2006;86:68–73. doi:10.1016/j.tube.2005.07.002.
198. Lin PL, Flynn JL. Understanding latent tuberculosis: a moving target. J Immunol. 2010;185:15–22. doi:10.4049/jimmunol.0903856.
199. Cardona PJ. A dynamic reinfection hypothesis of latent tuberculosis infection. Infection. 2009;37:80–6. doi:10.1007/s15010-008-8087-y.
200. Chiang CY, Riley LW. Exogenous reinfection in tuberculosis. Lancet Infect Dis. 2005;5:629–36. doi:10.1016/S1473-3099(05)70240-1.
201. Kulka K, Hatfull G, Ojha AK. Growth of Mycobacterium tuberculosis biofilms. J Vis Exp. 2012;60 pii:3820. doi:10.3791/3820.
202. Orr MT, Ireton GC, Beebe EA, Huang PW, Reese VA, Argilla D, Coler RN, Reed SG. Immune subdominant antigens as vaccine candidates against Mycobacterium tuberculosis. J Immunol. 2014;193:2911–8. doi:10.4049/jimmunol.1401103.
203. Shanley CA, Ireton GC, Baldwin SL, Coler RN, Reed SG, Basaraba RJ, Orme IM. Therapeutic vaccination against relevant high virulence clinical isolates of Mycobacterium tuberculosis. Tuberculosis (Edinb). 2014;94:140–7. doi:10.1016/j.tube.2013.08.010.
204. Cohen T, Dye C, Colijn C, Williams B, Murray M. Mathematical models of the epidemiology and control of drug-resistant TB. Expert Rev Respir Med. 2009;3:67–79. doi:10.1586/17476348.3.1.67.
205. Vilaplana C, Gil O, Caceres N, Pinto S, Diaz J, Cardona PJ. Prophylactic effect of a therapeutic vaccine against TB based on fragments of Mycobacterium tuberculosis. PLoS One. 2011;6:e20404. doi:10.1371/journal.pone.0020404.
206. Cho LY, Yang JJ, Ko KP, Park B, Shin A, Lim MK, JK O, Park S, Kim YJ, Shin HR, Yoo KY, Park SK. Coinfection of hepatitis B and C viruses and risk of hepatocellular carcinoma: systematic review and meta-analysis. Int J Canc. 2011;128(1):176–84.
207. Murray P, Bell A. Contribution of the Epstein-Barr virus to the pathogenesis of Hodgkin Lymphoma. Curr Top Microbiol Immunol. 2015;390:287–313. doi:10.1007/978-3-319-22822-8_12.
208. Hilsop AD, Taylor GS. T-Cell Responses to EBV; in Current Topics in Microbiology and Immunology, Epstein Barr Virus Volume 2, 391. In: Münz C, editor. . Cham: Springer; 2015. p. 325–43. doi:10.1007/978-3-319-22834-1_11.
209. Lünemann A, Rowe M, Nadal D. Innate immune recognition of EBV. Curr Top Microbiol Immunol. 2015;391:265–87. doi:10.1007/978-3-319-22834-1_9.
210. Akhiani AA. The role of type-specific antibodies in colonization and infection by helicobacter pylori. Curr Opin Infect Dis. 2005;18:223–7.
211. Boer MC, Joosten SA, Ottenhoff TH. Regulatory T-cells at the Interface between human host and pathogens in infectious diseases and vaccination. Front Immunol 2015 May 11;6:217. doi: 10.3389/fimmu.2015.00217. eCollection 2015
212. Kleinnijenhuis J, Quintin J, Preijers F, Joosten LA, Ifrim DC, Saeed S, Jacobs C, van Loenhout J, de Jong D, Stunnenberg HG, Xavier RJ, et al. Bacille Calmette-Guérin induces NOD2-dependent nonspecific protection from reinfection via epigenetic reprogramming of monocytes. Proc Natl Acad Sci U S A. 2012;109:17537–42. doi:10.1073/pnas.1202870109.

Chapter 6
Cancer Biology: Severe Cumulative Delayed Type Hypersensitivity Reactions

All Diseases Pass through Allergies and Differential Bioenergetics-Histamine a Blue Print!

Common sense is not so common.

Voltaire

Abstract The outcomes of two centuries of repeated failed cancer research and therapy show that cancer has been made as an imaginary problem, a black box, not to be solved by the decision makers in the medical/cancer establishment for huge profit. In this chapter the 'Other Side of Political Darkness' in cancer science will be discussed by attempting to systematically analyze and integrate available data and demonstrate that growth of cancer cells is the results of severe, aggressive, and progressive aggregation of immune response alterations (immune tsunami or cancer tsunami) or accumulation of delayed hypersensitivity responses in tissues. Cancer cell growth is proposed to initiate as 'mild' (often sub-clinical) altered immune dynamics (immune disorder) and progress innately, genetically or be induced primarily in immune-responsive tissues. Severe altered immune-responses could also damage the immune-privileged tissues by shifting the architectural integrities and barriers of these oxidative-sensitive tissues to behave as immune-responsive and promote growth.

Evidence is provided that cancerous cells behave like pathogens altering host immune dynamics by hijacking and taking advantage of loss of balance in dual (pleiotropy) properties of Yin (tumoricidal) and Yang (tumorigenic) processes of effective immunity at multiple levels (e.g., cytoplasmic, vasculature, extracellular and intracellular membrane trafficking) with differential bioenergetics requirements to create immune suppression and demand tissue adaption that allow cancer cells to grow and thrive resulting in host destruction. Answer to cancer is proposed to be correcting the balance and differential bioenergetics of Yin-Yang of immunity. Future studies are proposed in focusing on systematic understanding of age-associated bioenergetics defects in Yin (tumoricidal) and Yang (tumorigenic) responses of effective immunity. Crucial dysfunction of mitochondria, through pyruvate shuttle mechanisms as well as high energy demands of biosynthesis of structural proteins from branched amino acids are among important studies for better understanding the cancer biology. Defects in mitochondria (mitophagy) have far more influence in

M. Khatami, *Inflammation, Aging and Cancer*,
https://doi.org/10.1007/978-3-319-66475-0_6

age-associated disease processes such as site-specific cancers and loss of cellular integrity than originally thought. A proposed working model for future studies demonstrates functionality of mitochondria after birth being intimately involved in maintenance or loss of Yin-Yang energy requirements in health or disease processes. Presence and accumulation of cancerous cells or other immune disruptors ('biological terrorists', oxidative stress) alter bioenergetics profiles in tissues, shifting the ratios of Yin vs. Yang of immune surveillance in favor of tissue growth and carcinogenesis. Role of circulating histamine is hypothesized among major factors involved in genesis of defective cancerous cells, induction of tolerance and differential energy consumption in promotion of wound healing events.

Keywords Adipocytes • Alanine • Alkaline • Anabolic • Anaphylaxis • Angiogenesis • Asthma • ATP/ADP/AMP • Autophagy • Biomarkers • Cancer bioenergetics • Cancer disorderly growth • Cancer microenvironment • Catabolic • Catecholamine • Cell surface molecules • Constituent and adaptive receptors • Decoy receptors • Differential energy requirements in Yin-Yang • Environmental hazards • Extrinsic factors • Fetus orderly growth • Fumarate • Glycolysis • Golgi apparatus • Heterogeneity • Histamine • Immune chaos • Immune tolerance • Immune Tsunami • Inflammation • Innate and adaptive immune cells • Intrinsic factors • IRAK-M • Isoleucine • 'Leaky' MCs • Leucine • Low level circulating histamine • 'Mild' • 'Moderate' or 'severe' immune disorders • Mitogen-activated protein kinase • mTOR/PI3K/AKT • Mitochondria • Mitophagy • Neoplasm • Oxidative stress • Pathogen pattern recognition • Polyps • Prostaglandins • Site-specific cancers • Somatic mutations • Succinate • TCA cycle • TNFR • Transporters • Vasoactive • Vasculogenesis • Warburg • Wound healing

1 Introduction

> While falsely-based science will not hide scientific truth at the end, it creates confusion benefiting those who direct chaotic science for financial gain at high cost of erosion of public health and trust and destruction of humanity.

Finding answers to biological laws that govern the complex interactions and synergies between host tissue and its surrounding environment require logical pursuit of systematic and integrated studies of the fascinating 'molecular village' that form the body's effective immunity for maintenance of health. However, logical and systematic approaches to understand disease processes are rarely applied in medicine, particularly with regard to studying cancer biology and how to control it.

The definitions of cancer remain elusive, and little variations on its biology have been presented to be beneficiary for resolving cancer or other age-associated chronic diseases for the last century. According to the cancer definitions presented by cancer community such as Nature and other organizations: "*cancer is a complex disease in which cells in a specific tissue are no longer fully responsive to the signals within the tissue that regulate cellular differentiation, survival, proliferation and death.*" Finally in its recent definition of cancer, the cancer community included the word of 'inflammation' that "*As a result, these cells accumulate within the tissue, causing local damage and inflammation…*" for applying and obtaining research funding for cancer or clinical trials including the immunotherapy [1–5].[1] The NCI describes the types of cancer as '*There are more than 100 types of cancer. Types of cancer are usually named for the organs or tissues where the cancers form...*'[2]

However, despite existence of more than 20 millions publications related to basic science of cancer molecular biology, epidemiology, pathophysiology, clinical studies and therapies, and despite reported documents on circumstantial evidence for a link between prior injuries and carcinogenesis, definitions of cancer or inflammation remain elusive [5–29]. The two centuries of studying age-associated chronic diseases, particularly cancer research and therapy resulted in investment of trillions of dollars and loss of millions of precious lives due to wrong approaches to treatment. Furthermore, because of continued reductionist and chaotic approaches to cancer science, we are far from understanding how the body's biological laws (effective immunity or immune surveillance) that police and arrest the growth of cancerous cells are violated in such a way that the cancer oncogenes (defective cells of body) would take over the machinery of host for their lawless enhanced growth requirements that kill the host [5, 10–15].

In this chapter, unlike the popularized notions that cancer is too 'complicated' to be solved, or cancer is 'several different diseases' (100 or 200 types)!, which make cancer an imaginary problem that cannot be solved, the author attempts to present a simple and logical argument that all age-associated diseases (e.g., asthma, emphysema, neurodegenerative, autoimmune disorders, diabetes and vascular complications) or site-specific cancers arise from different degrees of 'mild', 'moderate' (intermediate) or 'severe' immune response mismatches (immune disorders) toward intrinsic or extrinsic foreign elements in susceptible tissues. Evidence is presented that carcinogenesis is the ultimate cumulative form of 'severe' delayed hypersensitivity reactions (not reversible) that would create an 'immune tsunami' and destroy the amazingly ordered complex biological laws and bioenergetics of the body [5, 10].

We recently proposed that oxidative stress (unresolved inflammation) and the induction of multistage carcinogenesis is the results of accumulation of dysregulated (lawless or chaotic) molecular activities that create opportunities for cancer cell oncogenes to escape being arrested by ineffective immunity (loss of Yin and Yang of acute inflammation), which enable them to take control of the machineries of host immunity to satisfy their enhanced growth requirements at the cost of host

[1] Nature statement on cancer, accessed through Internet 12-2-15.

[2] National Cancer Institute, accessed January 27, 2017.

survival [5, 10–15]. A working model will be presented on the differential bioenergetics of Yin and Yang pathways that parallel the function of mitochondria at different stages of life, from fetus growth and development, to adulthood, aging and disease processes, with emphasis on cancer biology.

2 Highlights of Two Centuries of Cancer Research and Therapies: Neglected Common Sense on Fundamental Observations and Discoveries

A great deal of intelligence can be invested in ignorance when the need for illusion is deep.
Saul Bellow[3]

Table 6.1, shows examples of heavy investment on reductionist and chaotic approaches to cancer research and therapies for the last couple of centuries. It represents that claimed 'targeted' therapies, 'personalized' or 'precision' medicine produced failure rates of 90% (+/–5), costing millions of precious lives and heavy economic burden (several trillion dollars) to the society. Table 6.1 also reflects a contrast between peculiar absence of interest to support continuation of fundamental discoveries to systematically understand how the immune disruptors (e.g., antigens, pathogens, defective cells, biological, chemical or environmental hazards) would initiate altered immunity toward multistep diseases such as cancers [5, 10–15, 30–160].

Table 6.1 also reflects the disproportionate heavy investment on identification of too many genetic mutations in the chaotic and disorganized molecular defects in site-specific cancer as bases for drug development and clinical trials that repeatedly failed the patients. There is something fundamentally wrong with the current reductionist views on cancer research and therapy. With the tremendous funding that cancer community received for decades, cancer biology and all other chronic diseases should have been understood, prevented and/or treated by now, if the decision makers who control public health did not insist supporting too many expensive and out-of-focus projects that are considered 'medical/scientific ponzi schemes' for conducting phase I, II or III clinical trials [5, 10]. The information overload and lack of validation, regulation and integration of relevant data on disease processes are major factors in bias, misinformation, controversy and abuse of funds, particularly with regard to cancer research and therapy [5, 10, 159–162].

Examples of major neglected discoveries are shown shown (Table 1) in contrast with heavily support of too many out-of-focus projects with outcome failure rates of 90% (±5) for solid tumors (5).

[3] Saul Bellow. A Canadian-born American writer (1915–2005), he was awarded the Pulitzer Prize, and the Nobel Prize for Literature,... "The Adventures of Augie" (March, 1953) "http://en.wikipedia.org/wiki/Saul_Bellow" Wikipedia

Table 6.1 Highlights of two centuries of cancer-related research and therapy[a]
Many a small thing has been made large by the right kind of advertising. Mark Twain

Year	Discoveries and professional events	Comments, funding support
1863	Rudolph Virchow: cancer cell develops at site of inflammation	Ongoing debates, controversies and neglected support
1889	Stephen Paget: Seed and soil hypotheses	Cancer Metastasis–reasonable progress made; since 1951
	In the last decades investigators such as Rex, Comman, Fidler, Liotta, Nowell, Nicolson, Poste, Talmage, Wolman and others demonstrated cellular and molecular mechanisms of metastasis in various site-specific tissues.	
1901	Pasteur: parasitic theories of cancer	Pasteur institute –lack of support to understand molecular events that initiate altered immunity toward multistep carcinogenesis
1910/1911	Peyton Rous: discoveries on virus theory of cancer; virus-causing cancer in chicken; transmission of malignancy in cell-free filtrate;	Father of virology. Knowledge that viruses cause cancer. Heavy support on studies of trillions of viruses; heavy investment on structure and substructure of evolving viruses
		Neglect to systematically understand how viruses initiate immune dysfunction in favor of carcinogenesis
1914	Boveri: Chromosomal mutations in cancer.	Heavy investment on reductionist approaches to identify endless somatic mutations in site-specific cancers for drug development;
	Somatic mutations studies began	
1937	NCI: Established	Government control of public health
1942/1943	Panic of polio	Number of death announced heavily antibiotics used for sanitation
		Public panic and outrage
1944	Avery: Cell DNA transformations	Ongoing heavily supported studies
1950	Traditional cancer drugs (cisplastin, Adriamycin, 5-fluorouracil, vinblastine) available	Chemotherapy with some success
1953	Report on DNA structure	Continued heavy support to date;

(continued)

Table 6.1 (continued)

Year	Discoveries and professional events	Comments, funding support
1955–1963	Salk and Sabin-preparation of polio vaccines in monkey's kidneys. Cutter vaccines were contaminated with SV-40 viruses;	Million doses of prepared contaminated vaccines consumed as injections or sugar pills;
	Young generation inoculated with virus -contaminated polio vaccines, despite discovery and warnings of Bernice Eddy (NIH scientist) that contaminated vaccines could create cancer epidemic;	Americans (current 'baby boomers') paid highest price from virus-contaminated polio vaccines;
		American health status ranks last among other developed nations.
1955	Public outrage and law suits against NIH on virus-contaminated polio vaccines, after loss of many lives; or vaccine-induced paralysis;	NIH and HHS directors resigned;
1957	Mc Farland Burnet: Fundamental theory of immune surveillance for control of cancer growth;	Neglected and minimized to continue support for systematic understanding of immune surveillance
1961–todate	Genetic code reported, identification of somatic mutations in site-specific cancers;	Continued heavy support on identification of infinite number of mutations in site-specific cancers, claims of 'targeted' therapies, 'precision', 'personalized' medicine; failure rates of 90% (±5);
	1960′/1970's; discovery of DMSO (dimethyl sulfoxide) as an inexpensive and potential safe healing agent, alone or as potentiating chemotherapeutic effect of conventional drugs (e.g., cisplatin, Adriamycin, 5-fluorouracil, Vinblastine) for treating several diseases including cancer; controversies on DMSO effects deserve study;	Downplayed role of DMSO; FDA banned its use in USA
1970	Reverse transcriptase studies and cancer	Heavy support
1960s–1990s	Cancer-causing Semian virus-40 (SV-40) polio vaccines	Heavy support on reductionist approaches to structures and substructures of numerous microbiota or individual molecules for cancer research and treatment continued;
	Discovery of T cell receptor genes, immunoglobulin genes; major histocompatibility complex (MHC);	Absence of systematic study on immune dysregulation and how carcinogenesis is initiated;

(continued)

Table 6.1 (continued)

Year	Discoveries and professional events	Comments, funding support
1971	Cancer act: Pres. Nixon increased NCI funding to $1.6 B to solve cancer problem in 8 years-	De Vita, director of NCI, initiated new programs; increased employment;
		Absence of any systematic study on what initiate carcinogens, despite numerous circumstantial evidence on a role that infective agents, prior injuries or carcinogens and environmental hazardous material played in carcinogenesis;
1975–todate	Cancer tracking, Surveillance, Epidemiology, and End Results (SEER) and other cancer programs and networks initiated;	Cancer careers increased, heavy support on genomics;
		Lack of evidence on initial molecular events, including initial identification of damage to genetic and epigenetic modifications that lead to multistep tumorigenesis and angiogenesis;
1976	Retroviral oncogenes structure defined	Heavy support continue to date;
1981–1992	Mahin Khatami-research team at Univ. PA: Accidental discoveries; direct evidence for inflammation-induced tumor growth in models of allergies;	NIH funding discontinued;
1991–1992	James Watson (Nobel laureate) resigns as first director of National Human Genome Research Institute (NHGRI) or National Genome Project (NGP);	James Watson resigns over conflict of interest and ethical matters on patenting partial DNA sequences of human genome projects-during Bernadine Healey as NIH director;
	Francis Collins was appointed as NHGRI or HGP director, he is currently NIH director (2009–);	Michael Gottesman, acting director of NHGRI or HGP;

(continued)

Table 6.1 (continued)

Year	Discoveries and professional events	Comments, funding support
2006-to date	HPV vaccine development for vaccinating young public.	Lowy and colleagues hold patents, invested to develop vaccines with drug companies; HPV vaccines sale; disregard for conflict of interest;
	HPV vaccines headed by Douglas Lowy at NCI;	Absence of systematic studies on potential short- and long-term adverse health effects for next generation; serious concerns expressed by professionals around the world on safety of HPV vaccines;
	Douglas Lowy installed as acting director.	Absence of interest to develop a universal vaccine, a prophylactic agent to promote immunity;
	2015–2017;	
	Sixty nine (69) cancer centers urged to vaccinate young generation with HPV	
	2016- Moonshot initiative [VP Biden] increase funding for NCI by $1.6 B. Blue Ribbon Panel formed to justify priority projects,	
	Obamacare insurance to pay for preparation and heavily advertised HPV and meningitis vaccination of young generation	
1998–2009	Mahin Khatami joined NCI/NIH; submitted proposals on role of inflammation in cancer research; design of clinical trials;	Severe opposition, denial, rejection by DCP/NCI/NIH [1999];
	Involved in PLCO cancer screening clinical trials; standardized cancer biomarkers criteria [data elements] for a database; [Fed Reg, NCI invention-2005];	2005; NCI/CCR initiated an inflammation research laboratory;
	2006-submitted comprehensive proposals on extension of 'accidental' discoveries to CCR/NCI/NIH;	2006-CCR/NCI/NIH management requested Khatami for proposal; proposals reviewed by questionable review panel; opposition, denial and rejection to systematically study role of inflammation in tumorigenesis;
		2009, Khatami retired from NCI/NIH
1970s–to date	Identification of hundreds/thousands of growth and apoptotic mediators, enzymes, metabolites, hormones, genetic mutations on site-specific cancers; drug development, clinical trials, immunotherapy [e.g., DFs, ILs, PGs, GFs, checkpoints] and explosion of fields of Omics [proteomics, metabolomics, genomics, lipidomics, glycomics]; specific technologies and use of numerous experimental models of tumors to test drugs prior to clinical trials;	Heavy research investment on chaotic molecular environment of site-specific cancers; heavy investment on too many Omics projects and network activities;
		2003-exploded fields of inflammation in cancer;
		Absence of support for systematic studies on what initiate carcinogenesis;

(continued)

Table 6.1 (continued)

Year	Discoveries and professional events	Comments, funding support
Overall outcomes of 2 centuries of cancer research and therapy	Over 20 million publications; thousands of molecules identified, hundreds of clinical trials; hundreds of cancer drugs, claims of 'targeted' therapies, 'personalized' or 'precision' medicine; virus-contaminated vaccines consumed by public;	Over $30 trillion spent on research, therapy and cancer care;
	American health status lowest among other developed nations.	Specific vaccines (e.g., polio, swine flu, HPV, meningitis) caused more death and diseases than saving lives by vaccines;
		Heavy use of drugs by public;
		Over 50 million patients lost lives due to toxicities of cancer drugs (poisons).
		Therapies for solid tumors produced failure rates of 90% [±5]

[a]This table does not, by any mean, represent all discoveries and observations on a wide range of immunology or cancer topics [e.g., DiGeorgo followed by Robert Good et al (1965–1984) on role of thymus in immunity and definition of 2 arms of humoral (HI) or cell-mediated immune response (CMI) and attempts in bone marrow transplant of severe combined immunodeficiency (SCID); identification of migration inhibitor factors as first lymphokine/cytokine (initiated by Lewis and Rich in 1932 and extended in 1966), and many other pioneers who used immunosuppressive agents (1970s, cyclosporine A), etc.

3 Forgotten Common Sense to Systematically Study Cancer Science: Bases for Lack of Progress in Therapy or Prevention

> Take up one idea that you love enough to consumes and possesses you in all of your awakening moments and in your dreams. That is when you achieve real success and satisfaction in finding happiness and the purpose of your being. (?)

Despite documented historical information on fundamental observations, theories and discoveries of pioneers such as Paul Ehrlich, who discovered the role of inflammatory cells in controlling cancer growth; Peyton Rous, the Father of virology who discovered that viruses induce cancer; Sir McFarland Burnet, who theorized immune surveillance as the ability of body to monitor and control growth of cancer cells; and the work of others that stood the test of time, there is a peculiar absence of interest to support to systematically extend these important logical studies to understand and solve the cancer mystery [5, 10–15, 30–40].

A personal example on the absence of interest to support logical studies in cancer is noteworthy. When author joined NCI/NIH in 1998, during analyses of a large amount of cancer-related data, she found with much excitement that the results of the 'accidental' discoveries that her research team established in 1980s on experimental models of acute and chronic ocular inflammatory diseases were closely related to cancer research. The results of these studies were suggestive of a series of first and only evidence on direct association between inflammation and dysfunction of immune responses toward multistep tumorigenesis. Peculiarly, continuation of submitted proposals, concepts and lectures to systematically extend these fundamental studies met with severe opposition, denial, minimization and rejection by the NCI decision makers (see Chaps. 2 and 4) [5, 10–15, 161, 162]. However, in recent years, it appears that her challenging efforts to promote the essential role of immunity/inflammation in cancer research awakened the entire cancer community within and outside NCI/NIH. Significant increased in funded projects in basic and translational research are invested on numerous inflammatory mediators and therapeutic approaches including cancer immunotherapies reflected in numerous published articles, conferences and networks. However, it is alarming that researchers continue to follow the same reductionists and chaotic methods on endless identification of too many mutational-derived inflammatory molecules for cancer research and immunotherapy. Review of literature shows that the current heavily funded projects on inflammation research or immunotherapy are practically name-changing, using words of 'inflammation' or 'immunotherapy' that created additional confusion in all aspects of research and therapy. While the immunotherapeutic approaches appear more logical, they lack interest to systematically understanding the host tissue complexes of immune and non-immune interactions toward therapy. Such studies are based on identification of specific somatic mutations of defective 'inflammatory' molecules, checkpoints of immune cells (e.g., T cells, DCs or NKs) or activation of specific death factors in the lawless molecular landscape of site-specific cancers [4–6, 10–15, 161, 162].

Among other major factors in lack of progress in cancer research and therapy are endless funded projects on details of evolving structural and biological properties of pathogens/microbes (e.g., viral, bacterial or parasites oncogenes structures and substructures) that are trillions in number. The number of pathogens and their genomic structures and substructures out-number those of human cells and the information on details of evolving behaviors or potencies of the microorganisms proven to be of little value to benefit the public. Studying the evolving properties of pathogens is like identifying 'shifting sands' in the desert. Decision makers who direct such chaotic projects ignore that the biology and potencies of the microorganisms change from individual to individual, organ/tissue to organ/tissue and from time to time. These expensive and useless projects created more confusion in understanding why some antibiotics or drugs work under certain conditions but fail in others. As detailed below, such reductionist views apply to all aspects of cancer research and therapy, including development of pathogen-specific vaccines (e.g., polio, HPV, Swine flu, meningitis) that not only failed to protect public health, the cumulative presence of structures of pathogens is considered immune-overload for the body [5, 10, 161, 162].

4 American Tragedy of 1955s: Virus-Contaminated Polio Vaccines and Sharp Increase in Cancer Incidence and Mortality and Other Chronic Inflammatory Diseases in Baby Boomer Generation: A Sick Drug-Dependent Society

Loyalty to petrified opinion never yet broke a chain or freed a human soul. Mark Twain

In 1900s, one of every 20 individuals (5%) reported to have cancer. That statistic coincided for the genomic factor of cancer development in normal population. In the 1940s (during the polio epidemic and before vaccinating the American public) 1/16 individuals developed cancer. After 1955s and with the intentional introduction of virus-contaminated polio vaccines to the public, cancer incidence and mortality sharply increased to its current deadly epidemic for the baby boomer generation. In the 1970s, the rate of individuals reported to have cancer was 10% (doubled from 1900s). However, in 2013, the American Association for Cancer Research (AACR) announced that 1/3 (33%) of all women and 1/2 (50%) of all men develop cancer in their life time. American health status ranks last among other developed nations despite the tremendous investment for health care (see Chap. 5). In 1940s/1950s, during the polio virus scare, the establishment saw a major opportunity to increase and solidify its power and control public health when virus-contaminated polio vaccines [e.g., polyoma viruses or simian virus-SV-40 cancer-causing viruses] were injected or consumed as 'sugar pills' by the public, despite the warning of a competent microbiologist who discovered that vaccines were contaminated before vaccinating the population. This American health catastrophe was avoidable, if the motives of the establishment were to prevent the cancer epidemic and discarded the million doses of prepared vaccines when the decision makers learned that the vaccines were contaminated in 1955 [5, 161–175].

It is estimated that for every case of polio that was eradicated by vaccines, the virus-contaminated vaccines (small or large filterable viruses including SV-40 or perhaps other viral particles) initiated at least 15 different cases of B cell-derived lymphomas such as aggressive or non-aggressive forms of acute leukemia, lymphocytic leukemia, Burkett's lymphoma, myelocytic leukemia, EBV-positive large B cell lymphoma in elderly, germinal center lymphoma or Kaposi sarcoma-associated herpes virus-encoded proteins in lymphoma whose clinical features, morphologies and pathogenicities in site-specific tissues or how to control or prevent them are topics of numerous clinical and basic science investigations in the last six decades. Numerous death and diseases are associated with other pathogen-specific vaccines such as Swine flu, HPV, pneumonia, meningitis, measles, or other vaccines [5, 10, 161–187].

After 1955s, the percentage of individuals (current baby boomers) who suffer from a number of health conditions such as allergies, neurodegenerative and autoimmune diseases, hypertension, diabetes and cardiovascular diseases, stroke, Alzheimer's, and particularly site-specific cancers significantly increased in comparison with the previous generations, despite the fact that modern medicine and the introduction of antibiotics and better hygiene increased longevity of population in the developed nations (Table 6.2) [5, 10, 161, 162, 177–187].

Table 6.2 List of increased chronic diseases since 1940s and the influence of environmental hazards (see Chap. 5) [5, 10, 161–184].

Number of chronic diseases since 1940
Influence of environmental hazards
2.2 million women are living with breast cancer
7.2 million women have coronary disease
9.8 million women are afflicted with one of the following seven or more common autoimmune diseases:
Lupus
Scleroderma
Rheumatoid arthritis
Multiple sclerosis
Inflammatory bowl disease
Sjogren's
Type 1 diabetes

5 Maintenance of Health: Biological Laws in Policing Body's Health. Biphasic/Dual Roles of Yin and Yang Pathways in Acute Inflammation

> A believer, a mind whose faith is consciousness, is never disturbed because other persons do not yet see the fact which he sees. Ralph Valdo Emerson[4]

Details on fundamental observations that Virchow, Ehrlich and others documented on the role of immune cells in recognizing and eliminating the tumor cells in the nineteenth century and early twentieth century as well as, Burton' s theory of immune surveillance in 1957 are provided in Chaps. 1 and 2 (Table 6.1) [5, 10, 30–39]. The important theory of immune surveillance (effective immunity) was based on analyses of a large amount of diverse biological information in Burton era. It describes that the immune system is capable of monitoring and controlling the growth of cancer cells and protecting organ systems from being harmed by elements that are perceived useless or threaten body's survival throughout life. The ability of immune surveillance to encounter, fight, arrest and neutralize hazardous elements and maintain health is provided through the self-terminating and protective mechanisms of acute inflammation. Since 2008, this fundamental theory was extended by Khatami based on analyses of a large body of information on inflammatory responses and tissue-specific immune disorders including site-specific cancers [5, 10–15]. Khatami described that acute inflammation (effective immunity) is the balance between 2 highly regulated and biologically opposing arms, termed Yin (apoptosis, initiation, pro-inflammatory, growth-arrest or tumoricidal) and Yang (wound healing, post-inflammatory, termination, growth-promote or tumorigenic) of immune

[4] Ralph Valdo Emerson. [1803–1882] an American essayist, lecturer, poet and philosopher who led the Transcendentalist movement of the mid-19th century-author of 'Nature' and 'The Conduct of Life'. Wikipedia

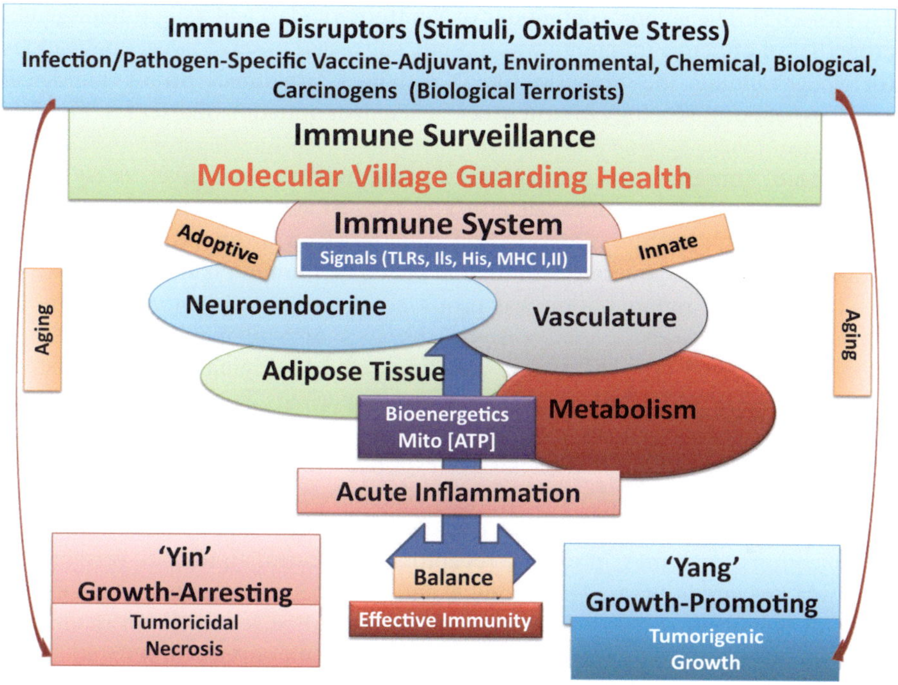

Fig. 6.1 Schematic representation of effective immunity provided through 'Yin' and 'Yang' of acute inflammation. It involves an elaborate crosstalk between immune and non-immune systems [(e.g., innate and adaptive immune cells, vasculature, neuroendocrine, metabolism, adipose tissue, mitochondria (bioenergetics)] to combat and destroy foreign elements such as infective agents, cancerous cells, pathogen-specific vaccines, environmental hazards, carcinogens, and injured host tissue and to resolve and terminate inflammation. Scheme also depicts that oxidative stress (stimuli, immune disruptors and aging) are biological terrorists that could alter the balance between Yin-Yang, leading to tissue necrosis (tumoricidal) or growth (tumorigenic) toward initiation and progression of chronic diseases or cancer. See text

cells that are intimately facilitated by crosstalk with non-immune systems (e.g., vasculature-metabolic-genomic-hormonal-neuronal pathways) to protect the body against all foreign elements (see Chaps. 2 and 4) (Fig. 6.1) [5, 10, 11].[5] In the last decade, the terms Yin and Yang have been increasing used in immunology-related literature for describing individual immune cells (e.g., MΦs) or inflammatory mediators/cytokines, redox regulation, autophagy or mitochondria, etc. [5, 10,

[5]The concept of Yin and Yang of acute inflammation was originally circulated to Nature journals; Nat. Rev. Cancer (NRC) and Nat Rev. Immunology (NRI), in 2006 [NRC-06-235 V 1] and 2007 respectively, followed by submission to Science. Editor of NRC rejected the article saying they were not interested in mast cells topic for cancer! In 2007, Editor of NRI stated that the article was potentially interesting to their readership but they cannot publish the article as they commissioned to publish a similar article! It should be noted that the Editor of NRI is no longer with the journal. Since then, the use of the terms Yin-Yang increased in immunology-related literature for describing individual immune cells (e.g., MΦs), various inflammatory mediators/cytokines, redox regulation, autophagy, mitochondria, etc.

11, 188–202]. The author's definitions of Yin (tumoricidal) and Yang (tumorigenic) properties of effective immunity was recently suggested to serve larger applications for understanding the biphasic (dual) activities (rhythmic, on-off biological switches) of body's biology in sustenance of health or initiation of diseases (Fig. 6.1) [5, 10].

Chronic (unresolved, subclinical) inflammation (oxidative stress) was hypothesized as the loss of balance in Yin-Yang of acute inflammation, accompanied by exaggerated expression and co-expression of apoptotic and wound healing factors that generate an immune chaos or immune tsunami in host tissues. Unresolved inflammation was proposed as a common denominator in the genesis of all age-associated chronic diseases or site-specific cancers. As recently described [10–15] among age-associated biological readjustments in tissues/organs, the sustained oxidative stress perhaps has the most adverse cumulative influence in immune and non-immune cells (e.g., APCs, T and B cells, epithelium, endothelium, GCs) responses that would damage cellular components (e.g., membrane, cytoplasm, chromosome, mitochondria, ER, lysosome, Golgi apparatus) and related molecules (e.g., DNA/RNA, epigenetic modifications, enzymes, proteins, receptors, cytokines, lipids) in vertebrates, invertebrates and humans. These logical and systematic concepts that are extensions of our original data on a series of 'accidental' discoveries on models of acute and chronic inflammatory diseases have been supported, directly and indirectly by numerous isolated and fragmented basic research, histopathological or clinical studies including treatment options for acute and chronic inflammatory diseases or site-specific cancers (see Chaps. 2 and 4) [5, 10–15, 78–90, 200–400].

As detailed throughout this book, for over a century compelling evidence demonstrated the roles that potent pathogens or severe trauma play in the induction of 'cytokine storm' that often lead to life-threatening acute inflammatory diseases (e.g., sepsis, pneumonia, meningitis) [5, 10–15, 204–226, 373–386]. Cancerous cells (defective cellular components) should be regarded as any other pathogens (viruses, bacteria, parasites) whose survival are dependent on the destruction of the host effective immunity; the amazingly ordered networks of immune and non-immune systems, whose job is to petrol and secure the body's health. Aging and persistence disruption or disturbance of immunity by frequent exposures to immune disruptors ('biological terrorists') could allow leaks in the highly orchestrated network of effective immunity that are provided through inherent dual function of Yin and Yang of acute inflammation. Further review of a large body of basic and clinical reports on acute and age-associated chronic inflammatory diseases and altered metabolism and function of tissues, we suggested that the induction of chronic diseases or site-specific cancers is the results of accumulation of heterogeneous degrees of body's hypo-, or hyper-sensitivity responses toward new or old antigens (see below) [5, 10–15, 355–510].

6 Hypersensitivity Reactions or Biological Terrorists: Tissue-Specific Immune Disorders or Cancers

Only she who attempts the absurd can achieve the impossible [?]

Ordinarily, innocuous substances and occasional exposures to a wide range of foreign elements are ignored by the immune system in tissues that are immune-responsive or immune-privileged, to various degrees. The condition is termed immune tolerance. The immune-privileged tissues (e.g., CNS, BBB, cornea, neuro-retina, reproductive organs) which are highly sensitive toward oxidative damage possess special features to ignore responses toward oxidative damage by foreign elements (stimuli). These tissues present higher and specific levels of immune tolerance, compared with those described for immune-response tissues (reviewed in Chap. 2) [5, 10–15]. However, the levels of immune tolerance are limited in both types of tissues. Under certain circumstances (acute or persistent tissue stimulation) the irritating components are deemed potential hazards (biological terrorists) to stimulate a wide range of immune responses leading to various degrees of acute or delayed hypersensitivity reactions or immune disorders (Fig. 6.2) [5, 10–15, 161, 162, 342–369].

Hypersensitivity reactions are generally classified as type I, II, III and IV immune/inflammatory reactions. Type I or immediate hypersensitivity reactions involve antigen-(immune-disrupter) induced activation of innate immune cells such as mast cells (MCs) acting as effector cells. The process initiates by stimuli- (allergen, parasites) activation of B/plasma cells and synthesis of antigen-specific IgE and IgG antibodies followed by sensitization of the mast cells (MCs) or basophils; synthesis of specific receptor and surface molecules involved in signaling and binding of IgE to MCs Fcε-R (receptor molecules). Upon re-exposure to sufficient amount of the same stimuli, antigen-IgE-fcεR-complex aggregates and the sensitized MCs become activated (pharmacologic effects) to degranulate and release vasoactive substances (e.g., histamine) and other preformed or newly synthesized mediators for producing rapid (within minutes) allergic symptoms (e.g., ocular, skin, gastrointestinal or lung airway reactions) (Yin events of acute inflammatory responses) [5, 10–15]. Depending on the nature and exposure frequency to stimuli, the process of MCs sensitization and activation takes about 9 days to a couple of weeks. Typical example of type 1 hypersensitivity reactions that often occur toward ordinary innocuous antigens is exposure to pollen. The IgE antibody production by B cells is often T cell-dependent and accompanied by expression of mediators such as IL-4 and involving CD4+ and TH2 (helper) cells, in an attempt to contribute/facilitate apoptosis and also to terminate and resolve acute inflammation (Yang events). The acute inflammatory responses (Yin and Yang processes) are facilitated by activation of vascular components, with the involvement of endothelial cells, vascular hyperpermeability, efflux of plasma proteins, infiltration of monocytes and blood components (see Chaps. 2 and 3) [5, 10–15, 342–375].

Review of literature on inflammation and multistep carcinogenesis demonstrate ongoing and controversial debates and misinformation about the role of inflamma-

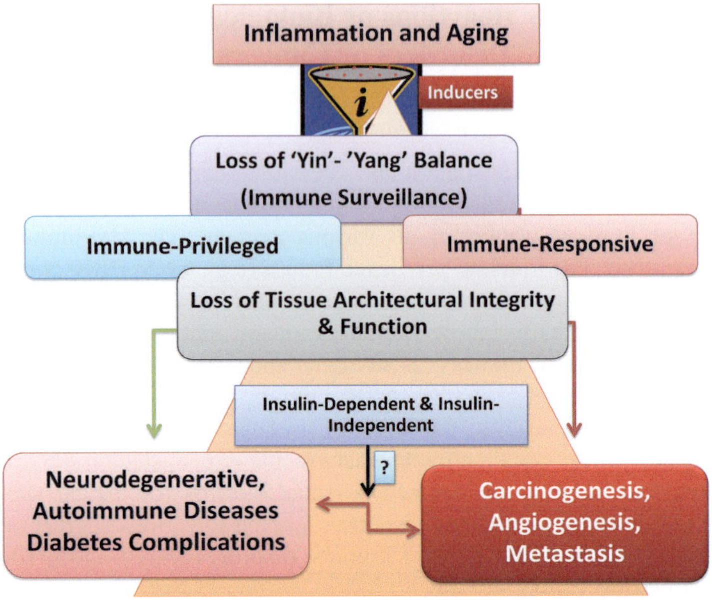

Fig. 6.2 Schematic representation that inflammation and aging (stimuli or inducers) result in loss of Yin-Yang balance of effective immunity. It depicts that oxidative stress differentially influence tissues that are immune-privileged, immune-responsive, or insulin-dependent and insulin-independent for glucose transport and metabolism. Altered tissue integrity and function could lead to initiation and manifestation of nearly all age-associated chronic diseases. See text

tion in allergies and chronic immune disorders and whether inflammation is protective in preventing cancer or it induces tumorigenesis and site-specific primary or secondary cancers [5, 10–15, 55, 56, 61, 285–371]. For example, several reports suggest the role of asthma, other allergies or circulating IgE as protective (decreasing) the risk of cancer, while IgE blocking antibodies or its receptor molecules are proposed to treat allergies or cancer along with other cancer drugs [5, 10, 157, 158, 344, 345, 351–354]. Analyses of data from a number of reported basic research and clinical studies including ours suggest that in general, aging process and repeated exposures of tissue to allergen, antigens, infective agents or biochemical and environmental or airborne hazards (e.g., dust mites, pet allergens, mold, nitrogen dioxide, ozone, sulfur dioxide, particulate matter, volatile organic agents), are 'immune disruptors' and would lead to expression of a combination of receptor molecules that would increase polarization of immune cells (Fig. 6.2). We demonstrated that altered immune response profiles during chronic inflammation (oxidative stress) change the protective role of acute inflammation (e.g., IgE-dependent tissue responses toward allergen) in preventing cancer [5, 10–15, 243, 361, 363].

Depending on the type of tissue and inflammatory conditions, stimuli-induced increased polarization of immune cells often accompany the following major events that would lead to immune suppression [5, 10–15, 329–339, 365–372] (Figs. 6.2 and 6.3):

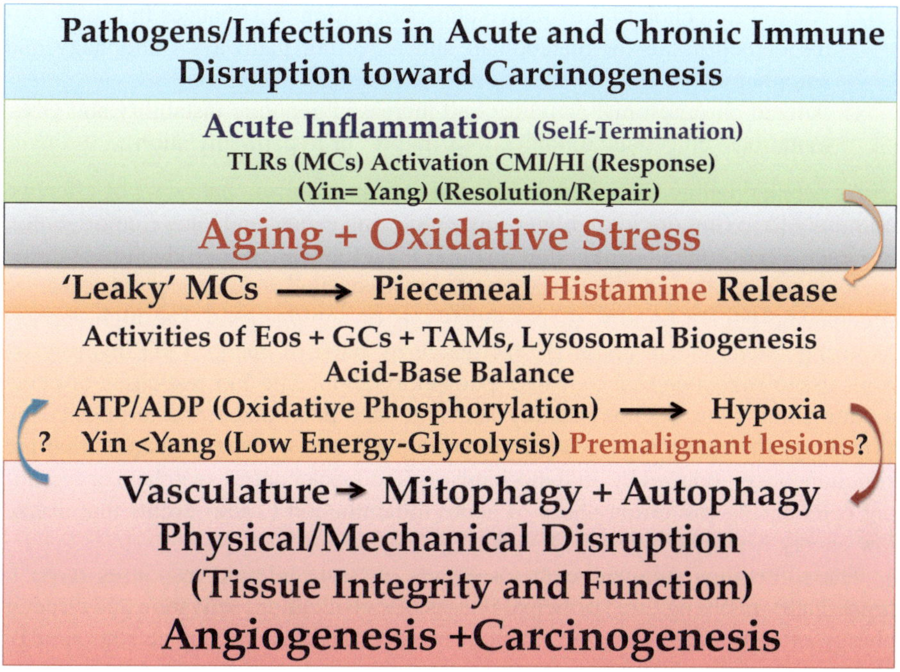

Fig. 6.3 Schematic representation that pathogens/infections induce acute or chronic inflammation toward carcinogenesis. The complex scheme shows that acute inflammation involves activation of MCs through toll-like receptors (TLRs) and responses from cell mediated or humoral immunity (CMI/HI) through activities of Yin and Yang pathways that lead to resolution of inflammation (self-terminating, protective). The scheme also represents that aging and unresolved inflammation (oxidative stress) lead to exhausted ('leaky') activities of MCs and release of low level histamine in surrounding tissue that contribute to infiltration, altered activity and polarization of other cells and components, such as Eos, GCs, TAM, lysosomal recycling pathways, acid-base balance, altered/reduced ratio of ATP/ADP (low energy) and induction of hypoxia. Loss of Yin and Yang balance is depicted to induce hypoxia and enhanced glycolysis that facilitate tissue growth and premalignant lesions. Multistep pathways in carcinogenesis and angiogenesis also involve altered activities of vasculature, mitochondria function (mitophagy) and autophagy that would further disrupt physical and mechanical behaviors and function of tissue. See text

(i) Development of 'leaky' MCs (TAMC) and release of low level histamine (piecemeal, independent from allergen-specific IgE-fcεR binding) into local (host) or distal tissue environment;
(ii) Increased infiltration of eosinophils;
(iii) Altered vasculature activities;
(iv) Increased ratios of mature/immature dendritic cells (DC2/DC1 or TADCs);
(v) Increased mucus secretion and synthesis of IgA;
(vi) Induction of M2/M1 (TAMs);
(vii) Altered activities of NK cells (NKs);
(viii) Increased polarization of T and B cell (Th1, Th2, Treg, B/plasma) phenotypes;

(ix) Altered mitochondrial oxidative phosphorylation and changes in energy status of cell/tissue for metabolism and recycling pathways (mitophagy and autophagy;
(x) Altered chromosomal activities and increased genomic instability and DNA mutations, epigenetic modifications (hypo-, or hypermethylation);

As detailed below, disturbed differential energy-requiring pathways of effective immunity [Yin (tumoricidal), high energy requiring events and Yang (tumorigenic), low energy requiring of acute inflammation] lay a foundation for induction of tissue necrosis or growth and manifestation of age-associated inflammatory diseases or site-specific benign tumors, cancer metastasis or angiogenesis. The high energy-requiring events in Yin phase are facilitated by burst of energy (ATP hydrolysis) from tissue mitochondrial oxidative phosphorylation. The Yin responses of acute inflammation must be immediately and precisely neutralized and terminated by expression of factors with growth promoting and anti-oxidant properties that are simultaneously induced by dual mechanisms (feedback control switches) or recruiting cells during resolution phase of acute inflammation (Yang) events that utilize low energy from glycolysis [5, 10–15].

The followings summarize major events in acute allergic responses (type I, immediate) involving three principal phases of sensitization, activation and effector phases, often initiated by involvement of mast cells (MCs) through activation of B/plasma cells during Yin responses and expression of pro-inflammatory or initiation factors (details in Chap. 2) [5, 10–15, 345–363, 381–397, 500–536]:

(i) **Sensitization phase:** involving B cells (act as innate immune cells for encountering antigen and the synthesis of IgE and sensitization of mast cells (MCs, act as effector cells), expression of antigen-specific receptor and surface molecules;
(ii) **Activation and Effector (pharmacological) phase:** binding of IgE antibodies to sensitized MCs-Fc receptor molecules (IgE-FcεR). Upon further exposure to the same stimuli, aggregation of antigen-IgE-FcεR-binding causes MCs degranulation and release of preformed or newly synthesized molecules. The most important mediators that are released during effector phase are histamine, heparin and prostaglandins, activation of vasculature complement cascade enzymes and a number of other pro-inflammatory cytokines and enzymes;
(iii) **Termination phase of acute inflammation:** involving expression of post-inflammatory mediators, such as growth factors, anti-oxidants, and cytokines with wound healing properties to terminate inflammation and repair any damage inflicted by hazardous agents and pro-inflammatory mediators (Yin events), and to reconstruct host tissue. Mediators that participate during wound healing (termination phase) of an acute inflammation often are facilitated through polarization of immune cells (e.g., leaky MCs, M2, Treg) induction of memory cells, vascular-derived growth factors, mucus secreting goblet cells, as well as endocrine hormonal regulation (epinephrine, thyroid hormones, cortisol).

It is noteworthy that the extent and complexity of immune response profiles depend on the function of the organs/tissues toward enteric (internal) and external exposures to biohazards. For example, in the complex composition of gut-associated lymphoid tissues (GALTs), the balance between Yin (tumoricidal) and Yang (tumorigenic) responses are protective of gut flora and maintenance of homeostasis of trillions of diverse microbial/microbiota (bacteria, fungi) in the gut flora (enteric microbiota) that are normally beneficial to health and facilitate food digestion and maintain acid-base balance of gastrointestinal track. Effective immunity in GALTs is additionally responsible for guarding the tissue against extrinsic harmful elements in food and ingested viruses or bacteria [5, 10, 66, 245–250, 252, 254, 262, 475, 519]. Significant imbalance in the enteric and external hazardous components are associated with a number of mild, moderate or severe compromised immunity in conditions such as allergies, autoimmunity, diabetes, autism, depression, Alzheimers, Yeast (fungi) overgrowth and site-specific cancers [5, 10, 66, 245–250, 252, 254, 262, 475, 519]. Therefore, effective immunity (composition and response profiles of immune and non-immune cells) in the GALTs, being the interface of external-internal environments, is expected to be more sophisticated than other organ systems (e.g., lymph nodes, skin or ocular tissues). In fact about 70% of body's complex immune system is in the crucial position of digestive/gastrointestinal track. The immune composition in GALTs also presents shared features with other tissues that are responsible for fighting against external harmful agents, such as the respiratory lung-associated lymphoid tissues (LALTs) or conjunctival-associated lymphoid tissues (CALTs) for early sensitization and tolerance (induction of Th2 phenotypes) against perennial allergens (e.g., dust mites or cat epithelium). The special features of immunity and tolerization in GALTs (e.g., increased numbers of plasma cells lining the gut epithelium for production of IgA and IgE, TLRs, enzymes and hormones) are required for maintenance of the homeostasis of gut microbiota (intrinsic foreign elements) and ingested foods. It should be also noted that the initial immunity and tolerance in respiratory and gastrointestinal tracts develop during fetal growth. Fetus immunological system, as detected in cord blood has Th2 phenotypes, is the basis for protection of 'graft-versus-host' reactions or tolerization [5, 10, 245–250, 495–497].

It is noteworthy that frequent exposure to stimuli including consumption of inactivated segments of infective agents and associated adjuvants (e.g., aluminum, mercury, L-histidine or stabilizers, chemicals) that are used in pathogen-specific vaccines (e.g., polio, measles, HPV, swine flu, shingle, BCG) could induce an 'antigen overload' or sustained oxidative stress and activation of a number of immunosuppressive pathways such as hyporesponsiveness of T cells (down-regulation of Th1), increased Th2 or regulatory cells (Treg), induction of antibodies [e.g., IgE, IgG isotypes (e.g., IgG1, IgG2, or IgG 4)] that would retard effective immunity toward increased allergies, autoimmune or neurodegenerative diseases or cancers, even in younger individuals [5, 10, 161, 162].

The sources of allergens/stimuli are diverse and include plants, fungi or fungal spores, parasites, pollen, house mites, foods such as milk, eggs, peanuts and cereals, insect venom, drugs, animal dander, as well as preserved or genetically altered food products (genetically modified organisms-GMOs), or perhaps frequent exposures to various environmental radio waves and electronic devices [5, 10–15, 161, 162, 246,

248, 249, 350, 355, 385, 388, 505]. It should be emphasized that many specific vaccines [e.g., inactivated high potency structures of human papilloma viruses (HPVs) or polio] or bacteria (mengiococcal, swine flu) that are used for prevention of certain infectious diseases or cancers should be considered as immune disruptors ('antigen overload') rather than immune promoters of the body. While pathogen-specific vaccines may provide some protection against specific infective agents, they often cause immediate clinical, subclinical or delayed hypersensitivity reactions. The long-term health hazards of many immune disruptors including pathogen-specific vaccines and potential shifts in immune response profiles in tissues that create an 'antigen overload' and contribute to multistep chronic diseases or site-specific cancers are discussed elsewhere [5, 10–15, 161, 162, 242, 363]. Furthermore, the need for developing universal vaccines and prophylactic agents that logically promote body's general immunity for prevention of diseases is yet to be seriously thought of [5, 161, 162].

As depicted in Fig. 6.4, depending on the type and susceptibility of target tissue and expression profiles of inflammatory mediators (accumulated mismatched immune responses), oxidative stress could induce tissue necrosis (growth-arrest) or tissue growth promotion toward multistep disease processes such as neurodegenerative or autoimmune diseases or tumorigenesis and angiogenesis [5, 10–15].

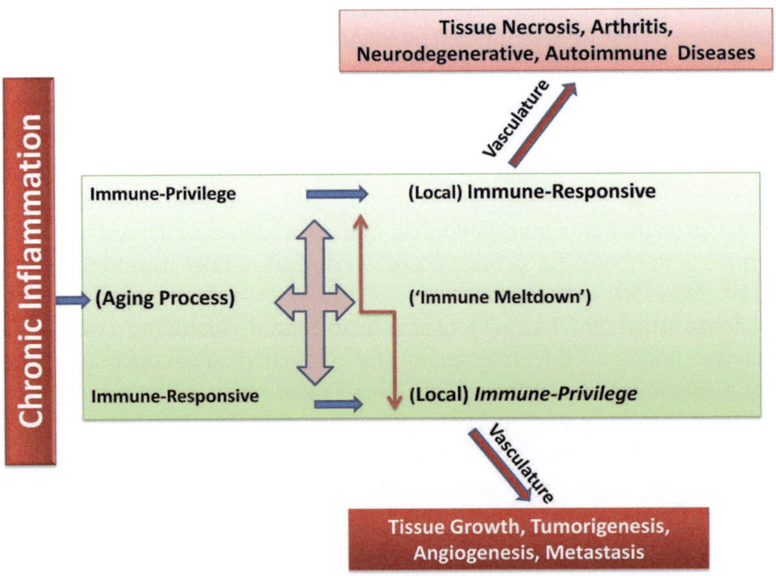

Fig. 6.4 Schematic representation that aging process and chronic inflammation would lead to response shifts ('immune meltdown' or 'immune tsunami') in immune-privileged or immune-responsive tissues toward tissue necrosis and/or growth. The scheme depicts that response switches in immune-privileged tissues cause local immune responsiveness toward necrosis and neurodegeneration of tissue. In contrast, in immune-responsive tissues, loss of Yin and Yang balance was hypothesized to induce expression of selective factors to cause local immune-privilege and facilitate tumor growth promotion and angiogenesis. See text

While there are a number of compensatory mechanisms to ensure maintenance of health, an 'antigen overload' could increase defects in any one of the complex cellular, metabolic, hormonal or genomics signals, enough to disturb the precise crosstalk between apoptotic and/or wound healing pathways causing exaggerated expression or co-expression of mediators that would lead to immune meltdown (immune chaos or immune tsunami) and adversely influence tissue function toward multistep disease processes in vulnerable tissues.

In summary, sustained unresolved inflammation ('antigen overload') or 'biological terrorists' would generate a spectrum of adverse or deleterious effects that could manifest as diverse allergies or immune disorders that were recently classified as 'mild', 'moderate' or 'severe' clinical symptoms. It is estimated that 20% of populations in USA suffer from some forms of allergies. Aging process and increased encounters with offending allergen and increased levels of free radicals in host tissues have been reported as rational for threshold effect of IgE and the increased allergies [e.g., asthma, skin eczema, hay fever, urticaria (hives), ocular inflammatory responses] or perhaps other health conditions such as gastritis, pancreatitis, hepatitis, or colitis in adults (see following sections) [5, 10–15, 161–183, 350–363, 384, 385, 445].

7 Immune Disorders: Common Denominators of 'Mild', 'Moderate' or 'Severe' Hypersensitivity Responses: Cancer a 'Severe' Cumulative Altered Immune Responses that Destroy Architectural Integrity of Tissue

7.1 Histamine a Blue Print? [An Idea Who's Time Has Come!]

Part of the secret of a success in life is to eat what you like and let the food fight it out inside.
Mark Twain

Aging is associated with biological rearrangements (biological senescence) accompanied by minor or major changes in immune and non-immune responses (immunosenescence) of tissues that would result in ineffective wear or tear (degeneration and regeneration) of organ systems. Longevity and repeated/frequent exposures to infective agents/microbiota or pathogens (e.g., viruses, bacteria, parasites or other microorganisms) or environmental, chemical or biological hazards (low level carcinogens) could cumulatively retard the immune response profiles in susceptible tissues to the extent that would damage the balance between tumoricidal (Yin) and tumorigenic (Yang) properties of protective immune surveillance to cause initiation and progression of chronic diseases including multistep carcinogenesis [5, 10–15] (details in Chaps. 2 and 4).

In the following sections an overview of the types of immediate and late phase inflammatory responses toward manifestation of disease processes will be presented. Comparison will be made that mediators that are identified in tissue-specific cancers share the biological features with those of other reported chronic inflammatory diseases. Such comparison is fundamental to the recently novel hypotheses that site-specific cancers are the results of 'severe' and aggressive (irreversible) forms of immune disorders that progressively destroy the inherent dual properties of immunity.

Scientifically it is logical to conclude that the molecular and functional defects in the complex biological network of effective immunity that guards the body's health, could lead to diverse manifestations of 'mild', 'intermediate' or 'severe' immune disorders or site-specific cancers. The importance of mitochondria and differential bioenergetics of Yin and Yang processes at different stages of life, from fetus organogenesis and development after birth, and throughout adulthood and aging process in the induction of chronic diseases or cancer will be overviewed. Site-specific cancers are considered as advanced and aggressive accumulation of immune disorders ('immune tsunami') that violate biological laws and disturb the amazingly ordered, precise and orchestrated crosstalk between immune and non-immune tumoricidal (Yin) and tumorigenic (Yang) arms of acute inflammation (Fig. 6.5).

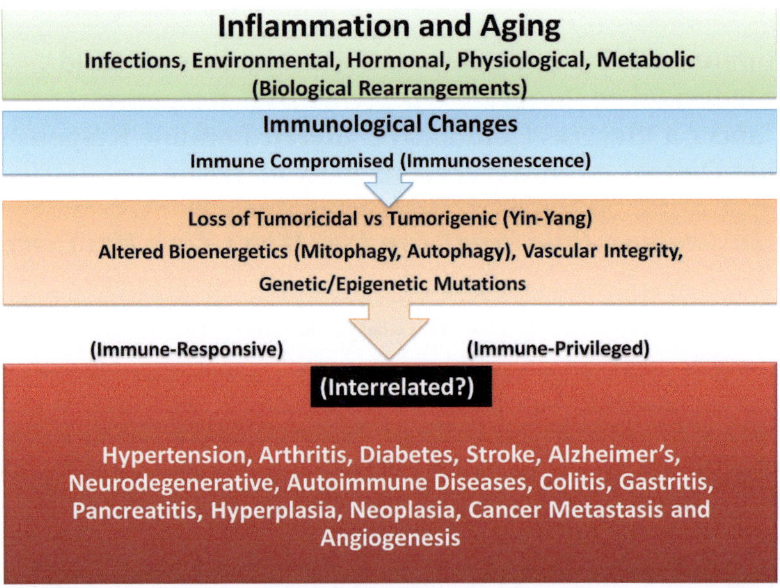

Fig. 6.5 Schematic representation that aging and chronic inflammation are interdependent cofactors in biological and immunological senescence that would increase the risk of age-associated chronic diseases and cancer. Loss of balance in Yin and Yang of immunity would lead to altered mitochondrial and lysosomal functions (mitophagy and autophagy) and other tissue components including vascular and chromosomal activities (e.g., genetic mutations and epigenetic modifications) that contribute to immune response mismatches in immune-responsive and immune-privileged tissues and induction of chronic diseases. The scheme represents that chronic inflammation is a common denominator in the genesis and progression of nearly all chronic disorders that are manifested as different diseases in tissues. See text

The intellectual exercise to integrate some of the available quality of information, while daunting, it is fundamental for comprehending the aging and disease processes and for developing useful biological roadmaps, and connecting the dots or identifying important missing data. Systematic understanding of the complex molecular network that uniquely guard effective immunity is expected to provide crucial clues of what constitutes the biology of health or diseases of aging and how to cost-effectively make decisions on diagnosis, prevention, accurate risk assessment or treatment of diseases.

7.2 *Interdependent Categories in Age-Associated Chronic Diseases*

In general, one should keep in mind that all diseases arise from the following medical/biological categories:

1. Congenital;
2. Hereditary;
3. Neonatal;
4. Induced;

In this book we primarily emphasize on the biological bases of 'induced' diseases. The important roles of biological hazards (e.g., pathogens and vaccines + ingredients)-induced expression of 'designer' or 'transient' receptor molecules that alter tissue bioenergetics and induction of immune disorders are the topics of discussion in this chapter.

Describing biological defects that contribute to other disease categories is beyond the scope of this monogram. However, it is likely that all other diseases possess, to varying degrees, shared features of defects in genetics-immune-hormonal-bioenergetics-metabolic-neuronal pathways with those that are described for induced diseases. It is also logical to consider that aging process is the outcomes of mixed innate+induced biological defects that would increase the risk of chronic diseases.

Special or shared biological complications of full-blown diseases that generally determine the outcomes of nearly all chronic conditions fall into three major interdependent categories:

(a) Vascular and lymphatic channels disorders;
(b) Tissue necrosis;
(c) Tissue growth.

There is little dispute that when the body ages, changes occur in the availability, transport, physiology or quality of hormones, metabolites, nutrients and associated receptor molecules and immune response dynamics in tissues (Fig. 6.5). These changes demand biological readjustments in organ systems (biological and immune-senescence) that accompany minor or major alterations in the function of immune and non-immune systems and altered (tardiness) inflammatory responses to old and new challenges and the initiation of a wide range of chronic diseases in immune-responsive or immune-privileged tissues [5, 10–15, 18, 72, 75, 183, 232, 233, 239–242, 259, 290–304, 334, 363, 367, 422–429, 489–491, 525, 535, 556, 558, 571]. We proposed that maintenance of health depends on the inherently precise expression and regulations of energy-requiring positive and negative biological control switches (biological rhythms or clocks) between the local (host) and distal contributions of innate and adaptive immune cells, vasculature, metabolic, genetic-epigenetic-neuroendocrine or neuro-hysiological pathways.

While the importance of individual genetic makeup (intrinsic factors) in longevity in the delayed onset of diseases is logical, how the confounding extrinsic factors such as the interactions of oxidative stress and aging process would lead to increased somatic mutations and the altered regulations of biological clocks and functions of organ systems in diseases are not understood. The degrees of interactions between the intrinsic (innate and enteric) factors that influence the physiological behaviors of the organs/tissues (e.g., vasculature, metabolic, hormonal, neuronal and immune response pathways) combined with those extrinsic factors (e.g., exposures to chemical, environmental, biological hazards, carcinogens, life styles, specific vaccines) would likely determine the outcomes of age-associated chronic conditions.

In brief, age-associated health conditions such as ocular or skin allergies, asthma, emphysema, hypertension, colitis, gastritis, hepatitis, thyroiditis, lupus, diabetes and cardiovascular complications, stroke, atherosclerosis, other autoimmune and neurodegenerative diseases such as Alzheimer's or Parkinson's and the site-specific cancers seem to be manifestations of different degrees of immune disorders. The challenging questions that may be addressed include to what extent the intrinsic and extrinsic biological heterogeneities and collective responses of organ systems are influenced by the age-induced altered hormonal, physiological, metabolic and immunological rearrangements that contribute to manifestation of specific diseases?

8 Metabolism and Function of Histamine (Catecholamine) in Acute and Chronic Inflammatory Diseases

The interdependent physiological and pharmacological properties of histamine in the induction of acute and chronic inflammatory diseases or carcinogenesis are overviewed in this section. Attempts were made to demonstrate that while different age-associated acute or chronic health problems are manifested in site-specific tissues as different pathological problems, they share molecular and immunobiological characteristics of one health problem- the loss of immune-surveillance, the biphasic properties of self-terminating acute inflammation (Yin-Yang) that is responsible for maintenance of health. We suggested that circulating levels of histamine, above normal, are major contributors in the maintenance of oxidative stress and induction of majority of acute or chronic age-associated disorders or tissue-specific cancers [5]. The biological and clinical effects of histamine that contribute to major immune disorders are summarized below.

8.1 Spectrum of Anaphylaxis and Inflammatory Diseases: When Beneficial Biphasic Yin and Yang of Immunity becomes Health Hazards

The term "anaphylaxis" was introduced by Paul Portiere and Charles Richet[6] in 1902 for explaining the results of their investigation and the mechanisms of marine invertebrate poisons on mammalian physiology. This was the first clinical example that the immune system could be harmful rather than protective or beneficiary to body's health [373–381]. In 1921, the passive transmission of hypersensitivity with human antibody by Prausnitz, known as the P-K reaction, was an important study of human allergy [378]. Originally, anaphylaxis was referred to as a serious and life-threatening form of acute hypersensitivity reactions during which release of vasoactive components (histamine or slow reacting substance of anaphylaxis-SRS-A) from mast cells induced a sudden drop in blood pressure to cause shock. Recent careful assessment of retrospective data from multicenter studies demonstrates that the risk and incidence of different degrees of anaphylaxis are increasing among the general population [5, 10, 350, 353–355, 363, 382–385, 445]. The clinical symptoms and severity of anaphylaxis vary among individuals. The symptoms include hypotension and shock (often fatal) or mild and moderate conditions such as itching, flushing, skin reactions, hives, mucosal and respiratory reactions such as cough, wheezing, dysphonia, chest tightness, shortness of breath, vomiting, cramp-like abdominal pain and diarrhea. The potential triggering factors in anaphylaxis include a wide range of prepared foods with preservatives or genetically modified organisms (GMOs), insect venoms, various drugs and pathogen-specific vaccines, rubber latex or even exercise. The biphasic reactions in anaphylaxis are known as primary or secondary (late) or protracted phases.

The roles that MCs activation and secretion of IgE isotypes (IgEα and IgEβ), their genomic promoter and receptor (e.g., IgE-fc epsilon/fcεR1), surface molecules (e.g., $CD25^{hi}$, CD69, Notch1 and 2,) and many inflammatory mediators (e.g., histamine, IL-1, IL-3, IL-10, Foxp3,...) play in the induction of acute and chronic hypersensitivity reactions or tumorigenesis, as well as the treatment options [e.g., use of corticosteroids or monoclonal antibodies for allergen immunotherapy (omalizumab), indications of graft-versus-host disease or the role of other innate (e.g., eosinophils, basophils, dendritic cells or macrophages) and adaptive immune cells, the formation of memory T and B or regulatory (Treg) cells have been the topics of extensive studies [5, 10–15, 386, 388, 389, 445–447, 453, 462–465, 473–475, 478, 484–544, 493–514, 517]. Analyses of data suggest that the development of

---

[6] In 1913, the Nobel Prize in Medicine and Physiology was awarded to Charles Richet, French physiologist for original experiments on induction of hypersensitivity ('anaphylaxis') reactions in collaboration with Paul Portiere.

immunity and sensitization toward allergen initiate during fetal growth. Our original observations on newborn sensitivity of ocular tissues toward antigen challenges support that the maternal/paternal atopy influences the newborn responses through mast cells activation and IgE production. Maternally transmitted genes (e.g., GSTP1 and IgE-FcεRIβ) are identified with lung airway function and mast cell sensitization. With regard to induction of asthma, the maternal effects on gene-environment interactions and epigenetic modifications were suggested to be greater than paternal influence [5, 10–15, 545–548]. However, due to complexity of the maternal/paternal interactions between ancestral and environmental influence on genetic and immunological make up of the offspring, our understanding of the methods of prediction and treatment remain fragmentary and present huge challenges to overcome.

Use of anti-histamine receptor-1 (HR1) or anti-inflammatory agents is common in treatment of anaphylaxis with different effectiveness. Depending on the severity of anaphylaxis, treatment options include use of neuroendocrine agents such as adrenaline (epinephrine) or intravenous, intramuscular or oral use of steroids or glucocorticoids with family variations of products (e.g., prednisone, prednisolone, methylprednisolone, betamethasone, solu-cortex, dexamethasone, triamcinolone). Use of drug often follows resuscitation. Anti-IgE antibodies (e.g., omalizumab) also have been used for severe allergies such as asthma [345–347, 367, 377, 380, 386, 389, 395, 396, 462, 464, 493–503]. The effectiveness of such interventions is controversial perhaps due to multiple factors including:

(i) Host immune response status to overcome the condition;
(ii) Time course kinetics of induction and clearance of primary or secondary phase of anaphylaxis;
(iii) Varied influence of histamine and receptor molecules (in addition to HR1) in diverse metabolic pathways;
(iv) Bioenergetics of host organ system to overcome shock and potential induction of 'cytokine storm';
(v) The stage of inflammatory reactions and potential contributions of other mediators during anaphylaxis episodes;

Furthermore, as discussed below, the long-term immune suppressive effects of treatment with steroids that contribute to wound healing events (Yang or tumorigenesis) and could potentially change the biphasic dynamics of immune responses toward induction of other health complications such as cell/tumor growth have not been seriously considered.

Severe inflammatory conditions such as sepsis, meningitis, pneumonia that are induced by potent pathogens, or major trauma are various forms of acute immune disorders and often cause induction of 'cytokine storm' or 'immune tsunami'. These severe inflammatory conditions, if not treated properly or immediately, could be life-threatening or may lead to chronic health problems [5, 10–15, 204–226]. Analyses and comparison of data between potent pathogen-induced severe molecular damage to organ system and those of current claimed cancer 'targeted' therapies, 'precision' or 'personalized' medicine, which use monoclonal antibodies against specific growth factors or potent apoptotic agents were recently reported [5, 10–15].

It was suggested that in conditions such as anaphylaxis, sepsis or many cancer drug-induced severe inflammatory reactions and sudden changes in energy demands from mitochondria that could significantly damage tissue oxidative metabolism in mitochondria would alter metabolism of branched amino acids and biosynthesis of structural proteins and other energy-requiring metabolic and physiological activities in target tissues. In brief, potent pathogen- (trauma or 'targeted' cancer drug-) induced internal biological trauma could cause activation of cellular components and secretion of inflammatory cytokines creating an environment that facilitate tissue damage and multiple organ failures (MOFs). The severe tissue damage is the results of a vicious cycle of immune cell activation leading to systemic or intraperitoneal expression of pro-inflammatory cytokines and damage-associated molecular pattern (DAMP), increased C-reactive protein (CRP), altered muscle F-actin filaments and high-mobility group box 1 (HMGB1), expression and co-expression of growth-arresting (Yin, tumoricidal) and growth-promoting (Yang, tumorigenic) cytokines such as TNF-α, ROS, interleukins (e.g., IL-4, IL-6, IL-8, IL-10, IL-12, IL-18), monocyte chemoattractant protein 1 (MCP-1), CXCR3, neutrophil extracellular traps (NETs), abnormal expression of vaculature components (e.g., P- and E-selectins, ICAM-1, VCAM-1) damage to mitochondrial oxidative metabolism and DNA and impaired energy production (ATP) from oxidative phosphorylation, induction of systemic inflammatory response syndrome. The severe inflammatory conditions, also known as immunoparesis or induction of 'immune tsunami', often accompany a range of seriously adverse outcomes for patients including frequent visits or long hospital stays and increased risk of mortality [5–15, 161, 162, 204–232, 265, 280, 285].

In brief, induction of 'immune tsunami' by potent pathogens or cancer 'targeted' or 'designer' drugs could result in the release and interactions of inflammatory mediators such as histamine and other pro-inflammatory mediators (above factors) and the activation and metabolism of membrane arachidonic acid pathways, biogenesis of prostaglandins and platelet metabolism, as well as compensatory mechanisms that would lead to drug-induced clinical complications (e.g., blood coagulation and thromboembolism, cancer relapse, sarcopenia, cachexia, fatigue), serious conditions that lead to severe damages to vital organ systems (e.g., liver, kidney, brain or heart) and multiple organ failures (MOFs) and death.

8.2 *Allergies and Induction of Diverse Diseases and Cancer*

In general, many allergies such as food allergies, asthma, ocular or skin allergies are clinically classified as symptoms of three types of tissue responses, IgE-mediated (acute or type 1), non-IgE-mediated (cellular or delayed type hypersensitivity) and mixed (IgE-mediated and delayed type responses). Analyses of relevant data on acute or chronic inflammatory conditions that were classically identified as Type I, II or III or delayed hypersensitivity responses seem to be the various degrees of loss of balance between the two biologically opposing arms (Yin and Yang) of acute inflammation. The proposed differential effects of inflammation in immune-privileged or immune-responsive tissues and manifestation of nearly all age-associated chronic diseases seem to be the collective consequences of altered metabolic, neuronal and cellular or humoral immune cell activities and directly or indirectly supported by numerous isolated basic research and clinical reports (see below) [5, 10–15, 61, 212–372, 490–600].

9 The Many Faces of Histamine: Friend and Foe!

Analyses and integration of data on biochemical and pharmacological properties of histamine and its direct or indirect influence on organ/tissue metabolism and function in the genesis and progression of nearly all acute hypersensitivity reactions, infections, pathogen-specific vaccines and their ingredients, age-associated chronic immune disorders or site-specific cancers are briefly discussed in the following sections to better appreciate the complexity of histamine role in health and diseases [5, 10–15, 178–184, 220–235, 328–357, 245–249, 275, 328, 345–363, 516, 517–560, 614, 628].

Catecholamine (histamine) stimulates contraction of smooth and cardiac muscles, or bronchoconstriction; the symptoms of anaphylactic shock and sudden change in blood pressure (see above). These life-threatening events required pharmaceutical industries to develop clinical antihistamine drugs. However, ongoing controversies on the effectiveness of drugs and continued search for more effective remedies are continued challenges for the industry perhaps due to the wide influence that histamine, its known receptor molecules and histamine biosynthesis and clearance pathways present in nearly all aspects of tissue metabolism and function (Table 6.3).

The primary source of histamine is tissue MCs, but basophile granules are also able to liberate preformed histamine when provoked. Data from several reports also demonstrate that other cells such as MΦs, smooth muscle, endothelial and fibroblasts are capable of releasing histamine [5, 10–15, 498–503]. Brain ischemic or hypoxic conditions also release histamine to cause changes in astrocytes function or limited normal histamine levels lrvrls, as likely the bases for certain conditions such as idiopathic hypersomnia, obstructive sleep apnea syndrome, as well as diseases such as Parkinson's or perhaps Alzheimer's [5, 10, 267, 275, 345–347, 523, 525–528, 578]. Muscle relaxants [e.g., anaestatic drugs (e.g., suxamethonium, opiods, plasma expanders) and adjuvant] or heavy exercise are also able to release histamine chemically (anaphylactoid) or immunologically (anaphylactic), while the clinical distinction and their mechanisms of actions are debatable [530–534, 569].

Histamine is an alkaline and a vasoactive component that is generated through the actions of the amino acid histidine decarboxylase (L-histidine decarboxylase) present throughout the body. The half-life of histamine is very short (<1 min) but pharmacologic effects of histamine last from 5 to 70 min. The short half-life of histamine in circulation, in all likelihood, is a required specific feature of

Table 6.3 Examples of antihistamine agents that are launched with some success [5, 345–347, 352, 355]

Year–Name	AKA, chemical name	Mode of action, comment
1933 Ethanolamine,	2-isopropyl-5-methyl phenoxyethyl diethylamine	Introduced by Fourneu and Bovet, Pasteur institute
1940s Diphenhydramine; diphenhydramine	N1Ndimethyl-N1-benzyl-N-phenyl-ethylenediamine;	Antergan, phenergan (other histamine receptors-varients—H1-H4- not known)
1940s Promethazine and chlorpromazine	Promethazine and chlorpromazine	Sedative effect, Thorazine – Rhone-Poulenc
1960s	H1 (anti-allergic) antagonists;	H1 antihistamines
Name changed for anti-histamine receptors	H2 antagonists	H2 antagonist gastric acid secretion and prevention of smooth muscle contraction
1970s- (?)	Cimetidine	Tagament-H2 receptor antagonist
1990s Olopatadine (Allelock1, oral), Patanol1, ophthalmic solution)	Olopatadine hydrochloride (11-[Z)-3(dimethylamino)-propylidine]-6,11-dihydrodibenzine[b,e]-oxepin-2acetic acid monohydrochloride)	H1 antagonist, inhibit AA metabolism, tryptase, LTs, PGD2, treatment of rhinitis, chronic urticaria, eczema dermatitis, purigo. Cutaneous pruritis, psoriasis vulgaris, erythma exudativum, allegic conjunctivitis.
1990s Astemisole Oxatomide Norastemisole	Ca2þ fluxes from intracellular stores, distort phase transition and fluidity of artificial membranes [L-alpha-dipalmitoyphosphotidyl choline liposome]	H1 antihistaminic, FcεIgE, inhibit Ca2þ fluxes, exocytosis in rat basophilic leukemia (RBL-2H3) biphasic effect on mediator release.

self-termination properties of acute (immediate) inflammation. In healthy individuals (normal conditions) the baseline levels of circulating histamine are approximately 0.3–1.0 ng/ml, perhaps contributing to the maintenance of acid-base homeostasis in tissues. However, the effective pharmacological levels of histamine to cause pro-inflammatory effects in ocular tissues, skin, gastrointestinal, lung respiratory or neuronal tissues are much greater, ranging from 3 to12 ng/ml. During stimulation of mucus secretion and skin irritation (pruritis), contraction of bronchial smooth muscle or vasodilatation, the histamine levels can reach as high as μM levels [275, 345–347, 350, 628].

Histamine metabolism and turnover occur through two enzymatic reactions of diamine oxidase (DAO) and histamine N-methyl transferase [HNMT, or HNT]. Activation of either enzyme is tissue location-dependent (e.g., peripheral or intracellular spaces). It has been suggested that the HNMT enzyme which is manufactured in a number of tissues (e.g., kidney, liver, brain) has a primarily role in allergic reactions. HNMT metabolizes histamine in the intracellular spaces within organ/

tissue-based responses (e.g., bronchial, skin or perhaps conjunctival epithelium) [10, 329–334, 498–505, 524–526].

Whether fluctuations of brain or other tissue histamine in vaccines (e.g., HPV), containing L-histidine (precursor of histamine) would induce alterations in the function of important histidine-proteins, as additional adverse effects of pathogen-specific vaccines in the induction of neurological or autoimmune disorders are important knowledge gaps [5, 10].

At least three or four types of histamine receptors (HRs, H1-H4) have been identified in producing various physiological effects such as vasodilatation, smooth muscle contraction, gastric acid secretion, brain/neuronal activation and cardiovascular actions [5, 10, 345–349, 362, 363, 516–522]. The most well characterized histamine receptors are H1 Rs. Histamine (H1) Rs are located on vascular endothelial and smooth muscle cells of the upper respiratory tract (bronchi and bronchioles). Release and binding of histamine to H1 Rs cause dilatation of capillaries and hyperpermeability of vasculature for influx of plasma fluids and infiltration of inflammatory cells to the site of target tissue. The actions induce rash or scratch, tearing and swelling (edema) of the skin or ocular inflammatory responses which are characteristics of clinical reactions of acute inflammation. If the vascular hyperpermeability and efflux of plasma fluid are extensive, sudden drop in blood pressure may result in shock (anaphylaxis) as noted above. H1R in smooth muscle contraction in airway tract often leads to breathing difficulties. Strong constriction of lung smooth muscle is perhaps part of defense mechanisms and exaggerated immune responses or tissue attempts to prevent influx/entry of allergen to lung airways. Studying experimental models of ocular acute and chronic inflammatory diseases, we noted that antigen-induced strong clinical ocular type 1 hypersensitivity reactions often accompanied by wheezing-like symptoms. It was suggested that circulating IgE binding caused sensitization of lung airways MCs FcεRs and activation (effector response), degranulation of MCs and release of histamine [5, 10–15, 357–363].

Histamine also binds to H2 receptors of the smooth muscle in the gastrointestinal tract and stimulates the release of stomach acid from the stomach mucosa, often resulting in cramps and severe diarrhea. Furthermore, depending on the location of the receptors, H2Rs stimulate nasal mucus secretion or they increase vascular permeability. As suggested above, the normal levels of circulating histamine, an alkaline agent, are required for contributing to the acid-base balance in different tissues via activation of appropriate receptor molecules [10, 345–347].

The possibility that inhibition of one or 2 histamine receptors or blocking the Ca^{+2} flux in MCs or basophils of local tissue could lead to the activation of altered or compensatory pathways (e.g., expression of decoy HRs or iso HRs) that are not inhibited by specific HRs inhibitors in the induction of immune disorders are yet to be discussed or understood. Furthermore, the roles that anti-histamine drugs play in retarding histamine clearance pathways or metabolic activities as well as the potential drug-, or inflammation-induced histamine biosynthesis and release that would facilitate cell growth or chronic allergic reactions are not understood (manuscript in preparation).

The results of a series of studies that we reported on experimental models of ocular acute and chronic inflammatory diseases in 1980's included massive lymphoid hyperplasia of conjunctival-associated lymphoid tissues (CALTs) as the first evidence for a direct link between inflammation and tumorigenesis and angiogenesis. Analyses of a series data on our 'accidental' discoveries in 1980s on models of acute and chronic inflammatory diseases in conjunctival-associated lymphoid tissues (CALTs) demonstrated at least three stages of interactions between resident (host) and recruited immune cells (details in Chap. 4) [5, 10–15, 360–362]:

(a) Acute phase; activation of mast cells (MCs), induction of IgE antibodies, release of histamine and synthesis of prostaglandins;
(b) Intermediate phase; down-regulation phenomenon, exhausted/degranulated MCs, heavy eosinophils (Eos) infiltrations into epithelia and goblet cells (GCs), tissue hypertrophy and neovascularization; and
(c) Chronic phase; induction of lymphoid hyperplasia, activated macrophages (Mϕs), increased (irregular size) B and plasma cells, loss of integrity of lymphoid tissue capsular membrane, presence of histiocytes, follicular and germinal center formation, increased ratios of local IgG1/IgG2, epithelial thickening (growth) and/or thinning (necrosis) and angiogenesis.

Activated MΦs (TAMs or M2) and eosinophils that are recruited in tissues (e.g., conjunctiva or perhaps lung airways) whose principal resident immune cells are MCs and lymphocytes were suggested to play crucial synergistic roles in enhancing the growth promoting capacities of host toward tumorigenesis. The release of low level histamine and down-regulation phenomenon toward induction of massive hyperplasia of CALTs and distinct phases of immune suppression were associated with increased number of 'leaky' (exhausted) MCs and activation of other inflammatory cells such as eosinophils and MΦs and expression of growth promoting mediators. For example, under oxidative stress, M-CSF could produce signals that are cumulative/synergistic with host mediators (e.g., low levels release of histamine), facilitating tumor-directed expression of decoy receptors and immune suppressive factors (e.g., dTNFR, IRAK-M, IL-5, IL-10, TGF-β, PGE2). We demonstrated that during down-regulation phenomenon, further challenges of conjunctiva with either antigen or MCs degranulating agents such as compound 48/80 produced minimal reaction supporting exhaustion of MCs. Furthermore, tissue challenge with histamine produced strong ocular reactions suggesting that HRs were functional (Fig. 6.6). However, repeated challenges with histamine led to down-regulation phenomenon of tissue [5, 10–15, 357–363]. It was suggested that exhausted MCs ('leaky' MCs) and the release of low level histamine (independent of MCs- IgE-FcεR degranulation) into host tissue environment contributed to infiltration of other immune cells such as eosinophils and recruitment of activated MΦs, that follow a sequence of interactions and synergies between altered (decreased) ratios of tumoricidal (Yin) vs. tumorigenic (Yang) phenotypes of MΦs (M1/M2 or TAMs) resulting cellular growth promotion (Fig. 6.6) [5, 15].

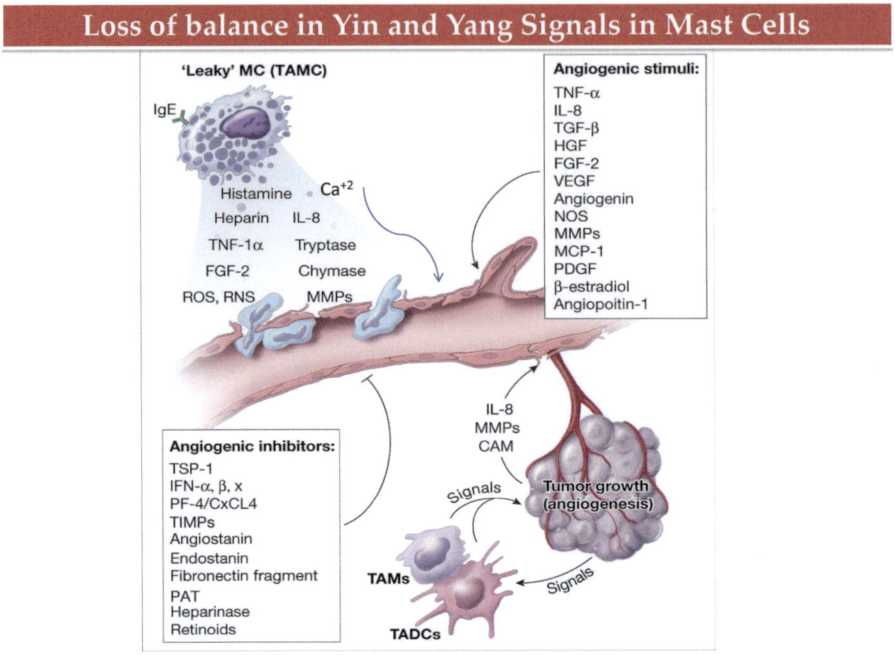

Fig. 6.6 Schematic representation of loss of balance in Yin and Yang signals in mast cells and induction of cell growth and angiogenesis. In acute inflammation, mature MCs are considered tumoricidal and IgE-dependent for degranulation and release of vasoactive components such as histamine. However, oxidative stress induces production of 'unscheduled' immature or partially degranulated or exhausted ('leaky') MCs. Leaky MCs could continuously and slowly release vasoactive mediators such as histidine, heparin, ROS, chymase or tryptase, expression of angiogenic factors from activated vasculature independent of IgE-fceR binding. The scheme depicts that oxidative stress promotes synthesis/expression of mediators that are involved in altered balance in angiogenic [e.g., VEGF, CAMs, hematopoitic growth factor, HGF-FGF-2 and membrane metaloproteases (MMPs), angiogenin 1 (ANG-1), etc] and anti-angiogenic (inhibitors of angiogenesis) factors [e.g., TSP-1 (thrombospondin 1),TPA (tissue plasminogen activator),TIMP (tissue inhibitor of membrane proateases), etc] contributing to activation of other immune cells (e.g., TAMs, TADCs) in the initiation and enhancement of tumor growth and angiogenesis (Adopted from Khatami (Ref. [11]) Exp Opin Biol Ther. with permission.)

In brief, normal levels of circulating histamine are likely required for contributing to the acid-base balance in different tissues via activation of appropriate receptor molecules. Stimuli-induced histamine release and biosynthesis of other pro-inflammatory mediators must be simultaneously and precisely removed and neutralized by expression of anti-inflammatory or wound healing factors, including cortisol or epinephrine, growth factors or enzymes to remove/decompose histamine and also digest histamine receptor molecules in Yang pathways [5, 10–15]. Under oxidative stress, understanding the details of histamine removal pathways or potential modifications of HRs that may lead to adverse health conditions deserve further investigations. Sustained oxidative stress could alter one or combination of the following pathways for histamine metabolism or removal:

(i) Altered or modified histaminases, tryptase or chymase activities;
(ii) Altered biosynthesis or functions of important histidine-related proteins/enzymes [e.g., histidine kinases (phosphorylation), histidine-rich glycoproteins or impaired activities of histidine decarboxylase or diamine oxidase (DAO);
(iii) Insufficient IgE digestion by proteases including tryptase;
(iv) Induction of histamine decoy- or iso-receptor molecules;
(v) Oxidative stress and heterogeneity in MCs biosynthesis leading to abnormal release of histamine in mastocytosis-like conditions in site-specific tissues (e.g., skin or bone);

9.1 Biological Gaps: Connecting Dots on Diverse Function of Histamine Under Oxidative Stress and Aging Process

Analyses of a wide range of basic and clinical data provoke the following questions that are interdependent biological knowledge gaps on the roles that histamine play in health and diseases and proposed future directions for systematic studies [4, 10, 344–347, 361, 388, 389, 501, 523–525]:

(i) Continued tissue stimulation or repeated use of traditional anti-histamine agents could promote cell growth in affected tissues by activating or inducing expression of histamine-like receptors (H-LRs), or histamine decoy receptors (HdRs). Allergic individuals who routinely consume anti-histamine drugs for conditions such as asthma, skin allergies or gastrointestinal tract problems seem to be at greater risk for developing site-specific or distal cancers, perhaps as the results of inhibition of specific HRs. The concept is indirectly supported by large clinical observations that asthmatic patients had higher risks for developing not only lung cancer, but they demonstrated to be at differential risk for other cancers (e.g., higher risk for stomach cancers and lower risk for soft tissue cancers or oral squamous cell carcinoma). The release of histamine or other pro-inflammatory mediators in circulation could potentially decrease the risk of soft-tissue cancers due to accessibility of these tissues to apoptotic mediators;
(ii) Oxidative stress or genetic factors could induce exaggerated and abnormal proliferation of MCs in organ systems and creation of a sub-group of heterogeneous clinical conditions known as mastocytosis affecting primarily the skin or bone marrow often involving systemic events in adults or children. Mastocytosis could enhance histamine release in large quantities that cannot be clinically treated or inhibited by anti-histamine agents or by histamine clearing mechanisms;
(iii) Aging process could impair/retard expression or activities of HRs, or histamine methyl transferase (HNMT) or diamine oxidase (DAO) that contribute to the progression of allergic reactions or histamine intolerance;

(iv) Whether reported increased in the incidence of replacement of a branched amino acid isoleucine 105 (Ile105) in the gene of enzyme histamine N-methyltransferase (HNMT) reported for Parkinson's would also apply to asthmatic patients or histamine intolerance individuals are not understood. The defective biosynthesis of HNMT could also influence mitochondrial oxidative metabolism and energy-requiring biosynthesis of architectural proteins that utilize branched amino acids such as Ile as potential altered activities of HNMT are important knowledge gaps for future investigation;

(v) Whether aging processes (immune-biological senescence) accompany alterations in cross reactivity of expression of HRs or induction of expression of histamine-like receptor molecules (H-LRs) that contribute to altered integrity and function of vasculature or inflammatory responses to old and new challenges are not understood.

10 Energy-Requiring Activation of Immune Cells in Health or Immune Disorders: Role of Mitochondrial Oxidative Phosphorylation and Autophagy

Stimuli-induced activation of innate immune cells such as MCs or MΦs, NKs and DCs requires burst of energy (ATP hydrolysis, high energy demands) from oxidative phosphorylation of mitochondria. For example, activation of MCs (effector pharmacological phase) leads to a decreased intracellular cAMP levels that allow calcium entry into the cell for degranulation processes. The effector phase of MCs activation is associated with the release of histamine and heparin and a number of preformed proteases (chymase or tryptase) followed by metabolism of membrane arachidonic acids (AAs) and activation of cyclooxygenase (COX) and lipooxygenase (LO) pathways and de novo synthesis of prostaglandins (PGs), as well as induction of inflammatory mediators and respective receptor molecules. The bioenergetics of these and other important cellular events including activation of several enzymes (e.g., NADH/NADPH oxidase) and expression of other oxidants, cytokines or mediators (e.g., TNF-α, IL-1, IL-6, IL-10, VEGF, complement cascades) in acute or chronic inflammation are important topics that are not fully understood (Figs. 6.3 and 6.6).

The major parallel and simultaneous on-off switches of response profiles during immune cell activation and complex pharmacological pathways involved in initiation (Yin or tumoricidal) and resolution (Yang or tumorigenic) of acute inflammation are briefly discussed below [5, 10–15].

Sensitization, differentiation, activation or effector functions of leukocytes are energy requiring metabolic events that are under increasing investigation in recent years, particularly with regard to T cell function. Similar to T cells, mast cells (effector cells within the innate immune cells) also undergo a dynamic and multistep metabolic reprogramming upon activation during early and late phase responses. An overview of the energy requiring complex inflammatory responses of degranulation or exocytosis of mast cells and release of a wide range of pre-formed or newly synthesized mediators in target tissue during apoptosis (Yin or tumoricidal) and wound healing (Yang or tumorigenesis) processes are summarized below. The role of chronic inflammation (loss of balance in Yin-Yang) in the developmental stages of age-associated diseases or carcinogenesis are also briefly proposed in the following [5, 10, 544, 557–615]:

(i) **Yin (tumoricidal – high energy consuming events): oxidative phosphorylation and mitochondrial role:** Involving burst of energy (ATP hydrolysis) required for secretory lysosomal activities, membrane fusion, exocytosis and ion fluxes, vascular hyperpermeability;
(ii) Acid-base homeostasis required for release of histamine and heparin during MCs degranulation and exocytosis processes;
(iii) Oxidative phosphorylation events (ATP hydrolysis) in the production of ROS from mitochondria to facilitate destruction of structure of foreign elements (e.g., allergen or parasites) and potential signals for activation of other immune cells (e.g., eosinophils, T or memory cells);
(iv) ROS-induced shut-down events in mitochondria for the TCA cycle regeneration;
(v) **Yang (tumorigenic-low energy consuming events): glycolysis Warburg effect:** Switching from oxidative phosphorylation (high energy demand from ATP hydrolysis of Yin) to low energy ATP production from glycolysis for termination of acute inflammation and wound healing or tissue repair. The events are similar to bioenergetics of cancer cells growth when mitochondrial function is impaired (see below);
(vi) Recycling of proteins and lipids of phagocytised materials, expression of lysosomal hydrolases and proteases in autophagy;
(vii) Termination/resolution of acute inflammation, wound healing, remodeling and repair of target tissue;

The precise sequences of events involved in simultaneous activities of Yin and Yang processes of acute inflammation that result in neutralization of foreign elements and repair of target/host tissues that include contributions from metabolic, neuronal and hormonal pathways are crucial biological gaps to be understood.

In a recently proposed working model, we hypothesized that the interdependent complex response dynamics of tissues toward external and internal stimuli require differential cellular bioenergetics. It was suggested that requirements for mitochondrial function to provide high energy at moment notice for combating foreign elements (pathogens, biological, chemical and environmental hazards) develop after birth for maintaining health and controlling diseases throughout life. Age-induced dysfunction of mitochondria could influence bioenergetic of Yin (tumoricidal) and Yang (tumorigenic) resulting in initiation of diverse health problems as 'mild', 'moderate' or 'severe' immune disorders, including site-specific cancers (see below) [5, 10].

11 Bioenergetics of Mast Cell Exocytosis, Secretory Lysosomes and Ca^{+2} Fluxes in Acute and Chronic Inflammation

Lysosomes play important roles in regulation of exocytosis and the breakdown of phagocytosed protein and lipid materials or cell debris for recycling processes. In general, degranulation of MCs and release of diverse charged molecules (e.g., histamine and heparin) or other mediators do not follow the 'all or none' pharmacological effects. For example, under a wide range of inflammatory conditions, allergen-induced membrane fusion often involves piecemeal release of mediators from MCs and lysosomal activities. The complex pathways during degradation, clearance and recycling of proteins, require energy-dependent biosynthesis of a number of acidic hydrolases or proteases and surface molecule signaling within endoplasmic reticulum (ER), Golgi apparatus and lysosomes. The review of relevant data demonstrates that these interdependent pathways are universal in living cells and influenced by aging and disease processes. The summarized events with emphasis on the role of MCs activation are provided below [5, 10–15, 275, 369, 370, 390, 393, 423–426, 436, 587–655].

The early events of FcεR aggregation and MCs degradation require membrane fusion for exocytosis of granules or the secretory lysosomes processes involving activation of a number protein receptor molecules at different stages of membrane fusion, requiring ATP hydrolysis and Ca^{+2} mobilization from intracellular stores. The lysosomal exocytic events are triggered following an increase in the free Ca^{2+} concentration acidified by protons (H^+/ATPase) for fusion and flux at the plasma membrane level. A number of studies using anti-allergic or antihistaminic agents (e.g., oxatomide, astemizole, olopatadine) demonstrated the role of IgE-fcεR, histamine and Ca^{+2} flux, as well as AA metabolism in several in vivo (e.g., rats) or in vitro models of allergies or basophilic leukemia cells (RBL-2H3) [49, 345–347]. Additionally, agents such as olopatadine hydrochloride were shown to inhibit inflammatory cytokines such as IL-4 expression by MCs both in vivo and in vitro. Olopatadine differentially inhibited Ca^{+2} influxes through receptor-operated channels (ROC) without affecting Ca^{+2} release from intracellular stores. The actions were associated with suppressed phosphorylation of P38 mitogen-activated protein kinase and c-Jun NH2-terminal kinase, pathways that are involved in IL-4 gene expression and tumorigenesis.

Earlier we suggested that under normal inflammatory conditions, stimuli-induced exocytosis of MCs and release of histamine or PGs (e.g., PGF-1α or PGI2) and oxidants or toxins (Yin, growth-arrest events) in the tissue environment would simultaneously signal for induction of neutralizing mediators and expression of anti-inflammatory mediators (e.g., IL-10, VEGF or PGE2) during Yang (growth-promote or tumorigenic) processes [5, 10–15] (details in Chaps. 2 and 4) (Figs. 6.3 and 6.6).

The overall analyses of relevant data using inhibitors of MCs degranulation, oxidative phosphorylation or glycolysis pathways (e.g., pyruvate oxidation), under a wide range of immune dysfunction or carcinogenesis suggest that MCs activation and release of histamine and other preformed or newly synthesized mediators, require activation of lysosomal exocytosis and Ca^{+2} flux from the stored-operated Ca^{+2} channels as part of effector function of MCs [5, 10–15, 345–364, 368–371, 373–385, 388, 561]. To what extent oxidative stress and low level release of histamine from 'leaky' MCs impair pathways that are involved in lysosomal activities and exocytosis or tissue acid-base homeostasis or expression of mediators from other immune cells (e.g., T cells, eosinophils or MΦs) to alter physiological behaviors of tissues and initiation of chronic diseases are among interdependent knowledge gaps. Another question is whether repeated activation of MCs (or MΦs) and release of low level histamine influence the level of free/stored Ca^{+2} in cells and associated induction of biosynthesis of immature or 'leaky' MCs or polarized M2 (TAMs) contribute to the multistep carcinogenesis (Figs. 6.6 and 6.7).

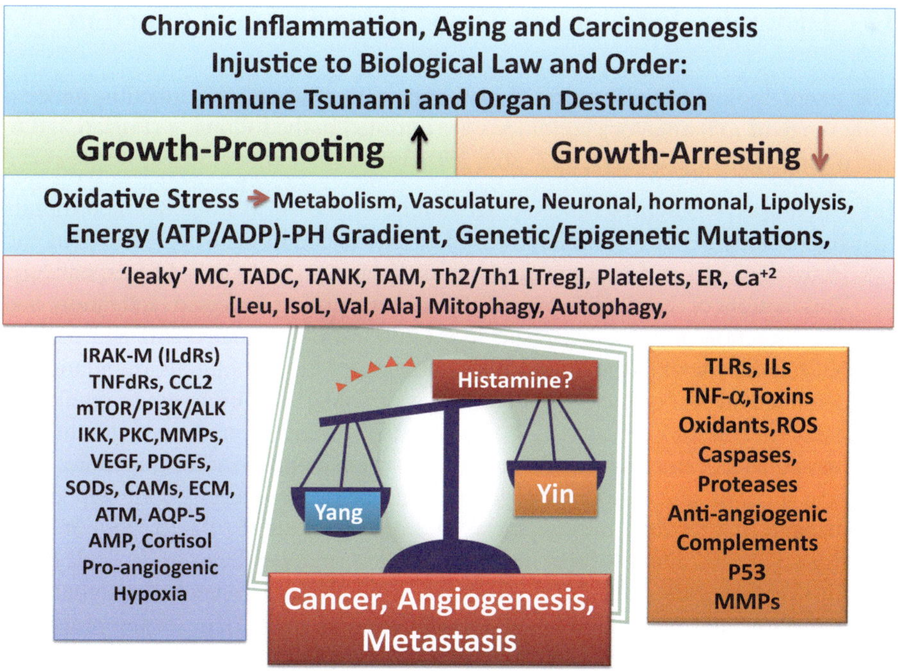

Fig. 6.7 Schematic representation that chronic inflammation and aging are biological injustices to molecular law and order in immunity that lead to immune tsunami and multistep carcinogenesis. The scheme shows that loss of balance in tumoricidal (Yin) and tumorigenic (Yang) properties of protective acute inflammation (effective immunity) is associated with mismatched and exaggerated expression and co-expression of apoptotic and wound healing factors. Circulating histamine release at low levels from 'leaky' MCs was hypothesized to play important roles in altered immune responses and induction of tumorigenesis and angiogenesis. See text (Adopted from Khatami (Ref. [10]) with permission.)

Depending on the level of antigen-receptor crosslinking, time-course kinetics of reformation/resynthesis of granules (maturation of MCs) or frequency of tissue stimulation, activated cells could release part or all of its granules content resulting in a wide range of immune/inflammatory responses. What we defined for the process of an acute inflammation; the balance between Yin-Yang properties of effective immunity, logically apply to the processes of exocytosis or effector phase of MCs, or basophils as well as NKs, MΦs or DCs or T and B cells. Therefore, activation and deactivation (Yin-Yang) of effective immunity require respective differential bioenergetics (high-low energy consumption).

Suggestions that oxidative stress-induced impaired activities of Ca^{+2} channels and altered lysosomal and mitochondrial functions during autophagy and mitophagy in the context of balance in Yin and Yang of immunity during aging or disease processes are among interdependent new concepts and deserve further investigation (manuscript in preparation).

12 Histamine Influence on Tissue Physiology and Function

The major biological influences of histamine on cellular/tissue function under a wide range of inflammatory conditions are outlined in the following (Figs. 6.3, 6.6, and 6.7) [5, 10–15, 344–347, 357–363, 370–385, 647–666]:

(a) **Chemotactic Factors (CCXs)**: Histamine is shown to influence neutrophils and eosinophils through the induction of expression of neutrophil chemotacttic factor (NCXF) and eosinophil chemotactic factor-A (ECXF-A), respectively. This action of histamine potentially occurs during repeated activation and degranulation of MCs that result in the infiltration of neutrophils and eosinophils at the site of tissue injury. We demonstrated that continuous stimulation of conjunctival-associated lymphoid tissues (CALTs) caused down-regulation phenomenon and exhausted or 'leaky' MCs (reduced number of granulated/mature MCs); the events followed by heavy eosinophils infiltration along with activation of mucus-secreting goblet cells and MΦs during multistep tissue damage that resulted tumorigenesis and angiogenesis [5, 10–15, 357–363]. It was suggested that low level histamine release (independent of IgE-FcεR binding) from degranulated MCs into tissue environment sequentially signals for activation and infiltration of other inflammatory cells (e.g., eosinophils and polarized macrophgages, M2 or TAMs) in an attempt to terminate the inflammation. The presence of 'leaky' MCs could additionally induce factors such as IL5 and oxidants to create an immunological chaos for recruitment of TAMs or induction of Th2 immune profiles or Treg that lead to immune suppression and facilitating progressive damages of target tissue (details in Chaps. 2 and 4).

(b) **Heparin**: Heparin, a mucopolysaccharide is an acidic proteoglycan and a major component in the matrix of MCs that holds together (neutralize) the basic mediators such as histamine and serotonin within the cell granules. Upon MCs degranulation and release of histamine and other mediators, heparin is released to inhibit blood coagulation. Analyses of relevant data [10, 487, 647, 648, 650] suggest that protamine, an inhibitor of heparin-dependent MCs protease (β-tryptase) may also contribute to the resolution of inflammation. While heparin may not be directly involved in anaphylaxis, its action on platelets aggregations during vasculature permeability could be quite important. Detailed understanding of the heparin action on platelets is particularly crucial with regard to cancer drugs-induced venous thromboembolism and related complications that are life-threatening and often require additional medication.

(c) **Platelet activating factor (PAF)**. PAF is the most potent bronchoconstriction and vasodilatation factor, and in extremely low doses is capable of inducing shock symptoms within minutes. PAF activates platelets to release histamine and serotonin during hypersensitivity reactions [5, 10, 661–666]. While its action in microthrombus formation has not been fully understood, it seems the action of PAF, originating from vasculature, enhances and facilitates the histamine actions.

(d) **Bradykinin**: is a vascular nanopeptide and a somewhat weaker alkaline compared with histamine and acts similar to histamine with slower dynamics. Bradykinin has been detected in the individual blood during anaphylaxis, perhaps to contribute to the drop in blood pressure.

(e) **Serotonin**: Histamine causes the release of serotonin, a basic component of MCs and facilitates smooth muscle contraction and increases the vascular permeability in some species, such as rodents.

(f) ***de Novo* synthesis of inflammatory mediators expressed from activated MCs or other immune cells include** (Figs. 6.3 and 6.7):

    (i) **Prostaglandins and Thromboxanes**: Prostaglandins (PGF1-α or PGI2) are synthesized at very low levels from membrane arachidonic acid (AA) metabolism followed by activation of cyclooxygenase pathways. Their actions are somewhat similar and perhaps complementary to the action of histamine in promoting bronchoconstriction. Being chemotactic factors they seem to participate in recruiting other inflammatory cells such as neutrophils, eosinophils, basophils, and monocytes to the site of injury.

    (ii) **Leukotriens**: Leukotirens (LTs- 1-4) are synthesized at very low levels from activated MCs membrane AAs metabolism and activation of lipooxygenase pathways. Like PGs, the actions of LTs facilitate vasoconstriction, prolonged smooth muscle constriction and chemotaxis of inflammatory cells such as eosinophils.

    (iii) **Proteases:** MCs proteases (e.g., tryptase, MCP-6, β-tryptase) contribute to the clearance of parasitic infections and chronic infection with bacteria (e.g., *Trichinella spiralis* or *Klebsiella pneumonia*) by recruiting neutrophils and their degradation abilities to cleave IgE molecules; potentially contributing to the termination and resolution arm of inflammation (Yang). Whether MCs proteases are involved in degradation of histamine receptors at the termination phase of an acute inflammation are among important biological gaps to be understood.

(iv) **Cytokines**: A wide range of mediators are expressed from activated MCs and other immune or non-immune cells during acute inflammation. These cytokines are secreted upon required intercellular signals during Yin and Yang processes. The inflammatory cytokines are tumoricidal or tumorigenic and initiate or terminate and resolve an inflammatory condition. As noted above, production of cytokines and chemokines during MCs activation include pro-inflammatory mediators such as TLRs (e.g., TLR-4), IL-1, TNF, and post-inflammatory mediators (e.g., IL-5, IL-10, FoxP3+) and their interactions with T regulatory proteins (CD4 + CD25+) [5, 10–15, 345–347, 357–371].

12.1 Oxidative Stress and Low Level Circulating Histamine: Preparing Host for Induction of Tumorigenesis?

It's not the size of the dog in a fight; it's the size of the fight in a dog. Mark Twain

In general, late and delayed hypersensitivity reactions (immune disorders) are likely the result of unresolved and accumulated presence of inflammatory mediators from recruited immune cells, locally (host) or at distant tissue (e.g., activated vasculature or secondary immune cells) [5, 10–15]. The late phase responses often follow anaphylactic reactions within 4–8 h and can persist for several days. To what degrees immune responses subside (resolve) following an acute inflammation (self-terminating, protective immune mechanisms) or persist (oxidative stress) depend on several intrinsic or extrinsic conditions including the following (Figs. 6.3, 6.4, 6.5, 6.6 and 6.7):

(a) Frequency of subsequent exposures to the same or similar immune disruptors;
(b) Potency and nature of immune disruptors;
(c) Immune effectiveness and integrity and functionality of innate and adaptive immune responses and the corresponding signals generated from non-immune systems (e.g., vasculature, metabolic, neuronal, hormonal);
(d) Genomic susceptibility of site-specific target tissues;
(e) Types of host tissues (e.g., immune-responsive or immune-privileged, insulin-dependent or insulin-independent tissues for glucose transport and utilization);
(f) Presence of other chronic illnesses in complicating the immunobiological responses in organ systems, particularly in an aging body;

The above biological heterogeneities seem to be major factors involved in the observed wide responses of individuals toward pathogens or allergen and the induction of multistep diseases or site-specific cancers. We suggested that cancerous cells are intrinsic defective (useless) cells whose oncogenic growth are routinely monitored and arrested by body's effective immunity. However, as detailed below, accumulated delayed hypersensitivity reactions and expression of mismatched tumoricidal and tumorigenic factors provide opportunities for cancerous cells to utilize the machinery of dysfunctional immune responses and satisfy their enhanced growth requirements in the directions of tumorigenesis, hypoxic conditions, angiogenesis and metastasis [5, 10–15].

12.2 Asthma: Intermediate Inflammatory Responses: Increased Risk of Cancer

Asthma is the pulmonary airways (bronchial) hyperresponsiveness of immune system. Induction of asthma is an example of chronic inflammatory disease; an intermediate ('moderate') immune disorders and potentially reversible if the asthmatic episodes and clinical obstruction of lung airways are not extensive. However, repeated episodes and long-term asthma when the conditions progress to other immune disorders such as emphysema and increased risks of lung cancer may not be reversible. Physiologically, the bronchial hyperresponsiveness of asthma is associated with a decreased in bronchial airflow upon exposures to triggers (e.g., smoking, pathogens or allergen) or when experimentally provoked (bronchoprovocation) by agents such as histamine or methacholine or other inflammatory cytokines [5, 10–15, 344, 345, 353, 370, 380–382, 445, 447, 493, 499–509, 512, 532, 545–551, 654, 670, 673]. Due to the similarities between lung airways immune and non-immune cell composition (e.g., mast cells, lymphoid tissue, mucus secreting cells, epithelia) in lung-associated lymphoid tissues (LALTs) and those in conjunctival-associated lymphoid tissues (CALTs), the immune response profiles in these tissues are somewhat comparable. Stimuli such as allergen induce an early phase reaction by activation of B lymphocytes (acting as innate immune cells) for biosynthesis of allergen-specific immunoglobulin E (IgE) and sensitization of MCs and expression of IgE-fcεR molecules followed by activation and degranulation of MCs and release of histamine that mediate a decrease in bronchial airflow. Subsequent exposure to stimuli often induces late-phase reaction (4–8 h) with a further decrease in bronchial airflow. Clinical and immunopathological features of airways in asthmatic patients include lung hyperinflation, smooth muscle hypertrophy, lamina reticularis thickening, mucosal edema, epithelial cell sloughing, cilia cell disruption, mucus gland hypersecretion as well as increased numbers of eosinophils, neutrophils, different size lymphocytes, and plasma cells in the bronchial tissues, bronchial secretions, and the mucus secreting cells. The recruitment of leukocytes (e.g., eosinophils) from activated vasculature to the airway involves activation of CD_4 T-lymphocytes. While the sequence of early events in the lung airway are not clear, it appears that, as we described for CALTs [5, 10, 15], repeated MCs degranulation of lung airways and the release of low levels histamine induce the recruitment of eosinophil infiltration and induction of altered-polarization of Th1/Th2 (decreased CD4+/CD8+) toward immune suppression. Analyses of data on features of mediators that are identified from asthmatic patients or models of asthma suggest mixed expression and co-expression of apoptotic and growth factors including histamine, leukotrienes, interleukins (e.g., IL-4, IL-5, IL-13) and antibodies (IgG, IgM, IgE). Expression of IL-5 influences differentiation, activation and infiltration of eosinophils or lymphocytes and creates an oxidative stress in the tissue and perpetuation of inflammation leading to impaired termination of inflammation and tissue remodeling mechanisms. Furthermore, sustained oxidative stress along with aging process increases the risk for lung cancer [5, 227, 533, 550, 551].

Often, but not always, the elevated circulating levels of IgE or histamine are the best markers of allergies, as some patients become reactive to histamine ('histamine intolerance') suggesting impaired histamine metabolism and clearance and/or over-reactivity of cells for histamine production and altered genetic involvement [5, 531–533]. Alternatively, it is possible that the absence of circulating IgE, which we also observed in experimental models of ocular allergies, be due to the effectiveness of MCs sensitivities and activation (effector cells). Antigen/allergen-induced specific IgE-FcεR was proposed to bind and sensitize MCs locally/host (e.g., conjunctiva) and at distant sites (e.g., lung airways) where it would react upon allergen challenge to release higher levels of histamine. In our studies, animals with high ocular hypersensitivity reactions also produced wheezing- (asthma-) like symptoms, when the sensitized eyes were challenged with antigen, suggesting MCs activation and antigen-specific IgE-binding to MCs of lung airways [5, 10–15]. Further support for this mechanism came from studies on newborn babies from highly sensitized animals who produced high ocular reactivity toward the 1st or 2nd antigen challenge, much earlier reactions compared with time course for MCs sensitization and degranulation (9 days to a couple of weeks of challenges) (see Chap. 4).

In addition, interesting reports that compared the DNA sequence from 237 healthy individuals and 192 asthmatic patients demonstrated a significant increase in the incidence of Ile105 replacement in the asthmatic group or patients with Parkinson's [10, 523–525]. Integration and analyses of relevant data show that some H1 antihistamines, such as diphenhydramine are potent HNMT blockers when treating allergic patients [523–529]. Whether increased in the replacement of isoleucine 105 (Ile 105), a branched amino acid, reflects the biosynthesis of altered HNMT and/or its potential impact on energy-consuming biosynthesis of structural proteins within mitochondria that utilize branch amino acids (leucine, isoleucine, valine or alanine) are important biological gaps that require systematic studies [10]. Whether induction of histamine intolerance in patients previously treated with H1 antihistamine drugs correlates with inactivation of histamine metabolism and clearance by HNMT is also not understood. Furthermore, data on histamine intolerance and genetically-inherited defects in enzyme HNMT activity that were associated with tyrosine or threonine replacement with isoleucine (IL-105) indirectly support our observations of parental transfer of hypersensitivity reactions (genetic predisposition) and early responses toward antigen in newborn guinea pigs [5, 15].

12.3 Mediators of Late Phase Hypersensitivity Responses

The detection of mediators that are released in late phase hypersensitivity reactions, including thromboxanes, interleukins (e.g., IL-3, IL-5, IL-8, IL-10), eosinophils chemotactic factor of anaphylaxis (ECF-A) indicate the presence of unresolved inflammation (oxidative stress) in target tissue and surrounding tissue environment (e.g., vasculature, fibroblasts). Under a wide range of experimental conditions these mediators have been shown to directly or indirectly promote immune cell proliferation and growth, immune suppression and tumor growth [5, 10–15, 244, 393]. As noted above, these growth promoting mediators influence, to varying degrees, activation, infiltration and degranulation of eosinophils and release of eosinophilic cationic protein (ECP), leukotrienes, platelet activating factor (PAF), arylsulfatase and major basic protein (MBP). The combined presence and interactions of these factors could cause local tissue damage often promoting immune suppression and accumulation of growth promoting responses (wound healing pathways). For example, eosinophil-induced expression of MBP, not only destroys various parasites or helminthes (e.g., schistosomes/trematodes, A Suum) by inflicting surface damage that immobilize pathogens, but it is extremely toxic to the mammalian ocular tissues, respiratory tract or perhaps gastrointestinal and mucus secreting tissues [5, 10, 244, 393, 661–663]. Furthermore, another eosinophil mediator, ECP is a known neurotoxin and an antihelminthes mediator (helminthotoxin) and inflicts damages to the host tissue. Other studies show that combined actions of ECF-A and IL-8 provoke activation, phagocytosis and degranulation of neutrophils in the late phase reaction. The actions of these mediators further lead to the release of lysosomal enzymes, leukotrienes, platelet activating factor (PAF), and abnormal mitochondrial oxidative phosphorylation. Therefore, in all likelihood, if the inflammatory responses are not properly resolved, the presence of oxidants and toxins would additionally stimulate T and B cells for expression of immune cells mediators causing chemotaxis and enhanced immune suppression. Our original suggestion that the presence of circulating low level release of histamine from 'leaky' MCs (independent of antigen-specific IgE-fcεR binding and degranulation) could lead to multistep tumorigenesis deserves further studies under various inflammatory conditions [5, 10]. Our proposed mechanisms of MCs responses are directly and indirectly supported by several reports on basic and clinical studies and age-associated diseases such as asthma, Parkinson's or site-specific cancers [5, 344, 345, 361, 367–369, 521, 523–535].

Therefore, the late phase of inflammatory responses, ordinarily should be considered as protective part of immunity when targeted tissue is exposed to pathogens or parasitic infections or for removal of defective and useless complex proteins including cancerous cells. However, the late phase become damaging to the host when tissue stimulation is continued by frequent infections or innocuous substances such as pollen or other immune disruptors including exposures to low level environmental chemical or biological agents or carcinogens, particularly during aging process (Figs. 6.3, 6.4, and 6.7).

It should be emphasized that except for our 'accidental' discoveries that were established three decades ago, there is little/no report on early biological events that are identified as sequences of immunological and/or genomic alterations in the developmental phases of immune dysfunction toward multistep tumorigenesis and angiogenesis [5, 10]. As recent as 2016, in an article authored by several professionals from various cancer disciplines, including colleagues at DCP/NCI/NIH who witnessed the author's challenging efforts to promote the role of inflammation in cancer research since 1998, admitted that '*There has been increasing focus on the molecu-*

lar origins of cancer over the last several years....In contrast to studies in malignancy, however, genome-wide analyses of premalignancy have been rare' [463]. In this 'Special Report' the authors finally and indirectly admitted that despite numerous reports that are available on molecular genomics and biology of cancer metastasis, study on *'...the progression of genomic events and inflammatory microenvironment that drive premalignancy provide unprecedented possibilities...'* [463]. The authors however, continue to disregard the existence of our fundamental contributions on a series of 'accidental' discoveries and the first evidence for a direct association between inflammation and multistep immune dysfunction that resulted in tumorigenesis and angiogenesis.

13 Pattern Recognition Receptors (PRRs) in Biological Events: Constituent (Innate) and Induced ('Designer'). Crucial Roles in Circadian Rhythms and Immunity

There is a wide range of pattern recognition molecules or receptor molecules that play crucial roles in signal transduction mechanisms in all biological events and they contribute to the maintenance of health or induction of diseases. Several excellent articles describe the roles of numerous intracellular or extracellular membrane receptor and surface molecules in the regulation of hormones, growth factors, cytokines/chemokines, metabolites/nutrients, ion transport and related enzymes. These receptor molecules contribute to all aspects of cells/tissues functions such as visual transduction, bone and lipid biosynthesis, bioenergetics, cellular infiltration, differentiation and growth, nuclear/chromosomal or chromatin activities, neuronal pathways, tissue necrosis or growth in immune and non-immune systems [10, 599, 646, 656, 688, 689, 692, 695–697, 707–761].

The time course kinetics and biological behaviors of receptor molecules present a complex molecular universe with unique or shared features. As an example of how daunting the field of receptor molecules is, suffice to note that discussing only the role of insulin receptors in various tissues for maintenance of health or induction of major problems such as diabetes-related complications is a huge topic [267, 273, 529, 553, 646, 779, 787, 788].

While discussion of receptor molecules is not the focus of this chapter, it is noteworthy that despite the pivotal roles that receptors play in all phases of cell/tissue biology, little efforts have been directed to make an overall classification and distinction of these important molecular signatures in health or diseases. The highly regulated biological laws (feedback control switches or rhythmic cycles) that we defined as the balance between Yin (tumoricidal) and Yang (tumorigenic) of effective immunity extend to the biology of activating and deactivating expression of pattern recognition receptors (PRRs) that are required for binding to respective ligands and performing their widely different biological actions.

Below, we attempted to categorize the general features of a wide range of receptors and pattern recognition molecules that are involved in effective immunity, with emphasis on cancer biology. The overall classifications of these 'biological signalers' (constituent/innate and transient/induced) that follow or violate the biological laws in maintenance of health or induction of disease include the following [10, 109, 202, 267, 273, 582, 599, 619, 656, 688, 689, 692, 713–715, 723–729, 731–733, 737, 738, 757–761, 779]:

13.1 Constituent: Innate and Adoptive Receptors and Surface Molecules

Constituent receptors and surface molecules are predictable and essential (innate) members of the mammalian embryonic growth and development. They are required for postnatal survival and biological schedules of organs/tissues throughout life. These receptors are synthesized and/or regenerated for routine maintenance of enormous biological activities of living cells. Examples of such pattern recognition receptor molecules are the various insulin receptors for glucose transport or metabolism in insulin-dependent tissues (e.g., muscle, adipocytes or liver) for transport and metabolism of glucose, or those insulin receptors that are required for organ development and maintenance of health in tissues such as the brain, retina, endothelial or neuronal systems [267, 273, 529, 553]. Numerous other molecules may be categorized as constituent receptor molecules for actions of hormones, metabolites, cytoplasm, extracellular, intracellular signaling, or nuclear and genomic transporter/enzyme receptors, mitochondrial membrane receptors, neuronal transporters, or related surface molecules involved routinely in physiology of immune or non-immune cells.

However, after birth, each of these genetically-determined and diverse molecules are strongly and often immediately influenced by the signals they receive from the environment and become adaptable/malleable to the quality of nutrition (initiated from mother's milk) and upon exposures to a variety of bioactive agents, microorganisms, environmental chemical and biological hazards. Analyses of relevant data suggest that the constituent receptor molecules could mature or shift, to some degrees, particularly in the gastrointestinal and upper respiratory tracks and skin [267, 273, 529, 553, 691–705].

The mechanisms of gene-environmental interactions and the degrees of alterations/adaptations of innate receptor molecules or their interdependence with induced (transient) receptor molecules in organ systems for maintenance of health or induction of diseases remain to be understood.

13.2 Induced or Transient Receptors and Surface Molecules: 'Designer' Molecules

These are known as 'designer' receptors and are generally induced when tissue is exposed to specific foreign elements (stimuli) such as allergen, pathogens (viruses or bacteria), certain foods, chemicals, carcinogens and other biological, chemical or environmental hazards and often present transient functions. In this category a large number of toll-like receptor molecules (TLRs-1-9), immune disruptor-induced specific cytokine/chemokine receptors, as well as allergen-specific synthesis of receptor molecules for antibody bindings and sensitization of MCs, DCs, MΦs or mucus secreting cells (e.g., IgE-fcεR, IgGγRs, IgARs) and related surface molecules are included. There are other receptors with short half-lives whose function may fit the profile of either or both constituents and induced. These receptors include a wide range of molecules for ion channels, such as activation-induced enhanced Ca^{+2} permeability by expression of receptor potential channels such as TRPM4 (transient receptor potential cation channel, subfamily 4), TRPC 5, in combination with STIM1 and CRACM1that contribute to FcεRI-induced Ca^{2+} influx during MCs degranulation [5, 10, 91, 616–618, 701–705].

13.3 Pattern Recognition Receptors (PRRs) in Health and Immune Disorders: Toll-like Receptors (TLRs) and Inhibitors: Role in Multistep Carcinogenesis

With regard to allergies, several publications show the roles of pattern recognition receptors (PRRs) in sensing, recognizing and differentiating various molecular structures on pathogens/microbial for initiating the warning (danger) signals to immune systems for further actions. Mechanisms of actions on multistep presentation of processed pathogens (microbial) or hazardous materials for immune response and elimination/neutralization are detailed in several excellent reviews [712–729]. A brief analyses of relevant data on the importance of toll-like receptors or pattern recognition receptor molecules (PRRs) that are expressed upon tissue exposure to microbiota are summarized below for their crucial contributions in the induction of immune suppression and carcinogenesis.

The important roles of PRRs, primarily the toll-like receptors (TLRs) in the defense of body for activation of innate immune cells and generation of death factors and pro-inflammatory responses as well as polarization of cells during initiation processes (Yin, tumoricidal) have been extensively studied. However, data on the mechanisms of signal transduction and degradation or binding to inhibitors/regulators of PRRs that could lead to termination (Yang, wound healing, tumorigenic) of inflammation or the roles in the induction of age-associated inflammatory diseases or cancer are fragmentary and confusing [267, 273, 529, 553, 649, 682, 690, 695–705, 711–742]. A brief discussion on mechanisms of actions of these molecules is helpful for better understanding and integrating or comparing data on mechanisms of actions of induced and specialized surface molecules with a number of stimuli-specific receptor molecules such as immunoglobulins (e.g., MCs-IgE- FcεR; MΦRs, IgM Rs or IgGRs, mucus-secreting IgARs) or surface molecules (e.g., CD 11, CD22, CD40,CD80, CD83, CD86,CAIX, integrin, indolamine 2,3 dioxygenase, sialic acids, CAMs, ECMs) that directly or indirectly act as promoter or inhibitors of proliferation of immune cells or enzymes and contribute to the host defense and inflammatory response dynamics, immune homeostasis or tolerance in maintenance of health or multistep carcinogenesis [5, 10–15, 397, 406, 420, 423, 589, 617, 618, 624, 627, 630–632, 678, 712–745].

Initiation of inflammatory responses from antigen presenting cells (APCs) such as DCs, MΦs or NKs, toward microbial is mediated through a number of pathogen recognition molecules (danger signals) which include specialized toll-like receptors-TLRs (e.g., TLR1-9). Stimuli-induced expression of TLRs contributes to the differential recognition of molecular structures or sub-structures of pathogens (bacteria, viruses or parasites) and specific activation of APCs. For example, LPS-induced expression of TLRs to specific structures of the pathogen leads to activation of immature DCs and differentiation/polarization and migration from peripheral tissues to lymphoid organs to further activate naïve T cells (T^0) and up-regulate expression of major histocompatibility complexes (MHC I and II) and co-stimulatory surface molecules, followed by expression of other pro-inflammatory cytokines, oxidants and chemokines leading to destruction of microbial (Yin, tumoricidal events). Review of relevant data shows that the danger molecules or TLRs, together with interleukin-1 receptor (IL-1R) form a group of superfamily regulatory proteins with shared and special features for signaling to the intracellular domains under a wide range of immune responses [5, 10, 253, 607, 616, 618, 659, 690, 696, 697, 722–748]. The combined signals apparently further regulate expression of other cytokines at extra-, and intracellular levels for inducing and recruiting adaptor molecule response such as gene 88 (myeloid differentiation or MY 88) and formation of receptor-adaptor complex domains. Danger molecules such as TRL1 and TLR2 are known to recognize and bind to ligands of specific molecular patterns of microbioms such as the tri-acyl lipopeptides, lipoarabinomannan or bacterial wall peptidoglycan (PGN) and lipoteichoic acid (LTA), and phospholipomannan of the bacteria (e.g., mycobacterium tuberculosis, Staphylococcus aureus). Other receptors (e.g., TRL4) bind to LPS of gram-negative bacteria for initial activation of DCs, while TLR3 recognizes viral dsRNA. TRL 7 and TRL 8 primarily bind to substructures of viruses and often initiate responses from macrophages as primary APCs [712–714].

13.4 Pattern Recognition for Regulation (Tolerance) of Inflammation by IRAK-M: Special Features of Yin-Yang Events?

The reports on mechanisms of inhibition of some of the TLRs demonstrate their crucial roles in pattern recognition during initiation and termination of inflammatory responses or induction of tolerance. For example, it has been shown that treatment with bacterial lipoteichoic acid (LTA) induces tolerance in macrophages for LPS-induced activation of NF-κB and increases expression of immune responses by interleukin receptor activation of kinase-M (IRAK-M) that regulates (terminates) acute inflammation [716, 721–728, 741–743]. Review of similar reports on activation of TLRs in tissues during various bacterial or viral infections on models of liver injury or influenza infection-induced lung tissue damage and lysis of epithelial cells show exaggerated immune cell activation and increased expression of IRAK-M to protect tissue damage [269, 270, 712–714, 722–744]. The reported data suggest the limited immunopathology protection of IRAK-M in tissue without influencing or decreasing the viral clearance. Therefore, it seems that expression of IRAK-M protects, to some degrees, damaging the lung or perhaps other epithelial tissues and preventing complications of asthma. Expression of IRAK-M also limits neutrophils-induced damage to tissue while improved tissue remodeling. Data on TLR7-induced MΦs activation (Yin, M1 phenotype?) and tolerance (Yang, M2 phenotype ?) seem to accompany an elevated expression of IRAK-M and diminished production of TNF-α, while it induced expression of NF-κB, p38 and stress-activated protein kinase (SAPK) within the protein family of MAPKs. This suggests the induction of immune suppression that is also feature of Yang (tumorigenic) events in acute inflammatory responses.

Whether IRAK-M and induction of decoy receptors that have been described during polarization of MΦs to M2 phenotype for termination of acute inflammation or tumorigenesis are the same receptors or they operate on different regulatory pathways or as complementary processes are not clear. However, these regulatory molecules suggest that the induction of TLR7 and tolerance involve increased expression of IRAK-M and sulfhydryl domain-(SH2) containing protein-tyrosine phosphatase (SHP-1) activities including involvement of 2 subgroup of MAPKs, c-Jun- NH(2) N-terminal kinase (JNK) and p38 MAPK that signal for immune suppression [641, 642, 731–739]. Collectively, it seems that involvement of SH-containing proteins in IRAK-M activity and acting as anti-oxidants and scavengers of free radicals (oxidants) support the mechanisms of termination of inflammation (Yang events) we described for acute inflammation [5, 10–15]. TNF-α secreted from activated macrophages in response to LPS and CpG DNA treatment induced necrosis/apoptosis of hepatocytes. It was concluded that induction of tolerance ('tolerization') associated with elevated expression of IRAK-M likely serves to prevent liver cell death. LPS-induced TNF-α production is associated with a lack of IRAK-M induction in liver cirrhotic lymphocytes [716, 717, 735, 739–741]. Other data show that IRAK-M expression could be regulated by activation of cell surface molecules, such as triggering receptor expressed on myeloid cells 1 (TREM-1) [725, 738]. Lagler et al. [725] demonstrated that activation of TREM-1 during the early *Streptococcus pneumoniae* infection resulted in decreased expression of lung IRAK-M and elevated pro-inflammatory cytokines were suggestive of decreased expression of IRAK-M, mediated by TREM-1 and promoted efficient early bacterial clearance. It would be interesting to study if TREM-1 activation that is triggered by TLRs signaling in response to bacterial infection would modulate the early IRAK-M activation. Similar reports demonstrate that mannose receptors and C-type lectin-induced DCs-specific intercellular adhesion molecule-3-grabbing non-integrin (DC-SIGN) bind to *Mycobacterium* tuberculosis cell wall components called mannose-capped lipoarabinomannans (Man-LAMs) [602, 740]. Furthermore, Man-LAMs inhibit LPS-induced IL-12 p40 production, NF-κB activation, and IRAK-1-TRAF6 interaction. This is accompanied by increased IRAK-M expression [269, 716, 741]. Whether IRAK-M expression facilitates Man-LAM-induced macrophage deactivation or silencing of IRAK-M to restore LPS-induced IL-12 production in Man-LAM treated cells involving mannooligosaccharide caps of LAM as major factors in the induction of IRAK-M remain to be understood.

Additionally, as suggested above, whether induction of IRAK-M is similar, same or different from the actions of decoy receptor molecules that possess immune suppressive effects during termination arm of acute inflammation (Yang) and polarization of immune cells (e.g., immature DCs) to mature DCs (DC2 or TADC) or M2 phenotypes are yet to be understood. However, since the actions of these inhibitory molecules seem very similar to the known decoy receptors and facilitate termination of inflammatory reactions (e.g., IL1dR), it is possible that these molecules are the same factors with different nomenclature. It is also possible that the complexes of activation of interleukin (IL) receptor-associated kinase M (IRAK-M) could be different or complementary to IL decoy receptors (ILdR) to induce control/termination or regulation of acute inflammation (Yang) in MΦs (M2 or TAMs) and the immune suppression during multistep tumorigenesis. Therefore, stimuli-induced inflammatory processes could be initiated by biogenesis of specific transient pattern recognition receptors (PRRs) followed by expression of danger molecules/alarms (alarmins) during activation of constituent (innate) receptors for adaptation and induction of specific responses. As proposed below, induction of specific transient PRRs and generation of pro-inflammatory factors for initiation of events in acute inflammation (Yin) have different (higher) energy requirements (oxidative phosphorylation from mitochondria) compared with induction of termination (Yang) or tolerance (glycolytic pathways).

In summary, the molecular complexes associated with IRAK-M that lead to immune suppression, if not the same as decoy receptors, they likely follow the same biological principals for maintenance of health or initiation of diseases.

14 Regulatory Signaling Mechanisms of Soluble Hormones and Tumor Factors in Immune Tolerance: Role of IRAK-M in Violations of Biological Laws and Tumorigenesis!

An overview on the roles of some of the pattern recognition receptors (PRRs) in acute and chronic inflammatory responses are provided below. This is helpful when we present hypotheses that cancerous cells are:

(a) Defective host cellular components whose growth is routinely arrested by effective immunity (balance in Yin and Yang of acute inflammation);
(b) They behave as any other pathogens whose oncogenic components induce specific signals (e.g., decoy receptor molecules and antigenic agents) to misdirect

or 'confuse' the organized crosstalk between immune and non-immune systems and escape immune surveillance, induce hypoxia and low energy requirements for growth promotion in the direction of tumorigenesis and angiogenesis.

(c) Lawless growth of cancer cells are comparable to orderly (one way) fetus growth, in the absence of functional mitochondria or high energy-demand of Yin events.

In general, a variety of hormones [e.g., estrogen, α-melanocyte-stimulating hormone (MSH), insulin, TSH, cortisol, adiponectin] that are induced or secreted from respective tissues have anti-inflammatory (growth-promoting, post-inflammatory or tumorigenic) properties and often are involved in wound healing (Yang) events. The actions of these hormones are regulated by a number of receptor molecules and inhibitors. For example, review of several elegant reports demonstrate that growth promoting factors such as adiponectin, insulin or anti-infective mediators that induce IRAK-M expression require activation of phosphatidyl inositol 3-kinase (PI3K), protein kinase B (AKT/PKB/mTOR) or ERK pathways to induce macrophage endotoxin tolerance and signal for wound healing and immune suppression [5, 10–15, 323, 744–759].

Further analyses and integration of related data suggest that the inhibitory effects and induction of tolerance in innate or adaptive immune cells and activation of growth pathways support definitions of dual function of Yin (tumoricidal) and Yang (tumorigenic) of immunity for maintenance of health or induction of immune disorders. As noted above, during 'tolerization' of cells, IRAK-M is bound to IRAK-1, suggesting a role in tridecapeptide alpha-melanocyte-stimulating hormone (α-MSH)-induced macrophage tolerance (down-regulation or induction of M2 phenotypes) or perhaps as costimulatory molecules (e.g., CD40, CD86, ICAM-1) of mature DCs (DC2) [678, 695–699, 710, 722–729]. In specific, our evidence on inflammation-induced interactions and synergies between host immune and non-immune cells (e.g., MCs, B cells, mucus secreting cells) and those recruiting cells (e.g., M2-TAMs, DCs or eosinophils) during cell growth and tumorigenesis indirectly support the chain of events that lead to activation of IRAK-M-PI3K- AKT/PKB-ERK described for induction of Treg and central or peripheral tolerance [250, 254, 442–447, 590, 710, 716, 719, 721]. Induction of M2 phenotype by inflammatory mediators (e.g., IL-4, IL-13) involved Th2 (Treg) and down-regulation of inflammation [15, 189, 716, 721, 722]. In brief, induction of tolerance in innate or adaptive immune cells by hormones or GFs requires synergies between a numbers of interdependent growth promoting mediators.

With regard to cancer growth, several studies show that tumor-derived factors such as acidic gangliosides (sialic acid-containing glycosphingolipids), hyaluronan/glycosaminoglycan or C-type lectin that are produced in the extracellular matrix or plasma membrane of different cell types (e.g., chondriocytes, MΦ or DCs) are capable of stimulating expression of IRAK-M that would inhibit danger signals (e.g., TLRs) in monocytes leading to immune suppression [10, 423, 722, 729, 741–743]. The events in the induction of immune suppression are facilitated by a number of cytokines, receptor and surface molecules or transcription factors (e.g., GM-CSF,

CD44, TLR4 intermediates, PGE2, TGF-β, NF-kB, CAMs, PU.1) that are involved in growth promoting (tumorigenic) events during wound healing and termination of inflammation [5, 10, 75, 280, 322, 323, 361, 363, 367, 369]. The findings that NO donor molecule (S-Nitrosoglutathione-GSNO) induces IRAK-M in LPS-activated monocytes in the presence of TNF-α are intriguing [713, 714]. It is possible that stimuli-induced TLRs and expression of TNF-α followed by induction of IRAK-M are the early and simultaneous signaling events that we described for termination of inflammation (Yang). Related studies reported elevated levels of IRAK-M in blood monocytes from patients with chronic inflammatory bowel disease or myeloid leukemia and metastasis [722, 729, 768]. Similarly, monocytes co-cultured with tumor cells or supernatant of tumor cells demonstrated significant decrease in expression of apoptotic factors such as TNF-α, IL-12 and IRAK-1, and an increased expression of IRAK-M. Tumor inoculation studies of IRAK-M-deficient models showed resistant to melonoma and fibrosarcoma tumor growth suggesting enhanced anti-tumor function of effector lymphocytes (e.g., T or B cell) in the absence of IRAK-M [423, 722, 729, 741–743].

Therefore, it seems that IRAK-M has an important role in limiting immune responsiveness to repeated pathogen exposures (induction of oxidative stress) through down-regulation of pathogen-induced danger signaling molecules such as TLRs that are required for expression of pro-inflammatory mediators (Yin) in DCs (DC2, TADCs) or MΦs (M2, TAMs) for induction of tolerance or growth. Thus, expression of IRAK-M results in pathogen/endotoxin tolerance or induction of cell growth. In the immune-responsive tissues (e.g., epithelial, endothelial or mucus-secreting cells) it is possible that increased IRAK-M expression plays important regulating roles in a wide range in inflammatory conditions, including epithelial-mesenchymal transition and cell growth promotion. Whether in the immune-privileged tissues (e.g., CNS, BBB, cornea, retina, reproductive organs) the expression levels of IRAK-M is naturally high to protect these oxidative stress-sensitive cells against stimuli-induced inflammatory conditions or induction of natural tolerance are important biological gaps deserving future investigations.

In the gastrointestinal tract, tolerance against various GI bacteria (GI flora) is due to regulatory/inhibitory complex molecules such as the interleukin receptor associated kinases (IRAK-M) and related immune suppressive pathways [695, 719, 768, 769]. Interestingly, expression of regulatory receptor molecules (IRAK-M) in epithelial lung tissue of asthmatic patients suggests induction of immune suppression of chronic inflammatory conditions that also involves expression of adenosine receptors (A2A) and surface molecules of CD4+ T lymphocutes. In related studies IRAK-M were suggested to interact with CD80 and disassociates in response to stimulation with CD28-containing neutrophil lipid rafts. This would lead to a decreased in IRAK-M interactions with TRAF6 and contributes to the induction of lethal cytokine storm and pathological inflammation [10, 227, 382, 654, 670, 673, 695, 719, 768, 769]. These data further suggest that IRAK-M negatively regulate activation of NF-κB/AP-1 via CD80 signaling in addition to TLR/IL-1R signaling.

Therefore, expression of molecules such as IRAK-M is likely the results of sustained oxidative stress and induction of exaggerated expression of growth promoting factors. The events involving immune cell tolerance (induction of wound healing or immune suppression) have been implicated in clinical trials such as allograft acceptance in transplanted host tissues such as the skin in models of allograft or bone marrow or stem cell transplantation [136, 496, 695, 769]. However, IRAK-M complex pathways may not be the only mechanisms that are involved in the induction of immune suppression pathways. Other compensating factors may be activated in the processes of immune mediation involving specific monocytes for allograft acceptance or chemotherapy.

14.1 Receptor Recognition and Function in Autoimmune Diseases

Expression of immunoglobulins G (IgG) antibodies, and the family of Fc gamma receptor molecules (FcγRs) are features of humoral immunity (HI), known to facilitate activation and down-regulation of inflammatory processes. For example, induction of IgG receptors (FcγRI, FcγRIIa, FcγRIIb, FcγRIIc, FcγRIII) amplify the actions of other pro-, or anti-inflammatory mediator receptors (e.g., TLR ligands, TNFα, IL-10, Th17) and are crucial factors in antibody/protein cross-reactivity reactions for mediating and controlling cytokine production by cell-mediated immunity (CMI) or immune cells (e.g., DCs, MΦs, Th2) and for opsonizing bacteria and forming complexes to efficiently counteract local or systemic infections [5, 10, 500–504, 702–704, 770]. Although detailed mechanisms of action of these receptors are not understood, IgG-receptors are likely involved in inhibition of inflammasome activation; mechanisms that are comparable to the actions described for blocking antibodies. However, overuse or inappropriate activation of IgGFcγRs by persistent unresolved inflammation, repeated infections or aging process, could contribute to the development of autoimmune diseases such as systemic lupus erythematosus (SLE), rheumatoid arthritis (RA), systemic sclerosis (SS, scleroderma), Sjogren's syndrome, multiple sclerosis or pemphigus [5, 671, 672, 770–778]. In these complications it seems that the immune cells (e.g., DCs or MΦs) view bacteria-aggregated IgG-fcγRs complexes as opsonized bacteria and overreact by expressing death factors (e.g., TLRs, TNFα, IL-β) and autoantibodies against the host, damaging the tissue and causing necrosis, fibrosis or nuclear reactions [5, 671, 672, 771–777]. The general features of autoimmune diseases such as SLE and RA or SS are the presence of IgG autoantibodies. Immune cells view IgG-complexes as danger signals and are activated to express apoptotic factors to necrotize the target tissue seen in the pathology of joints (RA), or damage DNA/RNA and nuclear structures of organs (e.g., kidneys, skin, lungs, brain, heart), in SLE or inducing excessive fibrosis in connective tissues, skin or internal organs (SS) [775, 776].

In summary, there are numerous immune and non-immune factors with dual (positive and negative control switches) functions that contribute to the maintenance of immunity or facilitate the immune disorders or carcinogenesis. As noted above, examples of molecular components with dual regulatory functions are TLRs and inhibitors (e.g., ILdRs, IRAK-M), MCP-1-CCL2, M-CSF, TGF-β, GM-CSF, histamine, heparin, TNF-α/TNFR and NFkB, VEGF, CAMs, MMPs, prostaglandins), surface antigens, adaptor molecules or cell recognition molecules (e.g., CD2, CD11, CD18, CD22, CD25, CD 50, CD54, CD63, CD69, CD88), cytokine suppressor molecules (e.g., S100 family of calcium-binding proteins), enzymes (e.g., tryptase/chymase, neutrophil-derived serine proteases, indolamine 2,3-dioxygenase, lipases or membrane metalloproteases/MMPs), peroxynitrite, cytokines/chemokines, interleukins (e.g., CCL2, CXC, Il-2, IL-3, IL-5, IL-10, IL-12, IL-13) or interferons (e.g., IFN-γ), ECFA, SCF, c-kit, antibodies (e.g., IgE, IgG isotypes, IgA, IgM), platelet-derived growth factor (PDGF), as well as expression products of pathways in gene activation (e.g., p53, p27, p70, MAPKs, KRAS, BRAF, ALK, Myc, BCR, ABL, MGMT, TKIs, PI3ks) from mutated DNA, hypo-, hyper-methylation products (Figs. 6.3, 6.4, 6.5, 6.6 and 6.7), [5, 10, 706, 707, 762–765, 780]. The amazingly secretive success of the biogenesis and interactions or synergies of these molecules with their counterparts are regulatory signals to safeguard and control oxidative stress. However, under persistent or unresolved inflammation (oxidative stress) expression and co-expression of apoptotic and anti-apoptotic mediator result in creation of biological lawlessness and chaos (immune tsunami) and adversely affect target tissue in the direction of multistep disease processes.

15 Energy-Dependent Differential Role of Mitochondria in Maintenance of Yin and Yang Balance: mTOR/PI3K/AKT Complexes in Health or Immune Disorders and Cancer

The principal free energy source that is required for all body's biochemical pathways is the universally known molecule of ATP. In general, the normal function of organ system uses ATP as both an intracellular energy source and an extracellular messenger for energy requiring transmission of signals in tissues such as the central nervous system (CNS) or optic nerve or immune and non-immune cells and for exocytosis, formation of Golgi complex, delivery of vesicles, as well as active transport of nutrients (e.g., glucose, Ca^{+2}, ascorbate), enzymatic processes (e.g., oxidases, kinases, lipases, hydrolases) and other physiological pathways, as well as physical, thermodynamics, mechanical or locomotion of cellular/tissue/organ integrity and architecture [5, 10, 188, 214, 215, 483, 557–600, 624–637, 781–790].

Several theories suggest that longevity is associated with altered (decreased) activities of family of proteins known as phosphoinositide (phosphatidyl inositol)-3 kinase (PI3K)-AKT- mechanistic (mammalian) Target Of Rapamycin (mTOR) or PI3K/AKT/mTOR pathways (biological senescence?) [585, 586, 627, 750, 754–759, 781–791].

As discussed above, under unresolved inflammation, expression of a wide number of growth factors, anti-oxidants, hormones and hormone-like mediators including activation of mTOR/AKT/IP3K pathways (Yang processes) are required to neutralize the toxic effects of stimuli-induced expression of pro-inflammatory and oxidants (Yin processes) in an attempt to terminate inflammation and tissue repair or to induce tolerance.

15.1 Mechanisms of mTOR-Kinase Complexes in Metabolism, Hormonal Regulation, Cell Growth and Immunity

The mammalian/mechanistic target of rapamycin (mTOR) is a serine/threonine kinase (also referred to as DRAK2) and a member of the phosphoinositide 3-kinase (PI3K)-family of kinases (PIKK). The super-family of mTOR/PIKK pathways is directly and indirectly involved in regulation of a wide range of tissue activities such as metabolism, proliferation, differentiation, lipid metabolism, growth and development, autophagy and immune cell responses [72, 196, 423, 455, 585, 587, 591–601, 604–606, 627, 657, 750, 754–758, 784, 789–793]. The two major constitutive (innate) and induced complexes of mTORC1 and mTORC2 seem to contribute to healthy tissue function and longevity. However, molecular defects (over-, or under-expression, genetic mutations) of any members of these complex pathways are reported to be involved in initiation of a wide range of metabolic disorders, infectious diseases (e.g., tuberculosis), neurological disorders (e.g., autism, epilepsy), cancer and other age-associated chronic illnesses.

In general, data on animal models of longevity demonstrate that growth hormones (GHs) modulate glucose uptake in insulin-dependent tissues (e.g., muscle). The growth hormones promoting signals involve IGF-1-independent pathways and the mTORC1 complex to activate Rag-GTPase family of enzymes and lipid metabolism. Low levels of plasma lipid were suggested to promote insulin sensitivity and signaling of PI3K/AKT/mTOR [476, 585, 757, 785, 786, 792].

Type 2 diabetes (adult onset) accompanied by expression of pro-inflammatory mediators (e.g., IL-6) and insulin-insensitivity increase the risk of several cancers. Related reports show that PI3K/AKT pathways are involved in glucose transporter-1 (GLUT-1) trafficking/activities. These pathways are also associated with cell growth and carcinogenesis and increased glucose consumption of cancerous cells through glycolysis (Warburg effect). Use of diabetes agents such as sulfonylurea and metformin are reported to directly influence ATP-sensitive k^+ channels for enhancing membrane depolarization of pancreatic beta cells and to stimulate exocytosis of insulin granules [361, 553, 585, 593, 744, 757, 784–786, 791–793]. While the suggested mechanisms and clinical values, efficacy or safety of such agents in diabetes are subjects of debates [553, 593, 784, 791, 793], it seems that these agents support other findings that cellular exocytosis is energy-dependent processes in many immune and non-immune cells/tissues with different functions. For example, we consider diabetes and related metabolic disorders as immune disorders that initially influence metabolic pathways and glucose transport and metabolism. Impaired glucose transport and utilization in these metabolic disorders, are associated with T cell activation and generation of memory or regulatory cells (Treg) and often require energy sources from fatty acid oxidation for glycolysis and glutaminolysis as additional or alternative pathways for tissue physiology. These pathways seem to be alternative or compensatory mechanisms to mitochondrial oxidative phosphorylation and generation of hypoxic conditions. Under these conditions, cell surface ligation and activation of membrane phospholipases (e.g., PLC) would allow mobilization of intracellular Ca^{+2} associated with loss of ER Ca^{+2} along with T cell plasma membrane influx of Ca^{+2} through ion channels [e.g., calcium release-activated channels (CRAC), also known as Ca release-activated Ca] signals to mediate regulation of Na/K ATPase and compensate for the Ca depletion of intracellular ER [329, 553, 592–599, 624–626, 752–754, 782–794].

Reported data on site-specific cancers such as renal cell carcinoma (RCC) suggest an association between up-regulation of hypoxia-inducible factor (HIF)-genes with growth factors such as platelet-derived growth factor (PDGF) and vascular endothelial growth factor (VEGF) and the binding to tyrosine kinase receptors as the result of activation of PI3K/AKT/ mTOR pathways. Other reports on genetic defects such as mutations in ras and von Hippel-Lindau (VHL) in tissues show activation of hypoxia-inducible factors (HIF-1 and HIF-2) and induction of VEGF expression and angiogenesis through PI3K/AKT/mTOR [767]. These and related reports demonstrate that oncogenes induce expression of vascular endothelial growth factor (VEGF), a key mediator in tumor angiogenesis [766, 767, 797]. Furthermore, radiation- or inflammation-induced mutations in any one of the interdependent pathways in PI3K/AKT/mTOR play important roles in outgrowth conditions in a variety of tissues (adipose, skeletal muscle, brain, lymphatic and vasculature) and cancer biology [686, 744, 753–759, 797]. It is also noteworthy that mTORC1 is sensitive to rapamycin and regulation of ribosomal protein recycling pathways and authophagy. However, chronic treatment with rapamycin inhibits mTORC2 pathways that mediate metabolism through FOXO and p38 MAPK pathways, crucial to oxidative stress resistance and lifespan in experimental animal studies [554, 555, 620–632, 646, 686, 744, 755, 759].

15.2 Role of mTOR in Metabolism and Immunity of Adipose Tissue (an Endocrine Organ)

Approximately 20% of genes that are expressed in adipocytes are hormones and growth factors for diverse functions. Examples of important metabolism of hormones and immune cell activities in adipose tissues and relations to mTOR signaling pathways in longevity are shown below (Fig. 6.8) [5, 10, 468, 544, 555, 646, 744–747, 752–759, 780, 782–784, 794, 795]:

(a) **Adiponectin Metabolism.** Adiponectin, secreted from adipose tissues is a hormone. Mediating through adiponectin receptors (AdipoR1 and AdipR2) the hormone involves activation of AMPK and PPARα signaling pathways and

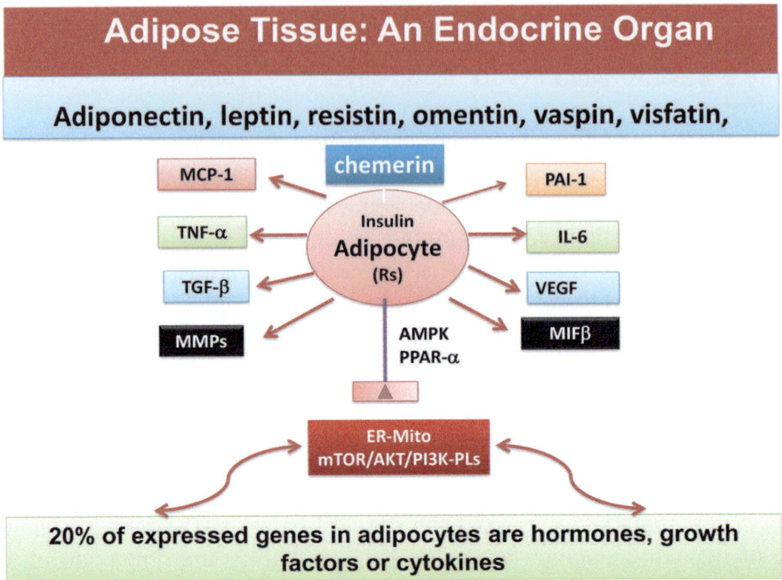

Fig. 6.8 Schematic representation of the roles that adipose tissue play in effective immunity. Adipose tissue is shown as an endocrine organ and an insulin-dependent tissue for glucose transport and metabolism. An integrated representation suggests that adipose tissue contributes to regulation of a wide range of immune-hormonal-metabolic activities in tissues in health or chronic diseases. See text

contributes to the regulation of tissue metabolism and lifespan. Its serum level is decreased in diabetes and increased upon weight loss [555, 744]. The AdipoR1 effects on insulin sensitivity are mediated through activation of AMPK and result in inhibition of mTORC1 complex and decreased activation of its substrate followed by inhibition of serine phosphorylation of IRS;

(b) **Leptin:** Leptin hormone produced by white adipose tissue is involved in regulation of energy balance for food intake and obesity. Leptin regulates neuronal and insulin signaling cascades through its receptors that mediate PI3K/AKT/mTOR-S6 K activities and involves SHP2-ERK and Jak2 mediation of insulin receptor phosphorylation and GH/IGF-1 pathways. Signaling pathways of leptin primarily influence the homeostasis of energy balance involving hypothalamic neurons (mediobasal) network. Altered leptin signaling pathways involving SOCS3, tyrosine phosphatase (PIP1B) and inflammatory mediators (IKK-NFkB and JNK) are suggested to be due to impaired ER-mitochondrial pathways in diseases such as obesity, diabetes and aging [755, 759];

(c) **Resistin:** Resistin, secreted in white adipocytes, decreases insulin sensitivity, affects cholesterol metabolism and regulation of LDL [468, 686];

(d) **Gherlin:** A neuropeptide (hunger hormone), released by the endocrine cells in empty stomach, antagonizes leptin function [554, 646];

(e) **Cholecystotokinin (CCK):** CCK is released by duodenal I-cells; stimulates gallbladder contraction and pancreatic exocrine secretion. CCK contributes to the regulation of glucose homeostasis and pancreatic acinar (beta) cells. CCK acts synergistically with leptin in promoting satiety perhaps by activation of AMPK in the hypothalamus and inhibition of mTORC1 complex [76, 77, 259, 439, 555];

(f) **Glucagan-like peptide 1 (GLP1):** GLP-1 is a hormone generated from proglucagan genes in the small intestine in response to nutrients and potentially stimulates insulin secretion. GLP1 agonists are being tested for treatment of chronic diseases such as Alzheimer's, stroke, Huntington's and Parkinson's diseases in various clinical studies [794]. However, the results are not conclusive.

(g) **Fibroblast growth factors (FGFs):** Several recent animal studies suggest the Klotho gene and FGF15/19, FGF21, FGF23 and related complexes play a role in glucose homeostasis or aging, involving also IGF1 activities mediated by PI3K/AKT pathways [780, 795].

(h) **Humanin:** Humanin is a short neuropeptide (23 residues) involved in mitochondrial (16S) or ribosomal RNA gene structure that binds to IGFBP-3. Humanin has a potential neuro-protective agent and a regulator of peripheral insulin sensitivity. It is also suggested that humanin increases the beta cell survival and glucose tolerance. Together with IGF-1-binding protein, humanin regulates apoptosis [795].

Therefore, it seems that PI3K/AKT/mTOR activities play interdependent crucial roles in growth and metabolism of tissues and influence the innate/intrinsic pathways. Related data on obesity show low-grade inflammation and impairment of insulin receptor signaling and insulin resistance, mediated through the complex and interdependent stress kinases [e.g., p38 MAPK (mitogen-activated protein kinase), c-Jun NH2-terminal kinase (inhibitor of NF-kB kinase - β-IKKβ), AMP-activated protein kinase, protein kinase C, Rho-associated coiled-coil containing protein kinase, and RNA-activated protein kinase] and phosphorylate the key regulators of glucose homeostasis in various tissues. The phosphorylation of serine residues in insulin receptors (e.g., IRS-1) results in diminished enzymatic activity of phosphatidylinositol 3-kinase (PI3K)/Akt pathway, the important mechanisms involved in insulin resistance and type 2 diabetes mellitus (T2-DM) or induction of cancer [267, 273, 529, 646, 686, 753–757]. A number of reports also suggest that insulin-insensitivity and hyperglycemia (high circulating glucose levels) alters mTOR complexes (mTORC1, mTORC2) signaling and mediate several interdependent pathways including metabolism, ribosomal biogenesis and autophagy. Whether caloric restriction (CR) and increased insulin sensitivity via decreased signaling through mTOR pathways, promotes endocrine factors and lifespan are subjects of recent debates and controversies [620–632, 646, 686, 744, 755, 759, 780, 794, 795].

As noted above, activation of PI3K/AKT is a common signaling pathway for oncogenes through hypoxia, a major stimulus for VEGF production. Effects of a selective PI3K inhibitor (LY294002) on HIF-1α and HIF-2α expression and endogenous VEGF response to hypoxia on breast cancer cell lines with different genetic changes suggest that use of PI3K inhibitors could inhibit synergistic and inducible effects of hypoxia with a wide range of common oncogenes, while basal hypoxia-inducible VEGF was partially inhibited [750, 790, 797, 830]. Analyses of relevant data also suggest the importance of these theories as linked to altered (increased) activities of signals in the chain of events in mTOR/AKT/kinases (e.g., mTORC2) pathways and loss of stress resistance and metabolism in tissues that contribute to cell growth and tumorigenesis.

In general, the various hormones or growth factors that are identified above seem to regulate glucose transport and metabolism by influencing insulin function in tissues and longevity or diseases of aging. The modes of actions of these hormones basically share involvement of the PI3K/AKT/mTOR signaling pathways via specific receptor molecules whose affect also differentially impact the sex hormones (e.g., 17b-estradiol) and longevity. Relevant experimental data also indirectly suggest that longevity is associated with growth hormone gene regulations such as IGFBP7 and influence tumor suppression. In all likelihood, the roles of adaptive/induced factors on the innate hormonal receptors (e.g., insulin, glucagon, estrogen, aldosterone, TSH) are important enough for maintenance of effective immunity and warrant further investigations. There are several recent clinical trials that aim to target mTOR for treatment of site-specific cancers (e.g., breast, renal cell carcinoma, NSCLC, anaplastic astrocytoma, mesothelioma, soft tissue sarcoma, cervical and uterine) [157, 750, 756, 758, 784, 785, 790, 811–814]. While the results are inconclusive the approaches support the fundamental roles of hormonal regulations in immunity and maintenance of health or metabolic diseases and tissue-specific cancers.

15.3 Bioenegetics of Chromatin Complexes: Remodeling of Nucleaosome

There are several studies that show the combined DNA double helix that spools around histone proteins to generate a somewhat stable nucleosome core particle involving clusters of weak contacts with hydrogen bonds and salts [17, 146, 578, 718, 796, 798, 799, 842]. The challenge to understand the regulatory factors in the assembly and integrity of genomic stability and DNA-histone proteins (octamers) within the parameters of nucleus in health and diseases has been noted in such studies. An overall analyses of data suggest that the bioenergetics (ATP utilization) and metabolic activities of nucleosome remodeling activities, de-association and re-association of DNA, repair enzymes and histone proteins follow the regulatory or control switches (positive and negative patterns) that are described for body's continually adapting to the environmental challenges via differential energy consuming activities of tumoricidal (Yin) and tumorigenic (Yang) events and influenced by oxidative stress or aging process. The fundamental processes of gene regulation and chromatin modifications involve cellular machinery for transcription and chromatin-associated histone proteins and integration of environmental inputs to mediate homeostatic responses through numerous intermediary metabolites and chromatin proteins that might be considered inherited transgenerational and tissue susceptibility toward injury or diseases of aging. The requirements for energy consumption and involvement of mitochondrial oxidative phosphorylation are fundamental to rapid movements of synthesized proteins (nucleosome sliding) and exchanges of sequences and interactions between specific DNA-binding proteins and regulatory factors during transcriptional events and assembly and maintenance of chromatin dynamics and the regulation of nuclei processes (e.g., replication of genome, transcription of genes, sensing and DNA repair, induction of genetic diversity or recombination processes) in all eukaryotic organisms [98–100, 139, 299, 300, 318, 472, 586, 627, 677, 681, 694, 762, 778]. These reports also suggest that the protective features that allow chromatin to remain inaccessible to the cellular environments require special DNA methylation and distinct patterns of histone modifications. Furthermore, accessibility of nucleaosomal genetic components and unfolding of highly ordered chromatin fiber by specific energy-dependent enzymatic and remodeling processes of nucleosome factors enable modulation of chromatin architecture for relocation of histone proteins and nucleosomal DNA during early 'sliding' events [98–100, 694, 778, 796–799, 827–829].

In brief, the energy-requirements for nucleosome remodeling serve to facilitate chromatin accessibility and unfolding, gene repression, chromatin assembly and maintenance of highly ordered structure of chromatin.

15.4 Inflammation-Hypothalamus-Adrenal Axis: Interdependent Acute Phase Response (APR) and Systemic Response

Within the spectrum of systemic reactions to internal or external stimuli, there are two major interdependent physiological responses associated with acute inflammation. The first involves alterations in the temperature set-point in the hypothalamus and the generation of the febrile response. The second involves alterations in the regulation of liver metabolism and genomic activities. Three major pro-inflammatory cytokines (e.g., IL-1, TNF and IL-6) that are expressed at the site of tissue injury or perhaps the induction of sepsis during combination cancer chemotherapy with radiation (cytokine storm, first response in Yin ?) involve the regulation of the febrile responses, possibly as protective mechanisms [5, 217–226, 528, 582, 601, 605, 657, 699, 701, 716, 741, 746, 747, 800–803, 822]. While the mechanisms of febrile responses are not fully understood, expression of pro-inflammatory cytokines of fever seems to follow through induction of anti-inflammatory mediators (e.g., PGE2, or IL-8 and IL-10) in tissue injury, sepsis or major brain trauma, as well as toxicity-(sepsis) induced by cancer chemotherapy and radiation (Yang?) often with life-threatening outcomes. The release of IL-1 and IL-6 perhaps act on adrenal-pituitary axis for signaling the production of adrenocorticotropic hormone (ACTH) to subsequently induce generation of corticosteroids and to offset (inhibit and terminate) the pro-inflammatory cytokine gene expression [5, 217–226, 528, 601, 605, 657, 699, 701, 716, 747, 800, 801]. The release of cytokines from activated macrophages proceeds by a complex sequences of events, involving signal transduction, nuclear-factor activation and transcription of various cytokine genes. The mechanisms of regulation of IL-1 and TNF synthesis are not well understood, partly due to the difficulty to work with isolated macrophage phenotype populations and lack of suitable macrophage cell-lines. However, detailed understanding on the mechanisms of initiation of acute phase reaction/response (APR) and progression to full blown systemic diseases requires better analyses and integration of data on multi-level communications between stimuli-induced inter-, intra-organ signaling pathways. For example, release of stored TNF and Ca^{+2} from activated mast cells (independent from degranulation or IgE-mediation) seem to accompany altered energy requirements, changes of $NADH/NAD^{+}$ ratios and acquired immune response profiles (e.g., NKs, Treg, MΦs, mucus secreting goblet cells and eosinophils) under a wide range of inflammatory conditions [e.g., familial Mediterranean fever-FMF), neurodegenerative and autoimmune diseases or site-specific cancers] [5, 238, 285, 351, 356, 369, 382, 391, 393, 461, 464, 471, 487, 521, 539, 540, 609, 615, 619, 628–630, 648, 699–701, 800–802].

As demonstrated below, the second wave of pro-inflammatory cytokine generation that is mediated through the action of IL-1 and TNF on stromal cells is better understood than the initiating wave of gene activation and expression of cytokines. The most detailed examination of sequences of expression of mediators is reported for the production of IL-6 by fibroblast cells. Analyses of relevant data suggest the two regions of the IL-6 gene appear to be important for the regulation of transcription as outlined below [9, 23, 50, 51, 210, 220, 367, 729, 746, 775, 776, 779]:

(a) One region comprises the serum-response element (SRE) and the binding site for the lymphocyte nuclear factor NF-IL-6;
(b) Second region is a binding site for an NF-B-like nuclear protein;

Co-operation between the two regions seems sufficient to upregulate transcription of the IL-6 gene. The IL-6 gene promoter also contains binding sites for other nuclear proteins, including the glucocorticosteroid receptor and AP-1 transcription. Furthermore, the likely stimulation of immune cells to express IL-6 occurs through at least three different signal-transduction pathways, including calcium mobilization, cAMP and diacylglycerol-activated protein kinases. Thus the initiation and progression of the APR involve a coordinated series of events, including cytokine release, endothelial-cell activation, leukocyte chemotaxis and alterations of the temperature set-point. Simultaneously, the adrenal-pituitary axis is activated to provide the necessary metabolic signals to the responding organs.

15.5 Inflammation- Hepatic Axis in Acute Phase Response (APR)

The liver is the principal target of systemic inflammatory mediators. It is also the organ responsible for determining the level of essential metabolites that are supplied to the organism during critical stages of stress. Moreover, the liver provides the necessary components for immediate defense at the site of tissue damage, as well as confining tissue destruction, clearing harmful agents and aiding tissue repair. Liver cells respond to several factors that are induced during the acute phase response via their cell-surface receptors. The liver response is characterized by prominent changes in the activities of most metabolic pathways, and in the co-ordinate stimulation of the acute phase plasma proteins (APPs) and potential involvement of energy requiring pathways in Wnt/b-catenin and Tbx3, IGFBP1-Bak activities and surface proteins (e.g., CD14/CD16) [7, 75, 77, 78, 80, 83, 85, 91, 92, 98, 105, 106, 112, 119, 120, 261, 262, 265, 266, 282, 409, 418, 425–432, 529, 732, 821].

15.6 Mitochondria and Immune Dysfunction: Activation of Oncogenes

Cancer is an induced disease of the Twentieth century, facilitated by medical establishment for corporate profit.

Definitions of the core 'genetic blueprint' for cancer cells growth and related epigenetics topics that are measured by OMICS platforms and specific detections technologies do not necessarily predict the cancer phenotypes or how to overcome growth of cancer cells [5, 10, 414, 419, 572, 573, 804, 805]. In general, cancer adaptive activities are likely the results of loss of balance between differential (mitochondrial-dependent) activities of high energy demand (tumoricidal or Yin) and low energy demand (tumorigenic or Yang) of effective immunity occurring through multiple pathways including mTOR/AKT/PI3K, Myc and Ras oncogenes altering activities of immune and non-immune cell components [5, 10–15, 572, 579, 585, 627, 628, 658, 750, 754]. Cancer cells induce alternative and adaptive metabolic pathways that bypass the limitations of mitochondrial oxidative phosphorylation for energy consumption and nutrition under hypoxic condition as part of their ability to escape immunity and resist stress. One of the important energy sources (ATP) for adaptation of cancer cell growth is the glucose-lactate metabolic pathways. To what extent altered mitochondrial function and ATP free energy source affect other cellular activities such as maturation and differentiation of cells or degeneration and regeneration (wear and tear) activities of tissues in aging and immune disorders are important topics that are not understood. The metabolic events and pro-growth signals seem to occur simultaneous and facilitate activation of oncogenes (wounds that do not heal) as loss of balance in tumoricidal vs tumorigenic (Yin-Yang) properties of immune surveillant that favor growth promoting pathways.

The reported mechanisms of activation of hypoxia-induced Warburg effect and increased aerobic glycolysis for energy requirements of growth of cancer cells seem controversial [412, 481, 559–566, 568, 570–576, 579–585]. The overall analyses of data suggest that in order to achieve their lawless growth and escape immune surveillance, the activated oncogenes with their increased evolving somatic mutations would impose the following major interdependent changes in metabolism and function of target (local) and distal tissues that destroy the body (Figs. 6.3 and 6.7) [5, 10–15, 196, 301, 419, 562, 579, 580, 585, 626–628, 644, 750–754, 784–787, 790, 793, 804, 805]:

(a) Altered immune cells polarity favoring growth promotion pathways. Expression of growth promoting cytokines, proteins and lipids leads to biological rearrangements at various cellular levels (e.g., ER and Golgi apparatus) and/or regulation of Ca^{2+} flux that facilitate growth enhancement signals;
(b) Depending on the composition of site-specific tissues, changes in immune cells polarity include induction of M1 to M2 (TAMs) phenotypes, DC1 (immature, tumoricidal) to DC2 (mature, TAM), or MCs (granulated) to 'leaky' MCs (degranulated, TAMCs);
(c) Overall growth promotion of tissues under hypoxic condition induces activation of low energy dependent pathways such as AMP-kinase and increased activities of PI3K-ser-thr kinase (AKT)-mTOR pathways for growth promotion (anabolic events). Warburg effect and activation of aerobic glycolysis is the preferred pathway for utilization of free energy (ATP) perhaps due to oxidative stress-induced impaired mitochondrial oxidative phosphorylation.
(d) Induction of neovacularization and exaggerated expression of growth promoting mediators such as PGE2, IL-8, IL-10, low level histamine (non-IgE-dependent), PKC, VEGF or HIFs;
(e) Oncogenes-induced oxidative stress leads to decreased signals for apoptotic mediators or reduced expression of pro-inflammatory mediators (tumoricidal, Yin);

Simply explained, the biological events that are inherent and normal for tissue metabolism during growth and development (Yin-Yang) are hijacked by increased activities of cancer oncogenes in favor of their enhanced lawless growth requirements. The reported data on immune cells dysregulation such as altered activities of TLRs, or PI3K/mTOR- induced growth of viral or bacterial genes are very likely similar and comparable to growth of cancer oncogenes in altering energy dynamics for induction of tolerance or immune suppression [5, 450–452, 455, 614, 637, 638, 709, 719, 747, 770].

Therefore, cancer oncogenes are viewed by the immune system as oxidative stress that cause induction of accumulated delayed type hypersensitivity in target tissue and demand continued signals for termination or repair [5, 10]. Aging process and frequent exposures to intrinsic and extrinsic unwanted/harmful elements drift the sharpness of immunity and provide opportunities for pathogens or oncogenes to take advantage of pleiotropic properties of immunity (positive and negative control switches in metabolic, apoptosis/wound healing, hormonal, neuronal and vasculature) that promote oncogenesis.

16 Bird's Eye View of Intrinsic (Innate) and Induced (Adaptive) Response Profiles in Initiation of 'Mild', 'Moderate' and 'Severe' Immune Disorders and Tumorigenesis: Differential Bioenergetics Requirement in Yin and Yang Events

As emphasized throughout this book, acute inflammation is a well orchestrated precise biological network or 'a molecular village of signals' and demands exact molecular participations from immune and non-immune systems, at the 'precise moments of need' for guarding, protecting and maintaining individual's health, after birth and throughout life (Figs 6.1 and 6.9). Serious disturbance in any of the

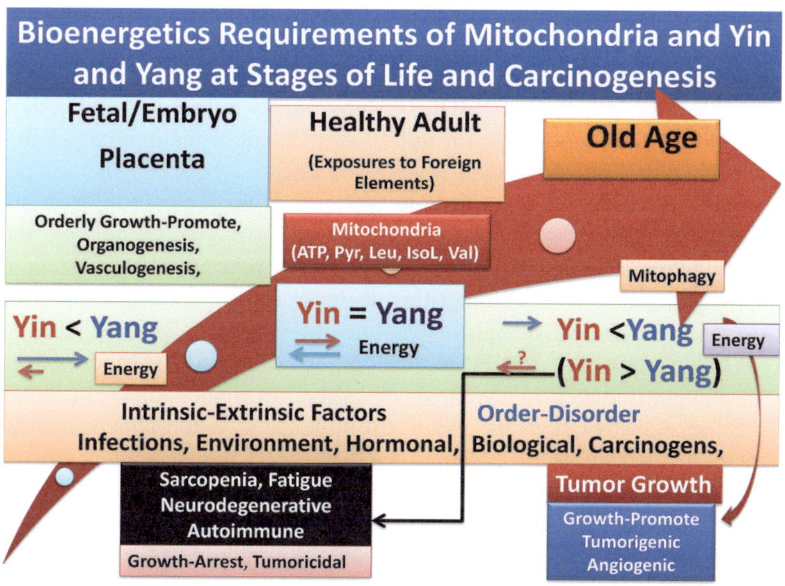

Fig. 6.9 Schematic representation of a working model hypothesis explaining parallel functionality of mitochondria and immune surveillance, or Yin (tumoricidal, growth-arrest) and Yang (tumorigenic, growth-promote) at different stages of life. It depicts that during orderly fetal growth there is limited need for high energy demands of a fully functional mitochondria or the requirements of an effective immune surveillance (balance in Yin-Yang) within the confined and protective environment of placenta. The scheme depicts that fully functional mitochondria along with highly regulated balance in Yin (tumoricidal, high energy demands from oxidative phosphorylation) and Yang (tumorigenic, low energy demands from glycolysis) of effective immunity are developed after birth and throughout adulthood for maintenance of health. The scheme also demonstrates comparable features of orderly fetus growth with that of disorderly (lawless) cancerous cells growth and impaired function of mitochondria. The role of oxidative stress-induced mitochondrial damage and induction of neurodegenerative and autoimmune diseases or cancer are depicted to lead to differential damages in immune-responsive and immune-privileged tissues. See text (Adopted from Khatami (Ref. [10]).)

many molecular organizations imposed by biological terrorists (oxidative stress or aging process) could shift such highly regulated communications between and among organ systems toward initiation and progression of a wide range of immune disorders.

Integration and analyses of data on tissue/organ development or information on age-induced increased neurodegenerative or autoimmune diseases or carcinogenesis suggest that age-associated immune-biological senescence and accumulation of oxidative stress induced by accumulation of pathogenic structural and genomic components or radiation and pathogen-specific vaccines and adjuvants (e.g., aluminum, mercury, L-histidine) would lead to alterations of mitochondrial energy-demands. The major altered activities of host tissues often involve cross-reactivity between pathogen-, or allergen-specific antibodies and modifications of a number of host surface molecules (e.g., TLRs, glycosylation of lipids or proteins, activities of membrane lipid-protein-enzymes, ion transports) along with conditions such as hypoxia, altered metabolism of branched amino acids (e.g., valine, leucine/isoleu and alanine) or aromatic amino acids (e.g., tyrosine, phenylalanine) in mitochondria and energy-dependent pathways of mTOR/PI3K/AKT [5, 10, 338, 483, 504, 557–563, 583, 584, 586, 747, 758, 759]. The oxidative stress-induced altered activities of tissues, are likely the foundations for initiation of minor or major changes in signal transduction and energy-dependent miscommunications between surface proteins and receptor molecules that contribute to tardiness of response profiles in immune and non-immune cells.

There are major knowledge gaps in understanding how altering crosstalk among these pathways lead to altered integrities or errors in host activities that influence active or passive transport of nutrients/solutes or ions (e.g., glucose transporters, Na^+/K^+ ATPase activities, Na^+/H^+ exchanges, Ca channels) or altered host and pathogen-allergen-induced biosynthesis of antibodies. Other important unknowns in disease processes relate to the extent of influence of external/extrinsic stimuli-(e.g., allergen, microbiota or environmental hazards) induced altered quality or nature of expression or co-expression of pattern recognition molecules and their influence on internal/intrinsic stimuli (e.g., accumulated senescence cells, cancerous or other defective cells or proteins, complex B lymphocytes, oxidized complex lipids or carbohydrates) that alter immune response profiles (e.g., histamine, oxidants or expression of respective receptor molecules). Time course kinetics for recognition or tolerance (ignoring) of external or internal foreign entities are likely different in genesis and outcomes of diseases. Furthermore, how aging processes skew the response qualities or interactions between constituent receptor molecules (e.g., insulin receptors, glucose active or passive transport) or induced receptor molecular expression are additional important knowledge gaps in understanding the aging process and host-pathogen interactions.

17 Is Cancer a Severe Late Hypersensitivity Reaction (Immune Tsunami) That Destroys Host Tissue for Immortal Life? The Precious Truth!!

> It is by the goodness of God that in our country we have those three unspeakably precious things: freedom of speech, freedom of conscience and the prudence never to practice either of them. Mark Twain

As discussed above (Sect. 7.1), nearly all full blown diseases seem to be the result of three major interdependent biological problems; (a) complications in vasculature and lymphatic channels; (b) tissue necrosis and atrophy; or (c) lawless tissue growth. The shared or special features of pathobiology of these complications contribute to a wide range of 'mild', 'moderate' (intermediate) or 'severe' allergic conditions or immune disorders (inflammatory diseases) and multistep carcinogenesis. For example, analyses of a large body of data on acute inflammatory diseases (e.g., sepsis or major trauma), or chronic illnesses such as neurodegenerative and autoimmune diseases and multistep carcinogenesis seem to support our suggestion [5, 10] that circulating low level histamine plays important roles in sustaining oxidative stress and alterations of vasculature function and the induction of vascular hyperpermeabily, neovascularization or angiogenesis [5, 10–15, 228, 237, 345–367, 516–528, 530–543, 552, 628, 629, 645, 668, 669].

Being the tree of life, the major function of vascular tissue for maintenance of health throughout life falls into the following energy-requiring categories:

1. Delivery of nutrients and oxygen to tissues/organs and removal of gases and waste products from the tissues from the early fetus growth, after birth and throughout life;
2. Gatekeeper of immune cell trafficking; involved in proliferation differentiation and infiltration of inflammatory cells into stimulated (infected or injured) targeted tissues, facilitating both apoptosis (Yin) and wound healing (Yang) processes;
3. Maintenance of precise crosstalk between the immune-hormonal-neuronal-metabolic pathways in organs/tissues;

Altered activities of vasculature are known features of nearly all disease processes including acute inflammatory diseases (e.g., anaphylactic shock, sepsis, meningitis, pneumonia), chronic illnesses such as hypertension, neurodegenerative and autoimmune diseases, lupus, diabetes, cardiovascular or stroke complications as well as multistep carcinogenesis.

In the original series of experiments, we reported that histamine is a potent vasoactive factor (messenger) and the primary mediator that is released from CALTs, followed by release of prostaglandin (PGF-1α, or prostacyclin) as secondary mediator release accompanied by vascular hyperpermeability [362]. Other data sugget that histamine release could stimulate gastrointestinal, respiratory, neuronal and skin causing vasodilatation, contractions of cardiac muscle or lung airways (bronchioles) (see above).

We recently described [5, 10] that the cancer growth and angiogenesis are late phase accumulation of exaggerated immune response disorders that create an 'immune tsunami' causing destruction of tissues that manifeste as site-specific primary cancers (e.g., lung, stomach, colon, breast, prostate, ovarian, pancreas) followed by cellular/molecular advances to metastasis to secondary sites according to the theory of "seed and soil" that was originally described by Paget in 1889 [41, 42] (Table 6.1). We proposed that the growth of cancerous cells is initiated from developmental phases of 'mild' to 'moderate' immune disorders such as asthma, emphysema, gastritis, pancreatitis and would advance to severe immune dysfunction that facilitate growth promotion. The development of cancers were hypothesized as the 'severe' degrees of accumulated immune response mismatches as the result of loss of tumoricidal (Yin) vs tumorigenesis (Yang) of acute inflammation (immune surveillance) or the loss of effective immunity [5, 10].

17.1 Cancer-Induced Oxidative Stress: Dysfunction of Genomic, Immune Response and Metabolism in Tissue

The natural control switches (positive or negative signals) that we originally defined as dual properties of Yin (tumoricidal) and Yang (tumorigenic) of acute inflammation seem to have wider applications in physiological behaviors of the organ systems and maintenance of health. However, age-induced tardiness of immunity and cumulative presence of cancerous cells, biological and environmental hazards could drastically disrupt the normal biological behaviors of tissues including genomic stability, physiology and immune response profiles. Tardiness of immunity would allow cancerous cells to escape being detected and destroyed (see above). Compromised immunity provides opportunity for cancer oncogenes to slowly or aggressively take over the machinery of host for its enhanced growth requirements.

As noted above, altered acid-base balance (altered proton-ATP) perhaps is accompanied by minor or major damages to oxidative metabolism of mitochondria and bioenergetics in tissues resulting in hypoxic conditions. The induction of hypoxia is associated with growth promotion pathways in target tissue and vasculature. The growth promotion events would eventually lead to altered or loss of functional integrity of extra-, and intra-cellular activities (e.g., membrane ion/nutrient transport, lysosomal exocytosis-ER, autophagy, mitochondria, nuclear reactions) resulting in cell growth, preneoplasia, precancer, tumorigenesis, cancer and angiogenesis (Fig. 6.9). The overall sequences of events in the induction of epithelial-mesenchymal transition in immune-responsive tissues and loss of tissue architectural integrity and function and bioenergetic requirements involved in disease processes and carcinogenesis are outlined below [5, 10–15, 21, 72, 196, 251, 258, 340, 423, 444, 445, 455, 483, 557–563, 587–594, 611–614, 636, 640, 667–680, 686–688, 707, 711, 738, 749, 750, 761, 766, 786-790, 797, 805–838]:

(a) In the tumor stroma, oxidative stress mimics the effects of tissue hypoxia that are present under aerobic condition, resulting in an excess production of reactive oxygen species (ROS). The oxidative stress-induced proinflammatory mediators (e.g., ROS, other oxidants) signal for expression of anti-inflammatory mediators in the environment of cancer cells causing an unequal (one way) inhibition of apoptotic factors (e.g., TNF-α, ILs, neurotoxins) that benefit cancer cells in being neutralized. Relevant data demonstrate that the production of ROS significantly contributes to altered genomic stability and anuploidity, as well as changes in centromere. Similarly, oxidative stress and accumulated presence of ROS in cancer environment is accompanied by alterations in mitochondrial oxidative phosphorylation and changes in ATP/ADP/AMP ratios and the induction of hypoxia;
(b) The epithelial-mesenchymal transition (EMT) processes are activated by a number of growth factors during sustained inflammatory processes that make tissue susceptible to tumor progression and metastasis. Expression of growth factors and receptor molecules (e.g., EGF-EGFR) are known contributors in the progression of cholangiocarcinoma (CCA) and the induction of EMT as key events in CCA progression. The EMT processes of cell transformation that often occur in immune-responsive tissues play crucial roles in the loss of cell contact control mechanisms and dysregulated cell growth promotion. Loss of epithelial cell features leads to adaptation of new characteristics of tissue that are typical of mesenchymal cells; lack of cell-cell adhesion properties;
(c) Data on epithelial-derived tumors (e.g., cholangiocarcinoma-CCA) further demonstrated that gene expression profile closely resemble features of mesenchymal cells, including increased expression of EMT-derived transcription factors (Snail), correlated with metastasis and inversely related to the level of E-cadherin adhesion molecules. The influence of TNF-α in enhancing migration and induction of Snail, while it reduces E-cadherin expression in cell line models of CCA (in vitro) support the role of impaired inflammatory responses in the induction of cancer;
(d) The bone marrow-derived mesenchymal stem cells (BMDMSCs) influence resolution of acute and chronic inflammation, in tissues such as the skin wounds by stimulation of collagen synthesis, deposition and induction of granulation process for improving MCs recovery or repair [826]. Although detailed mechanisms of stem cells function, after tissue injury (e.g., skin-metal implants) are not understood, it is possible that BMDMSCs being pleiotropic in nature, facilitate other immune cells (e.g., MCs, DCs) to improve function during remodeling of architectural integrity of target tissues;
(e) The mutagenic changes in tissues are referred to as retrotransposition or *de novo*retrotransposition events that would lead to heavy genomic methylation and inactivation of affected genes for transcription. It appears that the inactivation of genomic components (e.g., L1 retrotransposons) facilitate genomic instability by integrating into DNA and altering transduction. These are major contributors of insertion of misdirected expression of a number of functional proteins in the genesis of chronic diseases such as neuronal behaviors, as well

as altered growth pathways. Other data show that circulating abnormal micro RNAs [miR-21, miR-34, miR-126, miR-195, let-7a, miR-146a, and miR-155] are considered as 'inflamma-miRs' and modulate the NF-kB growth signaling network in aging, chronic inflammation and breast cancer [5, 251, 258, 718, 796, 826–829]). Whether these features of micro RNAs in persistent inflammation, cancer and aging are related to the heavy somatic mutations and manipulation of epigenetic methylation are among biological gaps that remain to be better understood;

(f) Aging process and the growth of cancerous cells often accompanied with accumulation of evolving and deleterious mutations in genomic components and abnormal expression or co-expression of pro-, or post-inflammatory mediators resulting the loss of maintenance of cell integrity, dysregulation of cell growth-death patterns and initiation of multistep chronic diseases or cancer.

17.2 *Tumor Lysis Syndrome and Tissue Metabolism*

In recent years tumor lysis syndrome (TLS) and treatment of patients with hematologic tumors (non-Hodgkin's lymphoma, B-cell lymphoma, Burkitt lymphoma, myeloid leukemia, lymphoblastic leukemia) has been the focus of several studies [7, 138, 228, 287, 465, 466]. The development of fatal TLS was established primarily in blood-born malignancies. However, TLS has also become a major concern in patients with solid tumors (e.g., hepatocellular carcinoma, lung squamous cell carcinoma, non-small cell lung cancer, metastatic lung adenocarcinoma, metastatic colon carcinoma, endometrial cancer, metastatic melanoma and androgen-dependent prostate cancer, germ cell tumors, gastric, breast or renal cancers) who received chemotherapies–'targeted' therapy, 'precision' or 'personalized' medicine with or without radiation [5, 466].

Among severe metabolic abnormalities, associated with TLS, which often result in life-threatening arrhythmia and/or multiple organ failure (MOF) are Ca^{+2} deficiencies and related tissue dysfunction as clinical symptoms are [465, 466]:

(a) Increased uric acid (UA) or hyperuremia and creatinine levels by 25%
(b) Increase potassium (hyperkalemia) level by 25%
(c) Increased phosphate, hyperphasphatemia (due to decline in calcium level) by 25%
(d) Reduced calcium level (hypocalcemia) by 25% and induction of fatal cardiac dysfunction (arrhythmia);

Tumor lysis syndrome (an induced cytokine storm in an already immune-compromised body) becomes serious and life-threatening perhaps by patient's health status. It is likely that, conditions such as kidney failure and abnormal filtration rate, hyper-, or hypotension, or diabetes-related complications and use of other drugs would intensify the effects of TLS.

18 Bioenergetics of Host-Immune Dynamics: Contribution of Mitochondria and Oxidative Metabolism

Whenever you find yourself on the side of the majority, it is time to pause and reflect. Mark Twain

Our recent hypotheses on the differential bioenergetics requirements of Yin-Yang of acute inflammation in health and diseases are extended in this section [5, 10]. Comparison on shared energy consumption of orderly fetal growth will be made with conditions of wound healing processes and the features of lawless growth of cancer cells. It will be shown that the high energy requirements of Yin events (utilizing oxidative phosphorylation from mitochondria) seem to be absent (not necessary and harmful) during fetal orderly growth and similarly impaired during lawless growth in carcinogenesis. In this context, mitochondrial function, and the pyruvate shuttle transporters and biosynthesis of structural proteins and metabolism of essential amino-acids (e.g., alanine, valine leucine, isoleucine) will be compared during fetal growth, normal adult biology (balance in Yin-Yang) and age-associated cancer growth. These new concepts and hypotheses for future studies include presentation of a working model on bioenergetics of cell function at distinct periods of life from fetus to post-birth, adulthood and aging process and carcinogenesis as detailed below [5, 10].

18.1 Differential and Parallel Bioenergetics Requirements of Mitochondria and Immune-Surveillance from Fetus Growth, and throughout Life: Features of 'Mild', 'Moderate' and 'Severe' Immunological Disorders and Cancer

Fetus growth is an orderly and almost one-way process of developing vasculogenesis and organogenesis. Growth of fetus utilizes low ATP energy from glycolytic pathways and under limited oxygen tension of placenta (hypoxic conditions) and in the absence of functional mitochondria for high energy production [5, 10, 677, 832–835]. Such growth features are somewhat comparable to the lawless growth of cancer cells as we recently proposed [5, 10]. Aging process and persistent unresolved inflammation was suggested to impair important functions of mitochondria for production of high energy oxidative phosphorylation to fight cancer cell growth. It was hypothesized that the impaired mitochondrial functions in aging parallel the tardiness of immune responses or the balance between high energy demands that are required during Yin (tumoricidal) and low energy consuming Yang (tumorigenic) processes [5, 10–15]. It was argued that the impaired mitochondrial function (mitophagy) would allow enhanced lawless growth of cancerous cells through increased cytosolic glycolysis and glucose utilization for production of low/

inefficient energy, under the hypoxic conditions or the Warburg effect. The roles that circulating low level histamine (sustained oxidative stress) play in the loss of balance between Yin-Yang events and induction of mitochondrial dysfunction (mitophagy) could lead to the initiation of different degrees of immune disorders that are manifested as 'mild', 'moderate' or 'severe' age-associated diseases or multistep carcinogenesis [5, 10].

Analyses of data on bioenergetics-related reports suggest that after birth drastic and simultaneous changes occur for adjusting the growth of newborn to the atmospheric pressure and high energy demands that are required for completion of development of organ systems (e.g., lung airways, cardiac muscle, brain, liver, eye, neuronal, lymphatic and vasculature) that are independent from maternal-placenta. Perhaps the most pronounced physiological changes in the newborn are the completion of mitochondrial development and function for supply of high energy demands (generation and hydrolysis of ATP via oxidative phosphorylation) from glucose oxidation and pyruvate-shuttle to the mitochondria. These biological events require biosynthesis of pyruvate carrier proteins/transporters and related enzymes for TCA cycle intermediates for oxidative phosphorylation, as well as metabolism of branched chain amino acids for biosynthesis of structural proteins [5, 10].

An stimuli-induced activation of immune cells, in a healthy individual, initially engage in rapid generation of energy (ATP hydrolysis) by utilizing the oxidative phosphorylation of mitochondria that otherwise is needed (reserved) for biosynthesis of tricarboxylic acid (TCA) cycle intermediates, biosynthesis of lipids and related enzymes and homeostasis of mitochondrial energy power for cells. Providing rapid energy (ATP hydrolysis) from oxidative metabolism, enables immune cells (e.g., M1, tumoricidal phenotype of MΦs) to express pro-inflammatory mediators and toxins and generate needed toxicity for killing/destroying pathogens or foreign elements (Fig. 6.1 Yin processes). However, Yang (wound healing) responses are involved in resolution of inflammation and simultaneously use activated immune cell phenotypes (e.g., M2 or TAMs phenotype) to produce growth promoting mediators by shifting the energy requirements toward aerobic glycolysis (Warburg effect). Therefore, unlike Yin events, the wound healing responses and the expression of HIF1 (VEGF) in the neighborhood of hypoxic neovasculature, to repair the tissue and return it to resting status, occur under the low energy and low oxygen requirements. The energy shifts from high ATP production in mitochondria to low energy consumption of aerobic glycolysis (Warburg effect) seem enable the cell to restore the Yin-induced rises in tricarboxylic acid (TCA) cycle intermediates (e.g., succinate, fumarate) in the mitochondria of activated immune cells. However, sustained oxidative stress or unresolved inflammation may increase utilization of aerobic glycolysis (Warburg effect) for energy consumption as the results of overuse (exhaustion) of oxidative phosphorylation pathways that cause dysfunction of mitochondria. The validity of this hypothesis seems supported by findings that angiogenesis and hypoxic conditions are primary features in tumor microenvironment and other inflammatory diseases.

In brief, the growth of cancer cells is the results of severe, aggressive, cumulative and progressive immune disorders (immune tsunami) that initiates slowly as mild (sub-clinical) alterations of immune responses in vulnerable/susceptible tissues. The altered immune responses differentially cause damages in the immune-responsive tissues (e.g., epithelial, endothelial, mucus-secreting cells or lymphocytes) or immune-privileged tissues (e.g., BBB, retina, CNS, reproductive organs) in multistep diseases.

18.2 Bases for Repeated Failed Cancer Therapeutics: Ignoring Nature of Compensating Biological Events!

The major problems with the repeatedly failed claimed 'targeted' therapies, 'precision' or 'personalized' medicine for solid tumors are the existence of numerous compensating and competing events that contribute to molecular chaos in the cancer environments (details in Chap. 5). Agents such as growth or kinase inhibitors and monoclonal antibodies or inhibitors or analogues of rapamycin (sirolimus) [e.g., everolimus or RAD001 (Afinitor®), AP23573 (CCI-779) and ester metabolite (temsirolimus), alone or in combination with other drugs (e.g., carboplatin, bevacizumab), that are used in Phase I, II or III clinical trials for treating and controlling growth and metastasis of solid tumors (e.g., breast, renal cell carcinoma, NSCLC, astrocytoma, mesothelioma, cervical and uterine cancers) produced little, if any success [5, 9, 14, 15, 26, 80, 152, 709, 782, 807–815, 839]. A major factor in lack of success in the claimed cancer therapies is that the mutated genes that are the bases of treatment (somatic mutations) possess features of heterogeneity and instability and capable of evolving to other mutations even during the therapy and not responsive to specific inhibition. In 2012, The Cancer Genome Atlas Network (TCGA) identified over 30,000 somatic mutations in breast cancer, and over 190,000 exons from over 18,000 genes in lung squamous cell carcinoma (lung SqCC) [816, 817]. In late phase of cancer growth and metastasis, the number of evolving mutations in solid tumors range from 10,000 to over 100,000 mutations and the chances of success at best are 0.001 to 0.03, under the 'conditions' that the somatic mutations do not further mutate. The interdependent factors are ignored when the therapies of solid tumors are decided and make such tremendously expensive trials worthless (details in Chap. 5) [5, 10, 14, 102, 128, 129, 136, 151–154, 161, 198, 203, 226, 265, 285, 331, 462, 463, 510, 514, 573, 574, 594]. These illogical and chaotic approaches are scientifically insane. The out-of-focus, reductionist, fuzzy and chaotic approaches to solid tumor therapy that repeatedly failed patients support our concerns that a century of cancer research and treatment are 'scientific/medical ponzi schemes' and remind us of the US Congressional debates on 'building too many expensive bridges to nowhere' or finding too many broken pieces of too many needles in a haystack and attempting to put them back [5, 13–15, 161, 162].

Recent attempts in cancer immunotherapies, while intellectually more logical compared with 'targeted' therapies that identify endless somatic mutations (growth factors) for drug development and clinical trials; they have the same basic flaws. For example, immunotherapeutic approaches use antibodies or inhibitors of checkpoint proteins on T cells for specific cancers or potentiate the apoptotic activities of program death (PD) factors of dendritic or other immune cells or targeting a particular inflammatory mediator or pathway [5, 6, 10, 150, 265, 507, 510, 708, 839]. Outcomes are measured whether inhibiting check point proteins or increasing death factors in specific innate immune cells would correct/prevent cancer growth. However, there are no serious attempts to understand that abnormal checkpoints on T cells are among hundreds or thousands of other molecular lawlessness that are present in the chaotic cancer molecular environment. Furthermore, in such expensive studies, little attention have been paid to measure how the inhibition of a checkpoint affects the ratios of apoptosis (tumoricidal) vs wound healing (tumorigenic) or the status of oxido-redox whose loss of balance initiate and progress to carcinogenesis [5, 10–15, 161 (Khatami, personal communications, NCI/NIH 2012–2014)].

19 Fundamental Questions for Future Considerations: Influence of Inflammatory Responses in Induction of Chronic Diseases or Cancer

The following are highlights of selected proposed biological gaps on early responses of tissues toward multistep cell growth with emphasis on histamine-related metabolic pathways and therapy in age-associate illnesses or tumorigenesis that deserve further studies. The overall observations and concepts on the influence of MCs in multistep tumorigenesis and angiogenesis described for conjunctival-associated lymphoid tissues (CALTs) may be extended to other cells/tissues with similar or different cell composition (details in Chaps. 2 and 4) [5, 10–15, 161, 162, 228, 236, 238, 288, 345, 351–354, 368, 391, 393, 471, 508, 516–528, 530–540, 541, 552, 628–635, 645, 648, 701, 801]:

(a) Older adults are immune compromised to varying degrees. In this context the role of mitochondrial function in supplying the energy for maintenance of balance between Yin (tumoricidal) and Yang (tumorigenic) of immune surveillance is fundamental. Age-associated immune compromises in susceptible tissues increase allergic conditions (e.g., asthma, emphysema, skin or ocular allergies) or other inflammatory conditions (e.g., colitis, gastritis, hepatitis) and carcinogenesis.
(b) The design of clinical trials, for assessment of disease risks and health status of public, is proposed to include determination of the baseline circulating histamine or histaminases as useful markers for the status of oxidative stress and acid–base levels in individuals over time. Developing cytokine chips that monitor early alterations of immune profiles may prove to be very effective for preventing chronic diseases.
(c) Among metabolic pathways whose levels are known to alter mitochondrial bioenergetics in favor of lawless cancer growth are metabolism of branched chained amino acids and biosynthesis of proteins in functional mitochondria

(perhaps after birth). Whether enhanced growth of cancer cells and associated loss of cell contact inhibition correlates with defective/loss of metabolism of branched chained amino acids (e.g., leucine, isoleucine or valine) and the dysfunction of mitochondria (mitophagy) awaits systematic studies. Furthermore, we proposed that the differences in energy demands during tumoricidal (Yin, high energy requiring) and tumorigenic (Yang, low energy from glycolysis) processes include asymmetry in bioelectricity of reaction processes and differential properties of pH gradients and respective ionic channels (e.g., H+/Na+ or Cl−/H+ exchangers), active transport systems or pumps (e.g., Na+/K+ ATPase, Ca+2 ATPase) or water channel (aquaporins) [5, 10]. Detailed understanding of the bioenergetics of mitochondria in maintaining the effective immunity should be among top research priorities for future studies.

(d) Whether stimuli-induced expression of histamine receptor molecules alter (induction of histamine decoy receptors or expression of mutated receptors) during developmental phases of immune dysfunction and multistep tumorigenesis. Our initial observations using histamine at the intermediate phase of ocular challenges (down regulation phenomena and observed MCs exhaustion with minimal clinical responses) demonstrated a strong type 1 reaction. The data suggested that histamine receptor molecules were intact, during down-regulation phenomenon (induction of exhausted or 'leaky MCs). Further experiments, using a MC degranulating agent (compound 48/80) also produced minimal clinical reaction, confirming that repeated challenge with antigen depleted MC degranulation capacity;

(e) The status of MCs granulation or degranulation in relation to B/plasma cells activation and challenge with antigen and onset of diseases are subjects of controversies. We reported that repeated antigen challenge in the chronic stages of ocular reactions that led to tumorigenesis was associated with altered ratios of IgG isotypes (IgG1/IgG2) in local/host tissue. Potential biosynthesis of immature MCs (defective granulation or unscheduled) or inappropriate/defective or insufficient synthesis of IgE-receptor molecules or surface proteins during response profiles are among interdependent biological gaps that require further investigations.

(f) The environmental effects of fetus growth and adaptation of host innate or adaptive immunity are the topic of intensive studies. We demonstrated that repeated ocular reactions could sensitize MCs in local or distal tissues including the ocular tissue MCs in new born guinea pigs of repeatedly sensitized ocular tissues of parents. Our data are suggestive of the first evidence that repeated stimulation of MCs influence the fetus immune dynamics altering the gene expression profiles and/or IgE paternal/maternal transfer of allergic responses and genomic predisposition in fetus;

(g) Immune-responsive or immune-privileged tissues and/or insulin-dependent or insulin-independent tissues for glucose transport may be differentially influenced by histamine or other inflammatory mediators. Several recent studies suggest that diabetes increases the risk of cancer in certain tissues. In addition to the increased level of cytokines such as IL-6, glucose toxicities may differentially influence the oxidative stress in tissues that are insulin-dependent (e.g., muscle, adipocytes or liver) or insulin-independent (e.g., vasculature, retina, CNS) for glucose transport and utilization.

(h) Metabolism of adenosine release and receptor. Adenosine and proton (H+) gradient in tissues may act synergistically to regulate, for example, the cerebral blood flow. Adenosine production is enhanced under various experimental conditions due to an imbalance between oxygen supply and oxygen need. Direct application of adenosine dilates the pial vessels, but changes in cerebral vascular resistance are not observed when adenosine is infused intra-arterially;

(i) Detailed understanding of the differential bioenergetics that are required in Yin-Yang processes for maintenance of health, or under oxidative stress, from fetal growth, organogenesis, after birth or in adulthood and aging processes involving intracellular behaviors of components such as mitochondrial function, ribosomal recycling pathways and nuclear activities;

(j) Influence of mitochondrial impaired function and shift to increased glycolytic pathways and adaption of cancer cells that would change mitochondrial-dependent activities of cMyc, Alt/PTEN or p53 and other pathways that contribute to apoptosis or pro-inflammatory (Yin) events that are high energy-consuming and voltage-dependent pathways for induction of apoptosis are important biological gaps. When redox-sensitive mitochondrial transition pore (MTP) opens to the cytoplasm, reaction is followed by depolarization, electron flux in the electron transport chain (ETC) and production of electron donors (NADH and FADH2) and increased level of reactive oxygen species (ROS).

20 Concluding Remarks and Future Perspectives

It takes a molecular village to maintain the effective immunity for protecting and promoting health. It is anticipated that systematic approaches to basic and clinical studies of chronic diseases require comprehending the details of interdependent communications of the amazing and secretive success of effective immunity in maintenance of health and how minor or major changes in such well orchestrated biological crosstalk or aging process influence initiation of disease processes.

The early events in the disruption of the balance between Yin and Yang properties of acute inflammation remain as a black box when it comes to understanding the cancer biology. The ‘normal’ health status in adulthood could be established by routine blood tests or other genetic diagnostic tools to determine the oxidative stress levels of individuals during aging process. Attempts in design of effective therapeutics for chronic immune disorders or site-specific cancers as proposed throughout this book should be based on understanding the fundamental question of how the effective immunity become negatively influenced under molecular attacks by unwanted foreign elements in specific target tissues toward disease initiation.

Future directions for understanding of the biological events that occur during the early immune disruptors-(antigen)-induced alterations in the immune response profiles of host require systematic identification of special or shared features of immunity at site-specific tissues/organs for more effective decisions on prevention or treatment of diseases. Minor or major heterogeneities in intrinsic biology and genetic makeup of individuals often lead to heterogeneities in response profiles toward different biological insults (immune disruptors). These confounding factors present unique challenges and opportunities to overcome in future. However, the outcomes are expected to be rewarding as the truth in science has always advanced us to extraordinary achievements in many biomedical fields. Solving cancer problem is not an exception if the business of cancer did not cloud the facts and scientific logics.

References

1. "Defining Cancer". National Cancer Institute. Source: http://en.wikipedia.org/wiki/Cancer. Retrieved June 10, 2014. Updated: 2017–02-24T05:55Z.
2. "Cancer Fact sheet -N°297". World Health Organization. February 2014. Retrieved June 10, 2014.
3. American Cancer Society; Cancer Facts and Figures 2013. ACS, Atlanta.
4. Barrett AJ, Savani BN. Does chemotherapy modify the immune surveillance of hematological malignancies? Leukemia. 2009;23(1):53–8.
5. Khatami M. Cancer research and therapy: scam of century–promote immunity [Yin-Yang]. 2016; pp 1–166. ISBN-10:153043100X; ISBN-13: 978-1530431007; Amazon-Createspace. .https://www.createspace.com/6123573
6. Kammula US, Marincola FM. Cancer immunotherapy: is there real progress at last? BioDrugs. 1999;11(4):249–60.
7. Marcucci G, Baldus CD, Ruppert AS, et al. Overexpression of the ETS-related gene, ERG, predicts a worse outcome in acute myeloid leukemia with normal karyotype: a cancer and leukemia group B study. J Clin Oncol. 2005;23:9234–42.
8. Byrne WL, Mills KH, Lederer JA, O'Sullivan GC. Targeting regulatory T cells in cancer. Cancer Res. 2011;71(22):6915–20.
9. Dijkgraaf EM, Heusinkveld M, Tummers B, Vogelpoel LT, Goedemans R, Jha V, et al. Chemotherapy alters monocyte differentiation to favor generation of cancer-supporting M2 macrophages in the tumor microenvironment. Cancer Res. 2013;73(8):2480–92. doi:10.1158/0008–5472.CAN-12-3542. Epub 2013 Feb 22
10. Khatami M. Is cancer a severe delayed hypersensivitity reaction and histamine a blueprint? Clin Transl Med. 2016;5:35. doi:10.1186/s40169-016-0108-3.
11. Khatami M. "Yin and Yang" in inflammation: duality in innate immune cell function and tumorigenesis. Expert Opin Biol Ther. 2008;8:1461–72.
12. Khatami M. Inflammation, aging, and cancer: tumoricidal versus tumorigenesis of immunity: a common denominator mapping chronic diseases. Cell Biochem Biophys. 2009;55:55–79.
13. Khatami M. Unresolved inflammation:'immune tsunami' or erosion of integrity in immune-privileged and immune-responsive tissues and acute and chronic inflammatory diseases or cancer. Expert Opin Biol Ther. 2011;11:1419–32.
14. Khatami M. Unresolved inflammation and cancer: loss of natural immune surveillance as the correct 'target' for therapy! Seeing the 'elephant' in the light of logic. Cell Biochem Biophys. 2012;62:501–9.
15. Khatami M. Chronic inflammation: synergistic interactions of recruiting macrophages (TAMs) eosinophils (Eos) with host mast cells (MCs) and tumorigenesis un CALTs. MCSF, suitable biomarker for cancer diagnosis! Cancers (Basel). 2014;6:297–322.

16. Jemal A, Bray F, Center MM, Ferlay J, Ward E, Forman D. Global cancer statistics. CA Cancer J Clin. 2011;61:69–90.
17. Whang-Peng J, Triche TJ, Knutsen T, et al. Chromosome translocation in peripheral neuroepithelioma. N Engl J Med. 1984;311:584–5.
18. Prattichizzo F, Bonafe M, Ceka A, Giuliani A, Rippo MR, Re M, Antonicelli R, Procopio AD, Olivieri F. Endothelial cell senescence and inflammaging: microRNAs as biomarkers and innovative therapeutic tools. Curr Drug Targets. 2015;3. [Epub ahead of print]
19. Hipkiss AR. Does chronic glycolysis accelerate aging? Could this explain how dietary restriction works? Ann N Y Acad Sci. 2006;1067:361–8.
20. Bianchi G, Borgonovo G, Pistoia V, Raffaghello L. Immunosuppressive cells and tumour microenvironment: focus on mesenchymal stem cells and myeloid derived suppressor cells. Histol Histopathol. 2011;26(7):941–51.
21. Brivio S, Cadamuro M, Fabris L, Strazzabosco M. Epithelial-to-mesenchymal transition and cancer invasiveness: what can we learn from cholangiocarcinoma? J Clin Med. 2015;4(12):2028–41. doi:10.3390/jcm4121958.
22. Cătană CS, Calin GA, Berindan-Neagoe I. Inflamma-miRs in aging and breast cancer: Are they reliable players? Front Med (Lausanne). 2015;2:85. doi:10.3389/fmed.2015.00085. eCollection 2015
23. Felger JC, Haroon E, Woolwine BJ, Raison CL, Miller AH. Interferon-alpha-induced inflammation is associated with reduced glucocorticoid negative feedback sensitivity and depression in patients with hepatitis C virus. Physiol Behav. 2015; doi:10.1016/j.physbeh.2015.12.013. pii: S0031–9384(15)30210–9. [Epub ahead of print]
24. Powell DR, Huttenlocher A. Neutrophils in the tumor microenvironment. Trends Immunol. 2015; doi:10.1016/j.it.2015.11.008. pii: S1471–4906(15)00291–4. [Epub ahead of print]
25. Haslett C. Resolution of acute inflammation and the role of apoptosis in the tissue fate of granulocytes. Clin Sci (Lond). 1992;83(6):639–48. Misunderstood inflammation
26. Yuryev A. Gene expression profiling for targeted cancer treatment. Expert Opin Drug Discov. 2015;10(1):91–9. doi:10.1517/17460441.2015.971007. Epub 2014 Oct 13.---MKC
27. Pauwels EK, Foray N, Bourguignon MH. Breast cancer induced by x- ray mammography screening? Med Princ Pract: A review based on Recent understanding of low-dose radiobiology; 2015. [Epub ahead of print]
28. Colotta F, Allavena P, Sica A, Garlanda C, Mantovani A. Cancer-related inflammation, the seventh hallmark of cancer: links to genetic instability. Carcinogenesis (review). 2009;30(7):1073–1081. ISSN 0143-3334. PMID 19468060. doi:10.1093/carcin/bgp127.
29. Kensler TW, Spira A, Garber JE, Szabo E, Lee J, Dong Z, Dannenberg AJ, Hait WN, Blackburn E, Davidson NE, Foti M, Lippman SM. Transforming cancer prevention through precision medicine and immune-oncology. Cancer Prev Res. 2016;9(1):2–10.
30. Virchow R. Cellular pathology. London: John Churchill; 1858.
31. Karnovsky ML. Metchnikoff in Messina: a century of studies on phagocytosis. N Engl J Med. 1981;304:1178–80.
32. Ehrlich P. Uber den jetzigen Stand der Karzinomforschung. Ned Tijdschr Geneeskd (German). 1909;5:273–90.
33. Rous P. A sarcoma of the fowl transmissible by an agent separable from the tumor cells. J Exp Med. 1911;13:397–411. doi:10.1084/jem.13.4.397.
34. Raju TN. The Nobel chronicles. 1966: Francis Peyton Rous (1879–1970) and Charles Brenton Huggins (1901–97). Lancet. 1999;354(9177):520. Erratum in: Lancet 1999 Sep 18;354(9183):1038
35. Rous P. A transmissible avian neoplasm (Sarcoma of the common fowl). J Exp Med. 1910;12(5):696–705. PMCID: PMC2124810
36. Rous P. The challenge to man of the neoplastic cell. Nobel Lecture. 1966;13
37. Rubin H. The early history of tumor virology: Rous, RIF, and RAV. Proc Natl Acad Sci U S A. 2011;108:14389–96. doi:10.1073/pnas.1108655108.
38. Burnet M. Cancer; a biologic approach. I The processes of control. Br Med J. 1957;1:779–86.

39. Burnet FM. Immunological recognition of self. Science. 1961;133:307–11.
40. Dvorak HF. Tumors: wounds that do not heal. Similarities between tumor stroma generation and wound healing. N Engl J Med. 1986;315:1650–9.
41. Zhong J, Chen Y, Wang LJ. Emerging molecular basis of hematogenous metastasis in gastric cancer. World J Gastroenterol. 2016;22(8):2434–40. doi:10.3748/wjg.v22.i8.2434.
42. Ribatti D, Mangialardi G, Vacca A. Stephen Paget and the 'seed and soil' theory of metastatic dissemination. Clin Exp Med. 2006;6(4):145–9.
43. Hawkins AJ, Golding SE, Khalil A, Valerie K. DNA double-strand break-induced pro-survival signaling. Radiother Oncol. 2011;101:13–7.
44. Khan HA, Alhomida AS. A review of the logistic role of L-carnitine in the management of radiation toxicity and radiotherapy side effects. J Appl Toxicol. 2011;31(8):707–13. doi:10.1002/jat.1716. Epub 2011 Aug 5
45. Hein AL, Ouellette MM, Yan Y. Radiation-induced signaling pathways that promote cancer cell survival (Review). Published online. 2014 Aug 20. doi: 10.3892/ijo.2014.2614.
46. Milas L, Raju U, Liao Z, Ajani J. Targeting molecular determinants of tumor chemo-radioresistance. Semin Oncol. 2005;32:S78–81.
47. Valerie K, Yacoub A, Hagan MP, et al. Radiation-induced cell signaling: inside-out and outside-in. Mol Cancer Ther. 2007;6:789–801.
48. Pellegriti G, Frasca F, Regalbuto C, Squatrito S, Vigneri R. Worldwide increasing incidence of thyroid cancer: update on epidemiology and risk factors. J Cancer Epidemiol. 2013:965212. Published online 2013 May 7. doi:10.1155/2013/965212.
49. Matsubara M, Masaki S, Ohmori K, Karasawa A, Hasegawa K. Differential regulation of IL-4 expression and degranulation by anti-allergic olopatadine in rat basophilic leukemia (RBL-2H3) cells. Biochem Pharmacol. 2005;67:1315–26. 0006–2952/$
50. Iguchi A, Kitajima I, Yamakuchi M, et al. PEA3 and AP-1 are required for constitutive IL-8 gene expression in hepatoma cells. Biochem Biophys Res Commun. 2000;279:166–71.
51. Kamimura D, Ishihara K, Hirano T. IL-6 signal transduction and its physiological roles: the signal orchestration model. Rev Physiol Biochem Pharmacol. 2003;149:1–38.
52. Nowell PC. The clonal evolution of tumor cell populations. Science. 1976;194:23–8.
53. Weber GF. Metabolism in cancer metastasis. Int J Cancer. 2015; doi:10.1002/ijc.29839. [Epub ahead of print]
54. Thomas DG, Ward AM, Williams JL. A study of 52 cases of adenocarcinoma of the bladder. Br J Urol. 1971;43:4–15.
55. Mostofi FK. Pathological aspects and spread of carcinoma of the bladder. JAMA. 1968;206:1764–9.
56. Bates AW, Baithun SI. Secondary neoplasms of the bladder are histological mimics of nontransitional cell primary tumours: clinicopathological and histological features of 282 cases. Histopathology. 2000;36:32–40.
57. Melicow MM. Tumors of the urinary bladder: a clinico-pathological analysis of over 2500 specimens and biopsies. J Urol. 1955;74:498–521.
58. Lopez-Beltran A, Martin J, Garcia J, Toro M. Squamous and glandular differentiation in urothelial bladder carcinomas. Histopathology, histochemistry and immunohistochemical expression of carcinoembryonic antigen. Histol Histopathol. 1988;3:63–8.
59. Holmang S, Aldenborg F. Stage T1 adenocarcinoma of the urinary bladder–complete response after transurethral resection and intravesical bacillus Calmette-Guerin. Scand J Urol Nephrol. 2000;34:141–3.
60. Siefker-Radtke A. Urachal adenocarcinoma: a clinician's guide for treatment. Semin Oncol. 2012;39:619–24.
61. Dadhania V, Czerniak B, Guo CC. Adenocarcinoma of the urinary bladder. Am J Clin Exp Urol. 2015;3(2):51–63. eCollection 2015
62. Wilson TG, Pritchett TR, Lieskovsky G, Warner NE, Skinner DG. Primary adenocarcinoma of bladder. Urology. 1991;38:223–6.

63. Zaghloul MS, Nouh A, Nazmy M, Ramzy S, Zaghloul AS, Sedira MA, Khalil E. Long-term results of primary adenocarcinoma of the urinary bladder: a report on 192 patients. Urol Oncol. 2006;24:13–20.
64. Rogers CG, Palapattu GS, Shariat SF, Karakiewicz PI, Bastian PJ, Lotan Y, Gupta A, Vazina A, Gilad A, Sagalowsky AI, Lerner SP, Schoenberg MP. Clinical outcomes following radical cystectomy for primary nontransitional cell carcinoma of the bladder compared to transitional cell carcinoma of the bladder. J Urol. 2006;175:2048–53.
65. Eble J, Sauter G, Epstein JI, Sesterhenn IA. Pathology and genetics of tumours of the urinary system and male genital organs. Lyon: IARC Press; 2004. World Health Organization Classification of Tumours
66. Smith AK, Hansel DE, Jones JS. Role of cystitis cystica et glandularis and intestinal metaplasia in development of bladder carcinoma. Urology. 2008;71:915–8.
67. Poore TE, Egbert B, Jahnke R, Kraft JK. Signet ring cell adenocarcinoma of the bladder: linitis plastica variant. Arch Pathol Lab Med. 1981;105:203–4.
68. Donhuijsen K, Schmidt U, Richter HJ, Leder LD. Mucoid cytoplasmic inclusions in urothelial carcinomas. Hum Pathol. 1992;23:860–4.
69. Black PC, Brown GA, Dinney CP. The impact of variant histology on the outcome of bladder cancer treated with curative intent. Urol Oncol. 2009;27:3–7.
70. Alam M, Ratner D. Cutaneous squamous-cell carcinoma. N Engl J Med. 2001;344:975–83.
71. DeVita VT Jr, Rosenberg SA. Two hundred years of cancer research. [200th A Nniversary Article]. N Engl J Med. 2012;366:2207–14. doi:10.1056/NEJMra1204479.
72. Gewirtz DA. Autophagy and senescence: a partnership in search of definition. Autophagy. 2013;9(5):808–12. doi:10.4161/auto.23922. Epub 2013 Feb 19
73. Bernardi MP, Ngan SY, Michael M, Lynch AC, Heriot AG, Ramsay RG, Phillips WA. Molecular biology of anal squamous cell carcinoma: implications for future research and clinical intervention. Lancet Oncol. 2015;16(16):e611–21. doi:10.1016/S1470-2045(15)00292-2.
74. Bosch FX, Ribes J, Diaz M, Cleries R. Primary liver cancer: worldwide incidence and trends. Gastroenterology. 2004;127:S5–S16.
75. Ramakrishna G, Rastogi A, Trehanpati N, Sen B, Khosla R, Sarin SK. From cirrhosis to hepatocellular carcinoma: new molecular insights on inflammation and cellular senescence. Liver Cancer. 2013;2(3–4):367–83. doi:10.1159/000343852.
76. Becker AE, Hernandez YG, Krucht H, Lucas AL. Pancreatic ductal adenocarcinoma: risk factors, screening, and early detection. World J Gastroenterol. 2014;20(32):11182–98.
77. Pitot HC. Altered hepatic foci: their role in murine hepatocarcinogenesis. Annu Rev Pharmacol Toxicol. 1990;30:465–500.
78. Calvisi DF, Thorgeirsson SS. Molecular mechanisms of hepatocarcinogenesis in transgenic mouse models of liver cancer. Toxicol Pathol. 2005;33:181–4.
79. Malumbres M, Barbacid M. RAS oncogenes: the first 30 years. Nat Rev Cancer. 2003;3:459–65.
80. Sakurai T, He G, Matsuzawa A, Yu GY, Maeda S, Hardiman G, Karin M. Hepatocyte necrosis induced by oxidative stress and IL-1 alpha release mediate carcinogen-induced compensatory proliferation and liver tumorigenesis. Cancer Cell. 2008;14:156–65.
81. Chen CH, Huang GT, Yang PM, Chen PJ, Lai MY, Chen DS, Wang JD, Sheu JC. Hepatitis B- and C-related hepatocellular carcinomas yield different clinical features and prognosis. Eur J Cancer. 2006; 42:2524–2529.
82. Boucher KM, Yakovlev AY. Estimating the probability of initiated cell death before tumor induction. Proc Natl Acad Sci U S A. 1997;94:12776–9.
83. Rebouissou S, Amessou M, Couchy G, Poussin K, Imbeaud S, Pilati C, Izard T, Balabaud C, Bioulac-Sage P, Zucman-Rossi J. Frequent in-frame somatic deletions activate gp130 in inflammatory hepatocellular tumours. Nature. 2009;457:200–4.
84. Eriksen KW, Kaltoft K, Mikkelsen G, Nielsen M, Zhang Q, Geisler C, Nissen MH, Ropke C, Wasik MA, Odum N. Constitutive STAT3-activation in Sezary syndrome: tyrphostin AG490

inhibits STAT3-activation, interleukin-2 receptor expression and growth of leukemic Sezary cells. Leukemia. 2001;15:787–93.
85. Fausto N. Mouse liver tumorigenesis: models, mechanisms, and relevance to human disease. Semin Liver Dis. 1999;19:243–52.
86. Haybaeck J, Zeller N, Wolf MJ, Weber A, Wagner U, Kurrer MO, Bremer J, Iezzi G, Graf R, Clavien PA, et al. A lymphotoxin-driven pathway to hepatocellular carcinoma. Cancer Cell. 2009;16:295–308.
87. Nakagawa H, Maeda S, Yoshida H, Tateishi R, Masuzaki R, Ohki T, Hayakawa Y, Kinoshita H, Yamakado M, Kato N, et al. Serum IL-6 levels and the risk for hepatocarcinogenesis in chronic hepatitis C patients; an analysis based on gender differences. Int J Cancer. 2009;125:2264–9.
88. Hedvat M, Huszar D, Herrmann A, Gozgit JM, Schroeder A, Sheehy A, Buettner R, Proia D, Kowolik CM, Xin H, et al. The JAK2 inhibitor AZD1480 potently blocks Stat3 signaling and oncogenesis in solid tumors. Cancer Cell. 2009;16:487–97.
89. Hennings H, Glick AB, Greenhalgh DA, Morgan DL, Strickland JE, Tennenbaum T, Yuspa SH. Critical aspects of initiation, promotion, and progression in multistage epidermal carcinogenesis. Proc Soc Exp Biol Med. 1993;202:1–8.
90. Karin M. Nuclear factor-kappaB in cancer development and progression. Nature. 2006;441:431–6.
91. Naugler WE, Sakurai T, Kim S, Maeda S, Kim K, Elsharkawy AM, Karin M. Gender disparity in liver cancer due to sex differences in MyD88-dependent IL-6 production. Science. 2007;317:121–4.
92. Ogata H, Kobayashi T, Chinen T, Takaki H, Sanada T, Minoda Y, Koga K, Takaesu G, Maehara Y, Iida M, Yoshimura A. Deletion of the SOCS3 gene in liver parenchymal cells promotes hepatitis-induced hepatocarcinogenesis. Gastroenterology. 2006;131:179–93.
93. Oka Y, Tsuboi A, Kawakami M, et al. Development of WT1 peptide cancer vaccine against hematopoietic malignancies and solid cancers. Curr Med Chem. 2006;13:2345–52.
94. El-Seragh HB, Marrero JA, Rudolph L, Reddy KR. Diagnosis and treatment of hepatocellular carcinoma. Gastroenterology. 2008;134:1752–63.
95. Yang L, Han Y, Saurez Saiz F, Minden MD. A tumor suppressor and oncogene: the WT1 story. Leukemia. 2007;21:868–76.
96. Morrison AA, Viney RL, Ladomery MR. The post-transcriptional roles of WT1, a multifunctional zinc-finger protein. Biochim Biophys Acta. 1785;2008:55–62.
97. Zhang D, Kaneda M, Nakahama K, Arii S, Morita I. Connexin 43 expression promotes malignancy of Huh7 hepatocellular carcinoma cells via the inhibition of cell-cell communication. Cancer Lett. 2007;252:208–15.
98. Oh BK, Kim H, Park HJ, et al. DNA methyltransferase expression and DNA methylation in human hepatocellular carcinoma and their clinicopathological correlation. Int J Mol Med. 2007;20:65–73.
99. Costa RH, Kalinichenko VV, Holterman A-XL, Wang X. Transcription factors in liver development, differentiation, and regeneration. Hepatology. 2003;38:1331–47.
100. Weisenberger HT. Genome-scale analysis of aberrant Dna methylation in colorectal cancer. Genome Res. 2012;22:271–82.
101. Tatsumi N, Oji Y, Tsuji N, et al. Wilms' tumor gene WT1-shRNA as a potent apoptosis-inducing agent for solid tumors. Int J Oncol. 2008;32:701–11.
102. Green CL, Khavari PA. Targets for molecular therapy of skin cancer. Semin Cancer Biol. 2004;14:63–9.
103. Miyoshi Y, Ando A, Egawa C, et al. High expression of Wilms' tumor suppressor gene predicts poor prognosis in breast cancer patients. Clin Cancer Res. 2002;8:1167–71.
104. Scharnhorts V, van der Eb A, Jochemsen AG. WT1 proteins: functions in growth and differentiation. Gene. 2001;273:141–61.
105. Berasain C, Herrero JI, García-Trevijano ER, et al. Expression of Wilms' tumor suppressor in the liver with cirrhosis: relation to hepatocyte nuclear factor 4 and hepatocellular function. Hepatology. 2003;38:148–57.

106. Sera T, Hiasa T, Mashibe T, et al. Wilms' tumor 1 gene expression is increased in hepatocellular carcinoma and associated with poor prognosis. Eur J Cancer. 2008;44:600–8.
107. Irizarry RA, Bolstad BM, Collin F, Cope LM, Hobbs B, Speed TP. Summaries of Affymetrix genechip probe level data. Nucleic Acid Res. 2003;31:e15.
108. Wettenhall JM, Smyth BM. Limma GUI: a graphical user interface for linear modeling of microarray data. Bioinformatics. 2004;20:3705–6.
109. Pham CG, Bubici C, Zazzeroni F, Papa S, Jones J, Alvarez K, Jayawardena S, De Smaele E, Cong R, Beaumont C, et al. Ferritin heavy chain upregulation by NF-kappaB inhibits TNFalpha-induced apoptosis by suppressing reactive oxygen species. Cell. 2004;119:529–42.
110. Pikarsky E, Porat RM, Stein I, Abramovitch R, Amit S, Kasem S, Gutkovich-Pyest E, Urieli-Shoval S, Galun E, Ben-Neriah Y. NF-kappaB functions as a tumour promoter in inflammation-associated cancer. Nature. 2004;431:461–6.
111. Castillo J, Erroba E, Perugorría MJ, et al. Amphiregulin contributes to the transformed phenotype of human hepatocellular carcinoma cells. Cancer Res. 2006;66:6129–38.
112. Berasain C, García-Trevijano ER, Castillo J, et al. Novel role for amphiregulin in protection from liver injury. J Biol Chem. 2005;280:19012–20.
113. Tsang WP, Kwok TT. Riboregulator H19 induction of MDR1-associated drug resistance in human hepatocellular carcinoma cells. Oncogene. 2007;26:4877–81.
114. Beck WT, Morgan SE, Mo Y-Y, Bhat UG. Tumor cell resistance to DNA topoisomerase II inhibitors: new developments. Drug Res Updates. 1999;2:382–9.
115. Ito K, Ozasa H, Nagashima Y, Hagiwara K, Horikawa S. Pharmacological preconditioning with doxorubicin: implications of heme oxygenase-1 induction in doxorubicin-induced hepatic injury in rats. Biochem Pharmacol. 2001;62:1249–55.
116. Gewirtz DA. A critical evaluation of the mechanisms of action proposed for the antitumor effects of the anthracycline antibiotics adryamycin and daunorubicin. Biochem Pharmacol. 1999;57:727–41.
117. Harper JW, Elledge SJ. The DNA damage response: ten years after. Mol Cell. 2007;28:739–45.
118. Zhang A, Lyu YL, Lin CP, et al. A protease pathway for the repair of topoisomerase II-DNA complexes. J Biol Chem. 2006;281:35997–6003.
119. Renard C-A, Labalette C, Armengol C, et al. Tbx3 is a downstream target of the Wnt/b-catenin pathway and a critical mediator of b-catenin survival functions in liver cancer. Cancer Res. 2007;67:901–10.
120. Leu JI-J, George DL. Hepatic IGFBP1 is a prosurvival factor that binds to bak, protects the liver form apoptosis, and antagonizes the proapoptotic actions of p53 at mitochondria. Genes Dev. 2007;21:3095–109.
121. Ewing J. Diffuse endothelioma of bone. Proc N Y Pathol Soc. 1921;21:17–24.
122. Janknecht R. EWS-ETS oncoproteins: the linchpins of Ewing tumors. Gene. 2005;363:1–14.
123. Petermann R, Mossier BM, Aryee DN, et al. Oncogenic EWS-Fli1 interacts with hsRPB7, a subunit of human RNA polymerase II. Oncogene. 1998;17:603–10.
124. Silk AW, Schuetze SM. Histology-specific therapy for advanced soft tissue sarcoma and benign connective tissue tumors. Curr Treat Options in Oncol. 2012;13(3):285–98. doi:10.1007/s11864-012-0194-4.
125. Melnikova VO, Ananthaswamy HN. Cellular and molecular events leading to the development of skin cancer. Mutat Res. 2005;571:91–106.
126. Chmielowski B, Federman N, Tap WD. Clinical trial end points for assessing efficacy of novel therapies for soft-tissue sarcomas. Expert Rev Anticancer Ther. 2012;12(9):1217–28. doi:10.1586/era.12.100.
127. Requena L, Kutzner H. Hemangioendothelioma. Semin Diagn Pathol. 2013;30(1):29–44. doi:10.1053/j.semdp.2012.01.003.
128. Cruz FD, Matushansky I. Solid tumor differentiation therapy – is it possible? Oncotarget. 2012;3:559–67.
129. Paulussen M, Frohlich B, Jurgens H. Ewing tumour: incidence, prognosis and treatment options. Paediatr Drugs. 2001;3:899–913.

130. Horowitz ME, Malawer MM, Woo SY, et al. Ewing's sarcoma family of tumors: Ewing's sarcoma of bone and soft tissue and the peripheral primitive Neuroectodermal tumors. In: Pizzo PA, Poplack DG, editors. Principles and practice of pediatric oncology. Philadelphia: Lippincott-Raven Publishers; 1997. p. 831–63.
131. Kimber C, Michalski A, Spitz L, et al. Primitive neuroectodermal tumours: anatomic location, extent of surgery, and outcome. J Pediatr Surg. 1998;33:39–41.
132. Grier HE. The Ewing family of tumors. Ewing's sarcoma and primitive neuroectodermal tumors. Pediatr Clin North Am. 1997;44:991–1004.
133. Kovar H. Ewing's sarcoma and peripheral primitive neuroectodermal tumors after their genetic union. Curr Opin Oncol. 1998;10:334–42.
134. Terrier P, Llombart-Bosch A, Contesso G. Small round blue cell tumors in bone: prognostic factors correlated to Ewing's sarcoma and neuroectodermal tumors. Semin Diagn Pathol. 1996;13:250–7.
135. Dahlin DC, Coventry MB, Scanlon PW. Ewing's sarcoma. A critical analysis of 165 cases. J Bone Joint Surg Am. 1961;43-A:185–92.
136. Peinemann F, Smith LA, Bartel C. Autologous hematopoietic stem cell transplantation following high dose chemotherapy for non-rhabdomyosarcoma soft tissue sarcomas. Cochrane Database Syst Rev. 2013;8:CD008216. doi:10.1002/14651858.CD008216.pub4.
137. Hart A, Melet F, Grossfeld P, et al. Fli-1 is required for murine vascular and megakaryocytic development and is hemizygously deleted in patients with thrombocytopenia. Immunity. 2000;13:167–77.
138. Ben-David Y, Giddens EB, Letwin K, et al. Erythroleukemia induction by friend murine leukemia virus: insertional activation of a new member of the ets gene family, Fli-1, closely linked to c-ets-1. Genes Dev. 1991;5:908–18.
139. Sharrocks AD. The ETS-domain transcription factor family. Nat Rev Mol Cell Biol. 2001;2:827–37.
140. Cavazzana AO, Magnani JL, Ross RA, et al. Ewing's sarcoma is an undifferentiated neuroectodermal tumor. Prog Clin Biol Res. 1988;271:487–98.
141. Jaishankar S, Zhang J, Roussel MF, et al. Transforming activity of EWS/FLI is not strictly dependent upon DNA-binding activity. Oncogene. 1999;18:5592–7.
142. Mao X, Miesfeldt S, Yang H, et al. The FLI-1 and chimeric EWS-FLI-1 oncoproteins display similar DNA binding specificities. J Biol Chem. 1994;269:18216–22.
143. Ouchida M, Ohno T, Fujimura Y, et al. Loss of tumorigenicity of Ewing's sarcoma cells expressing antisense RNA to EWS-fusion transcripts. Oncogene. 1995;11:1049–54.
144. Ohali A, Avigad S, Cohen IJ, et al. Association between telomerase activity and outcome in patients with nonmetastatic Ewing family of tumors. J Clin Oncol. 2003;21:3836–43.
145. Nakatani F, Tanaka K, Sakimura R, et al. Identification of p21WAF1/CIP1 as a direct target of EWS-Fli1 oncogenic fusion protein. J Biol Chem. 2003;278:15105–15.
146. Cremer M, Kupper K, Wagler B, et al. Inheritance of gene density-related higher order chromatin arrangements in normal and tumor cell nuclei. J Cell Biol. 2003;162:809–20.
147. van Doorninck JA, Ji L, Schaub B, et al. Current treatment protocols have eliminated the prognostic advantage of type 1 fusions in Ewing sarcoma: a report from the Children's Oncology Group. J Clin Oncol. 28:1989–94.
148. Zhou W, Liotta LA, Petricoin EF. Cancer metabolism: what we can learn from proteomic analysis by mass spectrometry. Cancer Genomics Proteomics. 2012;9(6):373–81.
149. DiFiore F, Sesboue R, Michel P, Sabourin JC, Frebourg T. Molecular determinants of anti-EGFR sensitivity and resistance in metastatic colorectal cancer. Br J Cancer. 2010;103:1765–72.
150. Wheeler DL, Dunn EF, Harari PM. Understanding resistance to EGFR inhibitors-impact on future treatment strategies. Nat Rev Clin Oncol. 2010;7:493–507.
151. Vigil D, Cherfils J, Rossman KL, Der CJ. Ras superfamily GEFs and GAPs: validated and tractable targets for cancer therapy? Nat Rev Cancer. 2010;10:842–57.
152. Normanno N, et al. Implications for KRAS status and EGFR-targeted therapies in metastatic CRC. Nat Rev Clin Oncol. 2009;6:519–27.

153. Gøtzsche PC. Deadly medicines and organised crime: in: how big pharma has corrupted health care. London: Radcliffe Publishing; 2013.
154. Faguet GB. In the war on cancer: an anatomy of failure-a blueprint for the future: Springer; 2005. 227 pages.
155. Grippo PJ, Sandgren EP. Highly invasive transitional cell carcinoma of the bladder in a simian virus 40 T-antigen transgenic mouse model. Am J Pathol. 2000;157:805–13.
156. Lou DQ, Molina T, Bennoun M, Porteu A, Briand P, Joulin V, Vasseur-Cognet M, Cavard C. Conditional hepatocarcinogenesis in mice expressing SV 40 early sequences. Cancer Lett. 2005;229(1):107–14.
157. Nagy E, Berczi I, Sehon AH. Growth inhibition of murine mammary carcinoma by monoclonal IgE antibodies specific for the mammary tumor virus. Cancer Immunol Immunother. 1991;34:63–9. doi:10.1007/BF01741326.
158. Daniels TR, Leuchter RK, Quintero R, Helguera G, Rodríguez JA, Martínez-Maza O, Schultes BC, Nicodemus CF, Penichet ML. Targeting HER2/neu with a fully human IgE to harness the allergic reaction against cancer cells. Cancer Immunol Immunother. 2012;61:991–1003. doi:10.1007/s00262-011-1150-z.
159. Klerings I, Weinhandl AS, Thaler KJ. Information overload in healthcare: too much of a good thing? Z Evid Fortbild Qual Gesundhwes. 2015;109(4–5):285–90. doi:10.1016/j.zefq.2015.06.005. Epub 2015 Jul 27
160. Thaler K, Kien C, Nussbaumer B, Van Noord MG, Griebler U, Klerings I. Gartlehner G; [UNCOVER project consortium]: inadequate use and regulation of interventions against publication bias decreases their effectiveness: a systematic review. J Clin Epidemiol. 2015;68(7):792–802. doi:10.1016/j.jclinepi.2015.01.008. Epub 2015 Jan 30
161. Khatami M. Safety concerns and hidden agenda behind HPV vaccines: another generation of drug-dependent society? Clin Transl Med. 2016;5(1):46. Epub 2016 Dec 5
162. Khatami M. Book review on cancer research and therapy: Safety concerns for HPV vaccination of young generation-Paid by Obamacare and V.P. Biden Moonshot Initiative. Global Vaccines Immunol. 2016;1(3):63–8. doi:10.15761/GVI.1000118.
163. Day A. 'An American tragedy', the cutter incident and its implications for the Salk polio vaccine in New Zealand 1955–1960. Health Hist. 2009;11:42–61.
164. Stewart SE. Leukemia in mice produced by a filterable agent present in AKR leukemic tissues with notes on a sarcoma produced by the same agent [abstract]. Anat Rec. 1953;117:532.
165. O'Hern EM. Sarah Elizabeth Stewart. In: Profiles of pioneer women scientists. Washington, DC: Acropolis; 1985. p. 161–9.
166. Morgan GJ. Ludwik Gross, Sarah Stewart, and the 1950s discoveries of Gross murine leukemia virus and polyoma virus. Studies in History and Philosophy of Biological and Biomedical Sciences. 2014. http://dx.doi.org/10.1016/j.shpsc.2014.07.013 1369–8486/2014. Elsevier Ltd. journal homepage: www.elsevier.com/locate/shpsc
167. Strickler HD, Goedert JJ. Exposure to SV40-contaminated poliovirus vaccine and the risk of cancer–a review of the epidemiological evidence. Dev Biol Stand. 1998;94:235–44.
168. Eddy BE, Stewart SE, Stanton MF, Marcotte JM. Induction of tumors in rats by tissue-culture preparations of SE polyoma virus. J Natl Cancer Inst. 1959;22:161–71.
169. Shimkin MB. As memory serves: an informal history of the National Cancer Institute, 1937–57. J Natl Cancer Inst. 1977;59(suppl):559–600.
170. Shahzad A. Time for a worldwide shift from oral polio vaccine to inactivated polio vaccine. Clin Infect Dis. 2009;49(8):1287–8.
171. Soltau AB. Acute poliomyelitis: with special reference to the outbreak in plymouth, stonehouse, and devonport. Br Med J. 1911;2(2653):1151–4.
172. Cutrone R, Lednicky J, Dunn G, Rizzo P, Bocchetta M, Chumakov K, et al. Some oral poliovirus vaccines were contaminated with infectious SV40 after 1961. Cancer Res. 2005;65(22):10273–9.
173. Barbanti-Brodano G, Sabbioni S, Martini F, Negrini M, Corallini A, Tognon M. Simian virus 40 infection in humans and association with human diseases: results and hypotheses. Virology. 2004;318(1):1–9.

174. Horvath BL, Fornosi F. Excretion of SV-40 virus after oral administration of contaminated polio vaccine. Acta Microbiol Acad Sci Hung. 1964;11:271–5.
175. Diamond B. Global polio campaign doomed to fail, experts warn. Nat Med. 2005;11:1260.
176. Pan American Health Organization/World Health Organization. Epidemiological alert – neurological syndrome, congenital malformations, and Zika virus infection – implications for Public Health in the Americas. Pan American Health Organization/World Health Organization, December 1, 2015. http://www.paho.org/hq/index.php?option=com_docman&task=doc_view&Itemid=270&gid=32405&lang=en
177. Neustadt RE, Fineberg HV, editors. The swine flu affair: decision-making on a slippery disease. Washington, DC: National Academies Press; 1978.
178. Toussirot É, Bereau M. Vaccination and induction of autoimmune diseases. Inflamm Allergy Drug Targets. 2015;14:94–8.
179. Lee SH, Vigliotti JS, Vigliotti VS, Joens W. From human papillomavirus (HPV) detection to cervical cancer prevention in clinical practice. Cancers. 2014;6:2072–99.
180. Stanely M. Prophylactic human papillomavirus vaccines: will they do their job? J Intern Med. 2010;267:251–8.
181. Einstein MH, Baron M, Levin MJ, Chatterjee A, Edwards RP, Zepp F. HPV-010 study group et al: comparison of the immunogenicity and safety of Cervarix and Gardasil human papillomavirus (HPV) cervical cancer vaccines in healthy women aged 18–45 years. Hum Vaccin. 2009;5:705–19.
182. Williams SE, Pahud BA, Vellozzi C, Donofrio PD, Dekker CL, Halsey N, et al. Causality assessment of serious neurologic adverse events following 2009 H1N1 vaccination. Vaccine. 2011;29:8302–8. doi:10.1016/j.vaccine.2011.08.093.
183. Grubeck-Loebenstein B, Della Bella S, Iorio AM, Michel JP, Pawelec G, Solana R. Immunosenescence and vaccine failure in the elderly. Aging Clin Exp Res. 2009:21, 201–229.
184. King DA, Matheson E, Chirina S, Shankar A, Broman-Fulks J. The status of baby boomers' health in the United States: the healthier generation? JAMA Intern Med. 2013;173(5):385–6.
185. Ricketts TC. The health care workforce: will it be ready as the boomers age? A review of how we can know (or not know) the answer. Annu Rev Public Health. 2011;32:417–30.
186. Gordon Duff. Is American medicine a war crime? Veterans Today, July 3, 2012. http://www.veteranstoday.com/2012/07/03/is-american-medicine-a-war-crime/
187. Gøtzsche PC. Deadly medicines and organised crime. In: How big pharma has corrupted health care. London: Radcliffe Publishing; 2013.
188. Baumann K. Ageing: the yin and yang of mitochondrial dysfunction. Nat Rev Mol Cell Biol. 2016;17(6):331. doi:10.1038/nrm.2016.71.
189. Allavena P, Sica A, Garlanda C, Mantovani A. The Yin-Yang of tumor-associated macrophages in neoplastic progression and immune surveillance. Immunol Rev. 2008;222:155–61. doi:10.1111/j.1600-065X.2008.00607.x.
190. Mantovani A. B cells and macrophages in cancer: yin and yang. Nat Med. 2011;17(3):285–6. doi:10.1038/nm0311-285. Olsen LF, Issinger OG, Guerra B: The Yin and Yang of redox regulation. Redox Rep. 2013;18(6):245–52. doi: 10.1179/1351000213Y.0000000059
191. Wu X, Hwang ST. Cutaneous T-cell lymphoma: the Yin and Yang of inflammation and neoplasia. J Investig Dermatol Symp Proc. 2015;17(1):34–5. doi:10.1038/jidsymp.2015.10.
192. Godson C, Perretti M. Novel pathways in the yin-yang of immunomodulation. Curr Opin Pharmacol. 2013;13(4):543–6. doi:10.1016/j.coph.2013.06.010. Epub 2013 Jul 16
193. Leança CC, Passarelli M, Nakandakare ER, Quintão EC. [HDL: the yin-yang of cardiovascular disease]. [Article in Portuguese] Arq Bras Endocrinol Metabol. 2010 Dec;54(9):777–784.
194. Azike CG, Charpentier PA, Hou J, Pei H, King Lui EM. The Yin and Yang actions of North American ginseng root in modulating the immune function of macrophages. Chin Med. 2011;6(1):21. doi:10.1186/1749-8546-6-21.
195. Malaguarnera L. Chitotriosidase: the yin and yang. Cell Mol Life Sci. 2006;63(24):3018–29.

196. Sherwood RK, Roy CR. Autophagy evasion and endoplasmic reticulum subversion: the Yin and Yang of legionella intracellular infection. Annu Rev Microbiol. 2016;70:413–33. doi:10.1146/annurev-micro-102215-095557.
197. Besold AN, Culbertson EM, Culotta VC. The Yin and Yang of copper during infection. J Biol Inorg Chem. 2016;21(2):137–44. doi:10.1007/s00775-016-1335-1. Epub 2016 Jan 20
198. Lauber K, Munoz LE, Berens C, Jendrossek V, Belka C, Herrmann M. Apoptosis induction and tumor cell repopulation: the yin and yang of radiotherapy. Radiat Oncol. 2011;6:176. doi:10.1186/1748-717X-6-176.
199. Tobin DM, Ramakrishnan L. TB: the Yin and Yang of lipid mediators. Curr Opin Pharmacol. 2013;13(4):641–5. doi:10.1016/j.coph.2013.06.007. Epub 2013 Jul 9
200. Mango R, Predazzi IM, Romeo F, Novelli G. LOX-1/LOXIN: the yin/yang of atheroscleorosis. Cardiovasc Drugs Ther. 2011;25(5):489–94. doi:10.1007/s10557-011-6333-6335.
201. Szala S. Angiogenesis and immune suppression: yin and yang of tumor progression? [Article in Polish]. Postepy Hig Med Dosw (Online). 2009;63:598–612.
202. Saika S. Yin and yang in cytokine regulation of corneal wound healing: roles of TNF-alpha. Cornea. 2007;26(9 Suppl 1):S70–4.
203. Karagiannis SN, Josephs DH, Karagiannis P, Gilbert AE, Saul L, Rudman SM, Dodev T, Koers A, Blower PJ, Corrigan C, et al. Recombinant IgE antibodies for passive immunotherapy of solid tumours: from concept towards clinical application. Cancer Immunol Immunother. 2012;61:1547–64. doi:10.1007/s00262-011-1162-8.
204. Osborn TM, Tracy JK, Dunne JR, Pasquale M, Napolitano LM. Epidemiology of sepsis in patients with traumatic injury. Crit Care Med. 2004;32:2234–40.
205. Hietbrink F, Koenderman L, Rijkers G, Leenen L. Trauma: the role of the innate immune system. World J Emerg Surg. 2006;1:15.
206. Maestro B, Sanz JM. Choline binding proteins from Streptococcus pneumoniae: a dual role as enzybiotics and targets for the design of new antimicrobials. Antibiotics (Basel). 2016;5(2). pii: E21) doi:10.3390/antibiotics5020021.
207. O'Brien KL, Wolfson LJ, Watt JP, Henkle E, Deloria-Knoll M, McCall N, Lee E, Mulholland K, Levine OS, Cherian T, et al. Burden of disease caused by *Streptococcus pneumoniae* in children younger than 5 years: global estimates. Lancet. 2009;374:893–902. doi:10.1016/S0140-6736(09)61204-6.
208. Johnson HL, Deloria-Knoll M, Levine OS, Stoszek SK, Freimanis HL, Reithinger R, Muenz LR, O'Brien KL. Systematic evaluation of serotypes causing invasive pneumococcal disease among children under five: the pneumococcal global serotype project. PLoS Med. 2010;7 doi:10.1371/journal.pmed.1000348.
209. Hazeldine J, Hampson P, Lord JM. The diagnostic and prognostic value of systems biology research in major traumatic and thermal injury: a review. Burns Trauma. 2016;4:33. doi:10.1186/s41038-016-0059-3. eCollection 2016
210. Hur J, Yang HT, Chun W, Kim JH, Shin SH, Kang HJ, et al. Inflammatory cytokines and their prognostic ability in cases of major burn injury. Ann Lab Med. 2015;35:105–10.
211. Bianchi ME. DAMPs, PAMPs and alarmins: all we need to know about danger. J Leukoc Biol. 2007;81:1–5.
212. Jeschke MG, Gauglitz GG, Finnerty CC, Kraft R, Mlcak RP, Herndon DN. Survivors versus nonsurvivors postburn: differences in inflammatory and hypermetabolic trajectories. Ann Surg. 2014;259:814–23.
213. Peltz ED, D'Alessandro A, Moore EE, Chin T, Silliman CC, Sauaia A, et al. Pathologic metabolism: an exploratory study of the plasma metabolome of critical injury. J Trauma Acute Care Surg. 2015;78:742–51.
214. Gu X, Yao Y, Wu G, Lv T, Luo L, Song Y. The plasma mitochondrial DNA is an independent predictor for post-traumatic systemic inflammatory response syndrome. PLoS One. 2013;8:e72834.
215. Simmons JD, Lee YL, Mulekar S, Kuck JL, Brevard SB, Gonzalez RP, et al. Elevated levels of plasma mitochondrial DNA DAMPs are linked to clinical outcome in severely injured human subjects. Ann Surg. 2013;258:591–6.

216. Lord JM, Midwinter MJ, Chen YF, Belli A, Brohi K, Kovacs EJ, et al. The systemic immune response to trauma: an overview of pathophysiology and treatment. Lancet. 2014;384:1455–65.
217. Ferreira LC, Regner A, Miotto KD, Moura S, Ikuta N, Vargas AE, et al. Increased levels of interleukin-6, -8 and -10 are associated with fatal outcome following severe traumatic brain injury. Brain Inj. 2014;28:1311–6.
218. Mann EA, Baun MM, Meininger JC, Wade CE. Comparison of mortality associated with sepsis in the burn, trauma, and general intensive care unit patient: a systematic review of the literature. Shock. 2012;37:4–16.
219. Kraft R, Herndon DN, Finnerty CC, Cox RA, Song J, Jeschke MG. Predictive value of IL-8 for sepsis and severe infections after burn injury: a clinical study. Shock. 2015;43:222–7.
220. Ozbalkan Z, Aslar AK, Yildiz Y, Aksaray S. Investigation of the course of proinflammatory and anti-inflammatory cytokines after burn sepsis. Int J Clin Pract. 2004;58:125–9.
221. Fitzpatrick M, Young SP. Metabolomics—a novel window into inflammatory disease. Swiss Med Wkly. 2013;143:w13743.
222. Feng Z, Shi Q, Fan Y, Wang Q, Yin W. Ulinastatin and/or thymosin α1 for severe sepsis: a systematic review and meta-analysis. J Trauma Acute Care Surg. 2016;80(2):335–40. doi:10.1097/TA.0000000000000909.
223. Xiao Z, Wilson C, Robertson HL, Roberts DJ, Ball CG, Jenne CN, Kirkpatrick AW. Inflammatory mediators in intra-abdominal sepsis or injury – a scoping review. Crit Care. 2015;19:373. doi:10.1186/s13054-015-1093-4.
224. Peng ZY, Wang HZ, Srisawat N, Wen X, Rimmele T, Bishop J, et al. Bactericidal antibiotics temporarily increase inflammation and worsen acute kidney injury in experimental sepsis. Crit Care Med. 2012;40:538–43. doi:10.1097/CCM.0b013e31822f0d2e.
225. Chiang TY, Tsao SM, Yeh CB, Yang SF. Matrix metalloproteinases in pneumonia. Clin Chim Acta. 2014;433:272–7. doi:10.1016/j.cca.2014.03.031. Epub 2014 Apr 8
226. Mirabile A, Numico G, Russi EG, Bossi P, Crippa F, Bacigalupo A, De Sanctis V, et al. Sepsis in head and neck cancer patients treated with chemotherapy and radiation: literature review and consensus. Crit Rev Oncol Hematol. 2015;95:191–213. doi:10.1016/j.critrevonc.2015.03.003. Epub 2015 Mar 19
227. Gomes M, Teixeira AL, Coelho A, Araújo A, Medeiros R. The role of inflammation in lung cancer. Adv Exp Med Biol. 2014;816:1–23. doi:10.1007/978-3-0348-0837-8_1.
228. Monczor F, Copsel S, Fernandez N, Davio C, Shayo C. Histamine H2 receptor in blood cells: a suitable target for the treatment of acute myeloid leukemia. Handb Exp Pharmacol. 2016;18. [Epub ahead of print]
229. Keibel A, Singh V, Sharma MC. Inflammation, microenvironment, and the immune system in cancer progression. Curr Pharm Des. 2009;15:1949–55.
230. Kim S, Miller BJ, Stefanek ME, Miller AH. Inflammation-induced activation of the indoleamine 2,3-dioxygenase pathway: relevance to cancer-related fatigue. Cancer. 2015;121:2129–36. doi:10.1002/cncr.29302. Epub 2015 Feb 27
231. Hashimoto J, Ito S. Central pulse pressure and aortic stiffness determine renal hemodynamics: pathophysiological implication for microalbuminuria in hypertension. Hypertension. 2011;58:839–46.
232. Arking R. The biology of aging: observation and principles. 2nd ed. Sunderland: Sinauer Associates Inc; 1998. p. 153–250.
233. Sehl ME, Eugene Yates F. Kinetics of human aging: I. Rates of senescence between ages 30 and 70 years in healthy people. J Gerontol A Biol Sci Med Sci. 2001;56:198–208.
234. Ignarro LJ, Balestrieri ML, Napoli C. Nutrition, physical activity, and cardiovascular disease: an update. Cardiovasc Res. 2007;73:326–40.
235. Croce K, Libby P. Intertwining of thrombosis and inflammation in atherosclerosis. Curr Opin Hematol. 2007;14:55–61.
236. Rafi A, Castle SC, Uyemura K, Makinodan T. Immune dysfunction in the elderly and its reversal by antihistamines. Biomed Pharmacol. 2003;57:246–50.

237. Chung HY, Cesari M, Anton S, Marzetti E, Giovannini S, Seo AY, Carter C, Yu BP, Leeuwenburgh C. Molecular inflammation: underpinning of aging and age-related diseases. Ageing Res Rev. 2008;8:18–30.
238. Chatterjee V, Gashev AA. Aging-associated shifts in functional status of mast cells located by adult and aged mesenteric lymphatic vessels. Am J Physiol Heart Circ Physiol. 2012;303:H693–702.
239. Davalos AR, Coppe JP, Campisi J, Desprez PY. Senescent cells as a source of inflammatory factors for tumor progression. Cancer Metastasis Rev. 2010;29:273–83.
240. Zheng B, Han S, Takahashi Y, Kelsoe G. Immunosenescence and germinal center reaction. Immunol Rev. 1997;160:63–77.
241. Intapad S, Tull FL, Brown AD, Dasinger JH, Ojeda NB, Fahling JM, Alexander BT. Renal denervation abolishes the age-dependent increase in blood pressure in female intrauterine growth-restricted rats at 12 months of age. Hypertension. 2013;61:828–34.
242. Harman D. Aging: a theory based on free radical and radiation chemistry. J Gerontol. 1956;11:298–300.
243. Thompson PA, Khatami M, Baglole CJ, Sun J, Harris SA, Moon EY, Al-Mulla F, Al-Temaimi R, et al. Environmental immune disruptors, inflammation and cancer risk. Carcinogenesis. 2015;1(Suppl):S232–53. doi:10.1093/carcin/bgv038.
244. Davis BP, Rothenberg ME. Eosinophils and cancer. Cancer Immunol Res. 2014;2(1):1–8. doi:10.1158/2326-6066.CIR-13-0196.
245. Vighi G, Marcucci F, Sensi LG, Frati F. Allergy and the gastrointestinal system. Clin Exp Immunol. 2008;153(Suppl 1):3–6. doi:10.1111/j.1365-2249.2008.03713.x. PMCID: PMC2515351
246. Lilja G, Dannaeus A, Falth-Magnusson K, et al. Immune response of the atopic woman and foetus: effects of high- and low-dose food allergen intake during late pregnancy. Clin Allergy. 1988;18:131–4.
247. Adlerberth I, Hansson LÅ, Wold AE. The ontogeny of the intestinal flora. In: Sanderson IR, Walker WA, editors. Development of the gastrointestinal tract. Hamilton: BC Decker; 1999. p. 279–92.
248. Wold AE. The hygiene hypothesis revised: is the rising frequency of allergy due to changes in the intestinal flora? Allergy. 1998;53:20–5.
249. Gillian H, Vance S, Holloway JA. Early life exposure to dietary and inhalant allergens. Pediatr Allergy Immunol. 2002;13(Suppl 15):14–8.
250. Faria AM, Weiner HL. Oral tolerance. Immunol Rev. 2005;206:232–59.
251. Rathinam VA, Vanaja SK, Fitzgerald KA. Regulation of inflammasome signaling. Nat Immunol. 2012;13:333–42.
252. Minns LA, Menard LC, Foureau DM, et al. TLR9 is required for the gut-associated lymphoid tissue response following oral infection of *Toxoplasma gondii*. J Immunol. 2006;176:7589–97.
253. Akira S, Takeda K. Toll-like receptor signalling. Nat Rev Immunol. 2004;4:499–511.
254. Mowat AM. Anatomical basis of tolerance and immunity to intestinal antigens. Nat Rev Immunol. 2003;3:331–41.
255. Kaess BM, Rong J, Larson MG, Hamburg NM, Vita JA, Levy D, Benjamin EJ, Vasan RS, Mitchell GF. Aortic stiffness, blood pressure progression, and incident hypertension. JAMA. 2012;308:875–81. doi:10.1001/2012.jama.10503.
256. Napoli C, Hayashi T, Cacciatore F, Casamassimi A, Casini C, Al-Omran M, Ignarro LJ. Endothelial progenitor cells as therapeutic agents in the microcirculation: an update. Atherosclerosis. 2011;215:9–22. doi:10.1016/j.atherosclerosis.2010.10.039.
257. Renault V, Thornell LE, Butler-Browne G, Mouly V. Human skeletal muscle satellite cells: aging, oxidative stress and the mitotic clock. Exp Gerontol. 2002;37:1229–36. doi:10.1016/S0531-5565(02)00129-8.
258. Davis BK, Wen H, Ting JP. The inflammasome NLRs in immunity, inflammation, and associated diseases. Annu Rev Immunol. 2011;29:707–35.

259. Moir JA, White SA, Mann J. Arrested development and the great escape–the role of cellular senescence in pancreatic cancer. Int J Biochem Cell Biol. 2014;57:142–8. doi:10.1016/j.biocel.2014.10.018. Epub 2014 Oct 23
260. Tower J. Programmed cell death in aging. Ageing Res Rev. 2015:90–100.
261. Zimmermann HW, Seidler S, Nattermann J, Gassler N, Hellerbrand C, Zernecke A, et al. Functional contribution of elevated circulating and hepatic non-classical CD14CD16 monocytes to inflammation and human liver fibrosis. PLoS One. 2010;5:e11049.
262. Trehanpati N, Shrivastav S, Shivakumar B, Khosla R, Bhardwaj S, Chaturvedi J, et al. Analysis of notch and TGF-β signaling expression in different stages of disease progression during hepatitis B virus infection. Clin Transl Gastroenterol. 2012;3:e23.
263. Martinon F, Mayor A, Tschopp J. The inflammasomes: guardians of the body. Annu Rev Immunol. 2009;27:229–65.
264. Vitale G, Salvioli S, Franceschi C. Oxidative stress and the ageing endocrine system. Nat Rev Endocrinol. 2013;9:228–40. doi:10.1038/nrendo.2013.29.
265. Miller JF, Sadelain M. The journey from discoveries in fundamental immunology to cancer immunotherapy. Cancer Cell. 2015;27(4):439–49. doi:10.1016/j.ccell.2015.03.007. Epub 2015 Apr 6
266. Szabo G, Csak T. Inflammasomes in liver diseases. J Hepatol. 2012;57:642–54.
267. Ferreira ST, Clarke JR, Bomfim TR, De Felice FG. Inflammation, defective insulin signaling, and neuronal dysfunction in Alzheimer's disease. Alzheimers Dement. 2014;10(1 Suppl):S76–83. doi:10.1016/j.jalz.2013.12.010.
268. Miura K, Kodama Y, Inokuchi S, Schnabl B, Aoyama T, Ohnishi H, et al. Toll-like receptor 9 promotes steatohepatitis by induction of interleukin-1beta in mice. Gastroenterology. 2010;139:323–34.
269. Ganz M, Csak T, Nath B, Szabo G. LPS stimulation induces and activates the Nalp3 inflammasome in the liver. World J Gastroenterol. 2011;17:4772–8.
270. Burdette D, Haskett A, Presser L, McRae S, Iqbal J, Waris G. Hepatitis C virus activates interleukin-1β via caspase-1-inflammasome complex. J Gen Virol. 2012;93:235–46.
271. Petrasek J, Bala S, Csak T, Lippai D, Kodys K, Menashy V, et al. IL-1 receptor antagonist ameliorates inflammasome-dependent alcoholic steatohepatitis in mice. J Clin Invest. 2012;122:3476–89.
272. Henao-Mejia J, Elinav E, Jin C, Hao L, Mehal WZ, Strowig T, et al. Inflammasome-mediated dysbiosis regulates progression of NAFLD and obesity. Nature. 2012;482:179–85.
273. Svegliati-Baroni G, Faraci G, Fabris L, Saccomanno S, Cadamuro M, Pierantonelli I, et al. Insulin resistance and necroinflammation drives ductular reaction and epithelial-mesenchymal transition in chronic hepatitis C. Gut. 2011;60:108–15.
274. Falkowski O, An HJ, Ianus IA, Chiriboga L, Yee H, West AB, et al. Regeneration of hepatocyte 'buds' in cirrhosis from intrabiliary stem cells. J Hepatol. 2003;39:357–64.
275. Kanbayashi T, Kodama T, Kondo H, Satoh S, Inoue Y, Chiba S, Shimizu T, Nishino S. CSF histamine contents in narcolepsy, idiopathic hypersomnia and obstructive sleep apnea syndrome. Sleep. 2009 Feb;32(2):181–7.
276. Gouw AS, Clouston AD, Theise ND. Ductular reactions in human liver: diversity at the interface. Hepatology. 2011;54:1853–63.
277. Zhou H, Rogler LE, Teperman L, Morgan G, Rogler CE. Identification of hepatocytic and bile ductular cell lineages and candidate stem cells in bipolar ductular reactions in cirrhotic human liver. Hepatology. 2007;45:716–24.
278. Hanna RF, Aguirre DA, Kased N, Emery SC, Peterson MR, Sirlin CB. Cirrhosis-associated hepatocellular nodules: correlation of histopathologic and MR imaging features. Radiographics. 2008;28:747–69.
279. Asaumi N, Omoto E, Mahmut N, Katayama Y, Takeda K, Shinagawa K, Harada M. Very late antigen-5 and leukocyte function-associated antigen-1 are critical for early stage hematopoietic progenitor cell homing. Ann Hematol. 2001;80:387–92.

280. Goswami B, Rajappa M, Sharma M. Inflammation: its role and interplay in the development of cancer, with special focus on gynecological malignancies. Int J Gynecolnn. 2008;18:591–9.
281. Sasaki M, Ikeda H, Sawada S, Sato Y, Nakanuma Y. Naturally-occurring regulatory T cells are increased in inflamed portal tracts with cholangiopathy in primary biliary cirrhosis. J Clin Pathol. 2007;60:1102–7.
282. Karlmark KR, Weiskirchen R, Zimmermann HW, Gassler N, Ginhoux F, Weber C, et al. Hepatic recruitment of the inflammatory Gr1+ monocyte subset upon liver injury promotes hepatic fibrosis. Hepatology. 2009;50:261–74.
283. Josephs DH, Spicer JF, Corrigan CJ, Gould HJ, Karagiannis SN. Epidemiological associations of allergy, IgE and cancer. Clin Exp Allergy. 2013;43(10):1110–23. doi:10.1111/cea.12178.
284. Deleve LD, Wang X, Guo Y. Sinusoidal endothelial cells prevent rat stellate cell activation and promote reversion to quiescence. Hepatology. 2008;48:920–30.
285. Khatami M. Cyclooxygenase inhibitor ketorolac or mast cell stabilizers: immunological challenges in cancer therapy. Clin Cancer Res. 2005;11:1349–51.
286. Coussens LM, Werb Z. Inflammation and cancer. Nature. 2012;420:860–7.
287. Thompson BJ, Buonamici S, Sulis ML, Palomero T, Vilimas T, Basso G, Ferrando A, Aifantis I. The SCFFBW7 ubiquitin ligase complex as a tumor suppressor in T cell leukemia. J Exp Med. 2007;204:1825–35.
288. Guidolin D, Marinaccio C, Tortorella C, Annese T, Ruggieri S, Finato N, et al. Non-random spatial relationships between mast cells and microvessels in human endometrial carcinoma. Clin Exp Med. 2016; doi:10.1007/s10238-016-0407-4.
289. He G, Yu GY, Temkin V, Ogata H, Kuntzen C, Sakurai T, Sieghart W, Peck-Radosavljevic M, Leffert HL, Karin M. Hepatocyte IKKbeta/NF-kappaB inhibits tumor promotion and progression by preventing oxidative stress-driven STAT3 activation. Cancer Cell. 2010;17(3):286–97. doi:10.1016/j.ccr.2009.12.048.
290. Lin H, Yan J, Wang Z, Hua F, Yu J, Sun W, Li K, Liu H, Yang H, Lv Q, Xue J, Hu ZW. Loss of immunity-supported senescence enhances susceptibility to hepatocellular carcinogenesis and progression in toll-like receptor 2-deficient mice. Hepatology. 2013;57(1):171–82. doi:10.1002/hep.25991.
291. Kang TW, Yevsa T, Woller N, Hoenicke L, Wuestefeld T, Dauch D, et al. Senescence surveillance of pre-malignant hepatocytes limits liver cancer development. Nature. 2011;479:547–51.
292. Blackburn EH, Greider CW, Szostak JW. Telomeres and telomerase: the path from maize, tetrahymena and yeast to human cancer and aging. Nat Med. 2006;12:1133–8.
293. Sharpless NE, DePinho RA. Telomeres, stem cells senescence and cancer. J Clin Invest. 2004;113:160–8.
294. Lin WR, Lim SN, McDonald SA, Graham T, Wright VL, Peplow CL, et al. The histogenesis of regenerative nodules in human liver cirrhosis. Hepatology. 2010;51:1017–26.
295. Wright TL. Regenerating nodules – are they premalignant lesions? Hepatology. 1991;13:1254–5.
296. Ng CH, Chan SW, Lee WK, Lai L, Lok KH, Li KK, Luk SH, Szeto ML. Hepatocarcinogenesis of regenerative and dysplastic nodules in Chinese patients. Hong Kong Med J. 2011;17:11–9.
297. Hernandez-Gea V, Toffanin S, Friedman SL, Llovet JM. Role of the microenvironment in the pathogenesis and treatment of hepatocellular carcinoma. Gastroenterology. 2013;144:512–27.
298. Seitz HK, Stickel F. Risk factors and mechanisms of hepatocarcinogenesis with special emphasis on alcohol and oxidative stress. Biol Chem. 2006;387:349–60.
299. Di Gioia S, Bianchi P, Destro A, Grizzi F, Malesci A, Laghi L, et al. Quantitative evaluation of RASSF1A methylation in the non-lesional, regenerative and neoplastic liver. BMC Cancer. 2006;6:89.
300. Um TH, Kim H, Oh BK, Kim MS, Kim KS, Jung G, et al. Aberrant CpG island hypermethylation in dysplastic nodules and early HCC of hepatitis B virus-related human multistep hepatocarcinogenesis. J Hepatol. 2011;54:939–47.

301. Guichard C, Amaddeo G, Imbeaud S, Ladeiro Y, Pelletier L, Maad IB, et al. Integrated analysis of somatic mutations and focal copy-number changes identifies key genes and pathways in hepatocellular carcinoma. Nat Genet. 2012;44:694–8.
302. Huang J, Deng Q, Wang Q, Li KY, Dai JH, Li N, et al. Exome sequencing of hepatitis B virus-associated hepatocellular carcinoma. Nat Genet. 2012;44:1117–21.
303. Bose S, Sakhuja P, Bezawada L, Agarwal AK, Kazim SN, Khan LA, et al. Hepatocellular carcinoma with persistent hepatitis B virus infection shows unusual downregulation of Ras expression and differential response to Ras mediated signaling. J Gastroenterol Hepatol. 2011;26:135–44.
304. Yaswen P, Campisi J. Oncogene-induced senescence pathways weave an intricate tapestry. Cell. 2007;128:233–4.
305. Epstein JI, Amin MB, Reuter VE. Glandular lesions. In: Epstein JI, Amin MB, Reuter VE, editors. Biopsy interpretation of the bladder. 2nd ed. Philadelphia: Lippincott Williams; 2010. p. 180–213.
306. Grignon DJ, Ro JY, Ayala AG, Johnson DE. Primary signet-ring cell carcinoma of the urinary bladder. Am J Clin Pathol. 1991;95:13–20.
307. Sinard J, Macleay L Jr, Melamed J. Hepatoid adenocarcinoma in the urinary bladder. Unusual localization of a newly recognized tumor type. Cancer. 1994;73:1919–25.
308. Lopez-Beltran A, Luque RJ, Quintero A, Requena MJ, Montironi R. Hepatoid adenocarcinoma of the urinary bladder. Virchows Arch. 2003;442:381–7.
309. Jacobs LB, Brooks JD, Epstein JI. Differentiation of colonic metaplasia from adenocarcinoma of urinary bladder. Hum Pathol. 1997;28:1152–7.
310. McLean MH, Murray GI, Stewart KN, Norrie G, Mayer C. The inflammatory microenvironment in colorectal neoplasia. PLoS One. 2011;6:e15366.
311. Harlé A, Salleron J, Perkins G, Pilati C, Blons H, Laurent-Puig P, Merlin JL. Expression of pEGFR and pAKT as response-predictive biomarkers for RAS wild-type patients to anti-EGFR monoclonal antibodies in metastatic colorectal cancers. Br J Cancer. 2015;113(4):680–5. doi:10.1038/bjc.2015.250. Epub 2015 Jul 14
312. Matsuoka Y, Machida T, Oka K, Ishizaka K. Clear cell adenocarcinoma of the urinary bladder inducing acute renal failure. Int J Urol. 2002;9:467–9.
313. Gilcrease MZ, Delgado R, Vuitch F, Albores-Saavedra J. Clear cell adenocarcinoma and nephrogenic adenoma of the urethra and urinary bladder: a histopathologic and immunohistochemical comparison. Hum Pathol. 1998;29:1451–6.
314. Oliva E, Young RH. Nephrogenic adenoma of the urinary tract: a review of the microscopic appearance of 80 cases with emphasis on unusual features. Mod Pathol. 1995;8:722–30.
315. Luo W, Lindley SW, Lindley PH, Krempl GA, Seethala RR, Fung KM. Mammary analog secretory carcinoma of salivary gland with high-grade histology arising in hard palate, report of a case and review of literature. Int J Clin Exp Pathol. 2014;7(12):9008–22. eCollection 2014
316. Sumegi J, Nishio J, Nelson M, et al. A novel t(4;22)(q31;q12) produces an EWSR1-SMARCA5 fusion in extraskeletal Ewing sarcoma/primitive neuroectodermal tumor. Mod Pathol. 2010;24:333–42.
317. Cimino-Mathews A, Subhawong AP, Illei PB, Sharma R, Halushka MK, Vang R, Fetting JH, Park BH, Argani P. GATA3 expression in breast carcinoma: utility in triple-negative, sarcomatoid, and metastatic carcinomas. Hum Pathol. 2013;44(7):1341–9.
318. Zheng R, Blobel GA. GATA transcription factors and cancer. Genes Cancer. 2010;1:1178–88.
319. Reading CL, Hutchins JF. Carbohydrate structure in tumor immunity. Cancer Metastasis Rev. 1985;4:221–60.
320. Ellis IO, Cornelisse CJ, Schnitt SJ, et al. Invasive breast carcinoma. In: Tavassoli FA, Devilee P, editors. World Health Organization classification of tumours: tumours of the breast and female genital organs. Lyon: IARC Press; 2003. p. 37.
321. Bellow JP, Magro G. Fibroepithelial tumors. In: Tavassoli FA, Devilee P, editors. World Health Organization classification of tumours: tumours of the breast and female genital organs. Lyon: IARC Press; 2003. p. 99–103.

322. Cimino A, Halushka M, Illei P, et al. Epithelial cell adhesion molecule (EpCAM) is overexpressed in breast cancer metastases. Breast Cancer Res Treat. 2010;123:701–8.
323. Voduc D, Cheang M, Nielsen T. GATA-3 expression in breast cancer has a strong association with estrogen receptor but lacks independent prognostic value. Cancer Epidemiol Biomark Prev. 2008;17:365–73.
324. Subhawong AP, Subhawong T, Nassar H, et al. Most basal-like breast carcinomas demonstrate the same Rb–/p16+ immunophenotype as the HPV-related poorly differentiated squamous cell carcinomas which they resemble morphologically. Am J Surg Pathol. 2009;33:163–75.
325. Yan W, Cao QJ, Arenas RB, Bentley B, Shao R. GATA3 inhibits breast cancer metastasis through the reversal of epithelial-mesenchymal transition. J Biol Chem. 2010;285:14042–51.
326. Chu IM, Michalowski AM, Hoenerhoff M, et al. GATA3 inhibits lysyl oxidase-mediated metastases of human basal triple-negative breast cancer cells. Oncogene. 2012;31:2017–27.
327. Usary J, Llaca V, Karaca G, et al. Mutation of GATA3 in human breast tumors. Oncogene. 2004;23:7669–78.
328. Dydensborg AB, Rose AA, Wilson BJ, et al. GATA3 inhibits breast cancer growth and pulmonary breast cancer metastasis. Oncogene. 2009;28:2634–42.
329. Oh-hora M, Johmura S, Hashimoto A, Hikida M, Kurosaki T. Requirement for Ras guanine nucleotide releasing protein 3 in coupling phospholipase C-gamma2 to Ras in B cell receptor signaling. J Exp Med. 2003;198:1841–51.
330. Takeda M, Kasai T, Morita K, Takeuchi M, Nishikawa T, Yamashita A, Mikami S, Hosoi H, Ohbayashi C. Cytopathological features of mammary analogue secretory carcinoma–review of literature. Diagn Cytopathol. 2015;43(2):131–7. doi:10.1002/dc.23146. Epub 2014 Mar 21
331. Denkert C, Loibl S, Noske A, Roller M, Müller BM, Komor M, et al. Tumor-associated lymphocytes as an independent predictor of response to neoadjuvant chemotherapy in breast cancer. J Clin Oncol. 2010;28:105–13.
332. Becker C, Fantini MC, Wirtz S. IL-6 signaling promotes tumor growth in colorectal cancer. Cell Cycle. 2005;4:217–20.
333. Bennecke M, et al. Ink4a/Arf and oncogene-induced senescence prevent tumor progression during alternative colorectal tumorigenesis. Cancer Cell. 2010;18:135–46.
334. Stanilov N, Miteva L, Deliysky T, Jovchev J, Stanilova S. Advanced colorectal cancer is associated with enhanced IL-23 and IL-10 serum levels. Labmedicine. 2010;41:159–63.
335. Cacev T, Radosevic S, Krizanac S, Kapitanović S. Influence of interleukin-8 and interleukin-10 on sporadic colon cancer development and progression. Carcinogenesis. 2008;29:1572–80.
336. Galon J, Costes A, Sanchez-Cabo F, Kirilovsky A, Mlecnik B, Lagorce-Pagès C, Tosolini M, Camus M, Berger A, Wind P, Zinzindohoué F, Bruneval P, Cugnenc PH, Trajanoski Z, Fridman WH, Pagès F. Type, density, and location of immune cells within human colorectal tumors predict clinical outcome. Science. 1960–1964;2006:313.
337. Schreiber RD, Old LJ, Smyth MJ. Cancer immunoediting: integrating immunity's roles in cancer suppression and promotion. Science. 2011;331:1565–70.
338. Kharbanda S, Saleem A, Datta R, Yuan ZM, Weichselbaum R, Kufe D. Ionizing radiation induces rapid tyrosine phosphorylation of p34cdc2. Cancer Res. 1994;54:1412–4.
339. Nosho K, Baba Y, Tanaka N, Shima K, Hayashi M, Meyerhardt JA, et al. Tumour-infiltrating T-cell subsets, molecular changes in colorectal cancer, and prognosis: cohort study and literature review. J Pathol. 2010;222:350–66.
340. Ogino S, Nosho K, Irahara N, Meyerhardt JA, Baba Y, Shima K, Glickman JN, Ferrone CR, Mino-Kenudson M, Tanaka N, Dranoff G, Giovannucci EL, Fuchs CS. Lymphocytic reaction to colorectal cancer is associated with longer survival, independent of lymph node count, microsatellite instability, and CpG island methylator phenotype. Clin Cancer Res. 2009;15(20):6412–20.
341. Park SY, Lee HE, Li H, Shipitsin M, Gelman R, Polyak K. Heterogeneity for stem cell–related markers according to tumor subtype and histologic stage in breast cancer. Clin Cancer Res. 2010;16:876–87.

342. Kaplan HJ, Niederkorn JY. Regional immunity and immune privilege. Chem Immunol Allergy. 2007;92:11–26.
343. Davies T. Pathogenesis of Hashimoto's thyroiditis (chronic autoimmune thyroiditis). Uptodate.com. 2016. http://www.uptodate.com/contents/pathogenesis-of-hashimotos-thyroiditis-chronic-autoimmune-thyroiditis. Accessed 30 Aug 2016.
344. Vesterinen E, Oukkala E, Timonen T, Aromaa A. Cancer incident among 78000 asthmatic patients. Intl J Epidemiol. 1993;22:976–82.
345. Cundell DR, Mickle KE. Developing the perfect antihistamine for use in allergic conditions: a voyage in H1 selectivity. eBook, Front Clin Drug Res-Anti Allergy Agents; 2016.
346. Thurmond RL, Kazerouni K, Chaplan SR, Greenspan AJ. Peripheral neuronal mechanism of itch: Histamine and itch. In Itch: mechanisms and treatment. In: Carstens E, Akiyama T, editors. Frontiers in neuroscience. Boca Raton: CRC Press/Taylor & Francis; 2014. Chapt 10.
347. García-Martín E, Ayuso P, Martínez C, et al. Histamine pharmacogenomics. Pharmacogenomics. 2009;10:867–83.
348. Johansson SGO, Bieber T, Dahl R, Friedmann PS, Lanier BQ, Lockey RF, Motala C, Martell JAO, Platts-Mills TAE, Ring J, Thien F, Cauwenberge PV, Williams HC. Revised nomenclature for allergy for global use: report of the nomenclature review committee of the World Allergy Organization. J Allergy Clin Immunol. 2004;113:832–6.
349. Bakker RA, Schoonus SB, Smit MJ, Timmerman H, Leurs R. Histamine H(1)-receptor activation of nuclear factor-kappa B: roles for G beta gamma- and G alpha(q/11)-subunits in constitutive and agonist- mediated signaling. Mol Pharmacol. 2011;60:1133–42.
350. Ho MH, Wong WH, Chang C. Clinical spectrum of food allergies: a comprehensive review. Clin Rev Allergy Immunol. 2014;46(3):225–40. doi:10.1007/s12016-012-8339-6.
351. Grimbaldeston MA, Metz M, Yu M, Tsai M, Galli SJ. Effector and potential immunoregulatory roles of mast cells in IgE-associated acquired immune responses. Curr Opinion Immunol. 2006;18:751–60.
352. Krauth MT, Majlesi Y, Sonneck K, Samorapoompichit P, Ghannadan M, Hauswirth AW, Baghestanian M, Schernthaner GH, Worda C, Muller MR, Sperr WR, Valent P. Effects of various statins on cytokine-dependent growth and IgE-dependent release of histamine in human mast cells. Allergy. 2006;61:281–8. doi:10.1111/j.1398-9995.2006.00997.x.
353. Dulek DE, Peebles RS Jr. Viruses and asthma. Biochim Biophys Acta. 2011;1810:1080e90.
354. Stott-Miller M, Chen C, Doody DR, Carter JL, Galloway DA, Madeleine MM, Schwartz SM. A history of allergies is associated with reduced risk of oral squamous cell carcinoma. Cancer Causes Control. 2012;23(12):1911–9. doi:10.1007/s10552-012-0068-x. Epub 2012 Sep 26
355. Boden SR, Wesley Burks A. Anaphylaxis: a history with emphasis on food allergy. Immunol Rev. 2011;(1):242, 247–57. doi:10.1111/j.1600-065X.2011.01028.x. Review.
356. Burnet FM. The probable relationship of some or all mast cells to the T-cell system. Cell Immunol. 1977;30:358–60.
357. Khatami M, Donnelly JJ, John T, Rockey JH. Vernal conjunctivitis. Model studies in guinea pigs immunized topically with fluoresceinyl ovalbumin. Arch Ophthalmol. 1984;102:1683–8.
358. Khatami M, Donnelly JJ, Rockey JH. Induction and down-regulation of conjunctival type-1 hypersensitivity reactions in guinea pigs sensitized topically with fluoresceinyl ovalbumin. Ophthalmic Res. 1985;17:139–47.
359. Haldar JP, Khatami M, Donnelly JJ, Rockey JH. Experimental allergic conjunctivitis: production of different isotypes of antibody by conjunctival-associated lymphoid tissue in culture. Regional Immunol. 1988;1:92–9.
360. Khatami M, Donnelly JJ, Haldar JP, Rockey JH. Massive follicular lymphoid hyperplasia in experimental chronic recurrent allergic conjunctivitis. Arch Ophthalmol. 1989;107:433–8.
361. Khatami M. Developmental phases of inflammation-induced massive lymphoid hyperplasia and extensive changes in epithelium in an experimental model of allergy: implications for a direct link between inflammation and carcinogenesis. Am J Ther. 2005;12:117–26.

362. Helleboid L, Khatami M, Wei Z-G, Rockey JH. Histamine and prostacyclin: primary and secondary release in allergic conjunctivitis. Invest Ophthalmol Vis Sci. 1991;32:2281–9.
363. Khatami M. Inflammation, aging and cancer: Friend or Foe? In: Khatami M, editor. Inflammation, chronic diseases and cancer-cell and molecular biology, immunology and clinical bases. Rijeka: InTech; 2012. p. 3–30.; ISBN: 978–953–51-0102-4.
364. Khatami M. Standardizing criteria on cancer biomarkers as foundation of a database: Creating a common language (data elements) for cancer biomarkers tracking and utilization for professionals in oncology research. Federal Register; HHS Reference No. E-147-2005/0--Research Tool. Government-Owned Inventions; Availability for Licensing. 2005. Volume 70: No. 140, Page 42350–42351. July 22, 2005.
365. Khatami M. Standardizing cancer biomarkers criteria: data elements as foundation of a database. M-CSF (model marker) for early detection of cancer. Cell Biochem Biophys. 2007;47:187–98.
366. Jabaut J, Ckless K (2012) Inflammation, immunity and redox signaling. In: Khatami M (ed) inflammation, chronic diseases and cancer. Cell and molecular biology, immunology and clinical bases. InTech, Rijeka, pp 145–160.
367. Khatami M. Inflammation, chronic diseases and cancer-cell and molecular biology, immunology and clinical bases, pp-1–430, InTech., ISBN978-953-51-0102-4, 2012, Rijeka., http://www.intechopen.com/books/editor/inflammation-chronic-diseases-and-cancer-cell-and-molecular-biology-immunology-and-clinical-bases
368. Portales-Cervantes L, Haidl ID, Lee PW, Marshall JS. Virus-infected human mast cells enhance natural killer cell functions. J Innate Immun. 2017;9(1):94–108. doi:10.1159/000450576. Epub 2016 Nov 3
369. Oskeritzian CA. Mast cell plasticity and sphingosine-1-phosphate in immunity, inflammation and cancer. Mol Immunol. 2015;63(1):104–12. doi:10.1016/j.molimm.2014.03.018. Epub 2014 Apr 22
370. Ahmed T, D'Brot J, Abraham W. The role of calcium antagonists in bronchial reactivity. J Allergy Clin Immunol. 1988;81:133–44.
371. Daëron M, Lesourne R. Negative signaling in Fc receptor complexes. Adv Immunol. 2006;89:39–86.
372. Brusko TM, Putnam AL, Bluestone JA. Human regulatory T cells: role in autoimmune disease and therapeutic opportunities. Immunol Rev. 2008;223:371–90.
373. Richet C. Anaphylaxies. Liverpool: University Press; 1913.
374. Rosenau MJ, Anderson JF. Hypersusceptibility. JAMA. 1906;47:1007.
375. FER S, editor. Ancestors of allergy. New York: Global Medical Communications; 1994.
376. Megendie F. Lectures on blood. Philadelphia: Aswell, Barrington and Haswell; 1839.
377. Dale HH, Laidlaw PP. The physiological action of beta-imidazolylethylamine. J Physiol. 1910;41:318–44.
378. Prausnitz C, Küster H. Studien über die Überempfindlichkeit. Zbl Bakt Abt 1 Orig, 1921:86–160.
379. Arthus N-M. La séro-anaphylaxie du lapin. Arch Int Physiol. 1909;7:471.
380. Mueller HL. Diagnosis and treatment of insect sensitivity. J Asthma Res. 1966;3:331–3.
381. May CD. The ancestry of allergy: being an account of the original experimental induction of hypersensitivity recognizing the contribution of Paul Portier. J Allergy Clin Immunol. 1985;75:485–95.
382. Holgate ST, Church MK. Asthma. The mast cell. Br Med Bull. 1992;48(1):40–50.
383. Ring J, Grosber M, Brockow K, Bergmann KC. Anaphylaxis. Chem Immunol Allergy. 2014;100:54–61. doi:10.1159/000358503. Epub 2014 May 15
384. Sherman PW, Holland E, Sherman JS. Allergies: their role in cancer prevention. Q Rev Biol. 2008;83(4):339–62.
385. Toda M, Heilmann M, Ilchmann A, Vieths S. The Maillard reaction and food allergies: is there a link? Clin Chem Lab Med. 2014;52(1):61–7. doi:10.1515/cclm-2012-0830.

386. Wu D, Cao M, Peng J, Li N, Yi S, Song L, Wang X, Zhang M, Zhao J. The effect of trimethylamine N-oxide on helicobacter pylori-induced changes of immunoinflammatory genes expression in gastricepithelial cells. Int Immunopharmacol. 2017;43:172–8. doi:10.1016/j.intimp.2016.11.032. Epub 2016
387. Lin YW, Lee B, Liu PS, Wei LN. Receptor-interacting protein 140 orchestrates the dynamics of macrophage M1/M2 polarization. J Innate Immun. 2016;8:97–107.
388. Kinney SR, Carlson L, Ser-Dolansky J, Thompson C, Shah S, Gambrah A, Xing W, Schneider SS, Mathias CB. Curcumin ingestion inhibits mastocytosis and suppresses intestinal anaphylaxis in a murine model of food allergy. PLoS One. 2015;10:e0132467. doi:10.1371/journal.pone.0132467.
389. Kluin-Nelemans HC, Oldhoff JM, Van Doormaal JJ, Van't Wout JW, Verhoef G, Gerrits WB, van Dobbenburgh OA, Pasmans SG, Fijnheer R. Cladribine therapy for systemic mastocytosis. Blood. 2003;102:4270–6. doi:10.1182/blood-2003-05-1699.
390. Bot I, de Jager SC, Zernecke A, Lindstedt KA, van Berkel TJ, Weber C, Biessen EA. Perivascular mast cells promote atherogenesis and induce plaque destabilization in apolipoprotein E-deficient mice. Circulation. 2007;115:2516–25.
391. Metcalfe DD, Kaliner M, Donlon MA. The mast cell. Crit Rev Immunol. 1981;3:23–74.
392. Tkaczyk C, Okayama Y, Woolhiser MR, Hagaman DD, Gilfillan AM, Metcalfe DD. Activation of human mast cells through the high affinity IgG receptor. Mol Immunol. 2001;38:1289–93.
393. Gunin AG, Kornilov NK, Vasilieva OV, Petrov VV. Age-related changes in proliferation, the numbers of mast cells, eosinophils, and cd45-positive cells in human dermis. J Gerontol Biol Sci Med Sci. 2011;66:385–92.
394. Ribatti D, Crivellato E. Mast cell ontology: an historical overview. Immunol Lett. 2014;159:11–4. doi:10.1016/j.imlet.2014.02.003.
395. Okayama Y, Benyon RC, Rees PH, Lowman MA, Hillier K, Church MK. Inhibition profiles of sodium cromoglycate and nedocromil sodium on mediator release from mast cells of human skin, lung, tonsil, adenoid and intestine. Clin Exp Allergy. 1992;22:401–9.
396. Zhang T, Finn DF, Barlow JW, Walsh JJ. Mast cell stabilisers. Eur J Pharmacol. 2016;778:158–68. doi:10.1016/j.ejphar.2015.05.071. Epub 2015 Jun 27
397. Gong J, Yang NS, Croft M, Weng IC, Sun L, Liu FT, Chen SS. The antigen presentation function of bone marrow-derived mast cells is spatiotemporally restricted to a subset expressing high levels of cell surface FcepsilonRI and MHC II. BMC Immunol. 2010;11:34. doi:10.1186/1471-2172-11-34.
398. Glass CK, Witztum JL. Atherosclerosis. The road ahead. Cell. 2001;104:503–16.
399. Libby P, Ridker PM, Hansson GK. Progress and challenges in translating the biology of atherosclerosis. Nature. 2011;473:317–25.
400. Hansson GK, Libby P. The immune response in atherosclerosis: a double-edged sword. Nat Rev Immunol. 2006;6:508–19.
401. Lahoute C, Herbin O, Mallat Z, Tedgui A. Adaptive immunity in atherosclerosis: mechanisms and future therapeutic targets. Nat Rev Cardiol. 2011;8:348–58.
402. Zhou X, Nicoletti A, Elhage R, Hansson GK. Transfer of CD4(+) T cells aggravates atherosclerosis in immunodeficient apolipoprotein E knockout mice. Circulation. 2000;102:2919–22.
403. Daugherty A, Puré E, Delfel-Butteiger D, Chen S, Leferovich J, Roselaar SE, Rader DJ. The effects of total lymphocyte deficiency on the extent of atherosclerosis in apolipoprotein E−/− mice. J Clin Invest. 1997;100:1575–80.
404. Oh P, Lobry C, Gao J, Tikhonova A, Loizou E, Manent J, van Handel B, Ibrahim S, Greve J, Mikkola H, et al. In vivo mapping of notch pathway activity in normal and stress hematopoiesis. Cell Stem Cell. 2013;13:190–204.
405. Connolly MK, Bedrosian AS, Malhotra A, Henning JR, Ibrahim J, Vera V, et al. In hepatic fibrosis, liver sinusoidal endothelial cells acquire enhanced immunogenicity. J Immunol. 2010;185:2200–8.
406. Fiorini E, Merck E, Wilson A, Ferrero I, Jiang W, Koch U, Auderset F, Laurenti E, Tacchini-Cottier F, Pierres M, et al. Dynamic regulation of notch 1 and notch 2 surface expression dur-

ing T cell development and activation revealed by novel monoclonal antibodies. J Immunol. 2009;183:7212–22.
407. Artavanis-Tsakonas S, Rand MD, Lake RJ. Notch signaling: cell fate control and signal integration in development. Science. 1999;284:770–6.
408. Butler JM, Nolan DJ, Vertes EL, Varnum-Finney B, Kobayashi H, Hooper AT, Seandel M, Shido K, White IA, Kobayashi M, et al. Endothelial cells are essential for the self-renewal and repopulation of notch-dependent hematopoietic stem cells. Cell Stem Cell. 1999;6:251–64.
409. Peter K, O'Toole TE. Modulation of cell adhesion by changes in αL β2 (LFA-1, CD11a/CD18) cytoplasmic domain/cytoskeleton interaction. J Exp Med. 1995;181:315–26.
410. Jang S-W, Yang S-J, Srinivasan S, Ye K. Akt phosphorylates MstI and prevents its proteolytic activation, blocking FOXO3 phosphorylation and nuclear translocation. J Biol Chem. 2007;282:30836–44.
411. Lanier LL, Le AM, Civin CI, Loken MR, Phillips JH. The relationship of CD16 (Leu-11) and Leu-19 (NKH-1) antigen expression on human peripheral blood NK cells and cytotoxic T lymphocytes. J Immunol. 1986;136:4480–6.
412. Arnett TR, Gibbons DC, Utting JC, Orriss IR, Hoebertz A, Rosendaal M, Meghji S. Hypoxia is a major stimulator of osteoclast formation and bone resorption. J Cell Physiol. 2003;196:2–8.
413. Missiha SB, Ostrowski M, Heathcote EJ. Disease progression in chronic hepatitis C: modifiable and non-modifiable factors. Gastroenterology. 2008;134:1699–714.
414. Bataller R, North KE, Brenner DA. Genetic polymorphisms and the progression of liver fibrosis: a critical appraisal. Hepatology. 2003;37:493–503.
415. Powell EE, Edwards-Smith CJ, Hay JL, Clouston AD, Crawford DH, Shorthouse C, et al. Host genetic factors influence disease progression in chronic hepatitis. Hepatology. 2000;31:828–33.
416. Huang H, Shiffman ML, Friedman S, Venkatesh R, Bzowej N, Abar OT, et al. A 7 gene signature identifies the risk of developing cirrhosis in patients with chronic hepatitis C. Hepatology. 2007;46:297–306.
417. Marcolongo M, Young B, Dal Pero F, Fattovich G, Peraro L, Guido M, et al. A seven-gene signature (cirrhosis risk score) predicts liver fibrosis progression in patients with initially mild chronic hepatitis C. Hepatology. 2009;50:1038–44.
418. Minouchi K, Kaneko S, Kobayashi K. Mutation of p53 gene in regenerative nodules in cirrhotic liver. J Hepatol. 2002;37:231–9.
419. Calado RT, Brudno J, Mehta P, Kovacs JJ, Wu C, Zago MA, et al. Constitutional telomerase mutations are genetic risk factors for cirrhosis. Hepatology. 2011;53:1600–7.
420. Adams PD. Healing and hurting: molecular mechanisms, functions, and pathologies of cellular senescence. Mol Cell. 2009;36:2–14.
421. Krizhanovsky V, Yon M, Dickins RA, Hearn S, Simon J, Miething C, et al. Senescence of activated stellate cells limits liver fibrosis. Cell. 2008;134:657–67.
422. Wiemann SU, Satyanarayana A, Tsahuridu M, Tillmann HL, Zender L, Klempnauer J, et al. Hepatocyte telomere shortening and senescence are general markers of human liver cirrhosis. FASEB J. 2002;16:935–42.
423. Wang Z, Lin H, Hua F, Hu ZW. Repairing DNA damage by XRCC6/KU70 reverses TLR4-deficiency-worsened HCC development via restoring senescence and autophagic flux. Autophagy. 2013;9:925–7.
424. Iredale JP. Models of liver fibrosis: exploring the dynamic nature of inflammation and repair in a solid organ. J Clin Invest. 2007;117:539–48.
425. Timchenko NA. Aging and liver regeneration. Trends Endocrinol Metab. 2009;20:171–6.
426. Ramakrishna G, Anwar T, Angara RK, Chatterjee N, Kiran S, Singh S. Role of cellular senescence in hepatic wound healing and carcinogenesis. Eur J Cell Biol. 2012;91:739–47.
427. Schnabl B, Purbeck CA, Choi YH, Hagedorn CH, Brenner D, et al. Replicative senescence of activated human hepatic stellate cells is accompanied by a pronounced inflammatory but less fibrogenic phenotype. Hepatology. 2003;37:653–64.

428. Wang HL, Lu DW, Yerian LM, Alsikafi N, Steinberg G, Hart J, Yang XJ. Immunohistochemical distinction between primary adenocarcinoma of the bladder and secondary colorectal adenocarcinoma. Am J Surg Pathol. 2001;25:1380–7.
429. Rutkowski MJ, Sughrue ME, Kane AJ, Ahn BJ, Fang S, Parsa AT. The complement cascade as a mediator of tissue growth and regeneration. Inflamm Res. 2010;59(11):897–905. doi:10.1007/s00011-010-0220-6. Epub 2010 Jun 2
430. Robertson MJ, Ritz J. Biology and clinical relevance of human natural killer cells. Blood. 1990;76:2421–38.
431. Dempsey PW, Allison ME, Akkaraju S, Goodnow CC, Fearon DT. C3d of complement as a molecular adjuvant: bridging innate and acquired immunity. Science. 1996;271:348–50. doi:10.1126/science.271.5247.348.
432. Cole DS, Morgan BP. Beyond lysis: how complement influences cell fate. Clin Sci (Lond). 2003;104:455–66. doi:10.1042/CS20020362.
433. Thomas A, Gasque P, Vaudry D, Gonzalez B, Fontaine M. Expression of a complete and functional complement system by human neuronal cells in vitro. Int Immunol. 2000;12:1015–23. doi:10.1093/intimm/12.7.1015.
434. D'Ambrosio AL, Pinsky DJ, Connolly ES. The role of the complement cascade in ischemia/reperfusion injury: implications for neuroprotection. Mol Med. 2001;7:367–82.
435. Markiewski MM, Lambris JD. The role of complement in inflammatory diseases from behind the scenes into the spotlight. Am J Pathol. 2007;171:715–27. doi:10.2353/ajpath.2007.070166.
436. Herwald H. Egesten a: cells of innate and adaptive immunity: a matter of class? J Innate Immun. 2017;9:109–10. doi:10.1159/000457176.
437. Singh N, et al. Generation of T cell hybridomas from naturally occurring FoxP3+ regulatory T cells. Meth Mol Biol. 2011;707:39.
438. Ribot J, Romagnoli P, van Meerwijk JP. Agonist ligands expressed by thymic epithelium enhance positive selection of regulatory T lymphocytes from precursors with a normally diverse TCR repertoire. J Immunol. 2006;177(2):1101.
439. Wong J, Mathis D, Benoist C. TCR-based lineage tracing: no evidence for conversion of conventional into regulatory T cells in response to a natural self-antigen in pancreatic islets. J Exp Med. 2007;204(9):2039–45.
440. Mack DG, Falta MT, McKee AS, Martin AK, Simonian PL, Crawford F, Terry Gordon T, et al. Regulatory T cells modulate granulomatous inflammation in an HLA-DP2 transgenic murine model of beryllium-induced disease. Proc Natl Acad Sci U S A. 2014;111(23):8553–8. doi:10.1073/pnas.1408048111. PMCID: PMC4060652
441. Belkaid Y, Rouse BT. Natural regulatory T cells in infectious disease. Nat Immunol. 2005;6(4):353.
442. Cebula A, Seweryn M, Rempala GA, Pabla SS, McIndoe RA, Denning TL, Bry L, Kraj P, Kisielow P, Ignatowicz L. Thymus-derived regulatory T cells contribute to tolerance to commensal microbiota. Nature. 2013;497(7448):258–62. doi:10.1038/nature12079. Epub 2013 Apr 28
443. Rempala GA, Seweryn M. Methods for diversity and overlap analysis in T-cell receptor populations. J Math Biol. 2012; doi:10.1007/s00285-012-0589-7.
444. Cortés-Garcia JD, López-López C, Cortez-Espinosa N, García-Hernández MH, et al. Evaluation of the expression and function of the P2X7 receptor and ART1 in human regulatory T-cell subsets. Immunobiology. 2016;221(1):84–93. doi:10.1016/j.imbio.2015.07.018. Epub 2015 Jul 29
445. Kim KH, Jahan SA, Kabir E. A review on human health perspective of air pollution with respect to allergies and asthma. Environ Int. 2013;59:41–52. doi:10.1016/j.envint.2013.05.007. Epub 2013 Jun 12
446. Steinman RM, Hawiger D, Liu K, Bonifaz L, Bonnyay D, Mahnke K, Iyoda T, Ravetch J, Dhodapkar M, Inaba K, Nussenzweig M. Dendritic cell function in vivo during the steady state: a role in peripheral tolerance. Ann N Y Acad Sci. 2003;987:15–25.

447. Cardet JC, Israel E. Update on reslizumab for eosinophilic asthma. Expert Opin Biol Ther. 2015;15(10):1531–9. doi:10.1517/14712598.2015.1090972.
448. Gondois-Rey F, Chéret A, Mallet F, Bidaut G, Granjeaud S, Lécuroux C, Ploquin M, Müller-Trutwin M, Rouzioux C, Avettand-Fenoël V, De Maria A, et al. A mature NK profile at the time of HIV primary infection is associated with an early response to cART. Front Immunol. 2017.; https://doi.org/10.3389/fimmu.2017.00054
449. Ploquin MJ, Madec Y, Casrouge A, Huot N, Passaes C, Lecuroux C, et al. Elevated basal pre-infection CXCL10 in plasma and in the small intestine after infection are associated with more rapid HIV/SIV disease onset. PLoS Pathog. 2016;12(8):e1005774. doi:10.1371/journal.ppat.1005774.
450. Strauss-Albee DM, Fukuyama J, Liang EC, Yao Y, Jarrell JA, Drake AL, et al. Human NK cell repertoire diversity reflects immune experience and correlates with viral susceptibility. Sci Transl Med. 2015;7(297):297ra115. doi:10.1126/scitranslmed.aac5722.
451. Mela CM, Burton CT, Imami N, Nelson M, Steel A, Gazzard BG, et al. Switch from inhibitory to activating NKG2 receptor expression in HIV-1 infection: lack of reversion with highly active antiretroviral therapy. AIDS. 2005;19(16):1761–9. doi:10.1097/01.aids.0000183632.12418.33.
452. Hong HS, Eberhard JM, Keudel P, Bollmann BA, Ballmaier M, Bhatnagar N, et al. HIV infection is associated with a preferential decline in less-differentiated CD56dim CD16+ NK cells. J Virol. 2010;84(2):1183–8. doi:10.1128/JVI.01675-09.
453. DiPenta JM, Johnson JG, Murphy RJ. Natural killer cells and exercise training in the elderly: a review. Can J Appl Physiol. 2004;29(4):419–43.
454. Tomasec P, Braud VM, Rickards C, Powell MB, McSharry BP, Gadola S, et al. Surface expression of HLA-E, an inhibitor of natural killer cells, enhanced by human cytomegalovirus gpUL40. Science. 2000;287(5455):1031. doi:10.1126/science.287.5455.1031.
455. Paludan C, Schmid D, Landhalter M, Vockerodt M, Kube D, Tuschl T, Munz C. Endogenous MHC class II processing of a viral nuclear antigen after autophagy. Science. 2005;307:593–6.
456. Muntasell A, Berger AC, Roche PA. T cell-induced secretion of MHC class II-peptide complexes on B cell exosomes. EMBO J. 2007;26:4263–72.
457. Doucet-O'Hare TT, Rodić N, Sharma R, Darbari I, Abril G, Choi JA, Young Ahn J, et al. LINE-1 expression and retrotransposition in Barrett's esophagus and esophageal carcinoma. Proc Natl Acad Sci U S A. 2015;112(35):E4894–900. doi:10.1073/pnas. 1502474112. Epub 2015 Aug 17
458. Klinker MW, Lizzio V, Reed TJ, Fox DA, Lundy SK. Human B cell-derived lymphoblastoid cell lines constitutively produce Fas ligand and secrete MHCII(+)FasL(+) killer exosomes. Front Immunol. 2014;5:144.
459. Oliver G. Lymphatic vasculature development. Nat Rev Immunol. 2004;4:35–45.
460. Mills CD, Ley K, Buchmann K, Canton J. Sequential immune responses: the weapons of immunity. J Innate Immun. 2015;7:443–9.
461. Hoffmann HJ. News in cellular Allergology: a review of the human mast cell and basophil granulocyte literature from January 2013 to May 2015. Int Arch Allergy Immunol. 2015;168(4):253–62. doi:10.1159/000443960. Epub 2016 Feb 20
462. Tran TH, Mattheolabakis G, Aldawsari H, Amiji M. Exosomes as nanocarriers for immunotherapy of cancer and inflammatory diseases. Clin Immunol. 2015;160:46–58.
463. Kensler TW, Spira A, Garber JE, Szabo E, Lee JJ, Dong Z, Dannenberg AJ, Hait WN, Blackburn E, et al. Transforming cancer prevention through precision medicine and immune-oncology. Cancer Prev Res (Phila). 2016;9(1):2–10. doi:10.1158/1940-6207.CAPR-15-0406.
464. Molderings GJ, Haenisch B, Brettner S, Homann J, Menzen M, Dumoulin FL, Panse J, Butterfield J, Afrin LB. Pharmacological treatment options for mast cell activation disease. Naunyn Schmiedeberg's Arch Pharmacol. 2016;389(7):671–94. doi:10.1007/s00210-016-1247-1. Epub 2016 Apr 30
465. Cortes J, Moore JO, Maziarz RT, Wetzler M, Craig M, Matous J, et al. Control of plasma uric acid in adults at risk for tumor lysis syndrome: efficacy and safety of rasburicase alone and

rasburicase followed by allopurinol compared with allopurinol alone–results of a multicenter phase III study. J Clin Oncol. 2010;28:4207–13. doi:10.1200/JCO.2009.26.8896.
466. McBride A, Westervelt P. Recognizing and managing the expanded risk of tumor lysis syndrome in hematologic and solid malignancies. J Hematol Oncol. 2012;5:75. doi:10.1186/1756-8722-5-75.
467. Vidarsson G, Dekkers G, Rispens T. IgG subclasses and allotypes: from structure to effector functions. Front Immunol. 2014;5:520. doi:10.3389/fimmu.2014.00520.
468. Huh JY, Park YJ, Ham M, Kim JB. Crosstalk between adipocytes and immune cells in adipose tissue inflammation and metabolic dysregulation in obesity. Mol Cells. 2014;37(5):365–71. doi:10.14348/molcells.2014.0074. Epub 2014 Apr 30
469. Oehlke J, Lorenz D, Wiesner B, Bienert M. Studies on the cellular uptake of substance P and lysine-rich, KLA-derived model peptides. J Mol Recognit. 2005;18(1):50–9.
470. Cassisa A. Pathophysiology of subcutaneous fat. G Ital Dermatol Venereol. 2013;148:315–23.
471. Dichlberger A, Kovanen PT, Schneider WJ. Mast cells: from lipid droplets to lipid mediators. Clin Sci (Lond). 2013;125(3):121–30. doi:10.1042/CS20120602.
472. Gustafsson Asting A, Caren H, Andersson M, Lönnroth C, Lagerstedt K, Lundholm K. COX-2 gene expression in colon cancer tissue related to regulating factors and promotor methylation status. BMC Cancer. 2011;11:238.
473. Wiiliam CS, Mann M, Dubois RN. The role of cycloxygenases in inflammation, cancer and development. Oncogene. 1999;18:7906–16.
474. Greenhough A, Smartt HJ, Moore AE, et al. The COX-2/PGE2 pathway: key roles in the hallmarks of cancer and adaptation to the tumour microenvironment. Carcinogenesis. 2009;30:377–86.
475. Sostres C, Lanas A. Gastrointestinal effects of aspirin. Nat Rev Gastroenterol Hepatol. 2011;8:385–94.
476. Legan M. Cyclooxygenase-2, p53 and glucose transporter-1 as predictors of malignancy in the development of gallbladder carcinomas. Bosn J Basic Med Sci. 2010;10:192–6.
477. Romagnolo DF, Papoutsis AJ, Selmin O. Nutritional targeting of cyclooxygenase-2 for colon cancer prevention. Inflamm Allergy Drug Targets. 2010;9:181–91.
478. Ozerdem U, Stallcup WB. Early contribution of pericytes to angiogenic sprouting and tube formation. Angiogenesis. 2003;6:241–9.
479. Gao Q, Tang J, Chen J, Jiang L, Zhu X, Xu Z. Epigenetic code and potential epigenetic-based therapies against chronic diseases in developmental origins. Drug Discov Today. 2014;19:1744–50.
480. Folkman J. Angiogenesis. Ann Rev Med. 2006;57:1–18.
481. Liao D, Johnson RS. Hypoxia: a key regulator of angiogenesis in cancer. Cancer Metastasis Rev. 2007;26:281–90.
482. Saghiri MA, Asatourian A, Orangi J, Sorenson CM, Sheibani N. Functional role of inorganic trace elements in angiogenesis-Part I: N, Fe, Se, P, Au, and Ca. Crit Rev Oncol Hematol. 2015; doi:10.1016/j.critrevonc.2015.05.010.
483. Sutendra G, Dromparis P, Kinnaird A, Stenson TH, Haromy A, et al. Mitochondrial activation by inhibition of PDKII suppresses HIF1a signaling and angiogenesis in cancer. Oncogene. 2013;32:1638–50.
484. Jackson SP. The growing complexity of platelet aggregation. Blood. 2007;109:5087–95.
485. Fielding RA, Vellas B, Evans WJ, Bhasin S, Morley JE, Newman AB, et al. Sarcopenia: an undiagnosed condition in older adults. Current consensus definition: prevalence, etiology, and consequences. International working group on sarcopenia. J Am Med Dir Assoc. 2011;12:249–56.
486. Wagner DD, Frenette PS. The vessel wall and its interactions. Blood. 2008;111:5271–81.
487. Ribatti D, Ranieri G. Tryptase, a novel angiogenic factor stored in mast cell graules. Exp Cell Res. 2015;332:157–62.
488. Jiang L, Zhang J, Monticone RE, Telljohann R, Wu J, Wang M, Lakatta EG. Calpain-1 regulation of matrix metalloproteinase 2 activity in vascular smooth muscle cells facilitates age-associated aortic wall calcification and fibrosis. Hypertension. 2012;60:1192–9.

489. Minniti AN, Cataldo R, Trigo C, Vasquez L, Mujica P, Leighton F, et al. Methionine sulfoxide reductase a expression is regulated by the DAF-16/FOXO pathway in *Caenorhabditis elegans*. Aging Cell. 2009;8:690–705.
490. Emerit J, Edeas M, Bricaire F. Neurodegenerative diseases and oxidative stress. Biomed Pharmacother. 2004;58:39–46.
491. Tower J. Programmed cell death in aging. Ageing Res Rev. 2015; doi:10.1016/j.arr.2015.04.002.
492. Campisi J, Andersen JK, Kapahi P, Melov S. Cellular senescence: a link between cancer and age-related degenerative disease? Sem Cancer Biol. 2011;21:354–9.
493. Hilvering B, Xue L, Pavord ID. Evidence for the efficacy and safety of anti-interleukin-5 treatment in the management of refractory eosinophilic asthma. Ther Adv Respir Dis. 2015;9(4):135–45. doi:10.1177/1753465815581279. Epub 2015 Apr 21
494. Leung DY, et al. Effect of anti-IgE therapy in patients with peanut allergy. N Engl J Med. 2003;348:986–93.
495. Miyajima H, Abe K, Ushiyama C, Okumura K, Ovary Z, Hirano T. IgE allotypes in sera of mice with autoimmune diseases and in mice with graft-versus-host disease after transfusion or bone marrow transplantation. Int Arch Allergy Immunol. 1996;111(2):152–5.
496. Sevigny CP, Li L, Awad AS, Huang L, McDuffie M, Linden J, et al. Activation of adenosine 2A receptors attenuates allograft rejection and alloantigen recognition. J Immunol. 2007;178(7):4240–9.
497. Chhabra P, Wang K, Zeng Q, Jecmenica M, Langman L, Linden J, et al. Adenosine A(2A) agonist administration improves islet transplant outcome: evidence for the role of innate immunity in islet graft rejection. Cell Transplant. 2010;19(5):597–612. doi:10.3727/096368910X491806.
498. Samitas K, Delimpoura V, Zervas E, Gaga M. Anti-IgE treatment, airway inflammation and remodelling in severe allergic asthma: current knowledge and future perspectives. Eur Respir Rev. 2015;24(138):594–601. doi:10.1183/16000617.00001715.
499. Crystal RG, Randell SH, Engelhardt JF, Voynow J, Sunday ME. Airway epithelial cells: current concepts and challenges. Proc Am Thorac Soc. 2008;5:772e7.
500. Bansal G, Xie Z, Rao S, Nocka KH, Druey KM. Suppression of immunoglobulin E-mediated allergic responses by regulator of G protein signaling 13. Nat Immunol. 2008;9(1):73–80. Epub 2007 Nov 18
501. MacGlashan DW Jr, Bochner BS, Adelman DC, Jardieu PM, Togias A, McKenzie-White J, Hamilton RG, Lichtenstein LM. Down-regulation of Fc(epsilon)RI expression on human basophils during in vivo treatment of atopic patients with anti-IgE antibody J Immunol 1997;158(3):1438–1445. doi:https://doi.org/10.1186/s40169-017-0144-7.
502. Pelaia G, Vatrella A, Busceti MT, Gallelli L, Terracciano R, Maselli R. Anti-IgE therapy with omalizumab for severe asthma: current concepts and potential developments. Curr Drug Targets. 2015;16(2):171–8.
503. Pedersen SE, Hurd SS, Lemanske RF, et al. Global strategy for the diagnosis and management of asthma in children 5 years and younger. Pediatr Pulmonol. 2011;46(1):1–17.
504. Waldmann TA, Strober W, Blaese RM, Terry WD. Immunoglobulin metabolism in disease. Birth Defects Orig Artic Ser. 1975;11:87–94.
505. Kulig M, Bergmann R, Klettke U, Wahn V, Tacke U, Wahn U. Natural course of sensitization to food and inhalant allergens during the first 6 years of life. J Allergy Clin Immunol. 1999;103(6):1173–9.
506. Lemanske RF Jr, Jackson DJ, Gangnon RE, et al. Rhinovirus illnesses during infancy predict subsequent childhood wheezing. J Allergy Clin Immunol. 2005;116:571e7.
507. Katz Y, et al. Oral immunotherapy: ready for prime time? J Allergy Clin Immunol. 2011;127:289–90.
508. Kinet JP. The high-affinity IgE receptor (Fc epsilon RI): from physiology to pathology. Ann Rev Immunol. 1999;17:931–72. doi:10.1146/annurev.immunol.17.1.931.

509. Froidure A, Mouthuy J, Durham SR, Chanez P, Sibille Y, Pilette C. Asthma phenotypes and IgE responses. Eur Respir J. 2016;47(1):304–19. doi:10.1183/13993003.01824-2014. Epub 2015 Dec 17
510. Josephs DH, Spicer JF, Karagiannis P, Gould HJ, Karagiannis SN. IgE immunotherapy: a novel concept with promise for the treatment of cancer. MAbs. 2014;6(1):54–72. doi:10.4161/mabs.27029.
511. Chung CH, Mirakhur B, Chan E, Le QT, Berlin J, Morse M, Murphy BA, Satinover SM, Hosen J, Mauro D, et al. Cetuximab-induced anaphylaxis and IgE specific for galactose-alpha-1,3-galactose. N Engl J Med. 2008;358:1109–17. doi:10.1056/NEJMoa074943.
512. Robinson DS. Regulatory T cells and asthma. Clin Exp Allergy. 2009:39, 1314–1323. doi:10.1111/j.1365-2222.2009.03301.x. Epub 2009 Jun 17
513. Arnold JN, Radcliffe CM, Wormald MR, Royle L, Harvey DJ, Crispin M, Dwek RA, Sim RB, Rudd PM. The glycosylation of human serum IgD and IgE and the accessibility of identified oligomannose structures for interaction with mannan-binding lectin. J Immunol. 2004;173:6831–40.
514. Teo PZ, Utz PJ, Mollick JA. Using the allergic immune system to target cancer: activity of IgE antibodies specific for human CD20 and MUC1. Cancer Immunol Immunother. 2012;61:2295–309. doi:10.1007/s00262-012-1299-0.
515. Kershaw MH, Darcy PK, Trapani JA, Smyth MJ. The use of chimeric human Fc(epsilon) receptor I to redirect cytotoxic T lymphocytes to tumors. J Leukoc Biol. 1996;60:721–8.
516. McNeill JH, Verma SC, Tenner TE Jr. Cardiac histamine receptors. Adv Myocardiol. 1980;1:209–16.
517. Brunstein F, Rens J, van Tiel ST, Eggermont AM, ten Hagen TL. Histamine, a vasoactive agent with vascular disrupting potential, improves tumour response by enhancing local drug delivery. Br J Cancer. 2006;95:1663–9.
518. Sachs G, Spenney JG, Rehm WS. Gastric secretion. Int Rev Physiol. 1977;12:127–1271.
519. Chen D, Aihara T, Zhao CM, Håkanson R, Okabe S. Differentiation of the gastric mucosa. I. Role of histamine in control of function and integrity of oxyntic mucosa: understanding gastric physiology through disruption of targeted genes. Am J Physiol Gastrointest Liver Physiol. 2006;291:G539–44.
520. Ferrada C, Moreno E, Casadó V, Bongers G, Cortés A, Mallol J, Canela EI, Leurs R, Ferré S, Lluís C, Franco R. Marked changes in signal transduction upon heteromerization of dopamine D1 and histamine H3 receptors. Br J Pharmacol. 2009;157(1):64–75. doi:10.1111/j.1476-5381.2009.00152.x.
521. Palacios C, Pintado E. Effect of protein kinase C activation on mast cell histamine release. Biochem Int. 1987;15(2):441–7.
522. Huck V, Niemeyer A, Goerge T, Schnaeker EM, Ossig R, Rogge P, et al. Delay of acute intracellular pH recovery after acidosis decreases endothelial cell activation. J Cell Physiol. 2007;211:399–409.
523. Jiménez-Jiménez FJ, Alonso-Navarro H, García-Martín E, Agúndez JA. Thr105Ile (rs11558538) polymorphism in the histamine N-methyltransferase (HNMT) gene and risk for Parkinson disease: a PRISMA-compliant systematic review and meta-analysis. Medicine (Baltimore). 2016;95(27):e4147. doi:10.1097/MD.0000000000004147.
524. Petersen J, Raithel M, Schwelberger HG. Histamine *N*-methyltransferase and diamine oxidase gene polymorphisms in patients with inflammatory and neoplastic intestinal diseases. Inflamm Res. 2002;51(suppl):S91–2.
525. Palada V, Terzić J, Mazzulli J, et al. Histamine *N*-methyltransferase Thr105Ile polymorphism is associated with Parkinson's disease. Neurobiol Aging. 2012;33:836.e1–3.
526. Watanabe T, Taguchi Y, Shiosaka S, et al. Distribution of the histaminergic neuron system in the central nervous system of rats; a fluorescent immunohistochemical analysis with histidine decarboxylase as a marker. Brain Res. 1984;295:13–25.
527. Hu WW, Chen Z. Role of histamine and its receptors in cerebral ischemia. ACS Chem Neurosci. 2012;3(4):238–47. doi:10.1021/cn200126p. Epub 2012 Feb 10

528. Wada H, Inagaki N, Itowi N, Yamatodani A. Histaminergic neuron system in the brain: distribution and possible functions. Brain Res Bull. 1991;27:367–70.
529. Gorgisen G, Gulacar IM, Ozes ON. The role of insulin receptor substrate (IRS) proteins in oncogenic transformation. Cell Mol Biol (Noisy-le-grand). 2017;63(1):1–5. doi:10.14715/cmb/2017.63.1.1.
530. Moss J. Muscle relaxants and histamine release. Acta Anaesthesiol Scand Suppl. 1995;106:7–12.
531. Fisher MM. Severe histamine mediated reactions to intravenous drugs used in anaesthesia. Anaesth Intensive Care. 1975;3(3):180–97.
532. McCuaig S, Martin JG. How the airway smooth muscle in cystic fibrosis reacts in proinflammatory conditions: implications for airway hyper-responsiveness and asthma in cystic fibrosis. Lancet Respir Med. 2013;1(2):137–47. doi:10.1016/S2213-2600(12)70058-9. Epub 2013 Jan 30
533. Maintz L, Novak N. Histamine and histamine intolerance. Am J Clin Nutr. 2007;85(5):1185–96.
534. Sharpless NS, Muenter MD, Tyce GM. Effect of L-DOPA on endogenous histamine metabolism. Med Biol. 1975;53:85–92.
535. Shan L, Swaab DF, Bao AM. Neuronal histaminergic system in aging and age-related neurodegenerative disorders. Exp Gerontol. 2013;48(7):603–7. doi:10.1016/j.exger.2012.08.002. Epub 2012 Aug 11
536. Ogasawara M, Yamauchi K, Satoh Y, Yamaji R, Inui K, Jonker JW, Schinkel AH, Maeyama K. Recent advances in molecular pharmacology of the histamine systems: organic cation transporters as a histamine transporter and histamine metabolism. J Pharmacol Sci. 2006;101(1):24–30. Epub 2006 Apr 28
537. Lenman JA, Turnbull MJ, Reid A, et al. Urinary monoamine metabolite excretion in disorders of movement. Effects of amantadine and levodopa. J Neurol Sci. 1977;32:219–25.
538. Ashida H, Ogawa M, Mimuro H, Kobayashi T, Sanada T, Sasakawa C. Shigella are versatile mucosal pathogens that circumvent the host innate immune system. Curr Opin Immunol. 2011;23(4):448–55. doi:10.1016/j.coi.2011.06.001. Epub 2011 Jul 15
539. West G. 5-Hydroxytryptamine, tissue mast cells and skin oedema. Int Arch Allergy Appl Immunol. 1957;10:257–75.
540. Phong B, Avery L, Menk AV, Delgoffe GM. Cutting Edge: Murine mast cells rapidly modulate metabolic pathways essential for distinct effector functions. J Immunol. 2016.; pii: 1601150. [Epub ahead of print]
541. Haas HL. Histamine hyperpolarizes hippocampal neurones in vitro. Neurosci Lett. 1981;22:75–8.
542. Ovary Z. Immediate hypersensitivity. A brief, personal history. Arerugi. 1994;43(12):1375–85.
543. Nish S, Medzhitov R. Host defense pathways: role of redundancy and compensation in infectious disease phenotypes. Immunity. 2011;34:629–36. doi:10.1016/j.immuni.2011.05.009.
544. Bax BE, Bloxam DL. Energy metabolism and glycolysis in human placental trophoblast cells during differentiation. Biochim Biophys Acta. 1997;1319:283–92.
545. Wu CC, Chen RF, Kuo HC. Different implications of paternal and maternal atopy for perinatal IgEproduction and asthma development. Clin Dev Immunol. 2012;2012:132–42. doi:10.1155/2012/132142. Epub 2012 Jan 9
546. Spann K, Snape N, Baturcam E, Fantino E. The impact of early-life exposure to air-borne environmental insults on the function of the airway epithelium in asthma. Ann Glob Health. 2016;82(1):28–40. doi:10.1016/j.aogh.2016.01.007.
547. Bisgaard H, Bonnelykke K, Stokholm J. Immune-mediated diseases and microbial exposure in early life. Clin Exp Allergy. 2014;44:475e81.
548. Carraro S, Scheltema N, Bont L, Baraldi E. Early-life origins of chronic respiratory diseases: understanding and promoting healthy ageing. Eur Respir J. 2014;44:1682e96.
549. Barger LW, Vollmer WM, Felt RW, Buist AS. Further investigation into the recent increase in asthma death rates: a review of 41 asthma deaths in Oregon in 1982. Ann Allergy. 1988;60(1):31–9.

550. Ettinger DS, Baylin SB, Minaberry D, Abeloff MD, Mellits ED. Response of plasma histaminase activity to heparin in normal subjects and in patients with small cell carcinoma of the lung. J Natl Cancer Inst. 1978;60:1239–42.
551. Baylin SB, Abeloff MD, Wieman KC, Tomford JW, Ettinger DS. Elevated histaminase (diaminase) activity in small-cell carcinoma of the lung. New Engl J Med. 1975;293:1286–90.
552. Massari NA, Medina VA, Martinel Lamas DJ, Cricco GP, Croci M, Sambuco L, Bergoc RM, Rivera ES. Role of H4 receptor in histamine-mediated responses in human melanoma. Melanoma Res. 2011;21:395–404.
553. Lecarpentier Y, Claes V, Vallée A, Hébert J-L. Interactions between PPAR Gamma and the Canonical Wnt/Beta-Catenin Pathway in Type 2 Diabetes and Colon Cancer. PPAR Res. 2017;2017:5879090. Published online 2017 Feb 19. doi: 10.1155/2017/5879090 PMCID: PMC5337359
554. Yin Y, Zhang W. The role of ghrelin in senescence: a mini-review. Gerontology. 2016;62(2):155–62. doi:10.1159/000433533. Epub 2015 Jul 7
555. Steinberg GR, Kemp BE. AMPK in health and disease. Physiol Rev. 2009;89:1025–78.
556. Majumder S, Caccamo A, Medina DX, Benavides AD, Javors MA, Kraig E, et al. Life-long rapamycin administration ameliorates age-dependent cognitive deficits by reducing IL-1β and NMDA signaling. Aging Cell. 2012; doi:10.1111/j.1474-9726.2011.00791.x.
557. Murphy MP. How mitochondria produce reactive oxygen species. Biochem J. 2009;417:1–13.
558. Salminen A, Ojala J, Kaarniranta K, Kauppinen A. Mitochondrial dysfunction and oxidative stress activate inflammasomes: impact on the aging process and age-related diseases. Cell Mol Life Sci. 2012;69:2999–3013.
559. Sánchez-Aragó M, Formentini L, Cuezva JM. Mitochondria-mediated energy adaption in cancer: the H(+)-ATP synthase-geared switch of metabolism in human tumors. Antioxid Redox Signal. 2013;19(3):285–98. doi:10.1089/ars.2012.4883. Epub 2012 Sep 24
560. Melser S, Lavie J, Bénard G. Mitochondrial degradation and energy metabolism. Biochim Biophys Acta. 2015;1853(10 Pt B):2812–21. doi:10.1016/j.bbamcr.2015.05.010. Epub 2015 May 12
561. Bender T, Martinou J-C. The mitochondrial pyruvate carrier in health and disease: to carry or not to carry? BBA - Molecular Cell Research. 2016; doi:10.1016/j.bbamcr.2016.01.017.
562. Xu XD, Shao SX, Jiang HP, Cao YW, Wang YH, Yang XC, Wang YL, Wang XS, Niu HT. Warburg effect or reverse Warburg effect? A review of cancer metabolism. Oncol Res Treat. 2015;38(3):117–22. doi:10.1159/000375435. Epub 2015 Feb 19
563. Berge K, Tronstad KJ, Bohov P, Madsen L, Berge RK. Impact of mitochondrial beta-oxidation in fatty acid-mediated inhibition of glioma cell proliferation. J Lipid Res. 2003;44:118–27.
564. Cairns RA, Harris IS, Mak TW. Regulation of cancer cell metabolism. Nat Rev Cancer. 2011;11:85–95.
565. Moreno-Sánchez R, Marín-Hernández A, Saavedra E, Pardo JP, Ralph SJ, Rodríguez-Enríquez S. Who controls the ATP supply in cancer cells? Biochemistry lessons to understand cancer energy metabolism. Int J Biochem Cell Biol. 2014;50:10–23. doi:10.1016/j.biocel.2014.01.025. Epub 2014 Feb 7
566. Boström M, Ninham BW. Energy of an ion crossing a low dielectric membrane: the role of dispersion self-free energy. Biophys Chem. 2005;114:95–101. Epub 2004 Dec 8
567. Tyagi S, Gupta P, Saini AS, Kaushal C, Sharma S. The peroxisome proliferator-activated receptor: a family of nuclear receptors role in various diseases. J Adv Pharm Technol Res. 2011;2:236–40.
568. Cantó C, Menzies KJ, Auwerx J. NAD(+) metabolism and the control of energy homeostasis: a balancing act between mitochondria and the nucleus. Cell Metab. 2015;22(1):31–53. doi:10.1016/j.cmet.2015.05.023. Epub 2015 Jun 25
569. Halliwill JR, Sieck DC, Romero SA, Buck TM, Ely MR. Blood pressure regulation X: what happens when the muscle pump is lost? Post-exercise hypotension and syncope. Eur J Appl Physiol. 2014;114(3):561–78. doi:10.1007/s00421-013-2761-1. Epub 2013 Nov 7

570. Wallace DC. The mitochondrial genome in human adaptive radiation and disease: on the road to therapeutics and performance enhancement. Gene. 2005;354:169–80.
571. Wallace DC. Mitochondrial DNA mutations in disease and aging. Environ Mol Mutagen. 2010;51(5):440–50. doi:10.1002/em.20586.
572. Wallace DC, Fan W. Energetics, epigenetics, mitochondrial genetics. Mitochondrion. 2010;10(1):12–31. doi:10.1016/j.mito.2009.09.006. Epub 2009 Sep 29
573. Bost F, Decoux-Poullot AG, Tanti JF, Clavel S. Energy disruptors: rising stars in anticancer therapy? Oncogenesis. 2016;18(5):e188. doi:10.1038/oncsis.2015.46.
574. Ubah OC, Wallace HM. Cancer therapy: targeting mitochondria and other sub-cellular organelles. Curr Pharm Des. 2014;20(2):201–22.
575. Ying W. NAD+ and NADH in cellular functions and cell death. Front Biosci. 2006;11:3129–48.
576. Quintana A, Hoth M. Mitochondrial dynamics and their impact on T cell function. Cell Calcium. 2012;52(1):57–63. doi:10.1016/j.ceca.2012.02.005. Epub 2012 Mar 14
577. Hernández-Pedro N, Magana-Maldonado R, Ramiro AS, Pérez-De la Cruz V, et al. PAMP-DAMPs interactions mediates development and progression of multiple sclerosis. Front Biosci (Schol Ed). 2016;8:13–28.
578. Salminen A, Haapasalo A, Kauppinen A, Kaarniranta K, Soininen H, Hiltunen M. Impaired mitochondrial energy metabolism in Alzheimer's disease: impact on pathogenesis via disturbed epigenetic regulation ofchromatin landscape. Prog Neurobiol. 2015;131:1–20. doi:10.1016/j.pneurobio.2015.05.001. Epub 2015 May 19
579. Hargreaves DC, Crabtree GR. ATP-dependent chromatin remodeling: genetics, genomics and mechanisms. Cell Res. 2011;21(3):396–420. doi:10.1038/cr.2011.32. Epub 2011 Mar 1
580. Hirschberg CB, Robbins PW, Abeijon C. Transporters of nucleotide sugars, ATP, and nucleotide sulfate in the endoplasmic reticulum and Golgi apparatus. Annu Rev Biochem. 1998;67:49–69.
581. Haferkamp I, Fernie AR, Neuhaus HE. Adenine nucleotide transport in plants: much more than a mitochondrial issue. Trends Plant Sci. 2011;16(9):507–15. doi:10.1016/j.tplants.2011.04.001. Epub 2011 May 31
582. Kamata H, Honda S, Maeda S, Chang L, Hirata H, Karin M. Reactive oxygen species promote TNFalpha-induced death and sustained JNK activation by inhibiting MAP kinase phosphatases. Cell. 2005;120:649–61.
583. Palmer TN, Caldecourt MA, Snell K, Sugden MC. Alanine and inter-organ relationships in branched-chain amino and 2-oxo acid metabolism. Rev Biosci Rep. 1985;5(12):1015–33.
584. Neis EP, Dejong CH, Rensen SS. The role of microbial amino acid metabolism in host metabolism. Forum Nutr. 2015;7(4):2930–46. doi:10.3390/nu7042930.
585. Pedroso JA, Zampieri TT, Donato J Jr. Reviewing the effects of L-leucine supplementation in the regulation of food intake, energy balance, and glucose homeostasis. Forum Nutr. 2015;7(5):3914–37. doi:10.3390/nu7053914.
586. Cunningham JT, Rodgers JT, Arlow DH, Vazquez F, Mootha VK, Puigserver P. mTOR controls mitochondrial oxidative function through a YY1-PGC-1alpha transcriptional complex. Nature. 2007;450:736–40. doi:10.1038/nature06322.
587. Ohsumi Y. Historical landmarks of autophagy research. Cell Res. 2014;24:9–23.
588. Herwald H. · Egesten a: intracellular clearance by Nobel laureates. J Innate Immun. 2017;9:1–2. doi:10.1159/000453127.
589. Varki A. Evolutionary forces shaping the Golgi glycosylation machinery: why cell surface glycans are universal to living cells. Cold Spring Harb Perspect Biol. 2011;3(6):pii: a005462. doi:10.1101/cshperspect.a005462.
590. Podwyssotzki W. Autolysis and autophagism in endotheliomae and sarcomae, as a basis principle for the elaboration of a method of healing unoperated tumors. Beitr Pathol Anat. 1905;38:449–55.
591. Takeshige K, Baba M, Tsuboi S, Noda T, Ohsumi Y. Autophagy in yeast demonstrated with proteinase-deficient mutants and conditions for its induction. J Cell Biol. 1992;119:301–11.

592. Madeo F, Tavernarakis N, Kroemer G. Can autophagy promote longevity? Nat Cell Biol. 2010;9:842–6.
593. Wang Y, Martins I, Ma Y, Kepp O, Galluzzi L, Kroemer G. Autophagy-dependent ATP release from dying cells via lysosomal exocytosis. Autophagy. 2013;9(10):1624–5. doi:10.4161/auto.25873. Epub 2013 Aug 13
594. Kroemer G, Galluzzi L, Kepp O, Zitvogel L. Immunogenic cell death in cancer therapy. Annu Rev Immunol. 2013;31:51–72.
595. Martins I, Wang Y, Michaud M, Ma Y, Sukkurwala AQ, Shen S, Kepp O, Métivier D, et al. Molecular mechanisms of ATP secretion during immunogenic cell death. Cell Death Differ. 2014;21(1):79–91. doi:10.1038/cdd.2013.75. Epub 2013 Jul 12
596. Criollo A, Senovilla L, Authier H, Maiuri MC, Morselli E, Vitale I, Kepp O, Tasdemir E, Galluzzi L, et al. IKK connects autophagy to major stress pathways. Autophagy. 2010;6(1):189–91.
597. Dice JF. Chaperone-mediated autophagy. Autophagy. 2007;3:295–9.
598. Gomez-Cambronero J, Kantonen S. A river runs through it: how autophagy, senescence, and phagocytosis could be linked to phospholipase D by Wnt signaling. J Leukoc Biol. 2014;96(5):779–84. doi:10.1189/jlb.2VMR0214-120RR. Epub 2014 Jul 31
599. Deretic V. Autophagy as an innate immunity paradigm: expanding the scope and repertoire of pattern recognition receptors. Curr Opin Immunol. 2012;24:21–31.
600. Nixon RA. The role of autophagy in neurodegenerative disease. Nat Med. 2013;19:983–97.
601. Stranks AJ, Hansen AL, Panse I, Mortensen M, Ferguson DJ, Puleston DJ, Shenderov K, Watson AS, Veldhoen M, Phadwal K, Cerundolo V, Simon AK. Autophagy controls acquisition of aging features in macrophages. J Innate Immun. 2015;7:375–91. doi:10.1159/000370112.
602. Khan N, Pahari S, Vidyarthi A, Aqdas M, Agrewala JN. NOD-2 and TLR-4 signaling reinforces the efficacy of dendritic cells and reduces the dose of TB drugs against*Mycobacterium tuberculosis*. J Innate Immun. 2016;8:228–42.
603. Cardone RA, Casavola V, Reshkin SJ. The role of disturbed pH dynamics and the Na+/H+ exchanger in metastasis. Nat Rev Cancer. 2005;5:786–95.
604. Mortensen M, Soilleux EJ, Djordjevic G, Tripp R, Lutteropp M, Sadighi-Akha E, Stranks AJ, Glanville J, Knight S, Jacobson SE, Kranc KR, Simon AK. The autophagy protein Atg7 is essential for hematopoietic stem cell maintenance. J Exp Med. 2011;208:455–67.
605. Dengjel J, Schoor O, Fischer R, Reich M, Kraus M, Muller M, Kreymborg K, Altenberend F, Brandenburg J, Kalbacher H, Brock R, Driessen C, Rammensee HG, Stevanovic S. Autophagy promotes MHC class II presentation of peptides from intracellular source proteins. Proc Natl Acad Sci U S A. 2005;102:7922–7.
606. Bonilla DL, Bhattacharya A, Sha Y, Xu Y, Xiang Q, Kan A, Jagannath C, Komatsu M, Eissa NT. Autophagy regulates phagocytosis by modulating the expression of scavenger receptors. Immunity. 2013;39:537–47.
607. Gill R, Tsung A, Billiar T. Linking oxidative stress to inflammation: toll-like receptors. Free Radic Biol Med. 2010;48:1121–32.
608. Pearce EL, Pearce EJ. Metabolic pathways in immune cell activation and quiescence. Immunity. 2013;38:633–43.
609. Pearce FL. Effect of nedocromil sodium on mediator release from mast cells. J Allergy Clin Immunol. 1993;92(1 Pt 2):155–8.
610. Desman G, Waintraub C, Zippin JH. Investigation of cAMP microdomains as a path to novel cancerdiagnostics. Biochim Biophys Acta. 2014;1842(12 Pt B):2636–45. doi:10.1016/j.bbadis.2014.08.016. Epub 2014 Sep 7
611. Lecarpentier Y, Claes V, Vallée A, Hébert JL. Thermodynamics in cancers: opposing interactions between PPAR gamma and the canonical WNT/beta-catenin pathway. Clin Transl Med. 2017;6(1):14. https://doi.org/10.1186/s40169-017-0144-7. Epub 2017 Apr 12
612. Almahariq M, Mei FC, Cheng X. The pleiotropic role of exchange protein directly activated by cAMP 1 (EPAC1) in cancer: implications for therapeutic intervention. Acta Biochim Biophys Sin Shanghai. 2016;48(1):75–81. doi:10.1093/abbs/gmv115. Epub 2015 Nov 2

613. Stagg J, Smyth MJ. Extracellular adenosine triphosphate and adenosine in cancer. Oncogene. 2010;29(39):5346–58. doi:10.1038/onc.2010.292. Epub 2010 Jul 26
614. Repovic P, Mi K, Benveniste EN. Oncostatin M enhances the expression of prostaglandin E2 and cyclooxygenase-2 in astrocytes: synergy with interleukin-1beta, tumor necrosis factor-alpha, and bacterial lipopolysaccharide. Glia. 2003;42:433–46.
615. Suzuki Y, Yoshimaru T, Inoue T, Niide O, Ra C. Role of oxidants in mast cell activation. Chem Immunol Allergy. 2005;87:32–42.
616. Fischer M, Ehlers M. Toll-like receptors in autoimmunity. Ann N Y Acad Sci. 2008;1143:21–34. doi:10.1196/annals.1443.012.
617. Santoni G, Cardinali C, Morelli MB, Santoni M, Nabissi M, Amantini C. Danger- and pathogen-associated molecular patterns recognition bypattern-recognition receptors and ion channels of the transient receptor potential family triggers the inflammasome activation in immune cells and sensory neurons. J Neuroinflammation. 2015;12:21. doi:10.1186/s12974-015-0239-2.
618. Fukata M, Vamadevan AS, Abreu MT. Toll-like receptors(TLRs) and nod-like receptors (NLRs) in inflammatory disorders. Semin Immunol. 2009;21:242–53.
619. Verma PK, Bala M, Kumar N, Singh B. Therapeutic potential of natural products from terrestrial plants as TNF-α antagonist. Curr Top Med Chem. 2012;12(13):1422–35.
620. Hebert DN, Molinari M. In and out of the ER: protein folding, quality control, degradation, and related human diseases. Physiol Rev. 2007;87:1377–408.
621. Mingeot-Leclercq MP, Piret J, Tulkens PM, Brasseur R. Effect of acidic phospholipids on the activity of lysosomal phospholipases and on their inhibition induced by aminoglycoside antibiotics–II. Conformational analysis. Biochem Pharmacol. 1990; 40:499–506.
622. Lowry MC, Gallagher WM, O'Driscoll L. The role of exosomes in breast cancer. Clin Chem. 2015;61(12):1457–65. doi:10.1373/clinchem.2015.240028. Epub 2015 Oct 14
623. Thery C, Duban L, Segura E, Veron P, Lantz O, Amigorena S. Indirect activation of naive CD4+ T cells by dendritic cell-derived exosomes. Nat Immunol. 2002;3:1156–62.
624. Pohl S, Marschner K, Storch S, Braulke T. Glycosylation- and phosphorylation-dependent intracellular transport of lysosomal hydrolases. Biol Chem. 2009;390(7):521–7. doi:10.1515/BC.2009.076.
625. Parenti G, Pignata C, Vajro P, Salerno M. New strategies for the treatment of lysosomal storage diseases (review). Int J Mol Med. 2013;31:11–20. doi:10.3892/ijmm.2012.1187. Epub 2012 Nov 19
626. Coutinho MF, Prata MJ, Alves S. Mannose-6-phosphate pathway: a review on its role in lysosomalfunction and dysfunction. Mol Genet Metab. 2012;105(4):542–50. doi:10.1016/j.ymgme.2011.12.012. Epub 2011 Dec 23
627. Martina JA, Diab HI, Li H, Puertollano R. Novel roles for the MiTF/TFE family of transcription factors in organelle biogenesis, nutrient sensing, and energy homeostasis. Cell Mol Life Sci. 2014;71(13):2483–97. doi:10.1007/s00018-014-1565-8. Epub 2014 Jan 30
628. Johansen T. Energy metabolism in rat mast cells in relation to histamine secretion. Pharmacol Toxicol. 1987;61(Suppl 2):1–20.
629. Pearce FL. Non-IgE-mediated mast cell stimulation. Ciba Found Symp. 1989;147:74–87.
630. Phong B, Avery L, Menk AV, Delgoffe GM, Kane LP. Cutting edge: murine mast cells rapidly modulate metabolic pathways essential for distinct effector functions. J Immunol. 2017;198(2):640–4. doi:10.4049/jimmunol.1601150. Epub 2016 Dec 14
631. Mierke CT. The fundamental role of mechanical properties in the progression ofcancer disease and inflammation. Rep Prog Phys. 2014;77(7):076602. doi:10.1088/0034-4885/77/7/076602. Epub 2014 Jul 9
632. Mierke CT. Physical view on migration modes. Cell Adhes Migr. 2015;9(5):367–79. doi:10.1080/19336918.2015.1066958.
633. Mierke CT, Rösel D, Fabry B, Brábek J. Contractile forces in tumor cell migration. Eur J Cell Biol. 2008;87(8–9):669–76. doi:10.1016/j.ejcb.2008.01.002. Epub 2008 Mar 4

634. Friedl P, Brocker EB. The biology of cell locomotion within three-dimensional extracellular matrix. Cell Mol Life Sci. 2000;57:41–64.
635. Ishizaki T, Maekawa M, Fujisawa K, Okawa K, Iwamatsu A, Fujita A, Watanabe N, Saito Y, Kakizuka A, Morii N, Narumiya S. The small GTP-binding protein Rho binds to and activates a 160 kDa Ser/Thr protein kinase homologous to myotonic dystrophy kinase. EMBO J. 1996;15:1885–93.
636. Leanza L, Biasutto L, Managò A, Gulbins E, Zoratti M, Szabò I. Intracellular ion channels and cancer. Front Physiol. 2013;4:227. doi:10.3389/fphys.2013.00227.
637. Du Clos TW, Mold C. The role of C-reactive protein in the resolution of bacterial infection. Curr Opin Infect Dis. 2001;14:289–93. doi:10.1097/00001432-200106000-00007.
638. Mold C, Du Clos TW. C-reactive protein increases cytokine responses to Streptococcus Pneumoniae through interactions with Fc gamma receptors. J Immunol. 2006;176:7598–604. doi:10.4049/jimmunol.176.12.7598.
639. Bonner F, Borg N, Jacoby C, Temme S, Ding Z, Flogel U, et al. Ecto-5′-nucleotidase on immune cells protects from adverse cardiac remodeling. Circ Res. 2013;113(3):301–12. doi:10.1161/CIRCRESAHA.113.300180.
640. Zhao HF, Wang J, Tony To SS. The phosphatidylinositol 3-kinase/Akt and c-Jun N-terminal kinasesignaling in cancer: alliance or contradiction? (Review). Int J Oncol. 2015;47(2):429–36. doi:10.3892/ijo.2015.3052. Epub 2015 Jun 16
641. Cuadrado A, Nebreda AR. Mechanisms and functions of p38 MAPK signalling. Biochem J. 2010;429(3):403–17. doi:10.1042/BJ20100323.
642. Yong HY, Koh MS, Moon A. The p38 MAPK inhibitors for the treatment of inflammatory diseases and cancer. Expert Opin Investig Drugs. 2009;18(12):1893–905. doi:10.1517/13543780903321490.
643. Lei YY, Wang WJ, Mei JH, Wang CL. Mitogen-activated protein kinase signal transduction in solid tumors. Asian Pac J Cancer Prev. 2014;15(20):8539–48.
644. Hodgkinson CA, Moore KJ, Nakayama A, Steingrimsson E, Copeland NG, Jenkins NA, Arnheiter H. Mutations at the mouse microphthalmia locus are associated with defects in a gene encoding a novel basic-helix-loop-helix-zipper protein. Cell. 1993;74(2):395–404.
645. Kuna P, Kaplan AP. Relationship of histamine-releasing factors and histamine-releasing inhibitory factors to chemokine group of cytokine. Allergy Asthma Proc. 1996;17(1):5–11.
646. Lin L, Saha PK, Ma X, Henshaw IO, Shao L, Chang BH, Buras ED, Tong Q, et al. Ablation of ghrelin receptor reduces adiposity and improves insulin sensitivity during aging by regulating fat metabolism in white and brown adipose tissues. Aging Cell. 2011;10(6):996–1010. doi:10.1111/j.1474-9726.2011.00740.x. Epub 2011 Oct 12
647. Wang Y, Zheng QC, Kong CP, Tian Y, Zhan J, Zhang JL, Zhang HX. Heparin makes differences: a molecular dynamics simulation study on the human βII-tryptase monomer. Mol BioSyst. 2015;11(1):252–61. doi:10.1039/c4mb00381k. Epub 2014 Nov 4
648. Anower-E-Khuda MF, Habuchi H, Nagai N, Habuchi O, Yokochi T, Kimata K. Heparan sulfate 6-O-sulfotransferase isoform-dependent regulatory effects of heparin on the activities of various proteases in mast cells and the biosynthesis of 6-O-sulfated heparin. J Biol Chem. 2013;288(6):3705–17. doi:10.1074/jbc.M112.416651. Epub 2012 Dec 6
649. Motiani RK, Stolwijk JA, Newton RL, Zhang X, Trebak M. Emerging roles of Orai3 in pathophysiology. Channels (Austin). 2013;7(5):392–401. doi:10.4161/chan.24960. Epub 2013 May 21
650. Khorana AA. Cancer and coagulation. Am J Hematol. 2012;87(Suppl 1):S82–7. doi:10.1002/ajh.23143. Epub 2012 Mar 3
651. Sato A, Oe K, Yamanaka H, Yokoyama I, Ebina K. C-reactive protein specifically enhances platelet-activating factor-induced inflammatory activity in vivo. Eur J Pharmacol. 2014;745:46–51. doi:10.1016/j.ejphar.2014.10.020. Epub 2014 Oct 22
652. Chen C, Han X, Fan F, Liu Y, Wang T, Wang J, Hu P, Ma A, Tian H. Serotonin drives the activation of pulmonary artery adventitial fibroblasts and TGF-β1/Smad3-mediated fibrotic

responses through 5-HT(2A) receptors. Mol Cell Biochem. 2014;397(1–2):267–76. doi:10.1007/s11010-014-2194-0. Epub 2014 Sep 4
653. Kaplan AP. Bradykinin-mediated diseases. Chem Immunol Allergy. 2014;100:140–7. doi:10.1159/000358619. Epub 2014 May 22
654. Bijanzadeh M, Ramachandra NB, Mahesh PA, Savitha MR, Vijayakumar GS, Kumar P, et al. Soluble intercellular adhesion molecule-1 and E-selectin in patients with asthma exacerbation. Lung. 2009;187:315–20.
655. Lamkanfi M, Dixit VM. Inflammasomes and their roles in health and disease. Annu Rev Cell Dev Biol. 2012;28:137–61.
656. Takeuchi O, Akira S. Pattern recognition receptors and inflammation. Cell. 2010;140:805–20.
657. Salminen A, Kaarniranta K, Kauppinen A. Inflammaging: disturbed interplay between autophagy and inflammasomes. Aging (Albany NY). 2012;4(3):166–75.
658. Dvorak A, Seder R, Paul W, Morgan E, Galli S. Effects of interleukin-3 with or without the c-kit ligand, stem cell factor, on the survival and cytoplasmic granule formation of mouse basophils and mast cells in vitro. Am J Pathol. 1994;11:160–70.
659. Blasius AL, Beutler B. Intracellular toll-like receptors. Immunity. 2010;32:305–15.
660. Weng PH, Huang YL, Page JH, Chen JH, Xu J, Koutros S, Berndt S, Chanock S, et al. Polymorphisms of an innate immune gene, toll-like receptor 4, and aggressive prostate cancer risk: a systematic review and meta-analysis. PLoS One. 2014;9(10):e110569. doi:10.1371/journal.pone.0110569. eCollection 2014
661. Yeaman MR. Platelets: at the nexus of antimicrobial defence. Nat Rev Microbiol. 2014;12:426–37.
662. Schattner M. Platelets and galectins. Ann Transl Med. 2014;2(9):85. doi:10.3978/j.issn.2305-5839.2014.09.02.
663. Ware J, Corken A, Khetpal R. Platelet function beyond hemostasis and thrombosis. Curr Opin Hematol. 2013;20:451–6.
664. Rivera J, Lozano ML, Navarro-Núñez L, et al. Platelet receptors and signaling in the dynamics of thrombus formation. Haematologica. 2009;94:700–11.
665. Romaniuk MA, Croci DO, Lapponi MJ, et al. Binding of galectin-1 to $\alpha_{IIb}\beta_3$integrin triggers "outside-in" signals, stimulates platelet activation, and controls primary hemostasis. FASEB J. 2012;26:2788–98.
666. Etulain J, Negrotto S, Tribulatti MV, et al. Control of angiogenesis by galectins involves the release of platelet-derived proangiogenic factors. PLoS One. 2014;9:e96402.
667. Thijssen VL, Hulsmans S, Griffioen AW. The galectin profile of the endothelium: altered expression and localization in activated and tumor endothelial cells. Am J Pathol. 2008;172:545–53.
668. Bonner F, Borg N, Burghoff S, Schrader J. Resident cardiac immune cells and expression of the ectonucleotidase enzymes CD39 and CD73 after ischemic injury. PLoS One. 2012;7(4):e34730. doi:10.1371/journal.pone.0034730.
669. Kitamura Y, Oboki K, Ito A. Molecular mechanisms of mast cell development. Immunol Allergy Clin N Am. 2006;26(3):387–405.
670. Sharma AK, Laubach VE, Ramos SI, Zhao Y, Stukenborg G, Linden J, et al. Adenosine A2A receptor activation on CD4+ T lymphocytes and neutrophils attenuates lung ischemia-reperfusion injury. J Thorac Cardiovasc Surg. 2010;139(2):474–82. doi:10.1016/j.jtcvs.2009.08.033.
671. Tsokos GC. Systemic lupus erythematosus. N Engl J Med. 2011;365:2110–21. doi:10.1056/NEJMra1100359.
672. Choy E. Understanding the dynamics: pathways involved in the pathogenesis of rheumatoid arthritis. Rheumatology (Oxford). 2012;51(Suppl 5):v3–11. doi:10.1093/rheumatology/kes113.
673. Emaminia A, Lapar DJ, Zhao Y, Steidle JF, Harris DA, Laubach VE, et al. Adenosine A(2)A agonist improves lung function during ex vivo lung perfusion. Ann Thorac Surg. 2011;92(5):1840–6. doi:10.1016/j.athoracsur.2011.06.062.

674. Zhao Y, LaPar DJ, Steidle J, Emaminia A, Kron IL, Ailawadi G, et al. Adenosine signaling via the adenosine 2B receptor is involved in bronchiolitis obliterans development. J Heart Lung Transplant. 2010; 29(12):1405–1414 10.1016/j.healun.2010.07.005
675. Pommey S, Lu B, McRae J, Stagg J, Hill P, Salvaris E, et al. Liver grafts from CD39-overexpressing mice are protected from ischemia reperfusion injury due to reduced numbers of resident CD4(+) T cells. Hepatology. 2013;57(4):1597–606. doi:10.1002/hep.25985.
676. Pear WS, Tu L, Stein PL. Lineage choices in the developing thymus: choosing the T and NKT pathways. Curr Opin Immunol. 2004;16(2):167–73.
677. Gerhardt DM, Pajcini KV, D'altri T, Tu L, Jain R, Xu L, Chen MJ, Rentschler S, Shestova O, Wertheim GB, et al. The Notch1 transcriptional activation domain is required for development and reveals a novel role for Notch1 signaling in fetal hematopoietic stem cells. Genes Dev. 2014;28(6):576–93. doi:10.1101/gad.227496.113.
678. Huang EY, Gallegos AM, Richards SM, Lehar SM, Bevan MJ. Surface expression of Notch1 on thymocytes: correlation with the double-negative to double-positive transition. J Immunol. 2003;171:2296–304.
679. Tu L, Fang TC, Artis D, Shestova O, Pross SE, Maillard I, Pear WS. Notch signaling is an important regulator of type 2 immunity. J Exp Med. 2005;202(8):1037–42.
680. Weng AP, Aster JC. Multiple niches for notch in cancer: context is everything. Curr Opin Genet Dev. 2004;14:48–54.
681. McKinney-Freeman S, Cahan P, Li H, Lacadie SA, Huang HT, Curran M, Loewer S, Naveiras O, Kathrein KL, Konantz M, et al. The transcriptional landscape of hematopoietic stem cell ontogeny. Cell Stem Cell. 2012;11:701–14.
682. Palaga T. MieleL, Golde TE, OsborneBA: TCR-mediated notch signaling regulates proliferation and IFN-gamma production in peripheral T cells. J Immunol. 2003;171:3019–24.
683. Singh AK, Stock P, Akbari O. Role of PD-L1 and PD-L2 in allergic diseases and asthma. Allergy. 2011;66(2):155–62. doi:10.1111/j.1398-9995.2010.02458.x. Epub 2010 Aug 17
684. Hirotsu Y, Hirashima M, Hayashi H. The mediation of tissue eosinophilia in hypersensitivityreactions. III. Separation of two different delayed eosinophil chemotactic factors and transfer of these factors by serum or cells from sensitized guinea-pigs. Immunology. 1983;48(1):59–67.
685. Arneth B. Early activation of CD4+ and CD8+ T lymphocytes by myelin basic protein in subjects with MS. J Transl Med. 2015;13:341. doi:10.1186/s12967-015-0715-6.
686. Codoñer-Franch P, Alonso-Iglesias E. Resistin: insulin resistance to malignancy. Clin Chim Acta. 2015;438:46–54. doi:10.1016/j.cca.2014.07.043. Epub 2014 Aug 13
687. Dawson H, Serra S. Tumours and inflammatory lesions of the anal canal and perianal skin revisited: an update and practical approach. J Clin Pathol. 2015;68(12):971–81. doi:10.1136/jclinpath-2015-203056.
688. Hu W, Bassig BA, Xu J, Zheng T, Zhang Y, Berndt SI, Holford TR, Hosgood HD 3rd, et al. Polymorphisms in pattern-recognition genes in the innateimmunity system and risk of non-Hodgkin lymphoma. Environ Mol Mutagen. 2013;54(1):72–7. doi:10.1002/em.21739. Epub 2012 Oct 11
689. Plato A, Hardison SE, Brown GD. Pattern recognition receptors in antifungal immunity. Semin Immunopathol. 2015;37(2):97–106. doi:10.1007/s00281-014-0462-4. Epub 2014 Nov 25
690. Pradere JP, Dapito DH, Schwabe RF. The yin and Yang of toll-like receptors in cancer. Oncogene. 2014;33(27):3485–95. doi:10.1038/onc.2013.302. Epub 2013 Aug 12
691. Rakoff-Nahoum S, Foster KR, Comstock LE. The evolution of cooperation within the gut microbiota. Nature. 2016;533(7602):255–9. doi:10.1038/nature17626. Epub 2016 Apr 25
692. Kigerl KA, de Rivero Vaccari JP, Dietrich WD, Popovich PG, Keane RW. Pattern recognition receptors and central nervous system repair. Exp Neurol. 2014;258:5–16. doi:10.1016/j.expneurol.2014.01.001.
693. Rakoff-Nahoum S, Coyne MJ, Comstock LE. An ecological network of polysaccharide utilization among human intestinal symbionts. Curr Biol. 2014;24:40–9.

694. Steingrimsson E, Tessarollo L, Reid SW, Jenkins NA, Copeland NG. The bHLH-zip transcription factor Tfeb is essential for placental vascularization. Development. 1998;125(23):4607–16.
695. Hubbard LL, Ballinger MN, Thomas PE, et al. A role for IL-1 receptor-associated kinase-M in prostaglandin E(2)-induced immunosuppression post-bone marrow transplantation. J Immunol. 2010;184:6299–308.
696. Wang J, Hu Y, Deng WW, Sun B. Negative regulation of toll-like receptor signaling pathway. Microbes Infect. 2009;11:321–7.
697. Chuang TH, Ulevitch RJ. Triad3A, an E3 ubiquitin-protein ligase regulating toll like receptors. Nat Immunol. 2004;5:495–502.
698. Mathar I, Jacobs G, Kecskes M, Menigoz A, Philippaert K, Vennekens R. TRPM4. Handb Exp Pharmacol. 2014;222:461–87. doi:10.1007/978-3-642-54215-2_18.
699. Hájková Z, Bugajev V, Dráberová E, Vinopal S, Dráberová L, Janáček J, Dráber P, Dráber P. STIM1-directed reorganization of microtubules in activated mast cells. J Immunol. 2011;186(2):913–23. doi:10.4049/jimmunol.1002074. Epub 2010 Dec 15
700. Holowka D, Baird B. Nanodomains in early and later phases of FcεRI signalling. Essays Biochem. 2015;57:147–63. doi:10.1042/bse0570147.
701. Ashmole I, Duffy SM, Leyland ML, Bradding P. The contribution of Orai(CRACM)1 and Orai(CRACM)2 channels in store-operated Ca2+ entry and mediator release in human lung mast cells. PLoS One. 2013;8(9):e74895. doi:10.1371/journal.pone.0074895. eCollection 2013
702. Buttmann M, Kaveri S, Hartung HP. Polyclonal immunoglobulin G for autoimmune demyelinating nervoussystem disorders. Trends Pharmacol Sci. 2013;34(8):445–57. doi:10.1016/j.tips.2013.05.009. Epub 2013 Jun 21
703. Small AG, Al-Baghdadi M, Quach A, Hii C, Ferrante A. Complement receptor immunoglobulin: a control point in infection and immunity, inflammation and cancer. Swiss Med Wkly. 2016;146:w14301. doi:10.4414/smw.2016.14301. eCollection 2016
704. Jackson DA, Elsawa SF. Factors regulating immunoglobulin production by normal and disease-associated plasma cells. Biomol Ther. 2015;5(1):20–40. doi:10.3390/biom5010020.
705. Aroca R, Chamorro C, Vega A, Ventura I, Gómez E, Pérez-Cano R, Blanca M, Monteseirín J. Immunotherapy reduces allergen-mediated CD66b expression and myeloperoxidase levels on human neutrophils from allergic patients. PLoS One. 2014;9(4):e94558. doi:10.1371/journal.pone.0094558. eCollection 2014
706. Mantelli F, Argüeso P. Functions of ocular surface mucins in health and disease. Curr Opin Allergy Clin Immunol. 2008;8(5):477–83. doi:10.1097/ACI.0b013e32830e6b04.
707. Haworth KB, Leddon JL, Chen CY, Horwitz EM, Mackall CL, Cripe TP. Going back to class I: MHC and immunotherapies for childhood cancer. Pediatr Blood Cancer. 2015;62(4):571–6. doi:10.1002/pbc.25359. Epub 2014 Dec 18
708. Yang B, Jeang J, Yang A, Wu TC, Hung CF. DNA vaccine for cancer immunotherapy. Hum Vaccin Immunother. 2014;10(11):3153–64. doi:10.4161/21645515.2014.980686.
709. Nauts HC, Fowler GA, Bogatko FH. A review of the influence of bacterial infection and of bacterial products (Coley's toxins) on malignant tumors in man; a critical analysis of 30 inoperable cases treated by Coley's mixed toxins, in which diagnosis was confirmed by microscopic examination selected for special study. Acta Med Scand Suppl. 1953;276:1–103.
710. Gallegos AM, Bevan MJ. Central tolerance: good but imperfect. Immunol Rev. 2006;209:290–6.
711. Stone JD, Harris DT, Kranz DM. TCR affinity for p/MHC formed by tumor antigens that are self-proteins: impact on efficacy and toxicity. Curr Opin Immunol. 2015;33:16–22. doi:10.1016/j.coi.2015.01.003. Epub 2015 Jan 22
712. Kim HG, Kim NR, Gim MG, et al. Lipoteichoic acid isolated from lactobacillus plantarum inhibits lipopoly-saccharide-induced TNF-alpha production in THP-1 cells and endotoxin shock in mice. J Immunol. 2008;180:2553–61.

713. del Fresno C, Gomez-Garcia L, Caveda L, et al. Nitric oxide activates the expression of IRAK-M via the release of TNF-alpha in human monocytes. Nitric Oxide. 2004;10:213–20.
714. Gonzalez-Leon MC, Soares-Schanoski A, del Fresno C, et al. Nitric oxide induces SOCS-1 expression in human monocytes in a TNF-alpha-dependent manner. J Endotoxin Res. 2006;12:296–306.
715. Nigou J, Zelle-Rieser C, Gilleron M, et al. Mannosylated lipoarabinomannans inhibit IL-12 production by human dendritic cells: evidence for a negative signal delivered through the mannose receptor. J Immunol. 2001;166:7477–85.
716. Mages J, Dietrich H, Lang R. A genomewide analysis of LPS tolerance in macrophages. Immunobiology. 2007;212:723–37.
717. Kim YI, Park JE, Martinez-Hernandez A, Yi AK. CpG DNA prevents liver injury and shock-mediated death by modulating expression of interleukin-1 receptor-associated kinases. J Biol Chem. 2008;283:15258–70.
718. Du Y, Topp CN, Dawe RK. DNA binding of centromere protein C (CENPC) is stabilized by single-stranded RNA. PLoS Genet. 2010;6:e1000835. doi:10.1371/journal.pgen.1000835.
719. Takebayashi K, Hokari R, Kurihara C, et al. Oral tolerance induced by enterobacteria altered the process of lymphocyte recruitment to intestinal microvessels: roles of endothelial cell adhesion molecules, TGFbeta and negative regulators of TLR signaling. Microcirculation. 2009;16:251–64.
720. Fukao T, Koyasu S. PI3K and negative regulation of TLR signaling. Trends Immunol. 2003;24:358–63.
721. Hassan F, Islam S, Tumurkhuu G, et al. Involvement of interleukin-1 receptor-associated kinase (IRAK)-M in toll-like receptor (TLR) 7-mediated tolerance in RAW 264.7 macrophage-like cells. Cell Immunol. 2009;256:99–103.
722. Weersma RK, Oostenbrug LE, Nolte IM, et al. Association of interleukin-1 receptor-associated kinase M (IRAK-M) and inflammatory bowel diseases. Scand J Gastroenterol. 2007;42:827–33.
723. Janssens S, Beyaert R. Functional diversity and regulation of different interleukin-1 receptor-associated kinase (IRAK) family members. Mol Cell. 2003;11:293–302.
724. Kobayashi K, Hernandez LD, Galan JE, et al. IRAK-M is a negative regulator of Tolllike receptor signaling. Cell. 2002;110:191–202.
725. Lagler H, Sharif O, Haslinger I, et al. TREM-1 activation alters the dynamics of pulmonary IRAK-M expression in vivo and improves host defense during pneumococcal pneumonia. J Immunol. 2009;183:2027–36.
726. Seki M, Kohno S, Newstead MW, et al. Critical role of IL-1 receptor-associated kinase-M in regulating chemokinedependent deleterious inflammation in murine influenza pneumonia. J Immunol. 2010;184:1410–318.
727. Hayashi T, Gray CS, Chan M, et al. Prevention of autoimmune disease by induction of tolerance to toll-like receptor 7. Proc Natl Acad Sci U S A. 2009;106:2764–9.
728. Tazi KA, Quioc JJ, Saada V, et al. Upregulation of TNF-alpha production signaling pathways in monocytes from patients with advanced cirrhosis: possible role of Akt and IRAK-M. J Hepatol. 2006;45:280–9.
729. del Fresno C, Otero K, Gomez-Garcia L, et al. Tumor cells deactivate human monocytes by up-regulating IL-1 receptor associated kinase-M expression via CD44 and TLR4. J Immunol. 2005;174:3032–40.
730. Black AP, Ogg GS. The role of p53 in the immunobiology of cutaneous squamous cell carcinoma. Clin Exp Immunol. 2003;132:379–84.
731. Su J, Xie Q, Wilson I, Li L. Differential regulation and role of interleukin-1 receptor associated kinase-M in innate immunity signaling. Cell Signal. 2007;19:1596–601.
732. Wesche H, Gao X, Li X, et al. IRAK-M is a novel member of the Pelle/interleukin-1 receptor-associated kinase (IRAK) family. J Biol Chem. 1999;274:19403–10.
733. Dajee M, Lazarov M, Zhang JY, et al. NF-κB blockade and oncogenic Ras trigger invasive human epidermal neoplasia. Nature. 2003;421:639–43.

734. Seitz CS, Lin Q, Deng H, Khavari PA. Alterations in NF-κB function in transgenic epithelial tissue demonstrate a growth inhibitory role for NF-κB. Proc Natl Acad Sci U S A. 1998;95:2307–12.
735. Rincón M, Davis RJ. Regulation of the immune response by stress-activated protein kinases. Immunol Rev. 2009;228(1):212–24. doi:10.1111/j.1600-065X.2008.00744.x.
736. Hardy MP, O'Neill LA. The murine IRAK2 gene encodes four alternatively spliced isoforms, two of which are inhibitory. J Biol Chem. 2004;279:27699–708.
737. Meyer-Bahlburg A, Khim S, Rawlings DJ. B cell intrinsic TLR signals amplify but are not required for humoral immunity. J Exp Med. 2007;204:3095–101.
738. Bosco MC, Raggi F, Varesio L. Therapeutic potential of targeting TREM-1 in inflammatory diseases and cancer. Curr Pharm Des. 2016;22(41):6209–33. doi:10.2174/1381612822666160826110539.
739. Manieri E, Sabio G. Stress kinases in the modulation of metabolism and energy balance. J Mol Endocrinol. 2015;55(2):R11–22. doi:10.1530/JME-15-0146.
740. Mihret A. The role of dendritic cells in mycobacterium tuberculosis infection. Virulence. 2012;3(7):654–9. doi:10.4161/viru.22586. Epub 2012 Nov 15
741. Bernard NJ, O'Neill LA. Mal, more than a bridge to MyD88. IUBMB Life. 2013;65(9):777–86. doi:10.1002/iub.1201.
742. Gordon S. Pattern recognition receptors: doubling up for the innate immune response. Cell. 2002;111:927–30.
743. Takeda K, Kaisho T, Akira S. Toll-like receptors Annu. Rev Immunol. 2003;21:335–76.
744. Hotta K, Funahashi T, Arita Y, Takahashi M, Matsuda M, Okamoto Y, Iwahashi H, Kuriyama H, et al. Plasma concentrations of a novel, adipose-specific protein, adiponectin, in type 2 diabetic patients. Arterioscler Thromb Vasc Biol. 2000;20(6):1595–9. doi:10.1161/01.ATV.20.6.1595.
745. Odegaard JI, Chawla A. The immune system as a sensor of the metabolic state. Immunity. 2013;38(4):644–54. doi:10.1016/j.immuni.2013.04.001.
746. Turnbull AV, Rivier CL. Regulation of the hypothalamic-pituitary-adrenal axis by cytokines: actions and mechanisms of action. Physiol Rev. 1999;16:1–71.
747. Parks KR, Davis JM. Epinephrine, cortisol, endotoxin, nutrition, and the neutrophil. Surg Infect. 2012;13(5):300–6. doi:10.1089/sur.2012.161.
748. Faes S, Dormond O. PI3K and AKT: unfaithful partners in cancer. Int J Mol Sci. 2015;16(9):21138–52. doi:10.3390/ijms160921138.
749. Stark AK, Sriskantharajah S, Hessel EM, Okkenhaug K. PI3K inhibitors in inflammation, autoimmunity and cancer. Curr Opin Pharmacol. 2015;23:82–91. doi:10.1016/j.coph.2015.05.017. Epub 2015 Jun 18
750. Ciruelos Gil EM. Targeting the PI3K/AKT/mTOR pathway in estrogen receptor-positive breast cancer. Cancer Treat Rev. 2014;40(7):862–71. doi:10.1016/j.ctrv.2014.03.004. Epub 2014 Mar 26
751. Hsu K, Champaiboon C, Guenther BD, et al. Anti-infective protective properties of S100 calgranulins. Antiinflamm Antiallergy Agents Med Chem. 2009;8:290–305.
752. Marshall S. Role of insulin, adipocyte hormones, and nutrient-sensing pathways in regulating fuel metabolism and energy homeostasis: a nutritional perspective of diabetes, obesity, and cancer. Sci STKE. 2006;2006(346):re7.
753. Vigneri R, Goldfine ID, Frittitta L. Insulin, insulin receptors, and cancer. J Endocrinol Investig. 2016;39(12):1365–76. Epub 2016 Jul 1
754. Haissaguerre M, Saucisse N, Cota D. Influence of mTOR in energy and metabolic homeostasis. Mol Cell Endocrinol. 2014;397(1–2):67–77. doi:10.1016/j.mce.2014.07.015. Epub 2014 Aug 7
755. Maya-Monteiro CM, Bozza PT. Leptin and mTOR: partners in metabolism and inflammation. Cell Cycle. 2008;7(12):1713–7. Epub 2008 Jun 16
756. Peng Y, Li L, Huang M, Duan C, Zhang L, Chen J. Angiogenin interacts with ribonuclease inhibitor regulating PI3K/AKT/mTOR signaling pathway in bladder cancer cells. Cell Signal. 2014;26(12):2782–92.

757. Dibble CC, Manning BD. Signal integration by mTORC1 coordinates nutrient input with biosynthetic output. Nat Cell Biol. 2013;15:555–64.
758. Jewell JL, Russell RC, Guan KL. Amino acid signalling upstream of mTOR. Nat Rev Mol Cell Biol. 2013;14:133.
759. Kwon O, Kim KW, Kim MS. Leptin signalling pathways in hypothalamic neurons. Cell Mol Life Sci. 2016;73(7):1457–77. doi:10.1007/s00018-016-2133-1. Epub 2016 Jan 19
760. Trinchieri G, Pflanz S, Kastelein RA. The IL-12 family of heterodimeric cytokines. New players in the regulation of T cell responses. Immunity. 2003;19:641–4.
761. Kolb R, Liu GH, Janowski AM, Sutterwala FS, Zhang W. Inflammasomes in cancer: a double-edged sword. Protein Cell. 2014;5(1):12–20. doi:10.1007/s13238-013-0001-4. Epub 2014 Jan 29
762. Yagil Z, Hadad Erlich T, Ofir-Birin Y, Tshori S, Kay G, Yekhtin Z, Fisher DE, Cheng C, Wong WS, Hartmann K, Razin E, Nechushtan H. Transcription factor E3, a major regulator of mast cell-mediated allergic response. J Allergy Clin Immunol. 2012;129(5):1357–66. e1355
763. Bifulco C, McDaniel K, Leng L, Bucala R. Tumor growth-promoting properties of macrophage migration inhibitory factor. Curr Pharm Des. 2008;14(36):3790–801.
764. Swafford D, Manicassamy S. Wnt signaling in dendritic cells: its role in regulation of immunity and tolerance. Discov Med. 2015;19(105):303–10.
765. Sorci G, Giovannini G, Riuzzi F, et al. The danger signal S100B integrates pathogen- and danger-sensing pathways to restrain inflammation. PLoS Pathog. 2011;7:e1001315.
766. Balamurugan K. HIF-1 at the crossroads of hypoxia, inflammation, and cancer. Int J Cancer. 2016;138(5):1058–66. doi:10.1002/ijc.29519. Epub 2015 Apr 7
767. Blancher C, Moore JW, Robertson N, Harris AL. Effects of ras and von Hippel-Lindau (VHL) gene mutations on hypoxia-inducible factor (HIF)-1alpha, HIF-2alpha, and vascular endothelial growth factor expression and their regulation by the phosphatidylinositol 3′-kinase/Akt signaling pathway. Cancer Res. 2001;61(19):7349–55.
768. Hubbard LL, Moore BB. IRAK-M regulation and function in host defense and immune homeostasis. Infect Dis Rep. 2010;2(1):pii: e9.
769. Hubbard LL, Wilke CA, White ES, Moore BB. PTEN limits alveolar macrophage function against Pseudomonas aeruginosa after bone marrow transplantation. Am J Respir Cell Mol Biol. 2011;45(5):1050–8. doi:10.1165/rcmb.2011-0079OC. Epub 2011 Apr 28
770. Snapper CM. Mechanisms underlying in vivo polysaccharide-specific immunoglobulin responses to intact extracellular bacteria. Ann N Y Acad Sci. 2012;1253:92–101. doi:10.1111/j.1749-6632.2011.06329.x. Epub 2012 Jan 30
771. Gurevitz SL, Snyder JA, Wessel EK, Frey J, Williamson BA. Systemic lupus erythematosus: a review of the disease and treatment options. Consult Pharm. 2013;28(2):110–21. doi:10.4140/TCP.n.2013.110. Rheumatoid arthritis RA
772. Elhai M, Avouac J, Kahan A, Allanore Y. Systemic sclerosis: recent insights. Joint Bone Spine. 2015;82(3):148–53. doi:10.1016/j.jbspin.2014.10.010. Epub 2014 Dec 31
773. Kyriakidis NC, Kapsogeorgou EK, Tzioufas AG. A comprehensive review of autoantibodies in primary Sjögren's syndrome: clinical phenotypes and regulatory mechanisms. J Autoimmun. 2014;51:67–74. doi:10.1016/j.jaut.2013.11.001. Epub 2013 Dec 13
774. Liang Y, Yang Z, Qin B, Zhong R. Primary Sjogren's syndrome and malignancy risk: a systematic reviewand meta-analysis. Ann Rheum Dis. 2014;73(6):1151–6. doi:10.1136/annrheumdis-2013-203305. Epub 2013 May 17
775. Vogelpoel LT, Baeten DL, de Jong EC, den Dunnen J. Control of cytokine production by human fc gamma receptors: implications for pathogen defense and autoimmunity. Front Immunol. 2015;6:79. doi:10.3389/fimmu.2015.00079. eCollection 2015
776. Vogelpoel LT, Hansen IS, Rispens T, Muller FJ, van Capel TM, Turina MC, Vos JB, Baeten DL, et al. Fc gamma receptor-TLR cross-talk elicits pro-inflammatory cytokine production by human M2 macrophages. Nat Commun. 2014;5:5444. doi:10.1038/ncomms6444.
777. Levesque MC. Translational mini-review series on B cell-directed therapies: recent advances in B cell-directed biological therapies for autoimmune disorders. Clin Exp Immunol. 2009;157(2):198–208. doi:10.1111/j.1365-2249.2009.03979.x.

778. Huan C, Kelly ML, Steele R, Shapira I, Gottesman SR, Roman CA. Transcription factors TFE3 and TFEB are critical for CD40 ligand expression and thymus-dependent humoral immunity. Nat Immunol. 2006;7(10):1082–91.
779. Donato R, Cannon BR, Sorci G, Riuzzi F, Hsu K, Weber DJ, Geczy CL. Functions of S100 proteins. Curr Mol Med. 2013;13(1):24–57.
780. Riuzzi F, Sorci G, Donato R. S100B protein regulates myoblast proliferation and differentiation by activating FGFR1 in a bFGF-dependent manner. J Cell Sci. 2011;124:2389–400.
781. Lucia U, Ponzetto A, Deisboeck TS. A thermo-physical analysis of the proton pump vacuolar-ATPase: the constructal approach. Sci Rep. 2014;2014(4):6763–9.
782. Breier A, Barancík M, Sulová Z, Uhrík B. P-glycoprotein–implications of metabolism of neoplastic cells and cancer therapy. Curr Cancer Drug Targets. 2005;5(6):457–68.
783. Bryksin AV, Laktionov PP. Role of glyceraldehyde-3-phosphate dehydrogenase in vesiculartransport from golgi apparatus to endoplasmic reticulum. Biochemistry (Mosc). 2008;73(6):619–25.
784. Zoncu R, Efeyan A, Sabatini DM. mTOR: from growth signal integration to cancer, diabetes and ageing. Nat Rev Mol Cell Biol. 2011;12:21.
785. Fang J, Zhou SH, Fan J, Yan SX. Roles of glucose transporter-1 and the phosphatidylinositol 3kinase/protein kinase B pathway in cancer radioresistance- (review). Mol Med Rep. 2015;11(3):1573–81. doi:10.3892/mmr.2014.2888. Epub 2014 Nov 6
786. Adekola K, Rosen ST, Shanmugam M. Glucose transporters in cancer metabolism. Curr Opin Oncol. 2012;24(6):650–4. doi:10.1097/CCO.0b013e328356da72.
787. Linehan WM, Rouault TA. Molecular pathways: fumarate hydratase-deficient kidney cancer–targeting the Warburg effect in cancer. Clin Cancer Res. 2013;19(13):3345–52. doi:10.1158/1078-0432.CCR-13-0304. Epub 2013 Apr 30
788. Cheng Y, Chen G, Hong L, Zhou L, Hu M, Li B, Huang J, Xia L, Li C. How does hypoxia inducible factor-1α participate in enhancing the glycolysis activity in cervical cancer? Ann Diagn Pathol. 2013;17(3):305–11. doi:10.1016/j.anndiagpath.2012.12.002. Epub 2013 Feb 1
789. Kania E, Pająk B, Orzechowski A. Calcium homeostasis and ER stress in control of autophagy in cancer cells. Biomed Res Int. 2015;2015:352794. doi:10.1155/2015/352794. Epub 2015 Mar 3
790. Ghayad SE, Cohen PA. Inhibitors of the PI3K/Akt/mTOR pathway: new hope for breast cancerpatients. Recent Pat Anticancer Drug Discov. 2010;5(1):29–57.
791. Foroutan N, Muratov S, Levine M. Safety and efficacy of dipeptidyl peptidase-4 inhibitors vs sulfonylurea in metformin-based combination therapy for type 2 diabetes mellitus: systematic review and meta-analysis. Clin Invest Med. 2016;39(2):E48–62.
792. Soranna D, Scotti L, Zambon A, Bosetti C, Grassi G, Catapano A, La Vecchia C, Mancia G, Corrao G. Cancer risk associated with use of metformin and sulfonylurea in type 2 diabetes: a meta-analysis. Oncologist. 2012;17(6):813–22. doi:10.1634/theoncologist.2011-0462. Epub 2012 May 29
793. Saxton RA, Knockenhauer KE, Wolfson RL, Chantranupong L, Pacold ME, Wang T, Schwartz TU, Sabatini DM. Structural basis for leucine sensing by the Sestrin2-mTORC1 pathway. Science. 2016;351(6268):53–8. doi:10.1126/science.aad2087. Epub 2015 Nov 19
794. Smits MM, Tonneijck L, Muskiet MH, Kramer MH, Cahen DL, van Raalte DH. Gastrointestinal actions of glucagon-like peptide-1-based therapies: glycaemic control beyond the pancreas. Diabetes Obes Metab. 2016;18(3):224–35. doi:10.1111/dom.12593. Epub 2016 Jan 5
795. Xiao J, Kim SJ, Cohen P, Yen K. Humanin: functional interfaces with IGF-I. Growth Hormon IGF Res. 2016;29:21–7. doi:10.1016/j.ghir.2016.03.005. Epub 2016 Apr 7
796. Xie W, Ling T, Zhou Y, Feng W, Zhu Q, Stunnenberg HG, Grummt I, Tao W. The chromatin remodeling complex NuRD establishes the poised state of rRNA genes characterized by bivalent histone modifications and altered nucleosome positions. Proc Natl Acad Sci U S A. 2012;109:8161–6. doi:10.1073/pnas.1201262109.
797. Agani F, Jiang BH. Oxygen-independent regulation of HIF-1: novel involvement of PI3K/AKT/mTOR pathway in cancer. Curr Cancer Drug Targets. 2013;13(3):245–51.

798. Steiner FA, Henikoff S. Diversity in the organization of centromeric chromatin. Curr Opin Genet Dev. 2015;31:28–35. doi:10.1016/j.gde.2015.03.010. Epub 2015 May 16
799. Petty E, Pillus L. Balancing chromatin remodeling and histone modifications in transcription. Trends Genet. 2013;29(11):621–9. doi:10.1016/j.tig.2013.06.006. Epub 2013 Jul 16
800. Schusdziarra V. Somatostatin–physiological and pathophysiological aspects. Scand J Gastroenterol Suppl. 1983;82:69–84.
801. Theoharides TC. Neuroendocrinology of mast cells: challenges and controversies. Exp Dermatol. 2017; doi:10.1111/exd.13288. [Epub ahead of print]
802. Erer B, Demirkaya E, Ozen S, Kallinich T. What is the best acute phase reactant for familial Mediterranean fever follow-up and its role in the prediction of complications? A systematic review. Rheumatol Int. 2016;36(4):483–7. doi:10.1007/s00296-015-3413-z. Epub 2015 Dec 28
803. Yalçinkaya F, Cakar N, Acar B, Tutar E, Güriz H, Elhan AH, Oztürk S, Kansu A, Ince E, et al. The value of the levels of acute phase reactants for the prediction of familial Mediterranean fever associated amyloidosis: a case control study. Rheumatol Int. 2007;27(6):517–22. Epub 2006 Nov 14
804. Sun ZP, Zhang J, Shi LH, Zhang XR, Duan Y, Xu WF, Dai G, Wang XJ. Aminopeptidase N inhibitor 4cc synergizes antitumor effects of 5-fluorouracil on human liver cancer cells through ROS-dependent CD13 inhibition. Biomed Pharmacother. 2015;76:65–72. doi:10.1016/j.biopha.2015.10.023. Epub 2015 Nov 10
805. Shapira I, Lee A, Vora R, Budman DR. P53 mutations in triple negative breast cancer upregulate endosomal recycling of epidermal growth factor receptor (EGFR) increasing its oncogenic potency. Crit Rev Oncol Hematol. 2013;88(2):284–92. doi:10.1016/j.critrevonc.2013.05.003. Epub 2013 Jun 5
806. Chevet E, Fessart D, Delom F, Mulot A, Vojtesek B, Hrstka R, Murray E, Gray T, Hupp T. Emerging roles for the pro-oncogenic anterior gradient-2 in cancerdevelopment. Oncogene. 2013;32(20):2499–509. doi:10.1038/onc.2012.346. Epub 2012 Sep 3.
807. Perl A. mTOR activation is a biomarker and a central pathway to autoimmune disorders, cancer, obesity, and aging. Ann N Y Acad Sci. 2015;1346(1):33–44. doi:10.1111/nyas.12756. Epub 2015 Apr 23.
808. Meng LH, Zheng XF. Toward rapamycin analog (rapalog)-based precision cancer therapy. Acta Pharmacol Sin. 2015;36(10):1163–9. doi:10.1038/aps.2015.68. Epub 2015 Aug 24. temsirolimus and everolimus approved for treatment of breast and renal cancer
809. Peterson TR, Laplante M, Thoreen CC, Sancak Y, Kang SA, Kuehl WM, et al. DEPTOR is an mTOR inhibitor frequently overexpressed in multiple myeloma cells and required for their survival. Cell. 2009;137:873–86.
810. Hara K, Maruki Y, Long XM, Yoshino K, Oshiro N, Hidayat S, et al. Raptor, a binding partner of target of rapamycin (TOR), mediates TOR action. Cell. 2002;110:177–89.
811. Motzer RJ, Escudier B, Oudard S, Hutson TE, Porta C, Bracarda S, et al. Efficacy of everolimus in advanced renal cell carcinoma: a double-blind, randomised, placebo-controlled phase III trial. Lancet. 2008;372:449–56.
812. Don AS, Zheng XF. Recent clinical trials of mTOR-targeted cancer therapies. Rev Recent Clin Trials. 2011;6:24–35.
813. Llovet JM, Hernandez-Gea V. Hepatocellular carcinoma: reasons for phase III failure and novel perspectives on trial design. Clin Cancer Res. 2014;20:2072–9.
814. Hasskarl J. Everolimus. Recent Results Cancer Res. 2014;201:373–92. doi:10.1007/978-3-642-54490-3_23.
815. Schulze M, Stock C, Zaccagnini M, Teber D, Rassweiler JJ. Temsirolimus. Recent Results Cancer Res. 2014;201:393–403. doi:10.1007/978–3–642-54490-3_24.
816. Network CGA. Comprehensive molecular portraits of human breast tumours (357 collaborators). Nature. 2012;490(7418):61–70. doi:10.1038/nature11412. Epub 2012 Sep 23
817. Cancer Genome Atlas Research Network Hammerman PS, et al. Comprehensive genomic characterization of squamous cell lung cancers. Nature. 2012;489:513–25.

818. de la Haba G, Khatami M, Cooper GW, Backlund P, Flaks JG. Alanine or pyruvate is required for the development of myotubes from myoblasts and cortisol satisfies this requirement. Mol Cell Biochem. 1999;198(1–2):163–70.
819. Fedele CG, et al. Inositol polyphosphate 4-phosphatase II regulates PI3K/Akt signaling and is lost in human basal-like breast cancers. Proc Natl Acad Sci U S A. 2010;107:22231–6. doi:10.1073/pnas.1015245107.
820. Comes N, Serrano-Albarrás A, Capera J, Serrano-Novillo C, Condom E, Ramón Y, Cajal S, Ferreres JC, Felipe A. Involvement of potassium channels in the progression of cancer to a more malignant phenotype. Biochim Biophys Acta. 2015;1848(10 Pt B):2477–92. doi:10.1016/j.bbamem.2014.12.008. Epub 2014 Dec 14
821. Green CR, Wallace M, Divakaruni AS, Phillips SA, Murphy AN, Ciaraldi TP, Metallo CM. Branched-chain amino acid catabolism fuels adipocyte differentiation and lipogenesis. Nat Chem Biol. 2016;12(1):15–21. doi:10.1038/nchembio.1961. Epub 2015 Nov 16
822. Rubio R, Berne RM, Winn HR. Production, metabolism and possible functions of adenosine in brain tissue in situ. Ciba Found Symp. 1978;56:355–78.
823. Dunlop K, Cedrone M, Staples JF, Regnault TR. Altered fetal skeletal muscle nutrient metabolism following an adverse in utero environment and the modulation of later life insulin sensitivity. Forum Nutr. 2015;7:1202–16.
824. Sangar F, Schreurs AS, Umaña-Diaz C, Clapéron A, Desbois-Mouthon C, Calmel C, Mauger O, et al. Involvement of small ArfGAP1 (SMAP1), a novel Arf6-specific GTPase-activating protein, in microsatellite instability oncogenesis. Oncogene. 2014;33(21):2758–67. doi:10.1038/onc.2013.211. Epub 2013 Jun 10
825. Techasen A, Namwat N, Loilome W, Bungkanjana P, Khuntikeo N, Puapairoj A, Jearanaikoon P, Saya H, Yongvanit P. Tumor necrosis factor-α (TNF-α) stimulates the epithelial-mesenchymal transition regulator snail in cholangiocarcinoma. Med Oncol. 2012;29(5):3083–91. doi:10.1007/s12032-012-0305-x. Epub 2012 Aug 19
826. Isackson D, Cook KJ, McGill LD, Bachus KN. Mesenchymal stem cells increase collagen infiltration and improve wound healing response to porous titanium percutaneous implants. Med Eng Phys. 2013;35(6):743–53. doi:10.1016/j.medengphy.2012.08.002. Epub 2012 Aug 31
827. Baillie JK, Barnett MW, Upton KR, Gerhardt DJ, Richmond TA, De Sapio F, Brennan PM, Rizzu P, et al. Somatic retrotransposition alters the genetic landscape of the human brain. Nature. 2011;479(7374):534–7. doi:10.1038/nature10531.
828. Ostertag EM, Kazazian HH Jr. Biology of mammalian L1 retrotransposons. Annu Rev Genet. 2001;35:501–38.
829. Wong LH, Brettingham-Moore KH, Chan L, Quach JM, Anderson MA, Northrop EL, Hannan R, Saffery R, Shaw ML, Williams E, et al. Centromere RNA is a key component for the assembly of nucleoproteins at the nucleolus and centromere. Genome Res. 2007;17:1146–60. doi:10.1101/gr.6022807.
830. Maxwell PJ, Gallagher R, Seaton A, Wilson C, Scullin P, Pettigrew J, Stratford IJ, Williams KJ, et al. HIF-1 and NF-kappaB-mediated upregulation of CXCR1 and CXCR2 expression promotes cell survival in hypoxic prostate cancer cells. Oncogene. 2007;26:7333–45.
831. Lucia U, Ponzettob A, Deisboeck TS. A thermodynamic approach to the 'mitosis/apoptosis' ratio in cancer. Phys A. 2015;436:246–55.
832. Foidart JM, Hustin J, Dubois M, Schaaps JP. The human placenta becomes haemochorial at the 13th week of pregnancy. Int J Dev Biol. 1992;36(3):451e3.
833. Jauniaux E, Watson A, Burton G. Evaluation of respiratory gases and acid-base gradients in human fetal fluids and uteroplacental tissue between 7 and 16 weeks' gestation. Am J Obstet Gynecol. 2001;184(5):998e1003.
834. Murray AJ. Oxygen delivery and fetal-placental growth: beyond a question of supply and demand? Placenta. 2012; doi:10.1016/j.placenta.2012.06.006.

835. Tissot van Patot MC, Murray AJ, Beckey V, Cindrova-Davies T, Johns J, et al. Human placental metabolic adaptation to chronic hypoxia, high altitude: hypoxic preconditioning. Am J Physiol Regul Integr Comp Physiol. 2010;298(1):R16672.
836. Nakada T. Conversion of brain cytosol profile from fetal to adult type during the perinatal period: taurine-NAA exchange. Proc Jpn Acad Ser B Phys Biol Sci. 2010;86:630–42.
837. Dromparis P, Michelakis ED. Mitochondria in vascular health and disease. Annu Rev Physiol. 2013;75:95–126. doi:10.1146/annurev-physiol-030212-183804. Epub 2012 Nov 16.
838. Kinnaird A, Michelakis ED. Metabolic modulation of cancer: a new frontier with great translational potential. J Mol Med (Berl). 2015;93(2):127–42. doi:10.1007/s00109-014-1250-2. Epub 2015 Jan 14.
839. McWilliams RR, Allred JB, Slostad JA, Katipamula R, Dronca RS, Rumilla KM, Erickson LA, et al. NCCTG N0879 (Alliance): a randomized phase 2 cooperative group trial of carboplatin, paclitaxel, and bevacizumab ± everolimus for metastatic melanoma. Cancer. 2017 Oct 17. https://doi.org/10.1002/cncr.31072. [Epub ahead of print].

Index

M. Khatami, *Inflammation, Aging and Cancer*,
https://doi.org/10.1007/978-3-319-66475-0

B

K

L

P

MIX
Papier aus verantwortungsvollen Quellen
Paper from responsible sources
FSC® C105338

If you have any concerns about our products,
you can contact us on
ProductSafety@springernature.com

In case Publisher is established outside the EU,
the EU authorized representative is:
Springer Nature Customer Service Center GmbH
Europaplatz 3, 69115 Heidelberg, Germany

Printed by Libri Plureos GmbH
in Hamburg, Germany